Palladium Assisted Synthesis *of* Heterocycles

T0133529

Navjeet Kaur
Department of Chemistry
Banasthali Vidyapith,
Rajasthan, India

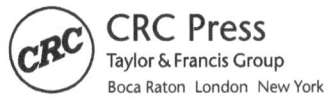

CRC Press
Taylor & Francis Group
Boca Raton London New York

CRC Press is an imprint of the
Taylor & Francis Group, an **informa** business

A SCIENCE PUBLISHERS BOOK

CRC Press
Taylor & Francis Group
6000 Broken Sound Parkway NW, Suite 300
Boca Raton, FL 33487-2742

First issued in paperback 2020

ISBN-13: 978-0-8153-7425-1 (hbk)
ISBN-13: 978-0-367-77987-0 (pbk)

Library of Congress Cataloging-in-Publication Data
Names: Kaur, Navjeet, author.
Title: Palladium assisted synthesis of heterocycles / Navjeet Kaur (Department of Chemistry, Banasthali Vidyapith, Rajasthan, India).
Description: Boca Raton, FL : CRC Press, 2019. | "A science publishers book." | Includes bibliographical references and index.
Identifiers: LCCN 2018058633 | ISBN 9780815374251 (hardback)
Subjects: LCSH: Heterocyclic compounds--Synthesis. | Palladium catalysts.
Classification: LCC QD400.5.S95 K38 2019 | DDC 547/.59--dc23
LC record available at https://lccn.loc.gov/2018058633

Visit the Taylor & Francis Web site at
http://www.taylorandfrancis.com

and the CRC Press Web site at
http://www.crcpress.com

Preface

In recent decades, a large number of reports related to the synthesis of *N*-, *O*- and *S*-containing heterocyclic compounds have appeared owing to a wide variety of their biological activity. The metal-catalyzed synthesis of heterocyclic compounds is becoming an important and highly rewarding method in organic synthesis. Heterocycles form by far the largest classical divisions of organic chemistry. Moreover, they are of immense importance not only both biologically and industrially but to the functioning of any developed human society as well. Heterocyclic compounds are prevalent in many natural products and pharmaceutically active compounds.

Development of newer approaches for heterocycle syntheses employing efficient and atom economical routes is popular research area nowadays. Among a variety of new synthetic transformations, transition metal-catalyzed reactions are the most attractive methodologies, since those reactions can directly construct multiply substituted molecules from readily accessible starting materials under mild conditions. Transition metal-catalyzed coupling transformations are now serving as one of the most useful and powerful tool in organic synthesis. Transition metal-catalyzed heteroannulation provides a useful and convenient tool for the construction of *N*-heterocycles.

The development of efficient, rapid and versatile routes for their synthesis has thus become a key area of research. To this end, protocols involving transition metal catalysis have gained prominence. Employing such tactic presents a departure from traditional approaches, in which harsh conditions, long reaction times and limited substrate scopes are common. Palladium is one of the most commonly used transition metal as it enables a number of very different reactions, including reactions that form C-C, C-O, C-N and C-S bonds. Palladium tolerates a wide range of functional groups and thus avoids protecting group chemistry. Moreover, most palladium-based methodologies proceeded stereo- and regioselectively in excellent yields. These advantages have led to significant growth in organopalladium chemistry over the last two decades, thus palladium catalysts are now known to be extremely active and reliable reagents for the syntheses of heterocycles.

The palladium-catalyzed transformations have seen a fascinating development in recent years. The importance of palladium in synthesis is evident from the huge number of name reactions in connection with this in the formation of carbon-carbon, carbon-nitrogen, carbon-oxygen and even carbon-sulfur bonds in the mildness of most of these processes, tolerating various functional groups. Palladium-catalyzed carbon-nitrogen, carbon-carbon, and carbon-oxygen bond forming reactions have recently being gained popularity among the scientific community for different discovery drug development programs.

Heterocyclic synthesis involving transition metal complexes has become of common use in the past decade because a metal-catalyzed reaction can directly build complicated molecules from readily accessible starting materials under mild conditions. This book focuses on the use of palladium for the synthesis of heterocylces. It describes the formation of different types of heterocyclic rings.

Dr. Navjeet Kaur
Department of Chemistry, Banasthali Vidyapith
Banasthali-304022 (Rajasthan), India
Email: *nvjithaans@gmail.com*

Contents

List of Abbreviations

AAC: azide alkyne cycloaddition
ACCI: amidation-coupling-cycloisomerization
AHA: asymmetric hydroamination of alkenes
BBEDA: N,N-bis-(benzylidene)ethylene-diamine
9-BBN: 9-borabicyclo[3.3.1]nonane
BDPP: (2S,4S)-2,4-bis(diphenylphosphino)
BINAM: 1,1-binaphthyl-2,2-diamine
BINAP: 2,2-bis(diphenyl-phosphanyl)-1,1-binaphthyl
BINOL: 1,1'-bi-2-naphthol
BOP: N,N-bis(2-oxo-3-oxazolidinyl)phosphine
BOXAX: 3,3'-disubstituted 2,2'-bis(oxazolyl)-1,1'-binaphthyls
BQ: benzoquinone
COD: cyclooctadiene
CoMFA: comparative molecular field analysis
4-CR: four-component reaction
DABCO: 1,4-diazabicyclo[2.2.2]octane
DBA: dibenzylideneacetone
DBU: 1,8-diazabicyclo[5.4.0]undec-7-ene
DCC: N,N'-dicyclohexylcarbodiimide
DCE: 1,2-dicholoethylene
DCM: dichloromethane
DDQ: 2,3-dichloro-5,6-dicyanobenzoquinone
DEAD: diethyl azodicarboxylate
DET: diethyltryptamine
DHQD: 3-dehydroquinate dehydratase
DHPs: 1,4-dihydropyridines
DIAD: diisopropyl azodicarboxylate
DIB: (diacetoxyiodo)benzene
DIBAL: diisobutylaluminum hydride
DIC: N,N'-diisopropylcarbodiimide
DIEA: diisopropylethylamine
DIPEA: N,N-diisopropylethylamine
DMA: dimethylaniline
DMAD: dimethyl acetylenedicarboxylate
DMAP: 4-dimethylaminopyridine

DME: dimethoxyethane
DMEDA: *N*,*N*′-dimethylethylenediamine
DMF: dimethylformamide
DMFDMA: *N*,*N*-dimethyl-formamide dimethyl acetal
DMP: Dess-Martin periodinane
DMS: dimethyl sulfide
DMSO: dimethylsulphoxide
DOPA: dopamine
DPEPhos: bis-[2-(diphenylphosphino)phenyl]ether
DPPA: diphenylphosphorylazide
DPPB: 1,4-bis(diphenylphosphino)butane
DPPE: 1,2-bis(diphenylphosphino)ethane
DPPF: 1,1′-bis(diphenylphosphino)ferrocene
DPPM: 1,2-bis(diphenylphosphino)methane
DPPP: 1,3-bis(diphenylphosphino)propane
DTBMP: 2,6-di-*tert*-butyl-4-methylpyridine
EDC: 1-ethyl-3-(3-dimethylaminopropyl)carbodiimide
EDDA: ethylenediamine-*N*,*N*′-diacetic acid
F-SPE: fluorous solid-phase extraction
GABA: *γ*-aminobutyric acid
HBTU: 2-(1*H*-benzotriazole-1-yl)-1,1,3,3-tetramethyluroniumhexafluorophosphate
HMPA: hexamethylphosphoramide
HOBt: 1-hydroxybenzotriazole
HWE: Horner-Wadsworth-Emmons
KHMDS: potassium hexamethyldisilazide
LAH: lithium aluminum hydride
LDA: lithium diisopropylamide
MBH: Morita-Baylis-Hillman
m-CPBA: *meta*-chloroperoxybenzoic acid
MCR: multi-component reaction
MOM: methoxymethyl ether
MONOPHOS: monodentate phosphoramidite
MWI: microwave irradiation
NBS: *N*-bromosuccinimide
NCS: *N*-chlorosuccinimide
NFBS: *N*-fluorobenzenesulfonimide
NHC: *N*-heterocyclic carbene
NMO: *N*-methylmorpholine-*N*-oxide
NMP: *N*-methyl-2-pyrrolidone
OTf: trifluoromethanesulfonate
OTs: *O*-tosyl
PCC: pyridinium chlorochromate
PEG: poly(ethylene glycol)
PHAL: 1,4-phthalazinediyl
S-PHANEPHOS: (*S*)-(+)-4,12-bis(diphenylphosphino)-[2.2]-paracyclophane
S-Phos: 2-dicyclohexylphosphino-2′,6′-dimethoxybiphenyl
PIFA: phenyliodine(III) bis(trifluoroacetate)
PMB: *p*-methoxybenzyl
PTSA: *p*-toluenesulfonic acid
RCM: ring-closing metathesis

SEM:	[2-(trimethylsilyl)ethoxy]methyl acetal
SIPr:	*N,N'*-bis(2,6-diisopropylphenyl)dihydroimidazol-2-ylidene
SPOS:	solid-phase organic synthesis
SPS:	solid-phase synthesis
TBAB:	tetrabutylammonium bromide
TBAC:	tetrabutylammonium chloride
TBAF:	tetrabutylammonium fluoride
TBAI:	tetrabutylammonium iodide
TBDMS:	*tert*-butyldimethylsilyl
TBS:	*tert*-butyldimethylsilyl ether
TBTH:	tributyltin hydride
TEA:	triethylamine
TEMPO:	(2,2,6,6-tetramethylpiperidin-1-yl)oxyl or
	(2,2,6,6-tetramethylpiperidin-1-yl)oxidanyl
TFA:	trifluoroacetic acid
TFAA:	trifluoroacetic anhydride
TFE:	tetrafluoroethylene
TFFH:	tetramethylfluoroformamidinium hexafluorophosphate
TFP:	tri(2-furyl)phosphine
THF:	tetrahydrofuran
TMB:	3,3',5,5'-tetramethylbenzidine
TMG:	1,1,3,3-tetramethylguanidine
TMM:	trimethylenemethane
TMOF:	trimethyl orthoformate
TMP:	3,4,7,8-tetramethyl-1,10-phenanthroline
TMS:	trimethylsilyl
TMSCN:	trimethylsilyl cyanide
TTMSS:	tris(trimethylsilyl)silane

CHAPTER 1

Five-Membered N-Heterocycles

1.1 Introduction

Nitrogen-containing heterocyclic compounds because of their presence in biologically active compounds and natural products are by far the most explored heterocycles. Five-membered nitrogen-containing heterocycles like indoles, pyrroles, and carbazoles are present in a number of biologically active compounds. Due to this synthetic chemists are continuously interested in the functionalization and generation of these heterocyclic compounds. Saturated five-membered *N*-heterocycles are significant not only for the preparation of pigments, drugs, and pharmaceuticals, but also for the development of organic functional materials [1]. Substituted pyrroles are very important compounds showing remarkable biological properties including anti-viral, anti-bacterial, anti-tumoral, anti-inflammatory, and anti-oxidant activities [2]. Therefore, a variety of methods have been investigated for the synthesis of pyrrolic ring. Among these procedures, Paal-Knorr reaction [3] is one of the most utilized protocol for the construction of pyrroles in which 1,4-dicarbonyl substrates are reacted with primary amines or NH_3 in the presence of many promoting agents [4]. Therefore, the preparation of these compounds has gained longstanding interest. Various protocols for the formation of these heterocyclic compounds involve carbon-nitrogen bond-forming reactions like reductive amination, nucleophilic substitution, or dipolar cycloaddition for ring closure. This chapter describes the approaches for the synthesis of five-membered nitrogen heterocycles with palladium [5-16].

1.2 Palladium assisted synthesis of five-membered heterocycles with nitrogen heteroatom

A novel sequential Pd/Ru-catalyzed four-component process for the synthesis of *C*-allyl-*N*-heterocycles was developed by Grigg et al. [17] in good yield which in turn can be used as an active dipolarophile in 1,3-dipolar cycloaddition. 1,6-Dienes underwent Ru-catalyzed ring-closing metathesis to give Δ3-pyrrolines (**Scheme 1**) [18a-b].

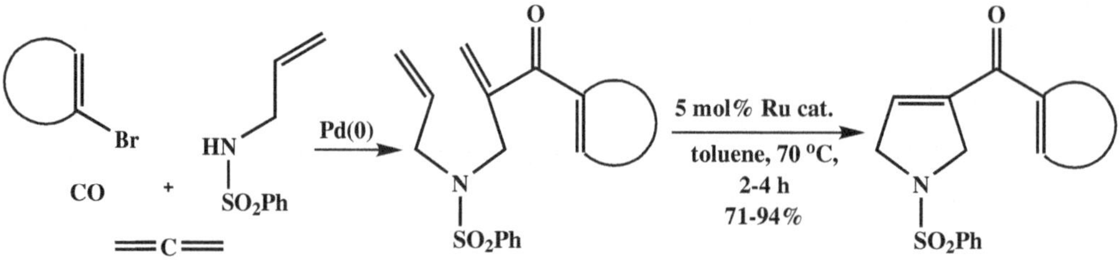

Scheme-1

Oximes have also been utilized in amino-Heck reactions to create nitrogen heterocycles. It has been reported that oximes underwent oxidative addition to Pd(0) complexes [19] which react with appended olefins to generate the corresponding heterocycles (**Scheme 2**). Other metal-catalyzed amino-Heck type reactions have been reported to produce pyrazolines, pyridines, pyrroles, azaazulenes, and isoquinolines [20-22].

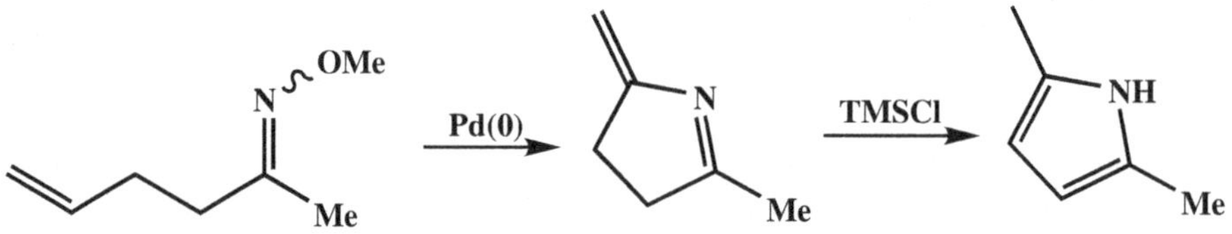

Scheme-2

The 2,3-*cis* selectivity was rationalized during pyrrolidine formation as shown in **Scheme 3**. The carbocyclization of a *p*-allyl Pd(II) intermediate occurred to form a conformer. However, this conformer was destabilized by an unfavorable steric interaction between phenyl group and pseudoaxial hydrogen atoms. Thus, the ring was formed preferably through more abundant conformers to produce *cis*-pyrrolidine as a single isomer [23].

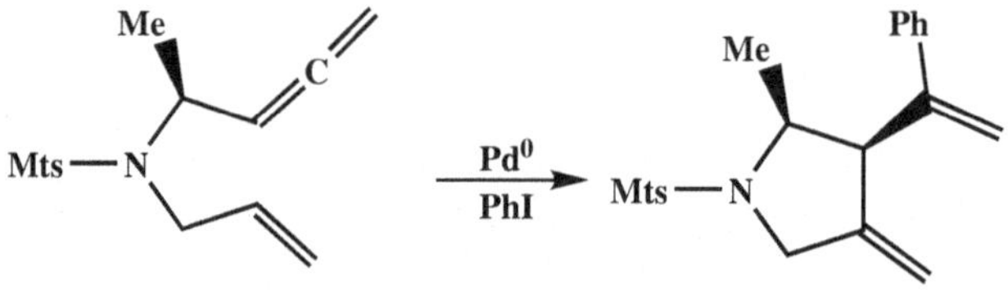

Scheme-3

The complex heterocycles were formed stereoselectively *via* Pd-catalyzed coupling reactions of γ-amino alkenes and γ-hydroxy alkenes with alkenyl and aryl halides [24]. For example, pyrrolidines, THF, piperazines, morpholines, isoxazolidines, pyrrazolidines and imidazoldin-2-ones [25-27] were prepared employing this strategy, which influenced the carbon-carbon and carbon-heteroatom bond formation in a single step (**Scheme 4**).

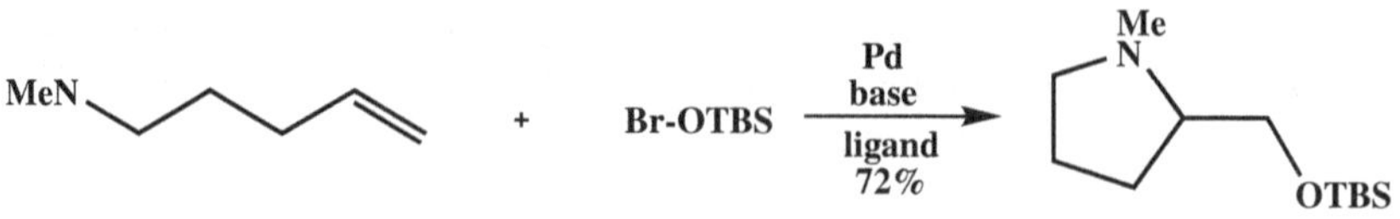

Scheme-4

The carboamination and carboetherification of substrates were examined using standard reaction conditions with various different ligands. Vinyl pyrrolidine was isolated rather than the desired product in the attempted carboamination reaction **(Scheme 5)** [28-29].

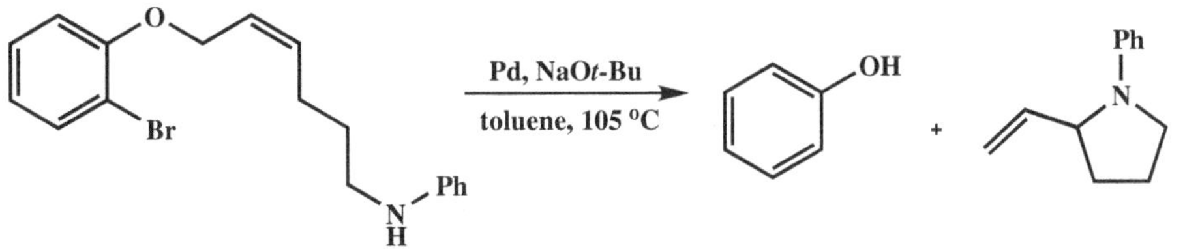

Scheme-5

The cyclization could be facilitated by substituting an iodide with bromide on arene, since the rate of oxidative addition was faster with iodides relative to bromides. However, upon subjection of amine substrate to carboamination conditions, vinyl pyrrolidine was formed again **(Scheme 6)** [30].

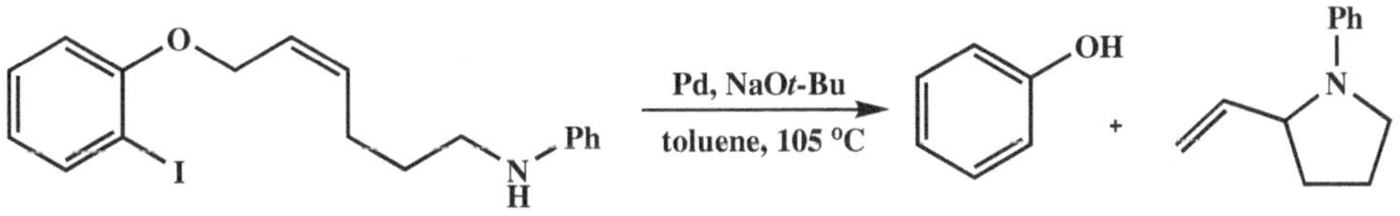

Scheme-6

A number of architectures were constructed through transition metal-catalyzed cycloisomerization of enynes [31]. The reaction products can be further functionalized due to the newly formed metal-carbon bonds which was the advantage of bismetalative cyclization of enynes. The palladium-catalyzed bismetalative cyclization of enynes proceeded efficiently with two different systems containing NHC as ligands in the presence of $Bu_3SnSiMe_3$. The vinylsilane and a homoallylstannane containing cyclized products were formed from *N*-bearing enynes in the presence of combination of $[Pd_2(dba)_3]$/imidazolium salt/cesium carbonate or $NaB[3,5-(CF_3)_2C_6H_4]_4$ **(Scheme 7)**. The formation of cyclopropanol derivatives from cyclized products has highlighted the synthetic applicability of this methodology [32-35].

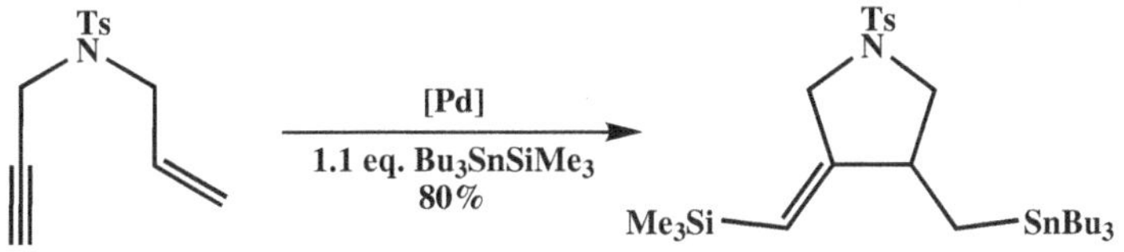

Scheme-7

In place of allenes and alkynes, CO also participated in insertion into carbon-metal bond and afforded lactams and lactones **(Scheme 8)** [36-39].

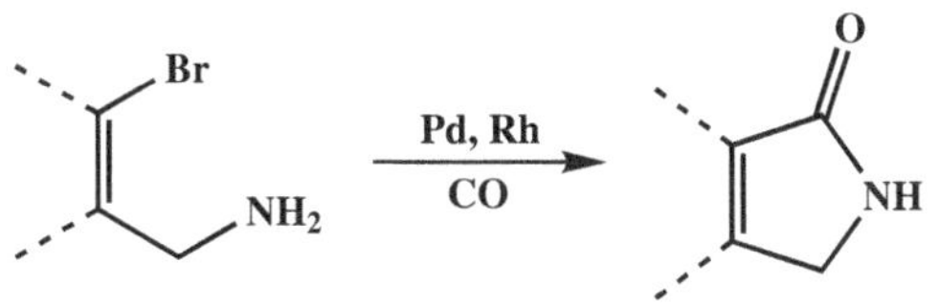

Scheme-8

Palladium-catalyzed asymmetric carboamination reactions for the synthesis of 2-(arylmethyl)- and 2-(alkenymethyl)pyrrolidines were developed [40-42]. However, asymmetric carboamination reactions of substituted *N*-Boc-pent-4-enylamines were unsuccessful. An enantioselective palladium-catalyzed carboamination reaction was explored and developed for the desymmetrization of starting compound and synthesis of enantiomerically enriched *cis*-2,5-disubstituted pyrrolidines, which generated 2 stereocenters and provided opportunities for further functionalization **(Scheme 9)**.

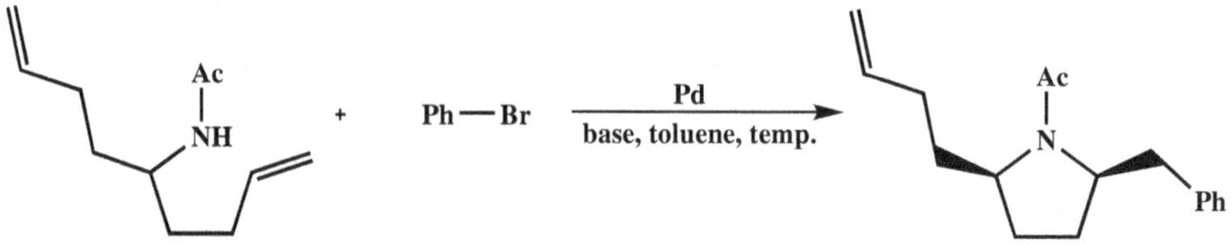

Scheme-9

The nature of substrate controlled the stereochemical outcome of these reactions, and was determined during the alkene *syn*-aminopalladation event. As shown in **Scheme 10**, the selective synthesis of *cis*-2,5-disubstituted 5-membered heterocycles proceeded through a transition state, where in the presence of nitrogen protecting group the axial orientation of group minimized the 1,3-strain [43-46].

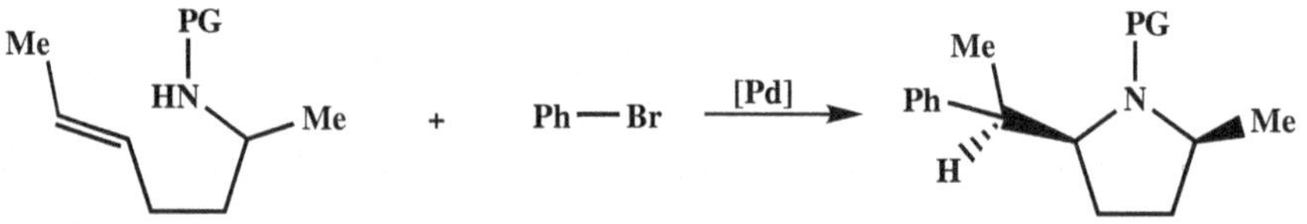

Scheme-10

Wolfe et al. [47-49] has developed a series of palladium-catalyzed alkene aminoarylation reactions for the synthesis of a variety of *N*-heterocycles including polycyclic guanidines, pyrazolidines and benzodiazepines **(Scheme 11)**. The uniqueness of these reactions was cross-coupling of simple aminoalkene substrates with alkenyl or aryl halides for the formation of heterocyclic ring with good to excellent stereocontrol through the formation of a carbon-nitrogen bond and carbon-carbon bond [43]. These processes were important for the formation of analogs of a particular scaffold, as a variety of aryl electrophiles were easily available.

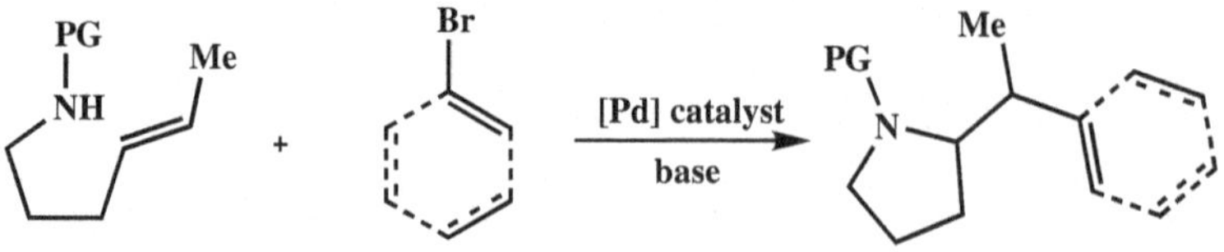

Scheme-11

Gabriele and co-workers [50] reported a related cycloisomerization of (*Z*)-2-en-4-ynyl amines to substituted pyrroles in the presence of a palladium(II) catalyst and potassium chloride in *N,N*-dimethylacetamide as shown in **Scheme 12**.

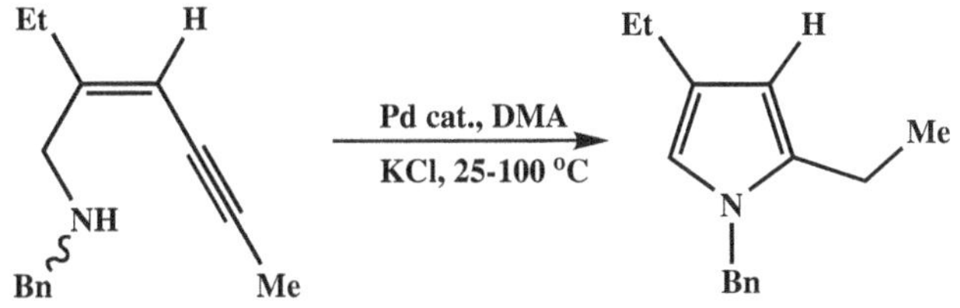

Scheme-12

Fix and co-workers [51] described an oxidative cyclization of aminoalkenes in the presence of Pd catalyst. A mixture of cyclic enamines was obtained from the reaction of terminal olefin containing aminoalkene (**Schemes 13**).

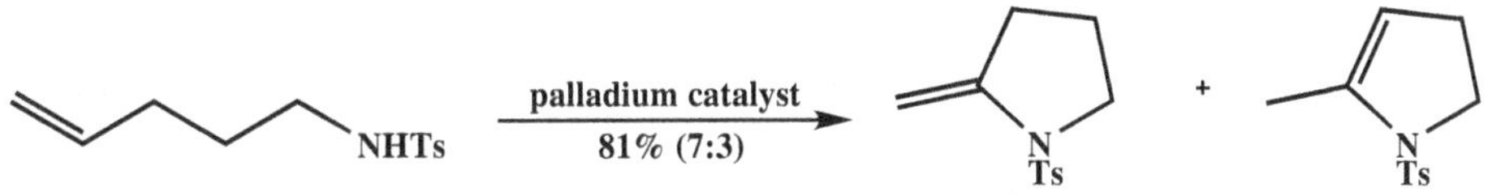

Scheme-13

Multiply substituted pyrroles were synthesized by a multi-component coupling of alkynes, imines and acid chlorides with Pd catalyst (**Scheme 14**) [52]. This method was based upon the ability of alkynes to underwent 1,3-dipolar addition with 1,3-oxazolium-5-oxides (münchnones) to produce pyrroles. The cycloaddition reactions of 1,3-dipoles münchnones with symmetrical and unsymmetrical substituted alkynes occurred easily. Arndtsen et al. [53-54] reported a four-component reaction of imines, acid chlorides, CO, and acetylene for the diversity-oriented formation of pyrroles. Pd-catalyzed coupling of imines, acid chlorides, and CO produced münchnones which underwent *in situ* [3+2] dipolar cycloaddition to form pyrroles [55-58].

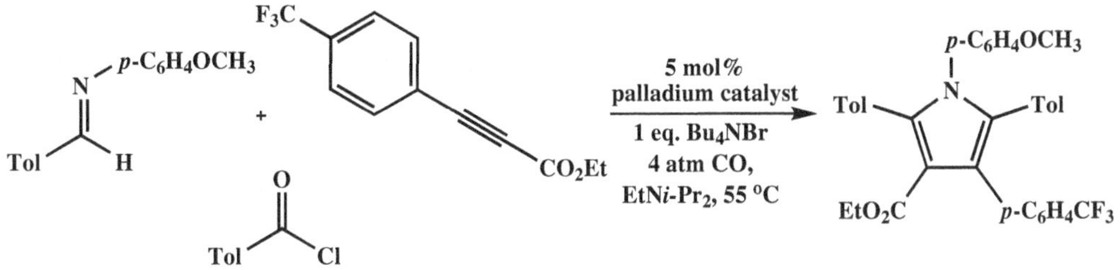

Scheme-14

The synthesis of pyrrole required a pre-assembled precursor(s) for cyclization [59-62]. This has imposed further steps on the overall synthesis as well as complicated the structural diversification. An ideal pathway to form complex molecules was the one which involved one-step, directly from easily available, easily varied and simple substrates, in a similar fashion to the Pauson-Khand reaction for carbocycle synthesis [63] and other multi-component reactions [52, 64-69]. The basic building blocks were utilized for assembling the pyrrole core *via* metal catalysis (**Scheme 15**).

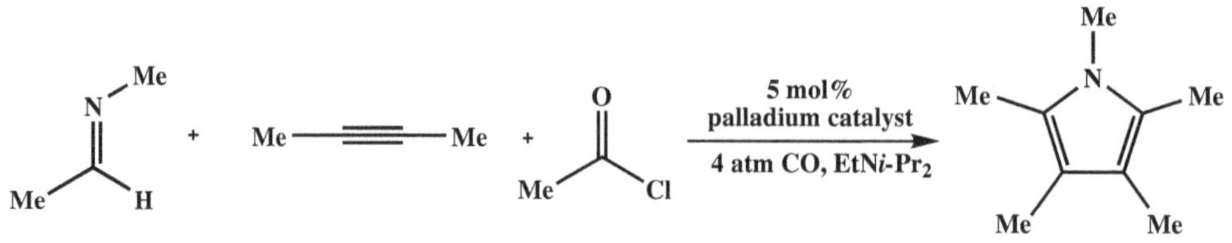

Scheme-15

The trimethylsilyl (TMS) enol ethers were synthesized *in situ* from aldehydes and ketones. This protocol was improved utilizing trimethylsilyl (TMS) enol ethers. Trimethylsilyl enol ethers of cyclic ketones were also suitable and diversity was increased by employing either thermodynamic or kinetic enol ether using methyl ketones as observed for benzyl methyl ketone. Thus, the product was formed by the reaction of "kinetic" TMS enol ether with aldehyde and dimethylbarbituric acid, whereas the isomer was formed from "thermodynamic" TMS enol ether **(Scheme 16-17)** [70].

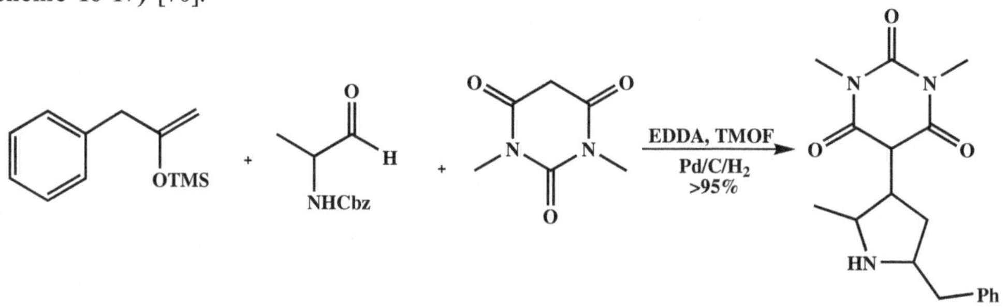

Scheme-16

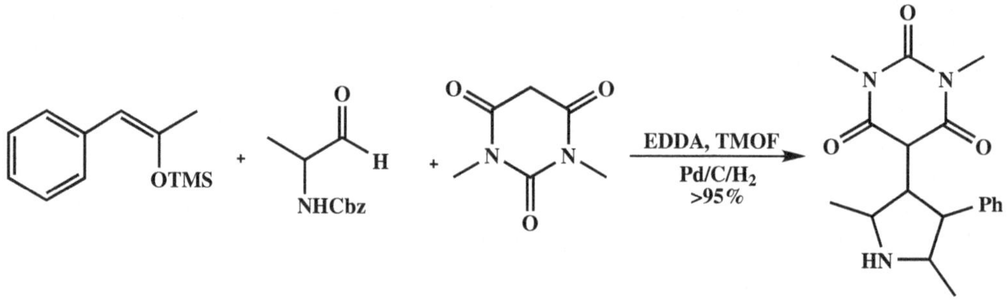

Scheme-17

De Kimpe and co-workers [71] described the synthesis of 1-isopropyl-3-methoxy-5,5-dimethylpyrrolidin-2-one through spontaneous cyclization of formed intermediate 2-methoxypentanoate from 2-alkoxy-4-amino-2-pentanoate. It happened by alkaline work-up of hydrogenated product of hydrochloride salt on silica gel **(Scheme 18)** [72].

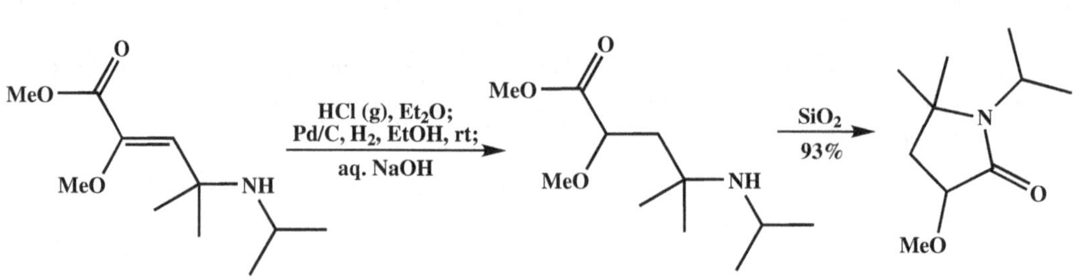

Scheme-18

The dibromo derivative was utilized for the *in situ* preparation of methyl 2-bromoacrylate and further was treated with NO_2 containing moiety to provide adduct **(Scheme 19)** [73]. The halogen was substituted with a hydroxyl group, subsequently the NO_2 group was reduced by catalytic hydrogenation to afford pyrrolidinone. This derivative by simple synthetic manipulations was transformed into aza-*iso*-nucleotide analogs. The same protocol was applied for the synthesis of 3,4-dihydroxy pyrrolidinones, which included the conjugate addition of nitroalkane to ethyl propynoate, formed *in situ*, and then dihydroxylation of formed unsaturated compound [74-75].

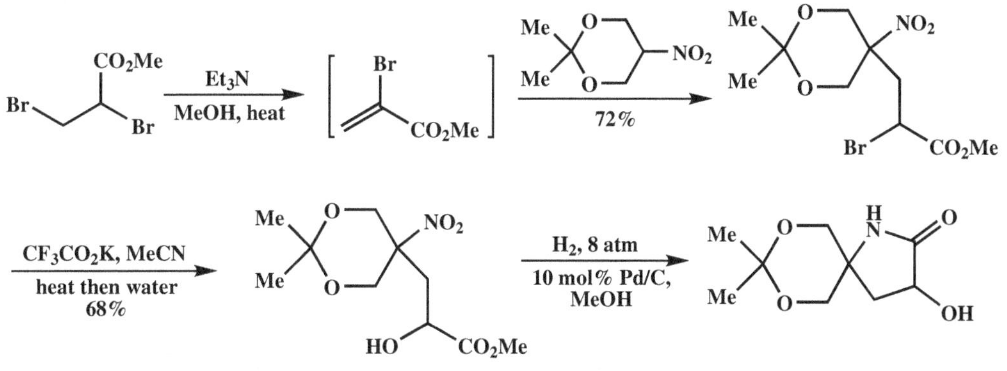

Scheme-19

Compounds with *syn* stereoisomer (predominantly) were formed by diastereoselective conjugate addition of nitroalkanes to chiral (Z)-enoate **(Scheme 20)** [76]. Good diastereoselection was observed with *E* isomer of compound [77]. The poor stereoselectivity was observed at carbon atom containing NO_2 group due to high acidity of hydrogen atom between the ester and NO_2 groups. Pyrrolidinones were synthesized upon reduction of NO_2 group and ring closure. Pyrrolidinones were utilized as synthetic intermediates for the preparation of many interesting compounds [75].

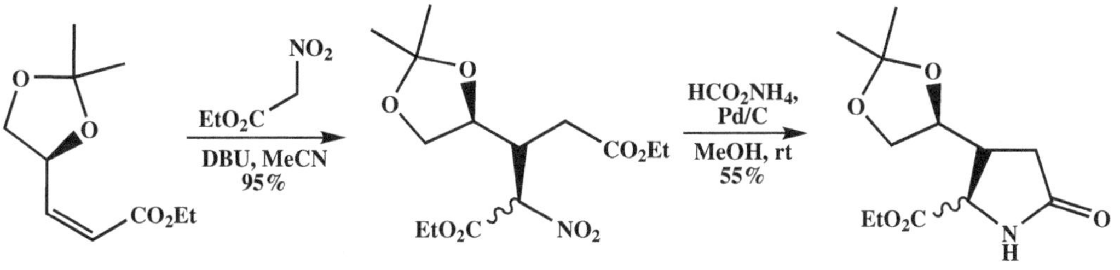

Scheme-20

The pyrrolidin-2-ones were reduced to prepare pyrrolidines. The reduction of NO_2 group formed a primary amine which reacted with other functional groups (like carbonyls, providing imino derivatives) and pyrrolidine ring was delivered upon further reduction. Adduct was formed when the unsaturated nitrile reacted with nitromethane, the formed adduct was catalytically hydrogenated with 10% palladium/carbon in methanol/acetic acid (9:1) and acylated to afford *N*-trifluoroacetylpyrrolidine **(Scheme 21)** [78]. The intermediate pyrrolidine was obtained when the primary amine was (produced by reduction of the NO_2 group) reacted with imine (synthesized by reduction of nitrile). Sinefungin is a nucleoside active against fungi, viruses, and parasites. Synthetic analogues of sinefungin were synthesized from *N*-trifluoroacetylpyrrolidine intermediate [75].

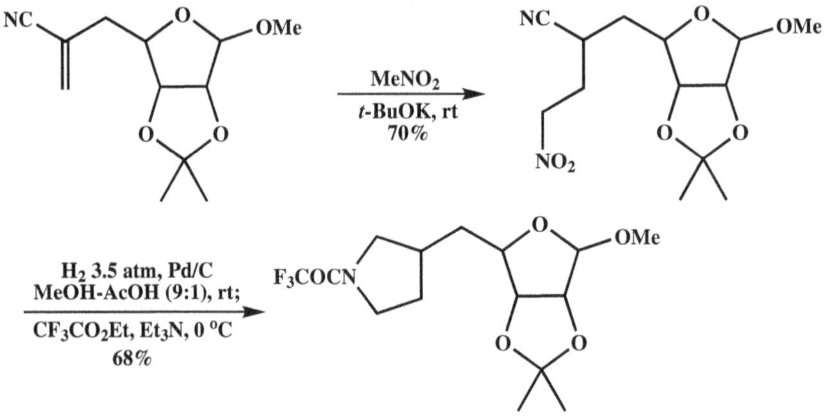

Scheme-21

The but-2-yne-1,4-diones and but-2-ene-1,4-diones through palladium/carbon-catalyzed hydrogenation of C-C double bond/triple bond followed by amination-cyclization afforded many aryl-substituted pyrrole derivates under MWI in one-pot synthetic strategy. Pyrrole was produced in less than 15% yield when the reaction was performed under traditional heating at 110 °C after 12 h (external oil bath 150 °C). Alkyl/aryl ammonium formates or HCOONH$_4$ were utilized both as sources of NH$_3$ and also as reducing agents in Pd-catalyzed transfer hydrogenation. For MW-assisted reaction poly(ethylene glycol)-200 (PEG-200) was used as the most convenient solvent due to its high boiling point (> 250 °C), high dielectric constant (ε = 20), and excellent H$_2$O miscibility **(Scheme 22)** [79].

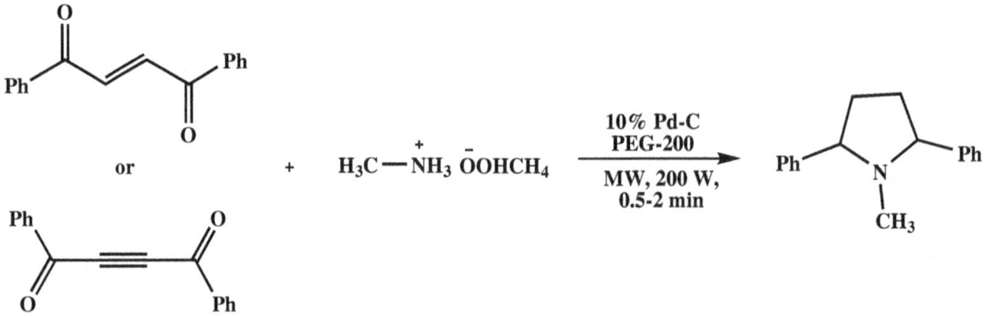

Scheme-22

Attempts were next diverted to check the possibility of an intermolecular olefin insertion *via* Heck reaction into the alkenylpalladium(II) intermediate. The A-H reaction followed by double bond insertion of methyl acrylate, was analyzed using different palladium catalysts including Pd(PPh$_3$)$_4$, Pd(dba)$_2$.P(*o*-tolyl)$_3$ and Pd(dba)$_3$.P(*t*-butyl)$_3$ **(Scheme 23)** [80-82].

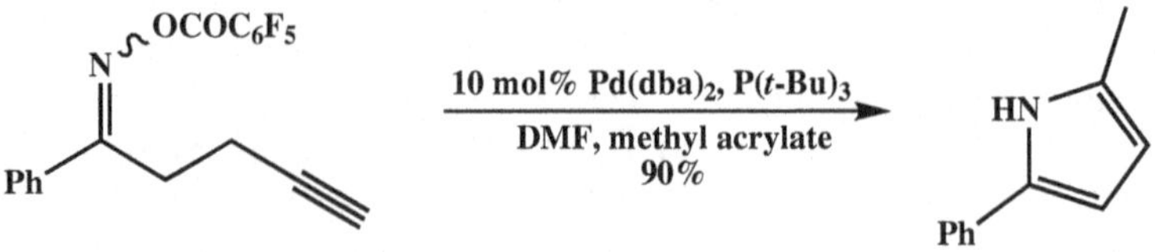

Scheme-23

The 1,3-dipolar cycloaddition reactions were used to form the carbon-heteroatom bonds under traditional conditions [83-88]. Dipolar cycloaddition reactions in the presence of Pd catalyst are rather rare. A few reports have described a palladium-catalyzed [3+2]-cycloaddition reactions of TMM with imines for the preparation of pyrrolidines [89-90]. Trost [91] produced enantioenriched pyrrolidine derivatives with an asymmetric variant of these reactions. For instance, the TMM precursor was reacted with imine to provide a product in 84% yield and 91% *ee* in the presence of Pd(dba)$_2$ and ligand **(Scheme 24)**.

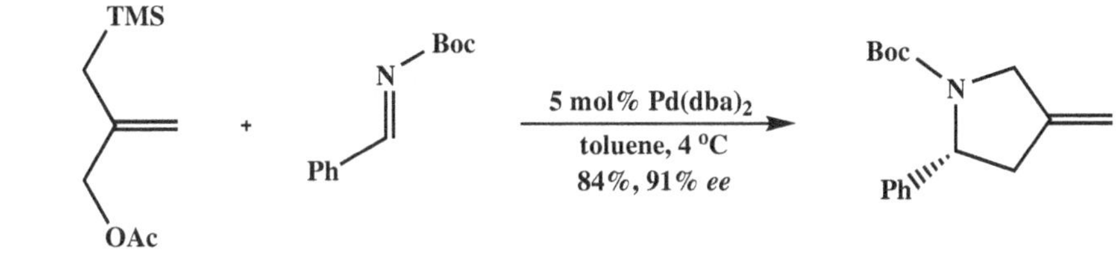

Scheme-24

The 5,5-divinyl oxazolidinones were converted into highly substituted pyrrolidines employing this methodology [92-93]. For instance, the product was afforded in 95% yield by reacting oxazole with activated alkene in the presence of palladium(0) catalyst. The allylpalladium complex was produced *via* oxidative addition followed by decarboxylation. An intermediate was formed by intermolecular conjugate addition and further the intramolecular trapping of allylpalladium moiety furnished the products **(Scheme 25)** [90].

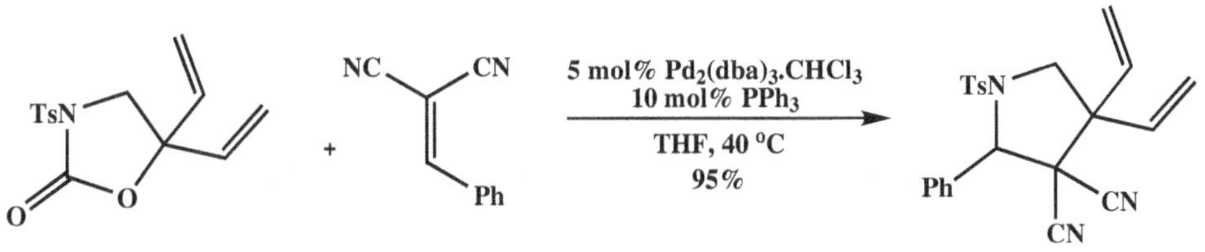

Scheme-25

The 1,1- and 1,2-disubstituted alkenes were examined for the coupling of 2-bromonaphthalene **(Scheme 26)**. Under optimized reaction conditions, no pyrrolidine product formation was observed. Efforts to employ a combination of weaker bases (cesium carbonate, potassium phosphate), ethereal solvents (dioxane, diglyme) and higher temperatures often led to low conversion to pyrrolidine products. Substitution on alkene seems to shut down alkene insertion in the asymmetric carboamination reaction. In these studies on intramolecular insertion of alkenes into palladium-nitrogen bonds, it was observed that 1,1′-bis(diphenylphosphino) ferrocene(palladium)(aryl)amido complexes that bear 1,1-disubstituted alkenes underwent slower *syn*-aminopalladation than the corresponding unsubstituted alkene 1,1′-bis(diphenylphosphino) ferrocene(palladium)(aryl)amido complexes [94-95].

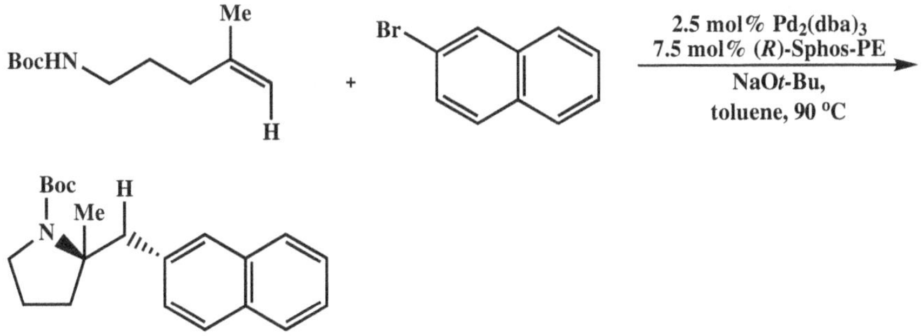

Scheme-26

In 2008 Yamamoto and Narisreddy [96] synthesized vinyl pyrrolidine derivatives *via* palladium-catalyzed intramolecular asymmetric hydroamination of internal alkynes **(Scheme 27)**. This group also reported similar conversions previously [97-98]. However, for improved reaction conditions and higher selectivities the methyl Norphos ligand was utilized. The enantioselectivities and yields up to 95% were reported although the substrate scope was limited to variations on alkyne [99].

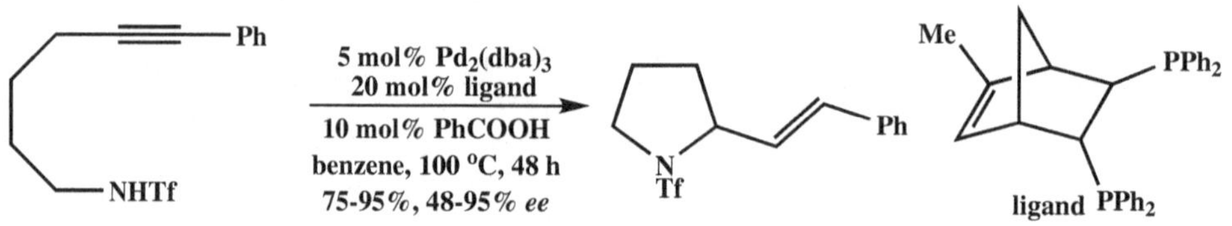

Scheme-27

Greau et al. [100] reported that *N*-heterocycle was formed by cyclization of 1,6-diyne with trimethylsilyltributyltin in the presence of Pd(0) catalyst. The *N*-heterocycle was formed in good yield with an uncommon (*Z,Z*)-geometry at *exo*-double bonds **(Scheme 28)**.

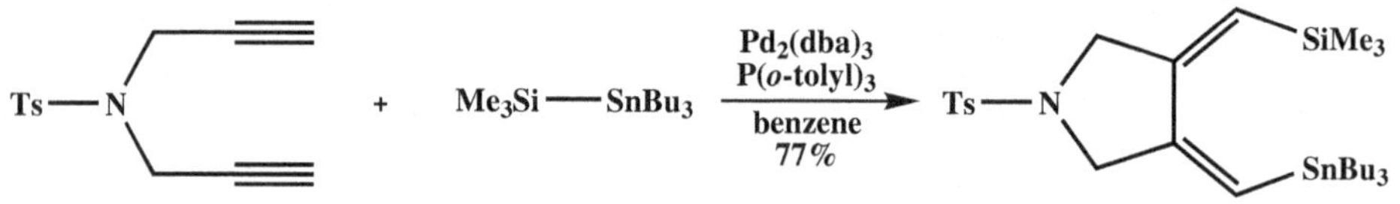

Scheme-28

Good yields of heterocycles were reported when an imine or an aldehyde group possessing allylic chlorides were reacted with allyltributylstannane in dimethylformamide in the presence of $Pd_2(dba)_3.CHCl_3$ **(Scheme 29)** [101-102].

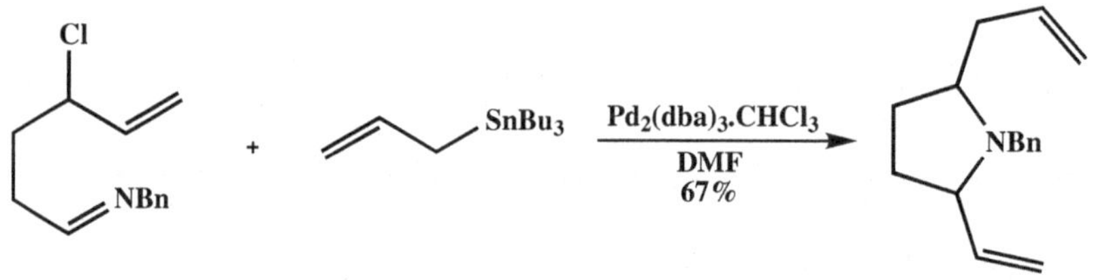

Scheme-29

Mori [103a] reported that propargyl ether containing amides underwent palladium(0)-catalyzed intramolecular cyclization in the presence of *N*-sulfonyl-substituted allenamides **(Scheme 30)**. The allenamides were obtained when monodentate ligand P-(*o*-tolyl)$_3$, for R = OTBS, was used. However, allenamides were further isomerized to dienamide when R = H [103b].

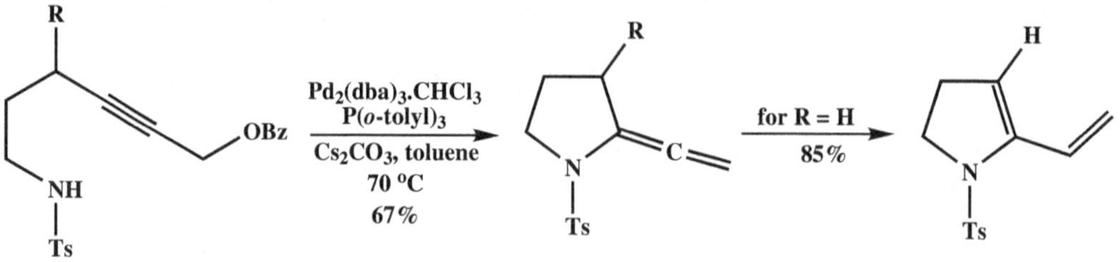

Scheme-30

The cyclization reaction of Boc-protected amine substrate was conducted under two sets of reaction conditions that provided both the *syn* and *anti*-addition products in carboetherification reactions: $Pd_2(dba)_3/PCy_3 \cdot HBF_4$ and $Pd_2(dba)_3/2,2$-bis(diphenyl-phosphanyl)-1,1-binaphthyl. When 2,2-bis(diphenyl-phosphanyl)-1,1-binaphthyl was used as a ligand, the cyclization yielded Boc-protected pyrrolidine (*anti*-addition) in modest yield and good diastereoselectivity (9:1 dr), whereas when PCy_3 was used as a ligand, the *syn*-addition product was generated in good yield and modest diastereoselectivity (2:1 dr) **(Scheme 31)** [104-106].

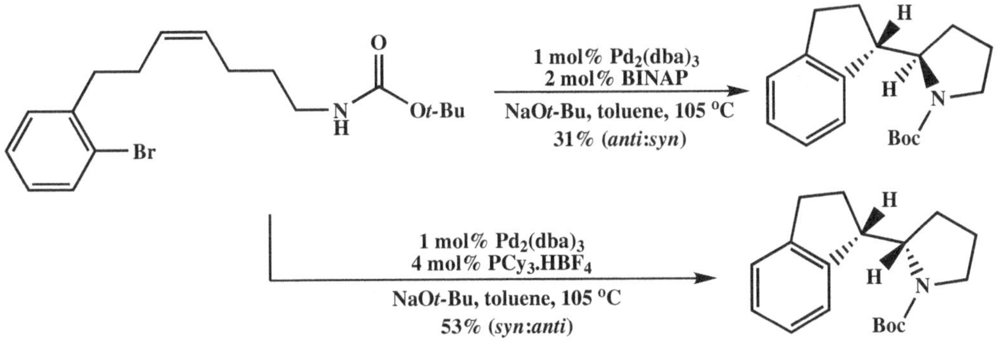

Scheme-31

The rolipram acted as a phosphodiesterase-4 inhibitor. The rolipram was synthesized by a three-component coupling in the presence of Pd catalyst. The alkenylboronate was generated in this method *via* palladium assisted three-component reaction further the Pd-mediated carbonylative cyclization reaction occurred. The rolipram was synthesized by hydrogenation of formed unsaturated lactam and removal of *N*-benzyl group **(Scheme 32)** [107-108].

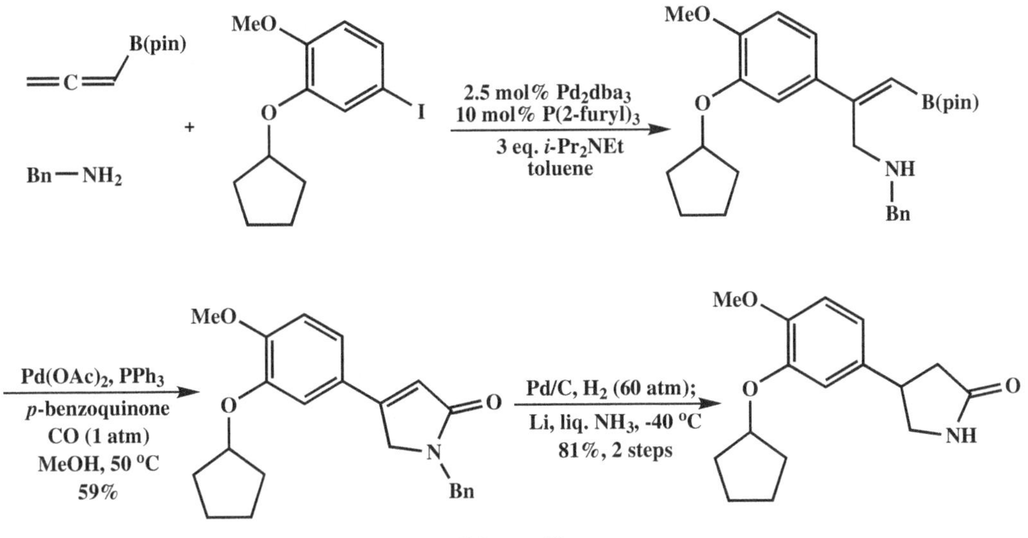

Scheme-32

The pyrrolidine cycloadducts were obtained with excellent selectivities and yields by an enantioselective [3+2]-cycloaddition of trimethylenemethane (TMM) with imines *via* Pd-catalyzed reaction in the presence of novel phosphoramidite ligands **(Scheme 33)** [109].

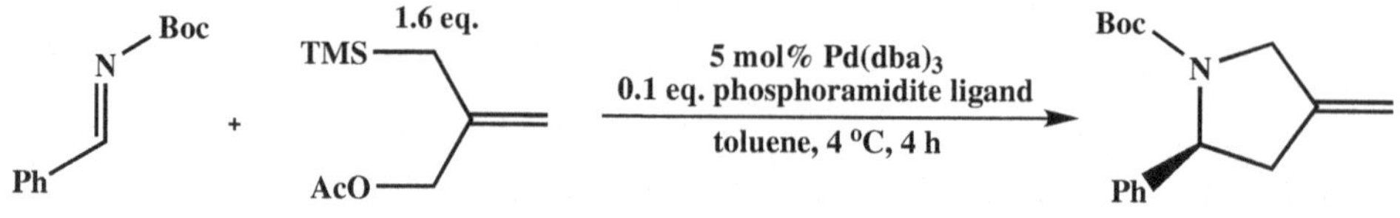

Scheme-33

Preliminary work on asymmetric palladium-catalyzed carboamination reactions was initially conducted by Dr. Qifei Yang, who was a former post-doctoral researcher in the Wolfe group [110]. After a brief survey of ligands, Dr. Yang found that treatment of *N*-phenylpent-4-enylamine and 2-bromonaphthalene with a catalyst system composed of Pd₂(dba)₃ and (*S*)-Quinap facilitated the formation of pyrrolidine in 30% yield and 10% *ee* (**Scheme 34**).

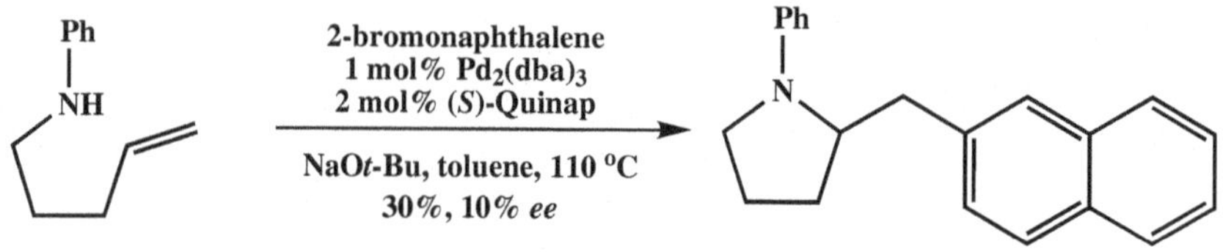

Scheme-34

Initial studies were conducted by Dr. Qifei Yang, a former post-doctoral researcher in the group, for the coupling of starting compound and 2-bromonaphthalene with Pd₂(dba)₃ and chiral ligands. As shown below in **Scheme 35**, monodentate phosphine ligand (*S*)-NMDPP provided product in 80% yield and 48% *ee*. Bis-phosphine ligands and MONOPHOS ligands such as (*R*)-2,2-bis(diphenyl-phosphanyl)-1,1-binaphthyl and (*R*)-monodentate phosphoramidite provided pyrrolidine product in low yields and enantioselectivities [111].

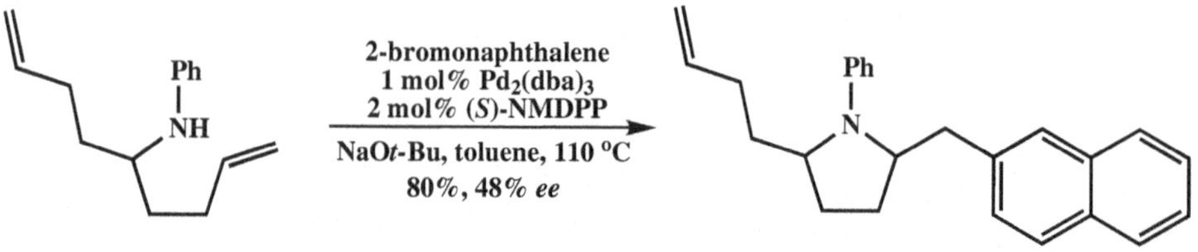

Scheme-35

The linear 4-pentenylamine and its derivatives underwent Pd-catalyzed amination reaction coupled with N-C bond-forming reaction for the stereoselective preparation of *N*-aryl-2-benzylpyrrolidines [112]. Two different aryl bromides were subsequently added to primary aliphatic amine with the help of Pd(0) catalyst. The palladium-catalyzed mono-*N*-arylation afforded γ-(*N*-arylamino)alkenes selectively followed by a carboamination reaction, after addition of the second aryl bromide [113a-b]. This cyclization/coupling reaction produced an intermediate when the organopalladium complex was reacted with γ-(*N*-arylamino) alkene. A *syn*-insertion of alkene into palladium-nitrogen bond in intermediate followed by reductive elimination formed the *N*-aryl-2-benzylpyrrolidines. In this protocol, Pd(0) was utilized as a catalyst in both reactions and the choice of phosphine ligand for carboamination reactions and *N*-arylation of amines was very important. To achieve the selective diarylation in good yields *in situ* modification of catalyst with phosphine ligand exchange was crucial (**Scheme 36**) [108].

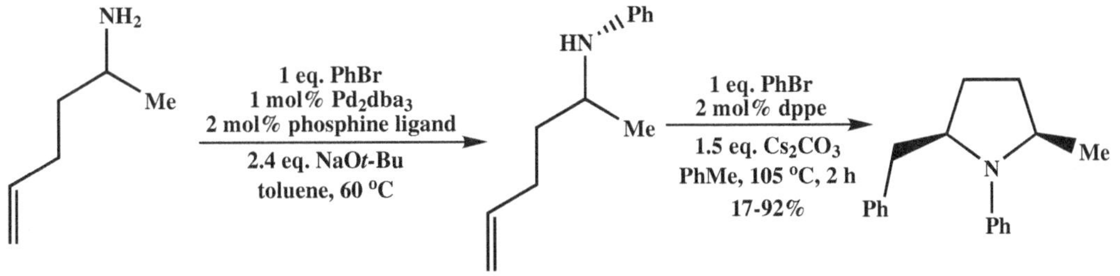

Scheme-36

Reactions completed with *syn*-selectivity with aniline containing substrates which were branched at C-1. For instance, product was provided in 5:1 diastereoselectivity and 55% yield when the *E*-alkene was reacted in the presence of catalytic amounts of $Pd_2(dba)_3/PCy_3 \cdot HBF_4$. The major product diastereomer contain 2,5-*trans*-disubstitution around the pyrrolidine ring; the minor diastereomer resulted from *syn*-addition with *cis*-pyrrolidine formation. In contrast, the 2,5-*cis*-disubstituted pyrrolidine products were obtained with high selectivity from analogous intermolecular carboamination reactions of γ-(*N*-arylamino)alkenes **(Scheme 37)** [113a-b].

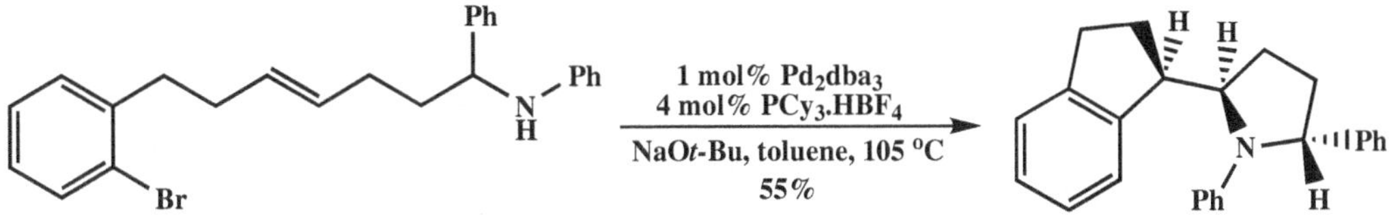

Scheme-37

The *N*-Boc- and *N*-acyl-protected pyrrolidines were synthesized stereoselectively when γ-(*N*-Boc-amino) alkenes and γ-(*N*-acylamino) alkenes were reacted with aryl bromides *via* palladium-catalyzed reaction and the reaction occurred with high levels of diastereoselectivity by the formation of two bonds in a single operation **(Scheme 38)** [114].

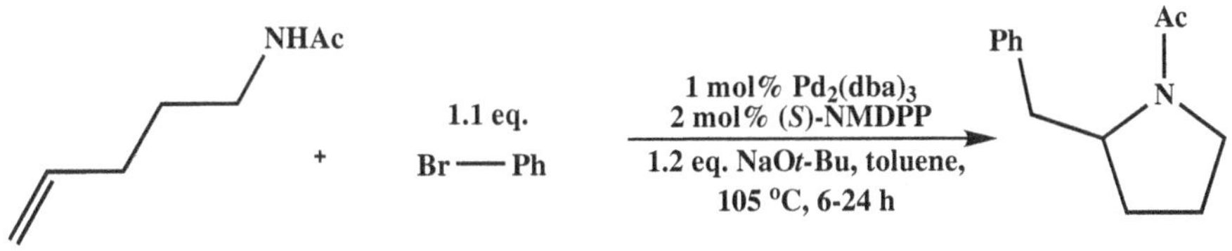

Scheme-38

The carboamination of amino olefin with 4-bromoanisole proceeded with high diastereo-selectivity for the formation of 2,5-*cis*-disubstituted pyrrolidine **(Scheme 39)** [113a,b-119].

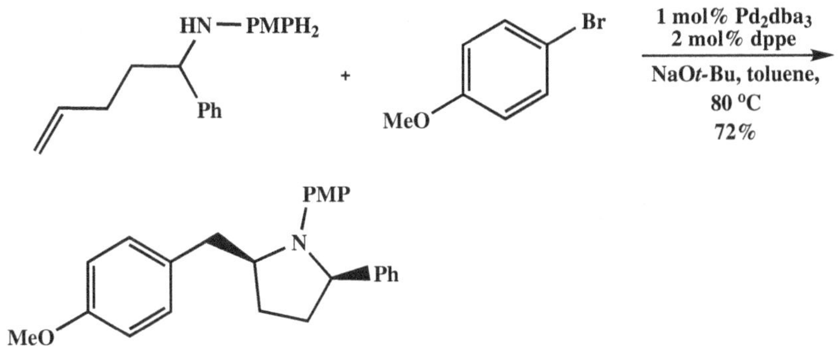

Scheme-39

Palladium-catalyzed carboamination of alkenes has become a useful method for the synthesis of a broad array of nitrogen-containing heterocycles [120]. In 2004, Wolfe [121] reported the palladium-catalyzed coupling of γ-aminoalkenes with aryl bromides to yield 2-benzylpyrrolidines **(Scheme 40)**. In addition to pyrrolidines being an interesting class of medicinally-relevant compounds [122], this carboamination method was demonstrated to involve a novel, intramolecular *syn*-aminopalladation step [113a-b].

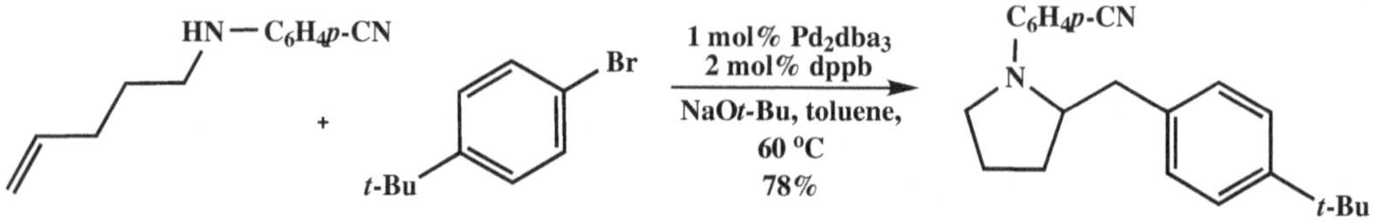

Scheme-40

A prominent goal in organic synthesis is control of product distribution by alteration of reaction parameters. Work of Wolfe group [24] has demonstrated that the relative rates of competing reaction pathways to desired carboamination can be influenced by both variance in group on the cyclizing nitrogen as well as though judicious choice of phosphine ligand. For example, Beaudoin Bertrand and Wolfe found that the relative ratio of Heck, carboamination, and *N*-arylation products in reactions of γ-aminoalkenes depends on the nature of functional group present on nitrogen. Groups such as Ac, Boc, and 4-MeO-Bz were utilized preferably for the desired cyclization to either *N*-arylation or Heck. In contrast, highly electron-poor groups such as Bz and 4-F$_3$C-Bz afforded a much higher percentage of Heck product. More electron-rich groups such as Bn and Ph allowed *N*-arylation to be competitive **(Scheme 41)** [123-126].

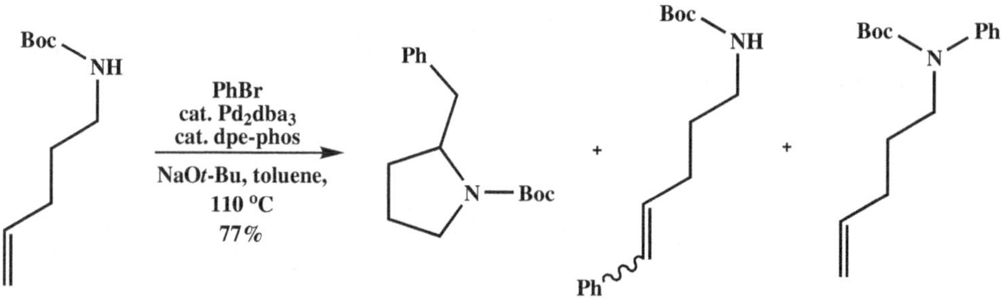

Scheme-41

Hara and co-workers [127] described that pyrrolidine was formed poorly when asymmetric metallo-ene reaction of bisallylamine was carried out in the presence of Pd$_2$(dba)$_3$-(S)-9-NapBN. The target compounds were obtained in low enantioselectivity and poor yield **(Scheme 42)** [72].

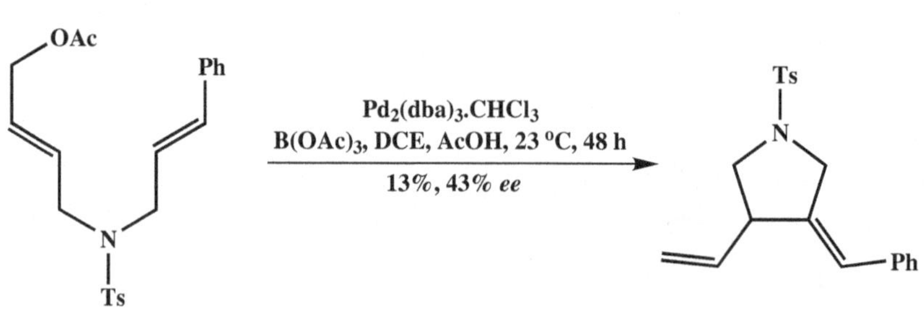

Scheme-42

Poli and co-workers [128] described that disubstituted γ-lactam was formed from *N*-acyl allylamine *via* a palladium-catalyzed intramolecular asymmetric allylic alkylation. The desired product was obtained with up to 84% *ee* in the presence of (*R*)-*t*-Bu-OMeBiphep ligand in a biphasic medium **(Scheme 43)**. DFT studies were performed for the rationalization of extent and direction of stereochemistry [72].

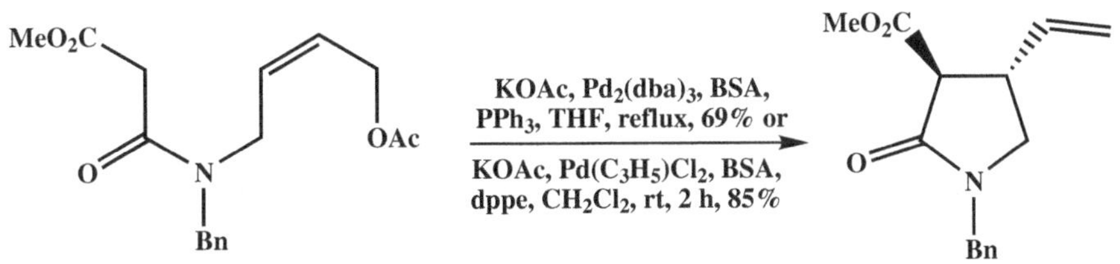
MeO2C
O
N
Bn
OAc
KOAc, Pd2(dba)3, BSA,
PPh3, THF, reflux, 69% or
KOAc, Pd(C3H5)Cl2, BSA,
dppe, CH2Cl2, rt, 2 h, 85%
MeO2C
O
N
Bn

Scheme-43

Wolfe [121] used two different aryl bromides and a terminally unsaturated amine for the formation of pyrrolidines **(Scheme 44)** [57, 123, 129].

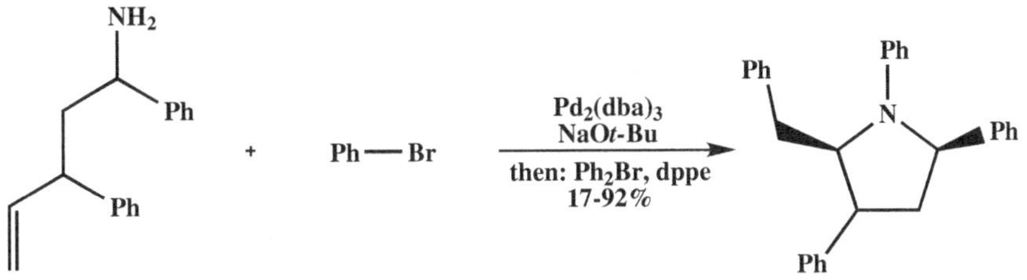
NH2
Ph
Ph
+
Ph—Br
Pd2(dba)3
NaOt-Bu
then: Ph2Br, dppe
17-92%
Ph
Ph
N
Ph
Ph

Scheme-44

The best enantioselectivities were obtained with β-bromostyrene (up to 94% *ee*) as electrophilic coupling partner. Alkenyl halides containing aliphatic chains were also effective coupling partners for the reaction. Two eq. of alkenyl coupling partner were required, since dimerization of alkenyl bromide can be problematic [130-131]. Low yields were obtained when low boiling alkenyl bromides such as 1-bromo-propene were employed in the reaction, even in excessive quantities **(Scheme 45)**.

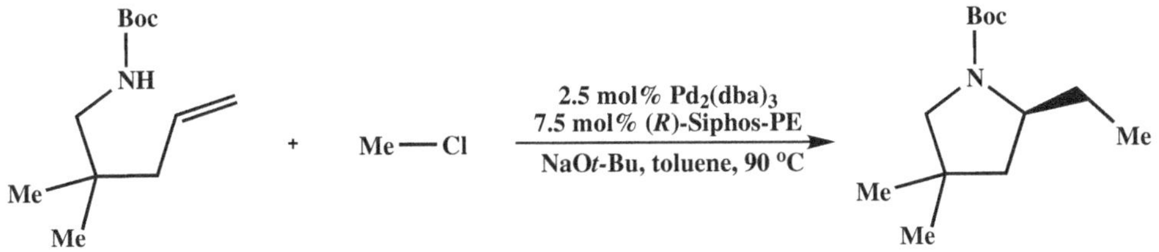
Boc
NH
Me
Me
+
Me—Cl
2.5 mol% Pd2(dba)3
7.5 mol% (R)-Siphos-PE
NaOt-Bu, toluene, 90 °C
Boc
N
Me
Me
Me

Scheme-45

Treatment of amine under typical carboamination conditions provided pyrrolidine in 50% yield and excellent diastereoselectivity. The yield of carboamination reaction of amine to pyrrolidine was higher. The inseparable mixture of olefin diastereomers complicated the analysis of reaction. The geometry of olefin was assigned by analogy to six-membered ring derivative on which a NOESY-2D was obtained. It appeared that one olefin isomer, which was assumed to be *E*-olefin reacted to provide pyrrolidine. The other olefin isomer also reacted, as evidenced by the lack of remaining starting material. Since the stereoselectivity of reaction was 22:1 dr, it was reasonable to assume that *Z*-olefin was not undergoing carboamination reaction under these reaction conditions and actually provided Heck product, which was also isolated. This example nicely illustrated a potential solution in complex molecule synthesis. In a situation such as this, when one olefin geometry does not undergo the desired transformation in an otherwise stereospecific cyclization, simply changing the catalyst in order to get the desired diastereomer was a very effective solution (**Scheme 46**) [132].

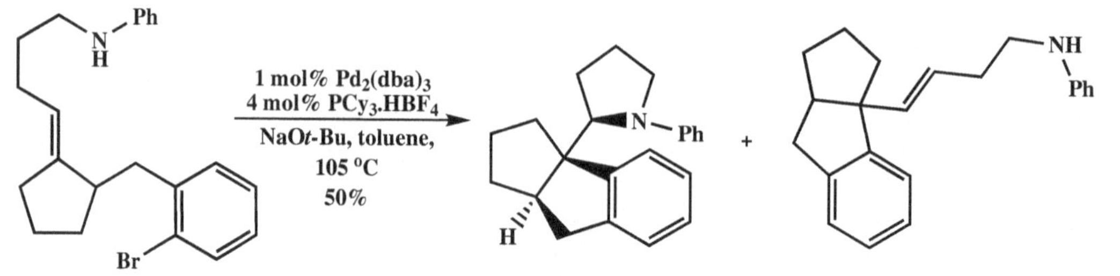

Scheme-46

The palladium-catalyzed cyclization occurred in a nonreversible manner (**Scheme 47**). To afford a selective product, cyclization would have to be slower than isomerization of the palladium-allyl complex and to avoid unnecessary purification, starting compound was utilized as a diastereomeric mixture. Furthermore, the cyclization of one diastereomeric intermediate should be kinetically faster than the other. The *trans* isomer was formed exclusively from diastereomer ratio of product. Although the C-cyclization was not observed, the successful isomerization of starting compound was encouraging. Lactams were formed in quantitative yield with lithium ethoxide (base) in ethanol. Unfortunately, equal amounts of diastereomers were formed [133-134].

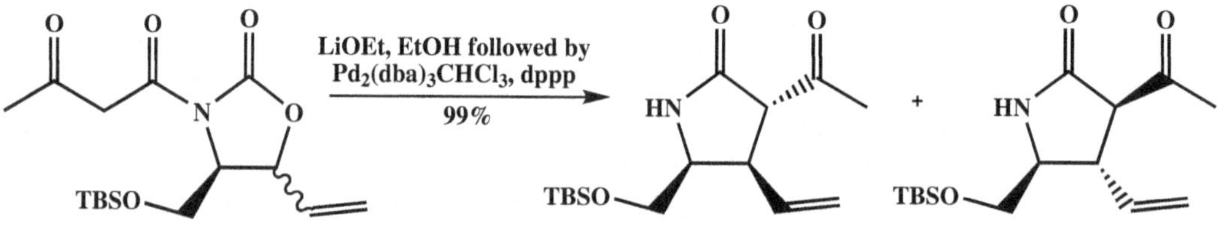

Scheme-47

Monocyclic heterocycles were synthesized by this strategy, though not to the degree of indoles and benzofurans. Either a saturated fragment or a double bond was placed in place of aryl spacer between amine and alkyne which was capable of elimination. Utimoto [135] reported in an early report, that many 2,4-substituted pyrroles were synthesized by cyclization of 1-amino-3-alkyn-2-ols with Pd(II) catalysts (**Scheme 48**).

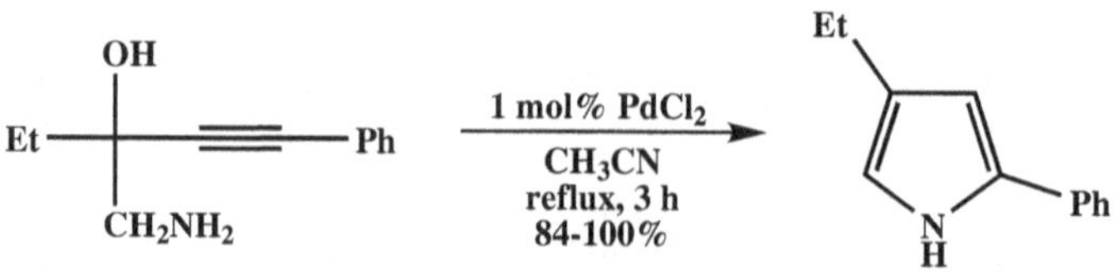

Scheme-48

α-Halo carbonyl compounds containing appropriately situated olefins underwent Heck-type cyclizations to afford the corresponding ring structure (**Scheme 49**) [136-141]. Such a cyclization involved the generation of a new stereocenter, although this was ultimately destroyed upon hydride elimination (and eventual double bond isomerization). It was hypothesized that if the alkylpalladium intermediate could be trapped prior to hydride elimination, possibly by some organometallic reagent or CO, then the newly formed stereocenter would be retained. Thus, if the cyclization could be conducted in an asymmetric fashion, then such a process could provide access to a number of enantioenriched heterocycles.

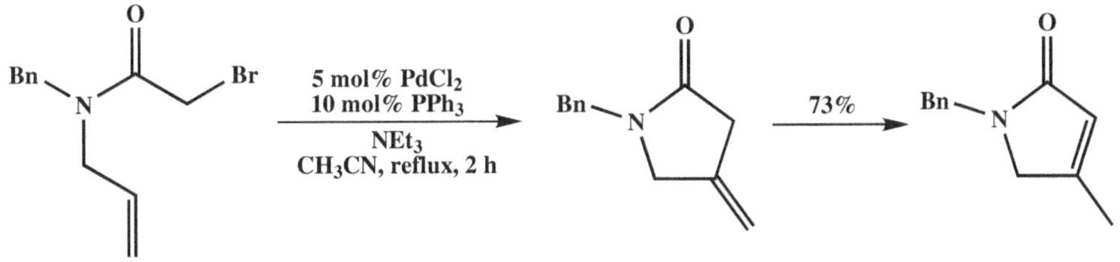

Scheme-49

The pyrrolidines were synthesized in this process [142]. For instance, the starting substrate was reacted with 15 mol% of $PdCl_2(PhCN)_2$ to synthesize the product as a single diastereomer in 77% yield [143]. The cyclization occurred without epimerization of amino ester stereocenter under mild reaction conditions (**Scheme 50**) [90].

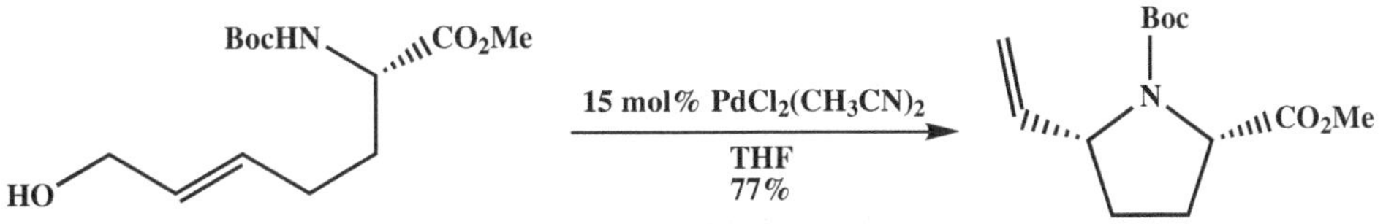

Scheme-50

Prandi and co-workers [144] used *N*-tosylalkoxydienylamines as starting compounds for the preparation of tri- and tetrasubstituted *N*-tosylpyrroles under dioxygen atmosphere *via* an aminopalladation reaction (**Scheme 51**) [72].

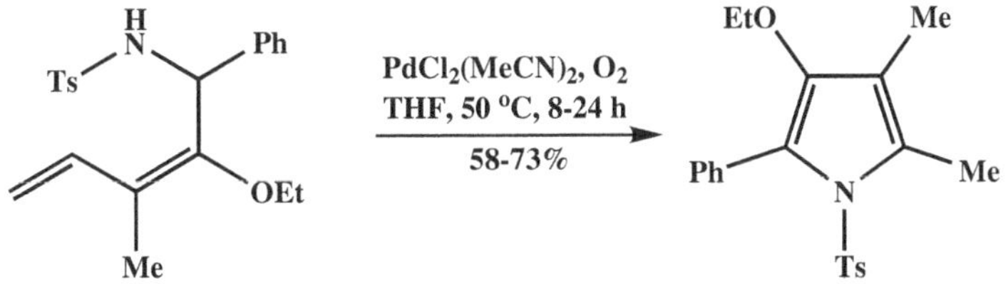

Scheme-51

Tosylated 2-hydroxy-3-butenylamines were utilized for the production of pyrrole derivatives (**Scheme 52**) [145-146]. For the cyclization reaction hydroxyl group was necessary. No addition occurred when palladium acetate was utilized instead of $PdCl_2(MeCN)_2$. In this cyclization chloride ion played a crucial role by allowing the addition of palladium chloride at C3-C4 followed by nucleophilic substitution of chlorine by nitrogen. Furans as well as pyrroles were prepared by this same synthetic protocol from keto-substituted alkenes [147-148]. In the first case, the enol forms of ketones underwent initial cyclization on double bond, followed by β-hydride elimination (and product rearrangement) and subsequent catalyst reoxidation by cupric chloride. Interestingly, the cyclization of alkyl-substituted ketone occurred with good selectivity for the synthesis of furan core over aryl-ketones, allowing for the generation of diversely substituted furans [149].

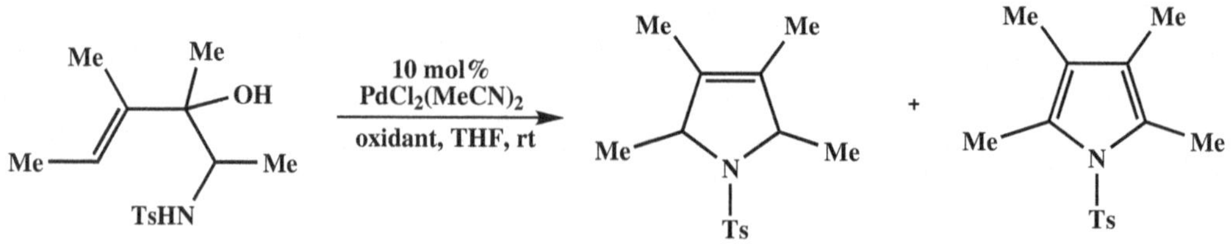

Scheme-52

An ester group possessing *cis*-1-n-butyl-2-carboalkoxy-3-methylaziridines underwent cycloaddition reaction. An efficient cycloaddition occurred to provide *cis*-l-n-butyl-3-(*p*-chlorophenyl)-4-carbomethoxy-5-methylimidazolidin-2-on in 80% yield when aziridine was reacted with *p*-chlorophenyl isocyanate in the presence of 10 mol% of bis-(benzonitrile)palladium dichloride at 120 °C in PhMe for 20 h. The reaction was stereo- as well as regiospecific, the cycloaddition took place with retention of stereochemistry at heterocyclic carbon centers containing substituent groups. Thiazolidinimines and imidazolidinones were afforded in good yields when aryl isothiocyanates and isocyanates were treated with aziridine in the presence of (PhCN)₂PdCl₂ (**Scheme 53**) [150-151].

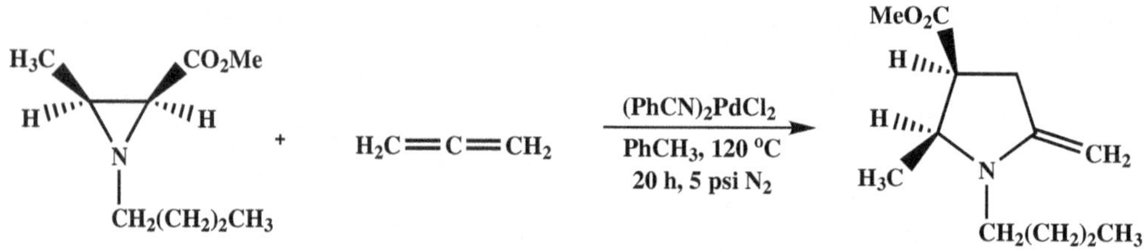

Scheme-53

This pathway [152] was utilized for the synthesis of disubstituted sulfinyl γ-lactams from substituted allylamines as shown in **Scheme 54**. The products with opposite diastereoselectivities were afforded from an enantiopure sulfinyl-derived substrate of defined absolute configuration under biphasic conditions (dichloromethane/water or toluene/water) in the presence of 2,2-bis(diphenyl-phosphanyl)-1,1-binaphthyl ligand [72].

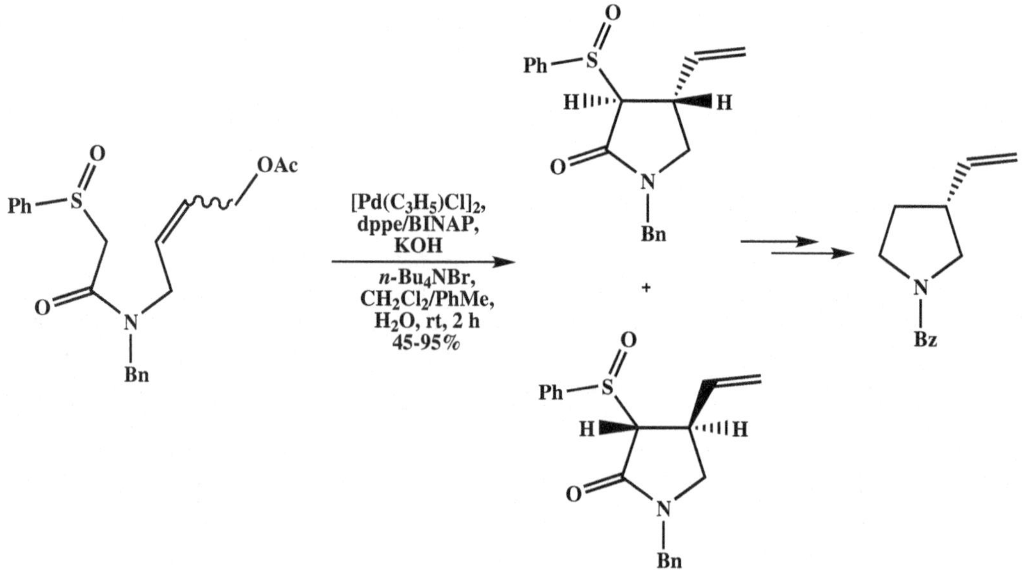

Scheme-54

Thuong and co-workers [153] manipulated the substituted allylamine for the synthesis of pyrrolidone derivative from allylic sulfone *via* intramolecular allylic alkylation in the presence of palladium catalyst (**Scheme 55**). The (-)-α-kainic acid was formed from pyrrolidone derivative [72].

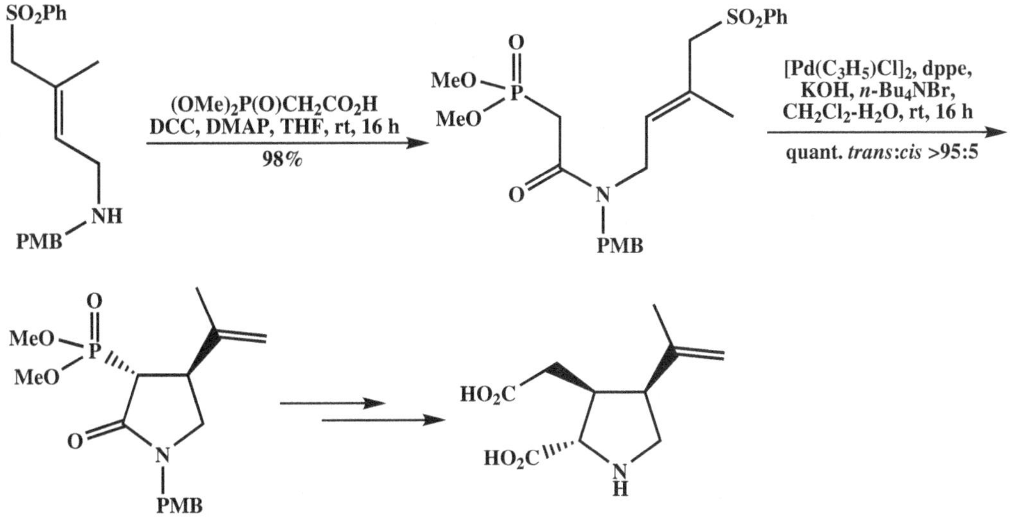

Scheme-55

The 2-alkenylpyrrolidine was synthesized in good to high yields by an intramolecular hydroamination of aminoallenes in the presence of Pd, CH_3COOH, and phosphine (**Scheme 56**) [154]. The oxidative addition of nitrogen-hydrogen bond to Pd(0) and subsequent hydropalladation of allene moiety produced a hydridopalladium species.

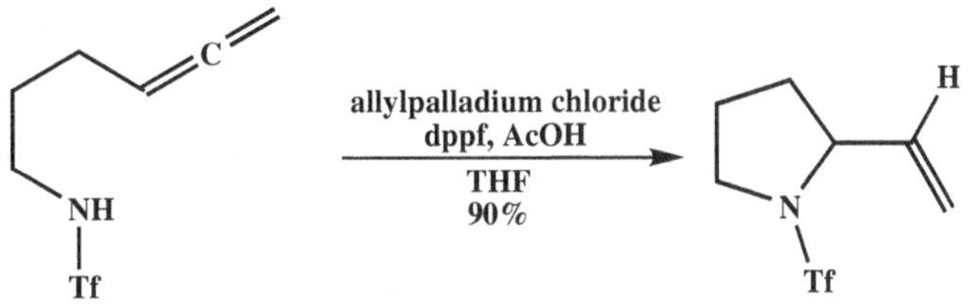

Scheme-56

Allylic alkylation reactions were conducted as asymmetric versions in the presence of palladium catalyst [155-158]. A class of ligands was developed by Trost [159] to afford excellent enantioselectivities and yields for many reactions. For example, the product was formed in 91% *ee* and 97% yield when allylic acetate was treated with 3 mol% of ligand and 1 mol% of allylpalladium chloride. Heterocyclic products were prepared by asymmetric desymmetrization reactions of *meso*-bis-carbamates (**Scheme 57**) [90, 160-161].

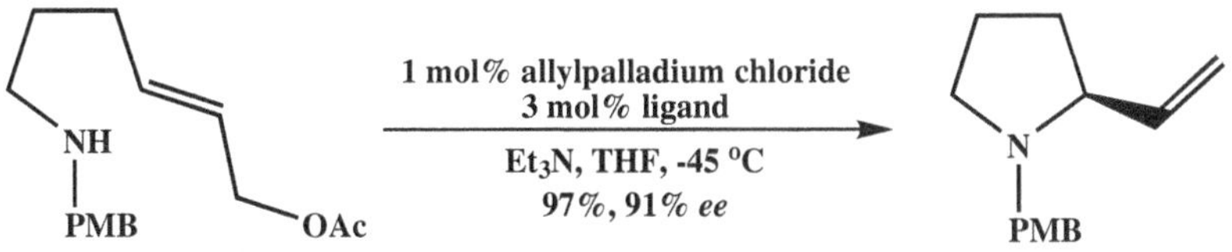

Scheme-57

Nitrogen-possessing heterocyclic compounds were synthesized in multi-component pathway initiated by an aza-Michael addition and terminated by a Pd-catalyzed ring-closure reaction. For example, Balme et al. [162] observed a three-component reaction of highly functionalized allyl- and 4-benzyl-pyrrolidines based on a combination of allylamines (converted to their sodium salts with sodium hydride), unsaturated halides (or triflate) and *gem*-diactivated alkenes as Michael acceptors in the presence of palladium catalyst. Three partners were reacted in equal amounts at rt with Pd(0) catalyst (prepared *in situ* by reduction of $PdCl_2(PPh_3)_2$ with *n*-BuLi). This one-pot conversion involved a palladium-catalyzed cyclofunctionalization of allyl moiety by carbopalladation/reductive elimination. The *N*-methyl- or *N*-allylpyrrolidines were reacted with 2-mercaptobenzoic acid in boiling acetonitrile to produce 3-sulfonylpyrolidin-2-ones (γ-lactams) as single *trans*-diastereomers in high yield. The γ-lactams were generated by acid-promoted synthesis of a ring-opened iminium salt intermediate, followed by hydrolysis and subsequent intramolecular attack of the released secondary amine onto ester group. Genet et al. [163] reported an unexpected conversion during palladium-catalyzed deallylation of *N*-allyl-3-sulfonylpyrrolidines in 2-mercaptobenzoic acid **(Scheme 58)**. Like other late transition metal compounds, co-ordinatively unsaturated palladium complexes revealed a pronounced carbophilic Lewis acidity [164]. This Pd mediated sequence was extended to allyl derivatives. Diastereomeric mixtures of tetrasubstituted pyrrolidines were formed in this 3-CR. Initially the allyl amine derivative was deprotonated and underwent an intermolecular Michael-addition to activated alkene. The stabilized carbanion with an alkene tether was used as a ligand for palladium species which triggered a 5-*exo-trig* cyclization after subsequent reductive elimination to afford the pyrrolidine [57, 108].

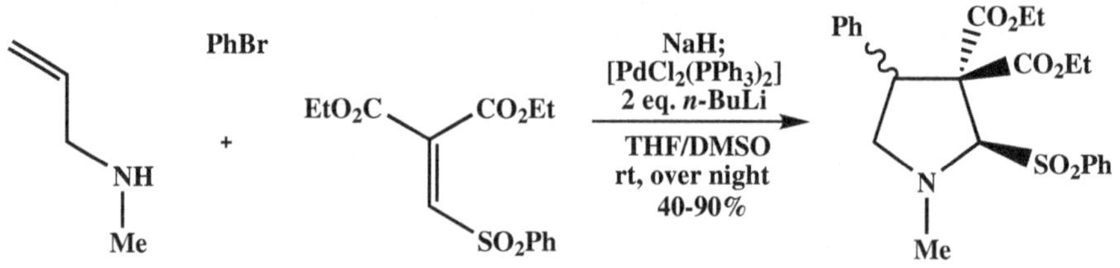

Scheme-58

The *N*-fluorobenzenesulfonimide was used as an aminating reagent for palladium-catalyzed diamination of unactivated alkenes. The substrate provided one nitrogen donor atom and other nitrogen was afforded by *N*-fluorobenzenesulfonimide to produce the cyclic diamine derivatives in a single step. The products were protected differentially at both the nitrogen which afforded maximum synthetic flexibility to method **(Scheme 59)** [165].

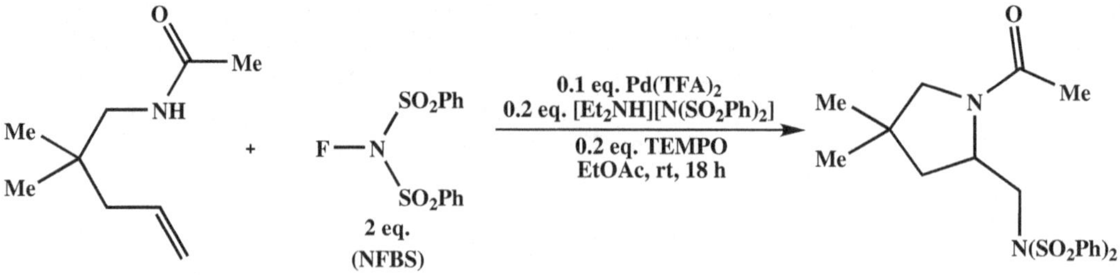

Scheme-59

The stoichiometric oxidant oxygen and (pyrox)Pd(II)(TFA)$_2$ catalyst was utilized for enantioselective intramolecular oxidative amidation of alkenes. The reactions occurred with high enantioselectivity and in very good yields at rt. For a number of chiral substrates, catalyst-controlled stereoselective cyclization reactions were demonstrated **(Scheme 60)** [166].

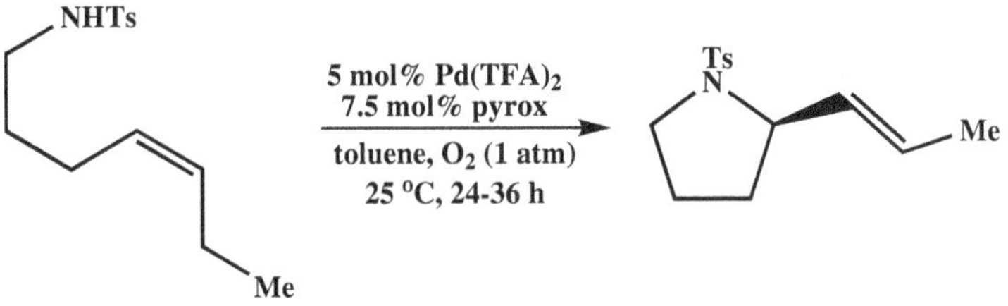

5 mol% Pd(TFA)$_2$
7.5 mol% pyrox

toluene, O$_2$ (1 atm)
25 °C, 24-36 h

Scheme-60

A highly enantioselective intramolecular Wacker-type oxidative cyclization of internal alkenyl sulfonamides was reported using (pyrox)Pd(II)(TFA)$_2$ as catalyst and oxygen as sole stoichiometric oxidant for the synthesis of enantioenriched pyrrolidines **(Scheme 61)** [167]. As shown below, substrates were converted to products in good to excellent yields and high enantioselectivities using a catalyst system of Pd(TFA)$_2$ and pyridine-oxazoline ligand. Preliminary computational studies have revealed that the reaction may proceed through a rate-limiting and enantio-determining transition state, where vinylic methyl group in transition state was oriented downward, away from the phenyl group, which led to differentiation of two enantiotopic faces of alkene in insertion step.

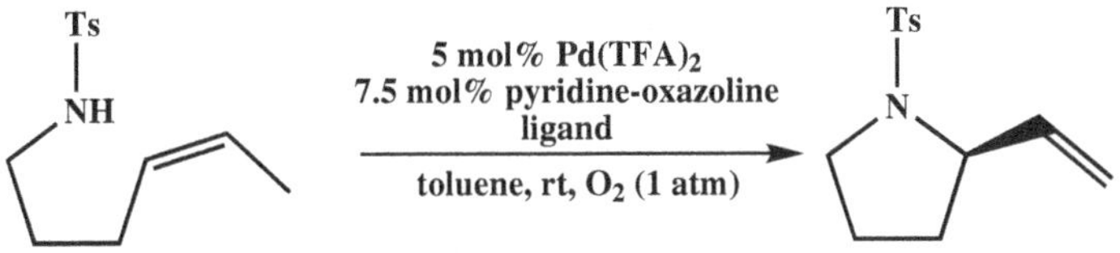

5 mol% Pd(TFA)$_2$
7.5 mol% pyridine-oxazoline
ligand

toluene, rt, O$_2$ (1 atm)

Scheme-61

Catalyst-controlled stereoselective cyclization was demonstrated for a number of chiral substrates **(Scheme 62)**. For example, treatment of chiral substrate with (*R*)- or (*S*)-enantiomer provided *cis*-2,4-disubstituted pyrrolidine or *trans*-2,4-disubstituted pyrrolidine respectively in good yield and high diastereoselectivity [168].

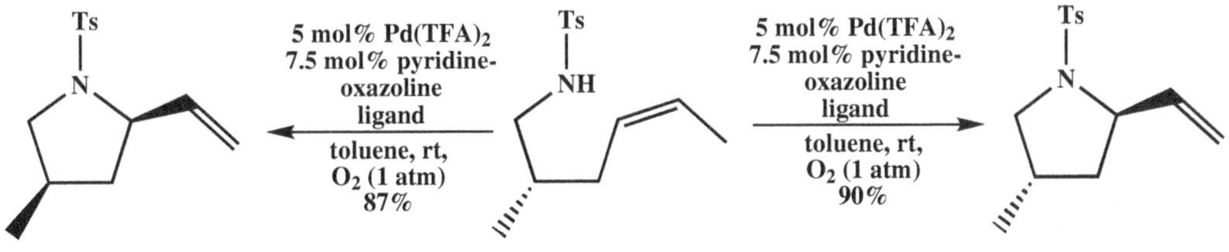

5 mol% Pd(TFA)$_2$
7.5 mol% pyridine-oxazoline
ligand

toluene, rt,
O$_2$ (1 atm)
87%

5 mol% Pd(TFA)$_2$
7.5 mol% pyridine-oxazoline
ligand

toluene, rt,
O$_2$ (1 atm)
90%

Scheme-62

The bridged bicyclic *N*-heterocycles were constructed in this pathway and has been employed for the preparation of alkaloid natural product (-)-ferruginine [169]. Sasai et al. [170] developed an asymmetric variant of this reaction. The sulfonamide was transformed into pyrrolidine in 60% *ee* and 95% yield in the presence of a catalyst composed of Pd(TFA)$_2$ and spiro bis(isoxazoline) ligand. Although this conversion needed very long reaction times (7 d) and high catalyst loadings, there was potential for achieving asymmetric induction in these systems, and development of new catalysts for these reactions was likely to be an area of future investigation **(Scheme 63)** [90].

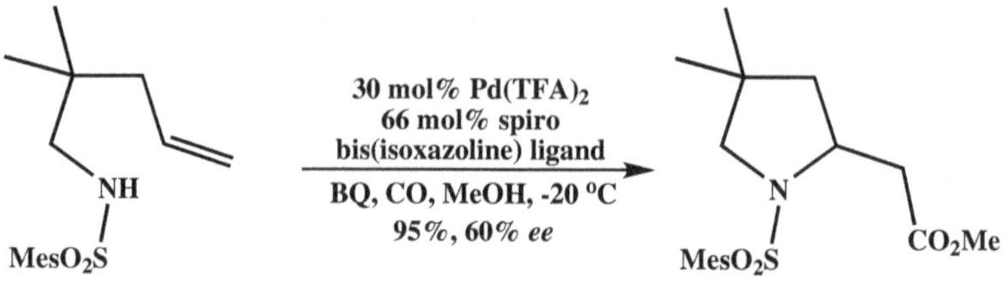

Scheme-63

Sperry and co-workers [171] synthesized 2-pyrrolidinone by palladium hydroxide-mediated hydrogenation of allylamine derivative to affect lactamization under acidic conditions **(Scheme 64)**. The natural product, (-)-berkeleyamide A, along with (-)-10-epiberkeleyamide A was produced from pyrrolidinone [72].

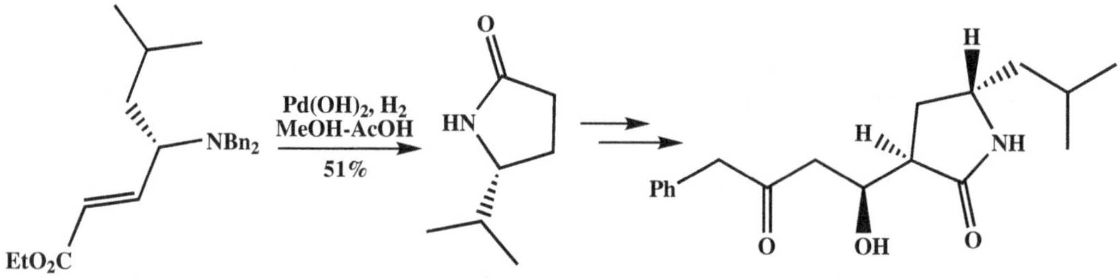

Scheme-64

Kim and co-workers [172] produced γ-lactams including diminolyxitol (a potent α-galactosidase inhibitor). The mechanism involved dihydroxylation of double bond followed by conversion into an isopropylidene group, which was then hydrogenated to induce a tandem reaction involving de-protection and lactamization **(Scheme 65)** [72].

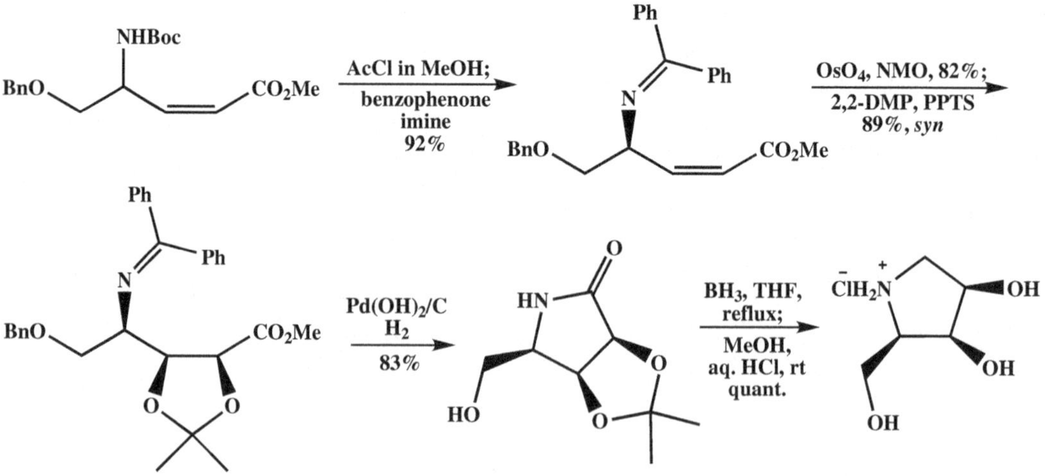

Scheme-65

Gabriele [50, 173] synthesized (Z)-(2-en-4-ynyl)amines which underwent cycloisomerization either under Pd-catalyzed conditions or spontaneously (with terminal or aryl-substituted alkynes) **(Scheme 66)**. Rearrangement to aromatic pyrrole occurred spontaneously through proton migration to afford good yields of tetrasubstituted pyrroles. The reaction occurred through a similar nucleophilic attack on terminal alkyne carbon in the presence of Pd catalyst, followed by proton migration and subsequent alcohol elimination allowing aromatization.

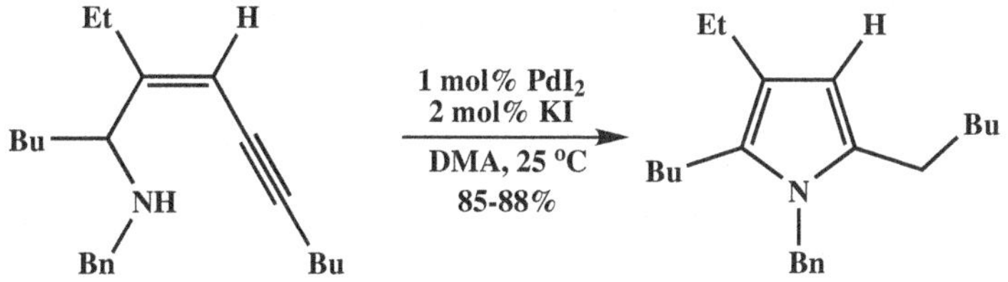

Scheme-66

Gabriele and co-workers [174-176] described the synthesis of 1,3-dihydroinol-2-one derivatives in good yields when *o*-ethynylanilines were reacted with CO, MeOH, and O_2 in the presence of Pd catalyst **(Scheme 67)**. The carbonylative nucleophilic trapping was also used for the interception of Pd intermediates. This protocol was employed to a variety of heterocyclic cyclizations, often in concert with alcohols to produce ester substituted products. The simple oxidant O_2 was employed in various examples. Gabriele and co-workers [177-178] explained the preparation of carbonyl derivatives, like pyrrole-2-acetic ester *via* palladium iodide-potassium iodide-catalyzed oxidative carbonylation of (*Z*)-(2-ene-4-ynyl)amines. Excess amounts of carbon dioxide were beneficial to the product selectivity as well as reaction rate [72].

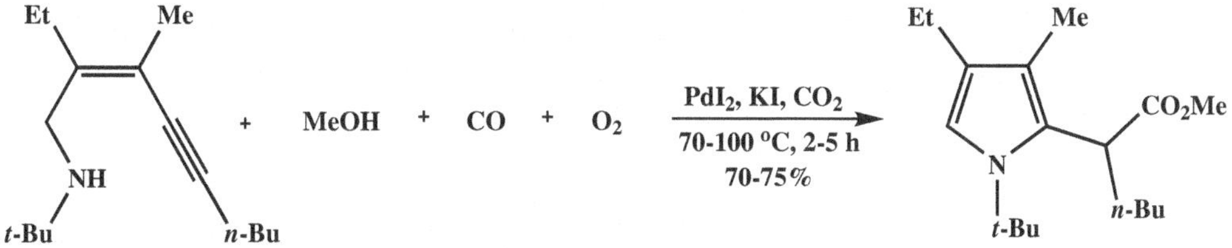

Scheme-67

O'Neil and Fuerstner [179] reported the synthesis of 2-substituted pyrrolidine from Boc-protected allylamine through a palladium-catalyzed boronate-alkyl Suzuki coupling and subsequent Michael reaction **(Scheme 68)**. Interestingly, the boronate was generated *in situ*, which participated in Suzuki coupling [72].

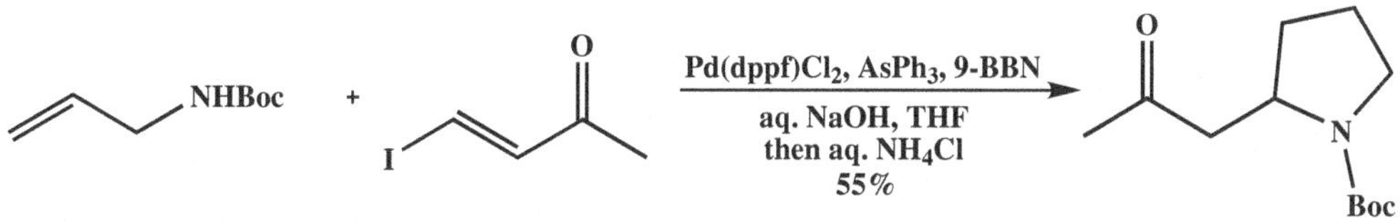

Scheme-68

This reductive cyclization reaction was performed in asymmetric version **(Scheme 69)**. The product was obtained with 82% *ee* in 63% yield when starting compound was reacted in the presence of [Pd(*S,S*-bdpp)(H$_2$O)$_2$](BF$_4$)$_2$ at rt in ethanol [180].

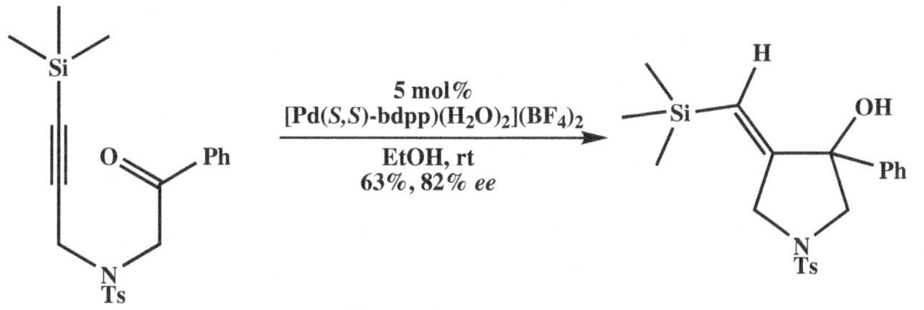

Scheme-69

Deuteriated ethanol was utilized in this reaction. The product was obtained in 97% yield without deuterium incorporation into product when starting compound underwent reductive cyclization in CH_3CH_2OD **(Scheme 70)**. However, product was obtained with a deuterium at vinyl position in 92% yield in the presence of CH_3CD_2OH **(Scheme 71)** [180].

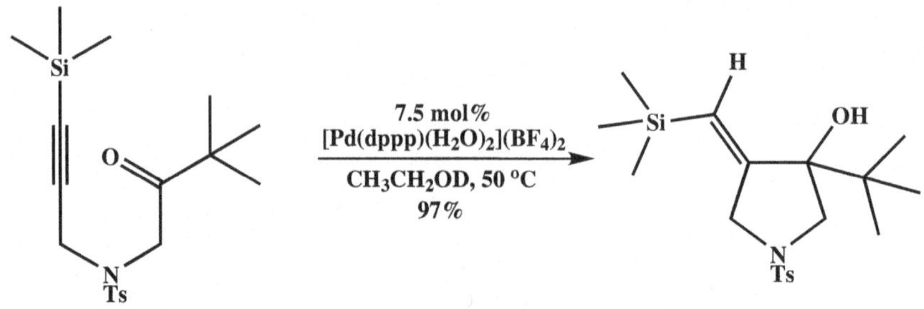

Scheme-70

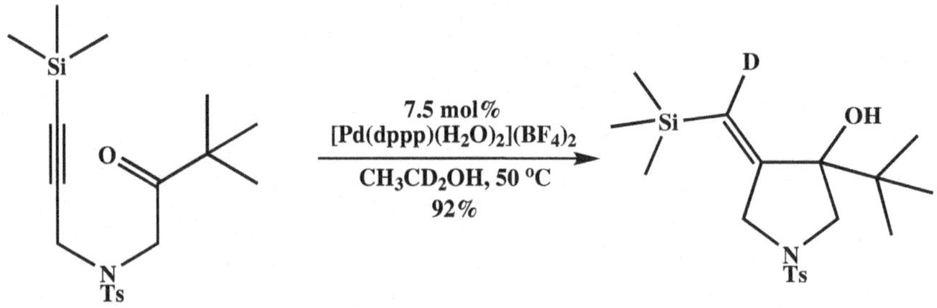

Scheme-71

In fluoropalladation step, a Pd-catalyzed tandem fluorination and cyclization of an enyne, the stereochemistry was investigated. The fluorinated 3-benzylidenyllactame with (*E*)-isomer was provided as major product in this reaction [181]. For the formation of Csp^2-F bond, the *cis*-aminopalladation of alkynes was a preferred strategy **(Scheme 72)** [182].

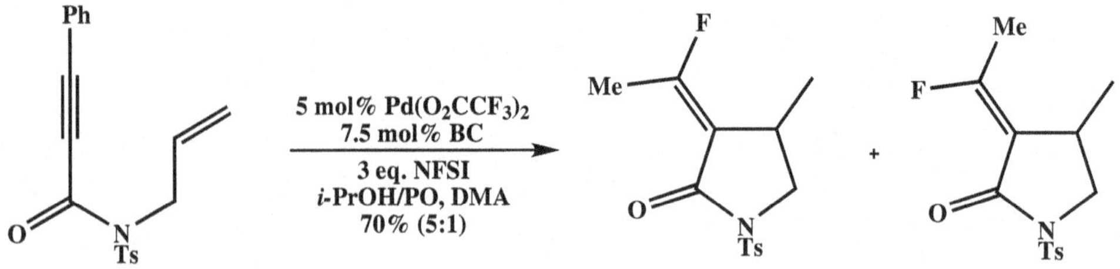

Scheme-72

REFERENCES

[1]   A. Fuerstner. 2003. Chemistry and biology of roseophilin and the prodigiosin alkaloids: a survey of the last 2500 years. Angew. Chem. Int. Ed. 42: 3582-3603.

[2]   J.S. Russel, E.T. Pelkey and S.J.P. Yoon-Miller. 2009. Five-membered ring systems: pyrroles and benzo analogs. In Prog. Heterocycl. Chem., Elsevier Ltd. 21: 145-178.

[3]   X. Jing, X. Pan, Z. Li, X. Bi, C. Yan and H. Zhu. 2009. Organic catalytic multicomponent one-pot synthesis of highly substituted pyrroles. Synth. Commun. 39: 3833-3844.

[4]   V. Amarnath, D.C. Anthony, K. Amarnath, W.M. Valentine, L.A. Wetterau and D.G. Graham. 1991. Intermediates in the Paal-Knorr synthesis of pyrroles. J. Org. Chem. 56: 6924-6931.

[5]   E.J. Kang and E. Lee. 2005. Total synthesis of oxacyclic macrodiolide natural products. Chem. Rev. 105: 4348-4378.

[6]   M. Saleem, H.J. Kim, M.S. Ali and Y.S. Lee. 2005. An update on bioactive plant lignans. Nat. Prod. Rep. 22: 696-716.

[7]   A. Bermejo, B. Figadere, M.-C. Zafra-Polo, I. Barrachina, E. Estornell and D. Cortes. 2005. Acetogenins from Annonaceae: recent progress in isolation, synthesis and mechanisms of action. Nat. Prod. Rep. 22: 269-309.

[8]   J.W. Daly, T.F. Spande and H.M. Garraffo. 2005. Alkaloids from amphibian skin: a tabulation of over eight-hundred compounds. J. Nat. Prod. 68: 1556-1575.

[9]   A.E. Hackling and H. Stark. 2002. Dopamine D3 receptor ligands with antagonist properties. Chem. Bio. Chem. 3: 946-961.

[10]   J.R. Lewis. 2001. Amaryllidaceae, *Sceletium*, imidazole, oxazole, thiazole, peptide and miscellaneous alkaloids. Nat. Prod. Rep. 18: 95-128.

[11]   N. Kaur. 2017. Methods for metal and non-metal catalyzed synthesis of six-membered oxygen containing poly-heterocycles. Curr. Org. Synth. 14: 531-556.

[12]   N. Kaur. 2017. Photochemical reactions: synthesis of six-membered *N*-heterocycles. Curr. Org. Synth. 14: 972-998.

[13]   F.-X. Felpin and J. Lebreton. 2003. Recent advances in the total synthesis of piperidine and pyrrolidine natural alkaloids with ring-closing metathesis as a key step. Eur. J. Org. Chem. 19: 3693-3712.

[14]   N. Kaur. 2017. Ionic liquids: promising but challenging solvents for the synthesis of *N*-heterocycles. Mini Rev. Org. Chem. 14: 3-23.

[15]   N. Kaur. 2016. Metal catalysts for the formation of six-membered *N*-polyheterocycles. Synth. React. Inorg. Metal-Org. Nano-Metal Chem. 46: 983-1020.

[16]   N. Kaur. 2017. Applications of gold catalysts for the synthesis of five-membered *O*-heterocycles. Inorg. Nano-Metal Chem. 47: 163-187.

[17]   R. Grigg, A. Hodgson, J. Morris and V. Sridharan. 2003. Sequential Pd/Ru-catalyzed allenylation/ olefin metathesis/1,3-dipolar cycloaddition route to novel heterocycles. Tetrahedron Lett. 44: 1023-1026.

[18]   (a) K.C. Majumdar, S. Muhuri, R.U. Islam and B. Chattopadhyay. 2009. Synthesis of five- and six-membered heterocyclic compounds by the application of the metathesis reactions. Heterocycles 78: 1109-1169.
        (b) K.C. Majumdar, S. Samanta and B. Sinha. 2012. Recent developments in palladium-catalyzed formation of five- and six-membered fused heterocycles. Synthesis 44: 817-847.

[19]   Y. Tan and J.F. Hartwig. 2010. Palladium-catalyzed amination of aromatic C-H bonds with oxime esters. J. Am. Chem. Soc. 132: 3676-3677.

[20]   M. Kitamura, S. Zaman and K. Narasaka. 2001. Synthesis of spiro imines from oximes by palladium-catalyzed cascade reaction. Synlett 974-976.

[21]   H. Tsutsui and K. Narasaka. 2001. Synthesis of pyridine and isoquinoline derivatives by the palladium-catalyzed cyclization of olefinic ketone *O*-pentafluorobenzoyloximes. Chem. Lett. 30: 526-527.

[22]   M. Kitamura, S. Chiba, O. Saku and K. Narasaka. 2002. Palladium-catalyzed synthesis of 1-azaazulenes from cycloheptatrienylmethyl ketone *O*-pentafluorobenzoyl oximes. Chem. Lett. 31: 606-607.

[23]   H. Ohno, K. Miyamura, Y. Takeoka and T. Tanaka. 2003. Palladium(0)-catalyzed tandem cyclization of allenenes. Angew. Chem. Int. Ed. 42: 2647-2650.

[24]   M.B. Hay and J.P. Wolfe. 2007. Stereoselective synthesis of isoxazolidines through Pd-catalyzed carboetherification of *N*-butenylhydroxylamines. Angew. Chem. Int. Ed. 46: 6492-6494.

[25]   J.S. Nakhla and J.P. Wolfe. 2007. A concise asymmetric synthesis of *cis*-2,6-disubstituted *N*-aryl piperazines *via* Pd-catalyzed carboamination reactions. Org. Lett. 9: 3279-3282.

[26]   M.L. Leathen, B.R. Rosen and J.P. Wolfe. 2009. New strategy for the synthesis of substituted morpholines. J. Org. Chem. 74: 5107-5110.

[27]   J.A. Fritz, J.S. Nakhla and J.P. Wolfe. 2006. A new synthesis of imidazolidin-2-ones *via* Pd-catalyzed carboamination of *N*-allylureas. Org. Lett. 8: 2531-2534.

[28] T.M. Meulemans, N.H. Kiers, B.L. Feringa and P.W.N.M. van Leeuwen. 1994. Catalytic oxidation of homoallylalcohols to α-alkoxytetrahydrofurans by a Pd-nitro complex and molecular oxygen. Tetrahedron Lett. 35: 455-458.

[29] T. Hosokawa, M. Hirata, S.-I. Murahashi and A. Sonoda. 1976. Palladium(II)-catalyzed cyclization of γ,δ-unsaturated alcohols synthesis of 2-vinyltetrahydrofurans. Tetrahedron Lett. 17: 1821-1824.

[30] H.J. Reich, J.M. Renga and I.L. Reich. 1975. Organoselenium chemistry. Conversion of ketones to enones by selenoxide *syn* elimination. J. Am. Chem. Soc. 97: 5434-5447.

[31] C. Aubert, O. Buisine and M. Malacria. 2002. The behavior of 1,n-enynes in the presence of transition metals. Chem. Rev. 102: 813-834.

[32] Y. Sato, N. Imakuni and M. Mori. 2003. Pd(0)-catalyzed bismetallative cyclization of enynes in the presence of $Bu_3SnSiMe_3$ using N-heterocyclic carbene as a ligand. Adv. Synth. Catal. 345: 488-491.

[33] M. Lautens and J. Mancuso. 2002. Silylstannation-cyclization of 1,6-enynes using palladium(0) and palladium(II) catalysis. Synlett 3: 394-398.

[34] Y. Sato, N. Imakuni, T. Hirose, H. Wakamatsu and M. Mori 2003. Further studies on palladium-catalyzed bismetallative cyclization of enynes in the presence of $Bu_3SnSiMe_3$. J. Organomet. Chem. 687: 392-402.

[35] S. Diez-Gonzalez, N. Marion and S.P. Nolan. 2009. N-Heterocyclic carbenes in late transition metal catalysis. Chem. Rev. 109: 3612-3676.

[36] L. Djakovitch and P. Rollet. 2004. Sonogashira cross-coupling reactions catalyzed by heterogeneous copper-free Pd-zeolites. Tetrahedron Lett. 45: 1367-1370.

[37] D.V. Kadnikov and R.C. Larock. 2000. Synthesis of coumarins *via* palladium-catalyzed carbonylative annulation of internal alkynes by *o*-iodophenols. Org. Lett. 2: 3643-3646.

[38] T. Morimoto, M. Fujioka, K. Fuji, K. Tsutsumi and K. Kakiuchi. 2003. Rhodium-catalyzed intramolecular aminocarbonylation of aryl halides using aldehydes as a source of carbon monoxide. Chem. Lett. 32: 154-155.

[39] R. Grigg, L. Zhang, S. Collard and A. Keep. 2003. Isoindolinones *via* a room temperature palladium nanoparticle-catalyzed 3-component cyclative carbonylation-amination cascade. Tetrahedron Lett. 44: 6979-6982.

[40] U.T. Strauss, U. Felfer and K. Faber. 1999. Biocatalytic transformation of racemates into chiral building blocks in 100% chemical yield and 100% enantiomeric excess. Tetrahedron: Asymmetry 10: 107-117.

[41] J.T. Mohr, D.C. Ebner and B.M. Stoltz. 2007. Catalytic enantioselective stereoablative reactions: an unexploited approach to enantioselective catalysis. Org. Biomol. Chem. 5: 3571-3576.

[42] A.P. Green and N.J. Turner. 2016. Biocatalytic retrosynthesis: redesigning synthetic routes to high-value chemicals. Perspect. Sci. 9: 42-48.

[43] D.M. Schultz and J.P. Wolfe. 2012. Recent developments in Pd-catalyzed alkene aminoarylation reactions for the synthesis of nitrogen heterocycles. Synthesis 44: 351-361.

[44] P.S. Hanley, D. Markovic and J.F. Hartwig. 2010. Intermolecular insertion of ethylene and octene into a palladium-amide bond. Spectroscopic evidence for an ethylene amido intermediate. J. Am. Chem. Soc. 132: 6302-6303.

[45] P.S. Hanley and J.F. Hartwig. 2011. Intermolecular migratory insertion of unactivated olefins into palladium-nitrogen bonds. Steric and electronic effects on the rate of migratory insertion. J. Am. Chem. Soc. 133: 15661-15673.

[46] J.S. Nakhla, D.M. Schultz and J.P. Wolfe. 2009. Palladium-catalyzed alkene carboamination reactions for the synthesis of substituted piperazines. Tetrahedron 65: 6549-6570.

[47] N.R. Babij and J.P. Wolfe. 2012. Asymmetric total synthesis of (+)-merobatzelladine B. Angew. Chem. Int. Ed. Engl. 51: 4128-4130.

[48] N.C. Giampietro and J.P. Wolfe. 2008. Stereoselective synthesis of *cis*- or *trans*-3,5-disubstituted pyrazolidines *via* Pd-catalyzed carboamination reactions: use of allylic strain to control product stereochemistry through N-substituent manipulation. J. Am. Chem. Soc. 130: 12907-12911.

[49] J.D. Neukom, A.S. Aquino and J.P. Wolfe. 2011. Synthesis of saturated 1,4-benzodiazepines *via* Pd-catalyzed carboamination reactions. Org. Lett. 13: 2196-2199.

[50] B. Gabriele, G. Salerno, A. Fazio and M.R. Bossio. 2001. Palladium-catalyzed cycloisomerization of (*Z*)-(2-en-4-ynyl)amines: a new synthesis of substituted pyrroles. Tetrahedron Lett. 42: 1339-1341.

[51] S.R. Fix, J.L. Brice and S.S. Stahl. 2002. Efficient intramolecular oxidative amination of olefins through direct dioxygen-coupled palladium catalysis. Angew. Chem. Int. Ed. 41: 164-166.

[52] R. Dhawan and B.A. Arndtsen. 2004. Palladium-catalyzed multicomponent coupling of alkynes, imines, and acid chlorides: a direct and modular approach to pyrrole synthesis. J. Am. Chem. Soc. 126: 468-469.

[53] B.A. Arndtsen. 2009. Metal-catalyzed one-step synthesis: towards direct alternatives to multistep heterocycle and amino acid derivative formation. Chem. Eur. J. 15: 302-313.

[54] R. Dhawan, R.D. Dghaym and B.A. Arndtsen. 2003. The development of a catalytic synthesis of münchnones: a simple four-component coupling approach to α-amino acid derivatives. J. Am. Chem. Soc. 125: 1474-1475.

[55] S.R. Neufeldt and M.S. Sanford. 2010. *O*-acetyl oximes as transformable directing groups for Pd-catalyzed C-H bond functionalization. Org. Lett. 12: 532-535.

[56] B.P. Coppola, M.C. Noe, D.J. Schwartz, R.L. Abdon and B.M. Trost. 1994. Intermolecular 1,3-dipolar cycloadditions of münchnones with acetylenic dipolarophiles: sorting out the regioselectivity. Tetrahedron 50: 93-116.

[57] D.M. D'Souza and T.J.J. Muller. 2007. Multi-component syntheses of heterocycles by transition-metal catalysis. Chem. Soc. Rev. 36: 1095-1108.

[58] N.T. Patil and Y. Yamamoto. 2007. Metal-mediated synthesis of furans and pyrroles. ARKIVOC (x): 121-141.

[59] C. Paal. 1885. Synthese von thiophen- und pyrrolderivaten. Ber. 18: 367-371.

[60] C.-F. Lee, L.-M. Yang, T.-Y. Hwu, A.S. Feng, J.-C. Tseng and T.-Y. Luh. 2000. One-pot synthesis of substituted furans and pyrroles from propargylic dithioacetals. New annulation route to highly photoluminescent oligoaryls. J. Am. Chem. Soc. 122: 4992-4993.

[61] C.A. Merlic, A. Baur and C.C. Aldrich. 2000. Acylamino chromium carbene complexes: direct carbonyl insertion, formation of münchnones and trapping with dipolarophiles. J. Am. Chem. Soc. 122: 7398-7399.

[62] G.S. Deng, N. Jiang, Z.H. Ma and J.B. Wang. 2002. $Rh_2(OAc)_4$-mediated diazo decomposition of δ-(*N*-tosyl)amino-β-keto-α-diazo carbonyl compounds: a novel approach to pyrrole derivatives. Synlett 11: 1913-1915.

[63] S.E. Gibson and A. Stevenazzi. 2003. The Pauson-Khand reaction: the catalytic age is here. Angew. Chem. Int. Ed. 42: 1800-1810.

[64] M. Beller and M. Eckert. 2000. Amidocarbonylation- an efficient route to amino acid derivatives. Angew. Chem. Int. Ed. 39: 1010-1027.

[65] J. Montgomery. 2000. Nickel-catalyzed cyclizations, couplings, and cycloadditions involving three reactive components. Acc. Chem. Res. 33: 467-473.

[66] R.D. Dghaym, R. Dhawan and B.A. Arndtsen. 2001. The use of carbon monoxide and imines as peptide derivative synthons: a facile palladium-catalyzed synthesis of α-amino acid derived imidazolines. Angew. Chem. Int. Ed. 40: 3228-3230.

[67] S. Kamijo, T. Jin, Z. Huo and Y. Yamamoto. 2003. Synthesis of triazoles from nonactivated terminal alkynes *via* the three-component coupling reaction using a Pd(0)-Cu(I) bimetallic catalyst. J. Am. Chem. Soc. 125: 7786-7787.

[68] B.M. Trost and A.B. Pinkerton. 2000. A Ru-catalyzed four-component coupling. J. Am. Chem. Soc. 122: 8081-8082.

[69] C. Cao, Y. Shi and A.L. Odom. 2003. A titanium-catalyzed 3-component coupling to generate α,β-unsaturated β-iminoamines. J. Am. Chem. Soc. 125: 2880-2881.

[70] L.F. Tietze and N. Rackelmann. 2004. Domino reactions in the synthesis of heterocyclic natural products and analogs. Pure Appl. Chem. 76: 1967-1983.

[71] Y. Dejaegher, M. D'Hooghe and N. De Kimpe. 2008. Synthesis of novel 3-oxopiperidin-2-ones from methyl 2-alkoxy-5-amino-2-pentenoates. Synlett 13: 1961-1964.

[72] S. Nag and S. Batra. 2011. Applications of allylamines for the syntheses of aza-heterocycles. Tetrahedron 67: 8959-9061.

[73] E. Mironiuk-Puchalska, E. Kołaczkowska and W. Sas. 2002. Synthesis of (±)-branched-chain azaisonucleosides *via* Michael addition of 5-nitro-2,2-pentamethylene-1,3-dioxane to methyl 2-bromoacrylate. Tetrahedron Lett. 43: 8351-8354.

[74] R. Kuciak and W. Sas. 1994. Synthesis of branched-chain azafuranose derivatives from secondary nitroalkanes. Facile synthesis of (±) 4-amino-4,4-bis(hydroxymethyl)-4-deoxythreonic-1,4-lactam. Tetrahedron Lett. 35: 8647-8648.

[75] R. Ballini and M. Petrini. 2009. Nitroalkanes as key building blocks for the synthesis of heterocyclic derivatives. ARKIVOC (ix): 195-223.

[76] J.L.O. Domingos, E.C. Lima, A.G. Dias and P.R.R. Costa. 2004. Stereoselective preparation of pyrrolidin-2-ones from a Z-enoate derived from D-(+)-MANNITOL. Tetrahedron: Asymmetry 15: 2313-2314.

[77] J.S. Costa, A.G. Dias, A.L. Anholeto, M.D. Monteiro, V.L. Patrocinio and P.R.R. Costa. 1997. *Syn*-selective Michael addition of nitromethane derivatives to enoates derived from (R)-(+)-glyceraldehyde acetonide. J. Org. Chem. 62: 4002-4006.

[78] A.M. Mouna, P. Blanchard, J.-L. Fourrey and M. Robert-Gero. 1990. Synthesis of adenine nucleosides related to sinefungin. Tetrahedron Lett. 31: 7003-7006.

[79] H.S.P. Rao, S. Jothilingam and H.W. Scheeren. 2004. Microwave mediated facile one-pot synthesis of polyarylpyrroles from but-2-ene- and but-2-yne-1,4-diones. Tetrahedron 60: 1625-1630.

[80] E.J. Corey and D. Enders. 1976. Applications of N,N-dimethylhydrazones to synthesis. Use in efficient, positionally and stereochemically selective C-C bond formation; oxidative hydrolysis to carbonyl compounds. Tetrahedron Lett. 17: 3-6.

[81] E.J. Corey and H.L. Pearce. 1979. Total synthesis of picrotoxinin. J. Am. Chem. Soc. 101: 5841-5843.

[82] D. Enders, L. Wortmann and R. Peters. 2000. Recovery of carbonyl compounds from N,N-dialkylhydrazones. Acc. Chem. Res. 33: 157-169.

[83] F. Bellina and R. Rossi. 2006. Synthesis and biological activity of pyrrole, pyrroline and pyrrolidine derivatives with two aryl groups on adjacent positions. Tetrahedron 62: 7213-7256.

[84] I. Coldham and R. Hufton. 2005. Intramolecular dipolar cycloaddition reactions of azomethine ylides. Chem. Rev. 105: 2765-2810.

[85] S.G. Pyne, A.S. Davis, N.J. Gates, J.P. Hartley, K.B. Lindsay, T. Machan and M. Tang. 2004. Asymmetric synthesis of polyfunctionalized pyrrolidines and related alkaloids. Synlett 15: 2670-2680.

[86] P.N. Confalone and E.M. Huie. 1988. The [3+2] nitrone-olefin cycloaddition reaction. Org. React. 36: 1-173.

[87] K.V. Gothelf and K.A. Jorgensen. 2000. Catalytic enantioselective 1,3-dipolar cycloaddition reactions of nitrones. Chem. Commun. 16: 1449-1458.

[88] S. Kanemasa. 2002. Metal-assisted stereocontrol of 1,3-dipolar cycloaddition reactions. Synlett 9: 1371-1387.

[89] M.D. Jones and R.D.W. Kemmitt. 1986. Reactions between trimethylenemethane metal complexes and the carbon-nitrogen double bond: nickel and palladium catalyzed synthesis of pyrrolidines. J. Chem. Soc. Chem. Commun. 15: 1201-1203.

[90] B.H. Oh, I. Nakamura, S. Saito and Y. Yamamoto. 2003. Synthesis of 3-methylenepyrrolidines by palladium-catalyzed [3+2] cycloaddition of alkylidenecyclopropanes with imines. Heterocycles 61: 247-257.

[91] B.M. Trost, S.M. Silverman and J.P. Stambuli. 2007. Palladium-catalyzed asymmetric [3+2] cycloaddition of trimethylenemethane with imines. J. Am. Chem. Soc. 129: 12398-12399.

[92] J.G. Knight, K. Tchabanenko, P.A. Stoker and S.J. Harwood. 2005. Synthesis of highly substituted pyrrolidines *via* palladium catalyzed formal [2+3] cycloaddition of 5-vinyloxazolidin-2-ones to activated alkenes. Tetrahedron Lett. 46: 6261-6264.

[93] J.G. Knight, P.A. Stoker, K. Tchabanenko, S.J. Harwood and K.W.M. Lawrie. 2008. Synthesis of highly substituted pyrrolidines *via* palladium-catalyzed cyclization of 5-vinyloxazolidinones and activated alkenes. Tetrahedron 64: 3744-3750.

[94] J.D. Neukom, N.S. Perch and J.P. Wolfe. 2010. Intramolecular alkene aminopalladation reactions of (dppf)Pd(Ar)[N(Ar^l)(CH$_2$)$_3$CH=CH$_2$] complexes. Insertion of unactivated alkenes into Pd-N bonds. J. Am. Chem. Soc. 132: 6276-6277.

[95] J.D. Neukom, N.S. Perch and J.P. Wolfe. 2011. Intramolecular insertion of alkenes into Pd-N bonds. Effects of substrate and ligand structure on the reactivity of (P-P)Pd(Ar)[N(Ar^l)(CH$_2$)$_3$CR=CHR′] complexes. Organometallics 30: 1269-1277.

[96] M. Narsireddy and Y. Yamamoto. 2008. Catalytic asymmetric intramolecular hydroamination of alkynes in the presence of a catalyst system consisting of Pd(0)-methyl norphos (or tolyl renorphos)-benzoic acid. J. Org. Chem. 73: 9698-9709.

[97] L.M. Lutete, I. Kadota and Y. Yamamoto. 2004. Palladium-catalyzed intramolecular asymmetric hydroamination of alkynes. J. Am. Chem. Soc. 126: 1622-1623.

[98] N.T. Patil, L.M. Lutete, H. Wu and Y. Yamamoto. 2006. Palladium-catalyzed intramolecular asymmetric hydroamination, hydroalkoxylation, and hydrocarbonation of alkynes. J. Org. Chem. 71: 4270-4279.

[99] Z. Lu and S. Ma. 2008. Metal-catalyzed enantioselective allylation in asymmetric synthesis. Angew. Chem. Int. Ed. 47: 258-297.

[100] S. Greau, B. Radetich and T.V. RajanBabu. 2000. First demonstration of helical chirality in 1,4-disubstituted (Z,Z)-1,3-dienes: R$_3$Si-SnR′$_3$-mediated cyclization of 1,6-diynes. J. Am. Chem. Soc. 122: 8579-8580.

[101] K. Nakamura, M. Ohtaka and Y. Yamamoto. 2002. Tandem nucleophilic allylation-alkoxyallylation of alkynylaldehydes *via* amphiphilic bis-π-allylpalladium complexes. Tetrahedron Lett. 43: 7631-7633.

[102] M. Bao, H. Nakamura, A. Inoue and Y. Yamamoto. 2002. Nucleophilic allylation-heterocyclization *via* bis-π-allylpalladium complexes: synthesis of five- and six-membered heterocycles. Chem. Lett. 31: 158-159.

[103] (a) Y. Kozawa and M. Mori. 2002. Synthesis of different ring-size heterocycles from the same propargyl alcohol derivative by ligand effect on Pd(0). Tetrahedron Lett. 43: 1499-1502.
      (b) T. Lu, Z. Lu, Z.-X. Ma, Y. Zhang and R.P. Hsung. 2013. Allenamides: a powerful and versatile building block in organic synthesis. Chem. Rev. 113: 4862-4904.

[104] L.V. Desai, K.L. Hull and M.S. Sanford. 2004. Palladium-catalyzed oxygenation of unactivated sp^3 C-H bonds. J. Am. Chem. Soc. 126: 9542-9543.

[105] B.S. Williams and K.I. Goldberg. 2001. Studies of reductive elimination reactions to form carbon-oxygen bonds from Pt(IV) complexes. J. Am. Chem. Soc. 123: 2576-2587.

[106] S.S. Stahl, J.A. Labinger and J.E. Bercaw. 1998. Homogenous oxidation of alkanes by electrophilic late transition metals. Angew. Chem. Int. Ed. 37: 2180-2192.

[107] K. Tonogaki, K. Itami and J.-I. Yoshida. 2006. Catalytic four-component assembly based on allenylboronate platform: new access to privileged allylic amine structures. J. Am. Chem. Soc. 128: 1464-1465.

[108] D. Bouyssi, N. Monteiro and G. Balme. 2011. Amines as key building blocks in Pd-assisted multicomponent processes. Beilstein J. Org. Chem. 7: 1387-1406.

[109] B.M. Trost and S.M. Silverman. 2012. Enantioselective construction of pyrrolidines by palladium-catalyzed asymmetric [3+2]-cycloaddition of trimethylenemethane with imines. J. Am. Chem. Soc. 134: 4941-4954.

[110] M.B. Bertrand, J.D. Neukom and J.P. Wolfe. 2008. Mild conditions for Pd-catalyzed carboamination of *N*-protected hex-4-enylamines and 1-, 3-, and 4-substituted pent-4-enylamines. Scope, limitations, and mechanism of pyrrolidine formation. J. Org. Chem. 73: 8851-8860.

[111] D.N. Mai and J.P. Wolfe. 2010. Asymmetric palladium-catalyzed carboamination reactions for the synthesis of enantiomerically enriched 2-(arylmethyl)- and 2-(alkenylmethyl)pyrrolidines. J. Am. Chem. Soc. 132: 12157-12159.

[112] Q. Yang, J.E. Ney and J.P. Wolfe. 2005. Palladium-catalyzed tandem *N*-arylation/carboamination reactions for the stereoselective synthesis of *N*-aryl-2-benzyl pyrrolidines. Org. Lett. 7: 2575-2578.

[113] (a) J.E. Ney and J.P. Wolfe. 2004. Palladium-catalyzed synthesis of *N*-aryl pyrrolidines from γ-(*N*-arylamino) alkenes: evidence for chemoselective alkene insertion into Pd-N bonds. Angew. Chem. Int. Ed. 43: 3605-3608.

     (b) J.S. Nakhla, J.W. Kampf and J.P. Wolfe. 2006. Intramolecular Pd-catalyzed carboetherification and carboamination. Influence of catalyst structure on reaction mechanism and product stereochemistry. J. Am. Chem. Soc. 128: 2893-2901.

[114] M.B. Bertrand and J.P. Wolfe. 2005. Carbamoylimidazolium and thiocarbamoylimidazolium salts: novel reagents for the synthesis of ureas, thioureas, carbamates, thiocarbamates and amides. Tetrahedron 61: 6447-6459.

[115] J.E. Ney and J.P. Wolfe. 2005. Selective synthesis of 5- or 6-aryl octahydrocyclopenta[*b*]pyrroles from a common precursor through control of competing pathways in a Pd-catalyzed reaction. J. Am. Chem. Soc. 127: 8644-8651.

[116] J.E. Ney, M.B. Hay, Q. Yang and J.P. Wolfe. 2005. Synthesis of *N*-aryl-2-allyl pyrrolidines *via* palladium-catalyzed carboamination reactions of γ-(*N*-arylamino)alkenes with vinyl bromides. Adv. Synth. Catal. 347: 1614-1620.

[117] K.G. Dongol and B.Y. Tay. 2006. Palladium(0)-catalyzed cascade one-pot synthesis of isoxazolidines. Tetrahedron Lett. 47: 927-930.

[118] M.B. Bertrand, M.L. Leathen and J.P. Wolfe. 2007. Mild conditions for the synthesis of functionalized pyrrolidines *via* Pd-catalyzed carboamination reactions. Org. Lett. 9: 457-460.

[119] J. Peng, W. Lin, S. Yuan and Y. Chen. 2007. Palladium-catalyzed highly stereoselective synthesis of *N*-aryl-3-arylmethylisoxazolidines *via* tandem arylation of *O*-homoallylhydroxylamines. J. Org. Chem. 72: 3145-3148.

[120] M. Eggersdorfer, D. Laudert, U. Létinois, T. McClymont, J. Medlock, T. Netscher and W. Bonrath. 2012. One hundred years of vitamins - a success story of the natural sciences. 51: 12960-12990.

[121] J.P. Wolfe. 2008. Stereoselective synthesis of saturated heterocycles *via* Pd-catalyzed alkene carboetherification and carboamination reactions. Synlett 19: 2913-2937.

[122] D. O'Hagan. 2000. Pyrrole, pyrrolidine, pyridine, piperidine and tropane alkaloids. Nat. Prod. Rep. 17: 435-446.

[123] D. Garcia-Cuadrado, A.A.C. Braga, F. Maseras and A.M. Echavarren. 2006. Proton abstraction mechanism for the palladium-catalyzed intramolecular arylation. J. Am. Chem. Soc. 128: 1066-1067.

[124] M.S. Driver and J.F. Hartwig. 1997. Carbon-nitrogen-bond-forming reductive elimination of arylamines from palladium(II) phosphine complexes. J. Am. Chem. Soc. 119: 8232-8245.

[125] J. Yin and S.L. Buchwald. 2002. Pd-catalyzed intermolecular amidation of aryl halides: the discovery that xantphos can be trans-chelating in a palladium complex. J. Am. Chem. Soc. 124: 6043-6048.

[126] M. Yamashita, J.V.C. Vicario and J.F. Hartwig. 2003. Trans influence on the rate of reductive elimination. Reductive elimination of amines from isomeric arylpalladium amides with unsymmetrical coordination spheres. J. Am. Chem. Soc. 125: 16347-16360.

[127] O. Hara, H. Fujino, K. Makino and Y. Hamada. 2008. Palladium-catalyzed asymmetric intramolecular metallo-ene reaction using monodentate phosphines, 9-PBN and 9-NapBN. Heterocycles 76: 197-202.

[128] X. Bantreil, G. Prestat, D. Madec, P. Fristrup and G. Poli. 2009. Enantioselective γ-lactam synthesis *via* palladium-catalyzed intramolecular asymmetric allylic alkylation. Synlett 9: 1441-1444.

[129] M. von Seebach, R. Grigg and A. De Meijere. 2002. Multicomponent queuing cascades of bicyclopropylidene, carbon monoxide and aryl iodides or aryl thiols. Eur. J. Org. Chem. 19: 3268-3275.

[130] R. Grigg, P. Stevenson and T. Worakun. 1985. Palladium catalyzed intra- and intermolecular coupling of vinyl halides. Regiospecific formation of 1,3-dienes. J. Chem. Soc. Chem. Commun. 14: 971-972.

[131] R. Grigg, P. Stevenson and T. Worakun. 1988. Regiospecific formation of 1,3-dienes by the palladium catalyzed intra- and inter-molecular coupling of vinyl halides. Tetrahedron 44: 2049-2054.

[132] J.P. Wolfe, R.A. Rennels and S.L. Buchwald. 1996. Intramolecular palladium-catalyzed aryl amination and aryl amidation. Tetrahedron 52: 7525-7546.

[133] G.R. Cook, P.S. Shanker and S.L. Peterson. 1999. Asymmetric synthesis of the balanol heterocycle *via* a palladium-mediated epimerization and olefin metathesis. Org. Lett. 1: 615-617.

[134] G.R. Cook and L. Sun 2004. Nitrogen heterocycles *via* palladium-catalyzed carbocyclization. Formal synthesis of (+)-α-allokainic acid. Org. Lett. 6: 2481-2484.

[135] K. Utimoto, H. Miwa and H. Nozaki. 1981. Palladium-catalyzed synthesis of pyrroles. Tetrahedron Lett. 22: 4277-4278.

[136] W. Cabri, I. Candiani, M. Colombo, L. Franzoi and A. Bedeschi. 1995. Non-toxic ligands in samarium diiodide-mediated cyclizations. Tetrahedron Lett. 36: 949-952.

[137] K. Jones, J. Wilkinson and R. Ewin. 1994. Intramolecular reactions using amide links: aryl radical cyclization of silylated acryloylanilides. Tetrahedron Lett. 35: 7673-7676.

[138] K. Jones and C. McCarthy. 1989. Chiral induction in aryl radical cyclizations. Tetrahedron Lett. 30: 2657-2660.

[139] W.R. Bowman, H. Heaney and B.J. Jordan. 1988. Synthesis of oxindoles by radical cyclization. Tetrahedron Lett. 29: 6657-6660.

[140] M. Mori, I. Oda and Y. Ban. 1982. Cyclization of α-halo amide with internal double bond by use of the low-valent metal complex. Tetrahedron Lett. 23: 5315-5318.

[141] S.-C. Yang and F.-R. Shea. 1995. Synthesis of γ-butyrolactams by the palladium-catalyzed cyclization of *n*-allylbromoacetamides. J. Chin. Chem. Soc. 42: 969-972.

[142] L. Banfi, A. Basso, V. Cerulli, G. Guanti and R. Riva. 2008. Polyfunctionalized pyrrolidines by Ugi multicomponent reaction followed by palladium-mediated S_N2' cyclizations. J. Org. Chem. 73: 1608-1611.

[143] J. Eustache, P. van de Weghe, D. Le Nouen, H. Uyehara, C. Kabuto and Y. Yamamoto. 2005. Controlled synthesis of *cis* or *trans* isomers of 1,3-disubstituted tetrahydroisoquinolines and 2,5-disubstituted pyrrolidines. J. Org. Chem. 70: 4043-4053.

[144] M. Blangetti, A. Deagostino, C. Prandi, S. Tabasso and P. Venturello. 2009. LIC-KOR-promoted synthesis of alkoxydienyl amines: an entry to 2,3,4,5-tetrasubstituted pyrroles. Org. Lett. 11: 3914-3917.

[145] M. Kimura, H. Harayama, S. Tanaka and Y. Tamaru. 1994. Palladium(II) catalyzed 5-endo-trigonal cyclization of 2-hydroxybut-3-enylamines: synthesis of five-membered nitrogen heterocycles. J. Chem. Soc. Chem. Commun. 26: 2531-2533.

[146] S. Igarashi, Y. Haruta, M. Ozawa, Y. Nishide, H. Kinoshita and K. Inomata. 1989. A convenient method for the preparation of furan and pyrrole derivatives *via* palladium(II)-catalyzed intramolecular cyclization of 3- and 4-alkenyl alcohol or amine derivatives. Chem. Lett. 18: 737-740.

[147] X. Han and R.A. Widenhoefer. 2004. Palladium-catalyzed oxidative alkoxylation of α-alkenyl β-diketones to form functionalized furans. J. Org. Chem. 69: 1738-1740.

[148] Z. Zhang, J. Zhang, J. Tan and Z. Wang. 2008. A facile access to pyrroles from amino acids *via* an aza-Wacker cyclization. J. Org. Chem. 73: 5180-5182.

[149] E.M. Beccalli, G. Broggini, M. Martinelli and S. Sottocornola. 2007. C-C, C-O, C-N Bond formation on sp^2 carbon by Pd(II)-catalyzed reactions involving oxidant agents. Chem. Rev. 107: 5318-5365.

[150] J.W. Coe, M.G. Vetelino and M.J. Bradlee. 1996. Convenient preparation of *N*-substituted indoles by modified Leimgruber-Batcho indole synthesis. Tetrahedron Lett. 37: 6045-6048.

[151] J.-O. Baeg, C. Bensimon and H. Alper. 1995. The first enantiospecific palladium-catalyzed cycloaddition of aziridines and heterocumulenes. Novel synthesis of chiral five-membered ring heterocycles. J. Am. Chem. Soc. 117: 4700-4701.

[152] S. Vogel, X. Bantreil, G. Maitro, G. Prestat, D. Madec and G. Poli. 2010. Palladium-catalyzed intramolecular allylic alkylation of α-sulfinyl carbanions: a new asymmetric route to enantiopure γ-lactams. Tetrahedron Lett. 51: 1459-1461.

[153] M.B.T. Thuong, S. Sottocornola, G. Prestat, G. Broggini, D. Madec and G. Poli. 2007. New access to kainic acid *via* intramolecular palladium-catalyzed allylic alkylation. Synlett 10: 1521-1524.

[154] M. Meguro and Y. Yamamoto. 1998. A new method for the synthesis of nitrogen heterocycles *via* palladium catalyzed intramolecular hydroamination of allenes. Tetrahedron Lett. 39: 5421-5424.

[155] B.M. Trost, M.R. Machacek and A. Aponick. 2006. Predicting the stereochemistry of diphenylphosphino benzoic acid (DPPBA)-based palladium-catalyzed asymmetric allylic alkylation reactions: a working model. Acc. Chem. Res. 39: 747-760.

[156] B.M. Trost and M.L. Crawley. 2003. Asymmetric transition-metal-catalyzed allylic alkylations: applications in total synthesis. Chem. Rev. 103: 2921-2944.

[157] B.M. Trost. 1996. Designing a receptor for molecular recognition in a catalytic synthetic reaction: allylic alkylation. Acc. Chem. Res. 29: 355-364.

[158] B.M. Trost and D.L. van Vranken. 1996. Asymmetric transition metal-catalyzed allylic alkylations. Chem. Rev. 96: 395-422.

[159] B.M. Trost, M.J. Krische, R. Radinov and G. Zanoni. 1996. On asymmetric induction in allylic alkylation *via* enantiotopic facial discrimination. J. Am. Chem. Soc. 118: 6297-6298.

[160] B.M. Trost and D.E. Patterson. 1998. Enhanced enantioselectivity in the desymmetrization of *meso*-biscarbamates. J. Org. Chem. 63: 1339-1341.

[161] S.-G. Lee, C.W. Lim, C.E. Song, K.M. Kwan and C.H. Jun. 1999. C_2-symmetric bisphosphinobioxazoline as a chiral ligand. Highly enantioselective palladium-catalyzed allylic substitutions and formation of P,N,N,P tetradentate palladium(II) complexes. J. Org. Chem. 64: 4445-4451.

[162] G. Balme, D. Bouyssi, T. Lomberget and N. Monteiro. 2003. Cyclizations involving attack of carbo- and heteronucleophiles on carbon-carbon π-bonds activated by organopalladium complexes. Synthesis 14: 2115-2134.

[163] S. Lemaire-Audoire, M. Savignac, J.-P. Genet and J.-M. Bernard. 1995. Selective de-protection of allyl amines using palladium. Tetrahedron Lett. 36: 1267-1270.

[164] L. Martinon, S. Azoulay, N. Monteiro, E.P. Kundig and G. Balme. 2004. Pd-catalyzed one-pot coupling of allylamines, activated alkenes, and unsaturated halides (or triflate): an atom efficient synthesis of highly functionalized pyrrolidines. J. Organomet. Chem. 689: 3831-3836.

[165] P.A. Sibbald and F.E. Michael. 2009. Palladium-catalyzed diamination of unactivated alkenes using *N*-fluorobenzenesulfonimide as source of electrophilic nitrogen. Org. Lett. 11: 1147-1149.

[166] R.I. McDonald, P.W. White, A.B. Weinstein, C.P. Tam and S.S. Stahl. 2011. Enantioselective Pd(II)-catalyzed aerobic oxidative amidation of alkenes and insights into the role of electronic asymmetry in pyridine-oxazoline ligands. Org. Lett. 13: 2830-2833.

[167] N. Kaur. 2015. Benign approaches for the microwave-assisted synthesis of five-membered 1,2-*N,N*-heterocycles. J. Heterocycl. Chem. 52: 953-973.

[168] K.-T. Yip, M. Yang, K.-L. Law, N.-Y. Zhu and D. Yang. 2006. Pd(II)-catalyzed enantioselective oxidative tandem cyclization reactions. Synthesis of indolines through C-N and C-C bond formation. J. Am. Chem. Soc. 128: 3130-3131.

[169] W.-H. Ham, Y.-H. Jung, K. Lee, C.-Y. Oh and K.-Y. Lee. 1997. A formal total synthesis of (±)-ferruginine by Pd-catalyzed intramolecular aminocarbonylation. Tetrahedron Lett. 38: 3247-3248.

[170] T. Shinohara, M.A. Arai, K. Wakita, T. Arai and H. Sasai. 2003. The first enantioselective intramolecular aminocarbonylation of alkenes promoted by Pd(II)-spiro bis(isoxazoline) catalyst. Tetrahedron Lett. 44: 711-714.

[171] J. Sperry, E.B.J. Harris and M.A. Brimble. 2010. Total synthesis and absolute configuration of (-)-berkeleyamide A. Org. Lett. 12: 420-423.

[172] J. Jeon, J.H. Lee, J.-W. Kim and Y.G. Kim. 2007. *syn*-Selective dihydroxylation of γ-amino-α,β-unsaturated (Z)-esters from D-serine: stereoselective synthesis of D-iminolyxitol. Tetrahedron: Asymmetry 18: 2448-2453.

[173] B. Gabriele, G. Salerno and A. Fazio. 2003. General and regioselective synthesis of substituted pyrroles by metal-catalyzed or spontaneous cycloisomerization of (Z)-(2-en-4-ynyl)amines. J. Org. Chem. 68: 7853-7861.

[174] B. Gabriele, G. Salerno, F. De Pascali, G.T. Sciano, M. Costa and G.P. Chiusoli. 1997. Novel synthesis of furan-2-acetic esters by palladium-catalyzed oxidative cyclization-alkoxycarbonylation of (Z)-2-en-4-yn-1-ols. Tetrahedron Lett. 38: 6877-6880.

[175] B. Gabriele, G. Salerno, A. Fazio and F.B. Campana. 2002. Unprecedented carbon dioxide effect on a Pd-catalyzed oxidative carbonylation reaction: a new synthesis of pyrrole-2-acetic esters. Chem. Commun. 13: 1408-1409.

[176] B. Gabriele, G. Salerno, F. De Pascali, M. Costa and G.P. Chiusoli. 1999. An efficient and general synthesis of furan-2-acetic esters by palladium-catalyzed oxidative carbonylation of (Z)-2-en-4-yn-1-ols. J. Org. Chem. 64: 7693-7699.

[177] B. Gabriele, G. Salerno, A. Fazio and L. Veltri. 2006. Versatile synthesis of pyrrole-2-acetic esters and (pyridine-2-one)-3-acetic amides by palladium-catalyzed, carbon dioxide-promoted oxidative carbonylation of (Z)-(2-en-4-ynyl)amines. Adv. Synth. Catal. 348: 2212-2222.

[178] B. Gabriele, G. Salerno, L. Veltri, M. Costa and C. Massera. 2001. Stereoselective synthesis of (E)-3-(methoxycarbonyl)methylene-1,3-dihydroindol-2-ones by palladium-catalyzed oxidative carbonylation of 2-ethynylanilines. Eur. J. Org. Chem. 24: 4607-4613.

[179] G.W. O'Neil and A. Fuerstner. 2008. β-alkyl Suzuki couplings for the stereoselective synthesis of substituted pyrans. Chem. Commun. 36: 4294-4296.

[180] K. Shen, X. Han and X. Lu. 2013. Cationic Pd(II)-catalyzed reductive cyclization of alkyne-tethered ketones or aldehydes using ethanol as hydrogen source. Org. Lett. 15: 1732-1735.

[181] H. Peng and G. Liu. 2011. Palladium-catalyzed tandem fluorination and cyclization of enynes. Org. Lett. 13: 772-775.

[182] G. Liu. 2012. Transition metal-catalyzed fluorination of multi carbon-carbon bonds: new strategies for fluorinated heterocycles. Org. Biomol. Chem. 10: 6243-6248.

CHAPTER 2

Five-Membered N-Polyheterocycles

2.1 Introduction

The heterocyclic compounds are widely used in biological, chemical, and industrial settings. Heterocyclic compounds form the central core of several pharmaceutical agents and biologically active natural products, and are applied in corrosion inhibitors and herbicides. Various naturally-occurring compounds possess benzo-fused heteroaromatic structures having a wide range of pharmaceutical applications like anti-microbial and anti-biotics agents [1a-e]. Many synthetic methods are employed for the synthesis of 5-, 6-, 7- and 8-membered benzo-fused heterocyclic compounds. These structures have a wide range of medicinal applications due to their ability to bind to multiple receptors with high affinity. These compounds are "bicyclic privileged structures" and are defined as "a single molecular framework able to provide ligands for diverse receptors" [2-7].

    The indole is one of the most commonly reported heterocyclic compounds. Indole is present in numerous natural products, which exhibit interesting biological activity, for instance reserpine, is one of the first drugs to treat diseases of central nervous system [8-11]. The introduction of an indole moiety into pharmacologically active amino acid tryptophan is further evidence of its implicit relevance to life. The indole scaffold is successfully used in many pharmaceutical agents, for instance new anti-migraine drugs and HIV-1 reverse transcriptase inhibitors (rescriptor). This indole moiety is used in other fields of chemistry such as polymer chemistry for the fabrication of micro pH sensors [12-16]. Therefore, there is an interest in these structures and this chapter describes the relevant examples of syntheses of these molecules.

2.2 Palladium assisted synthesis of five-membered polyheterocycles with nitrogen heteroatom

The drawback of cyclization-anion capture protocol was that most of the cascades were two-component processes. The relay phase was extended with introduction of both intra- and inter-molecular segments to avoid this shortcoming if poly-component processes could be achieved. The synthesis of ester was an example of a 3-CR **(Scheme 1)**. With carbon monoxide (1 atm) in combination with MR and anionic groups of capture agents Y a number of three-component processes occurred readily [17-20].

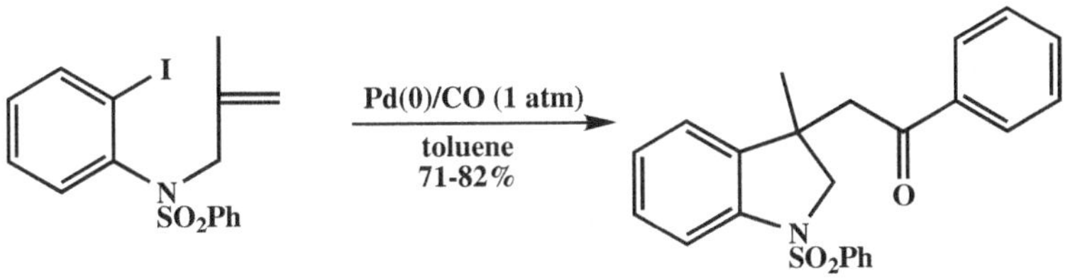

Scheme-1

Nakamura and co-workers [21] synthesized indoles from transannulation reaction of *N*-aroylbenzotriazoles with alkynes in the presence of Pd catalyst **(Scheme 2)**. The authors took advantage of closed/opened form equilibrium between acyltriazole and its diazonium isomer, which served as an equivalent of haloanilide that was employed in indole synthesis [22]. The benefits of this protocol as compared to Larock's classical indole synthesis were from an environmental standpoint including benign by-product (N_2) and base-free conditions of this transannulation reaction [23].

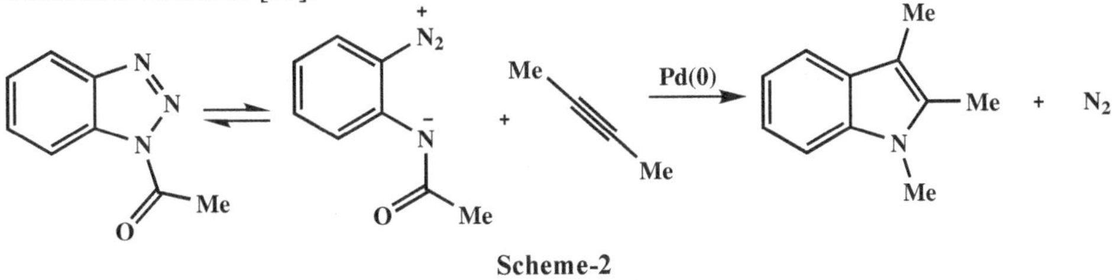

Scheme-2

The Pd-catalyzed carbon-nitrogen bond forming reaction from aryl triflates or halides and amides, amines, and carbamates, has attracted the much attention after pioneering work of Hartwig and co-workers [24-28]. The carbon-nitrogen bond forming reaction for the preparation of indole rings by intramolecular *N*-arylation was also observed. The *N*-aminoindoles were generated through Pd-catalyzed cyclization of *o*-chloroarylacetaldehyde *N,N*-dimethylhydrazones. Commercially accessible dimethylaminomethylferrocene was utilized for the preparation of 2-(dimethylaminomethyl)-1-(di-*tert*-butylphosphinyl)ferrocene ligand in one-step. Satisfactory results were reported in some cases where bulky electron-rich P(Bu-*t*)$_3$ was utilized. Rb$_2$CO$_3$ and cesium carbonate could also be used as bases. The chloroindoles were obtained in lower yields as compared to fluoroindoles or unsubstituted indoles because oxidative addition of chloroindoles to palladium(0) species occurred under reaction conditions. Since for increasing the molecular complexity of indole products the indole derivatives containing chloro substituents on carbocyclic ring were useful substrates, the authors investigated a domino process based on intramolecular cyclization to chloroindoles in the presence of Pd catalyst followed by Pd-catalyzed functionalization of their carbocyclic rings **(Scheme 3)** [29a-b].

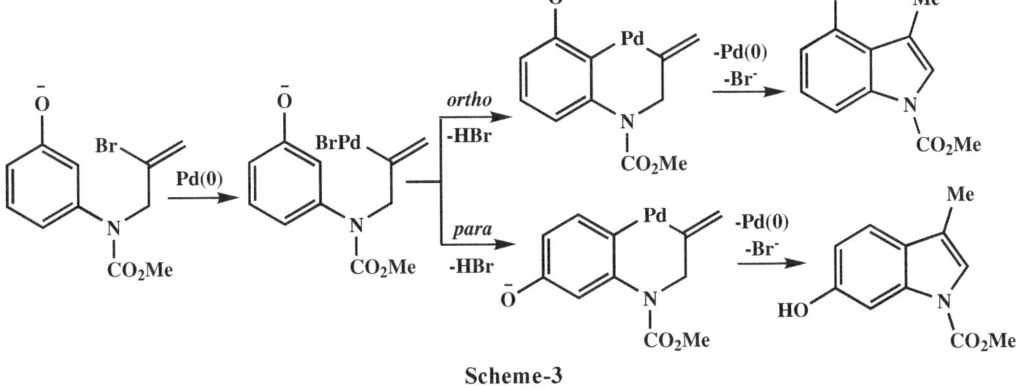

Scheme-3

Various heterocyclic compounds such as benzofurans, 1,2-dihydroisoquinolines, isocoumarins, and benzopyrans were synthesized by this method. The cycloaddition reactions of alkynes with transition metal are of great interest. The most widely used metal, for such processes [30], multiple alkyne insertions, or insertion and subsequent cyclization back on to a pre-existing aromatic ring, was Pd. The Pd-catalyzed heteroannulation of internal alkynes produced indoles regioselectively **(Scheme 4)**.

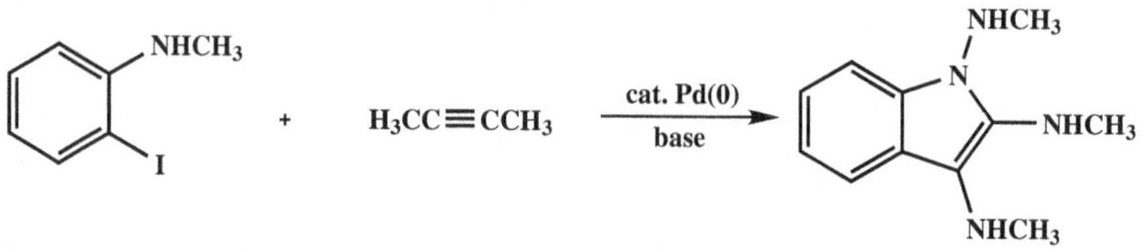

Scheme-4

The *o*-haloanilino enamine conjugated to an ester group (synthesized *via* a Wittig reaction) was utilized for the synthesis of 2-trifluoromethylated indoles [31-32]. The cyclization does not involve classical Heck sequence (*i.e.*, carbopalladation of the C-C double bond followed by a *syn*-β-elimination of hydridopalladium species) **(Scheme 5)** [29a-b].

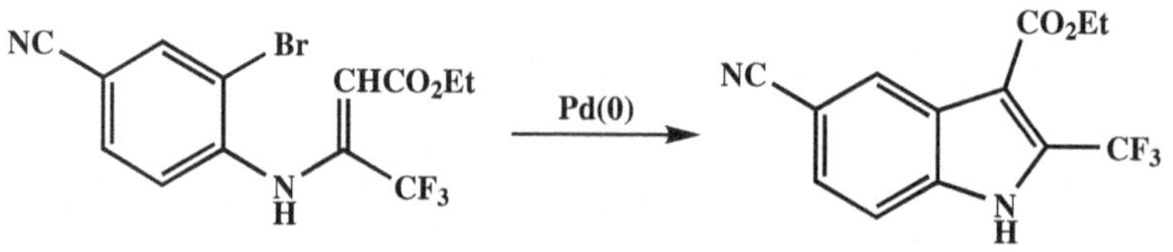

Scheme-5

In oxidative addition to palladium(0) centers the alkenyl halides were highly reactive as compared to aryl halides [33]. This interesting feature of palladium-catalyzed aminations was utilized to program several cascade palladium-catalyzed events, and eventually synthesized heterocyclic compounds. To see the feasibility of this characteristic **(Scheme 6)**, the reaction of *o*-haloanilines with alkenyl halides was selected. The initially produced enamine participated in an intramolecular Heck reaction [34] to synthesize a substituted indole directly in the presence of palladium catalyst [35].

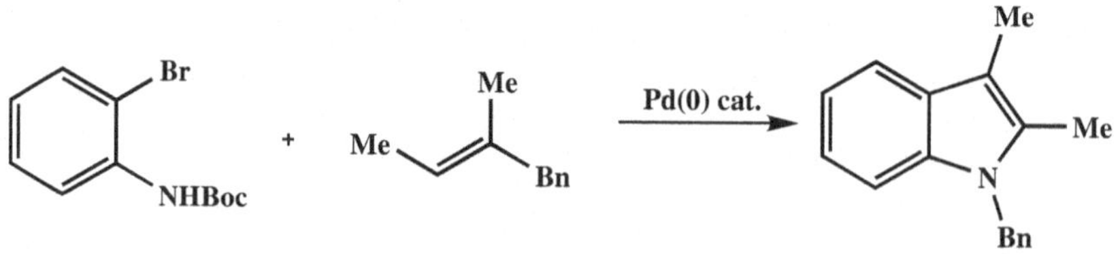

Scheme-6

Hartwig [36] took advantage of carbon-hydrogen functionalization using Pd(0) catalysis and oxime *O*-acetates as precursors for intramolecular reactions to form indoles. The proposed mechanism involved N-O bond insertion with tautomerization to yield an enamine intermediate **(Scheme 7)**. From this structure, carbon-hydrogen functionalization and reductive elimination of Pd(0) regenerated the catalyst and provided the product. Proof of N-O bond insertion came from isolation and characterization of an intermediate, which upon treatment under standard reaction conditions afforded expected indole **(Scheme 8)**.

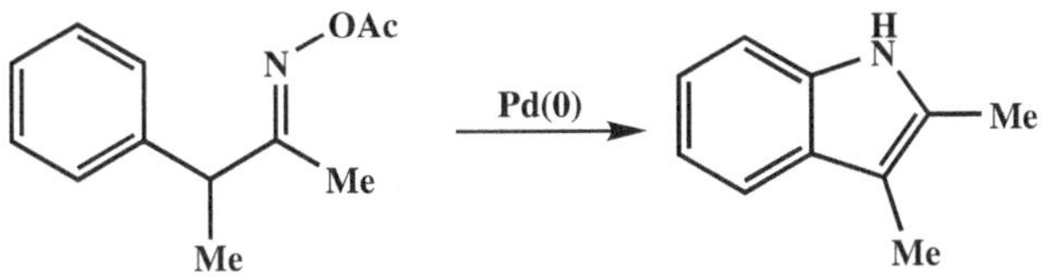

Scheme-7

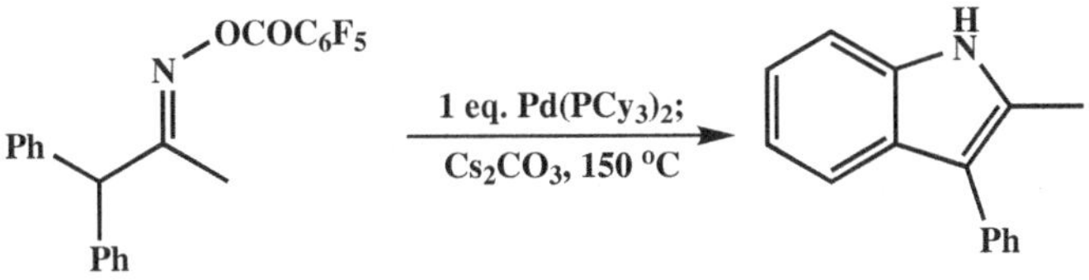

Scheme-8

Taylor and co-workers [37] provided a tolan functionality through a thallation reaction in which cyclization was carried out with PdCl$_2$. The cyclization of Pd intermediate with allyl chlorides in the presence of palladium(II) allowed Utimoto and co-workers [38] to introduce an allyl substituent in third position of indoles. Very often alkynyl group was introduced in *ortho* to amine *via* a coupling reaction and then the cyclization was performed. In second pathway the cyclization of diarylamines occurred *via* Buchwald-Hartwig coupling **(Scheme 9)** [39].

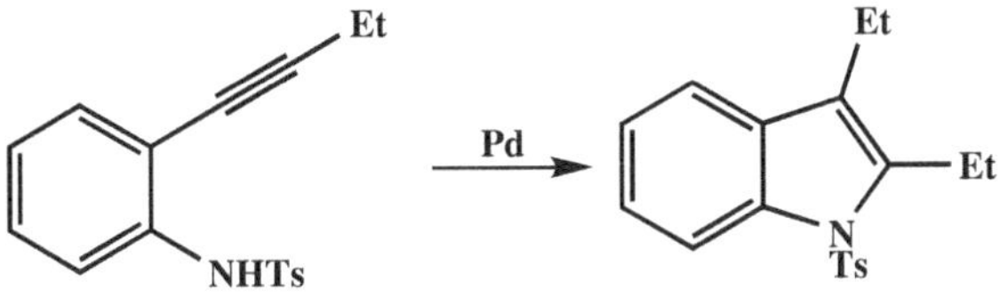

Scheme-9

Lautens et al. [40-42] utilized this method for the synthesis of indole derivatives with a high degree of modularity. In indole cyclization the tandem Pd-catalyzed protocols have used 1,1-dibromoalkenes, where one vinyl-bromide bond was available for Pd-catalyzed indole synthesis, and the second for subsequent functionalization **(Scheme 10)**.

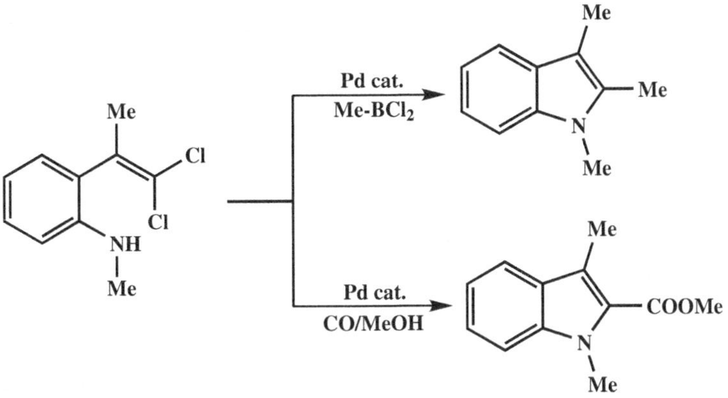

Scheme-10

For PhI the reactions occurred in short reaction time (15-30 min) at ambient temperature. But with aryl bromides 60 °C heating was needed for the reaction to occur and took long time to produce coupling product. This coupling was extended **(Scheme 11)** for the preparation of indole derivatives. The multi-catalytic system containing a NHC Pd complex and CuI was utilized [43] in reaction of *o*-dihaloarenes, terminal alkynes and many substituted amines for the formation of substituted indoles. Liang and co-workers [44] prepared polysubstituted furans in one-pot synthetic protocol through Pd-catalyzed, cyclization-coupling, three-component reaction of propargyl carbonate, β-keto esters and PhI [45-46].

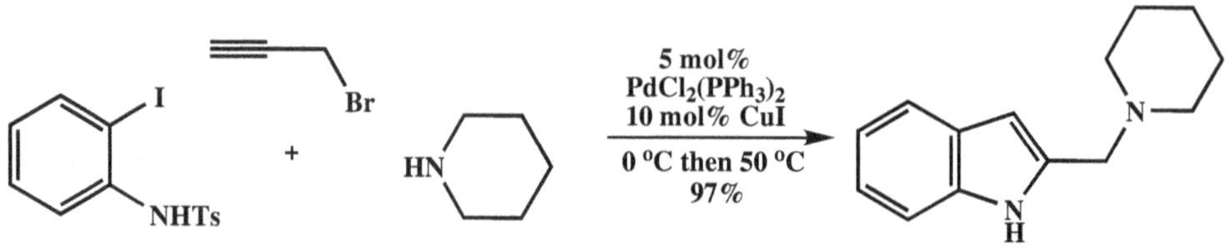

Scheme-11

A *gem*-dimethyl substrate was utilized for the synthesis of 2,3-dimethylindole. The cyclization of 2-ethylnitrobenzene was not successful as small amounts of respective aniline derivative and only starting material were recovered **(Scheme 12)**. These two results have indicated that a direct carbon-hydrogen bond amination mechanism does not occur in these cyclizations. More likely, the electrophilic palladium-nitroso or palladium-nitrene intermediate was quenched by pendent olefin which resulted in either a zwitterionic pyrrolidine or an aziridine-intermediate. Moderate yield of 2,3-dimethylindole was afforded upon subsequent 2,3-methyl and 1,3-hydride shifts [47].

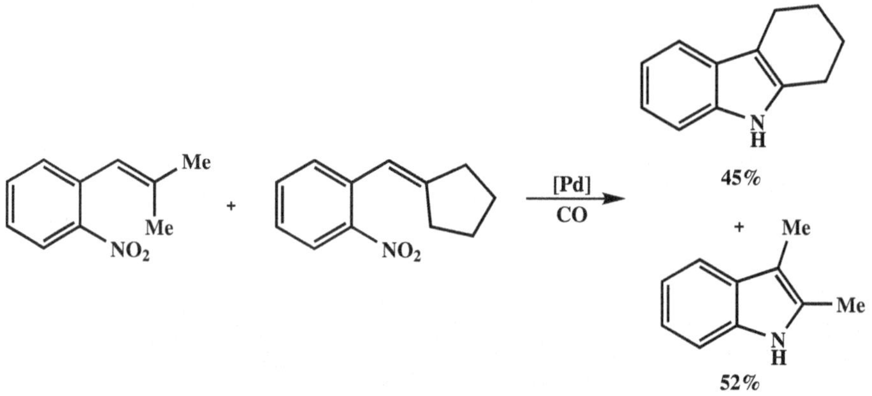

Scheme-12

Cenini et al. [48] continued to study this palladium-catalytic system and expanded the scope of reaction to include 2-nitrochalcones (affording 2-acyl indoles) and heteroaryl substituted *o*-nitrostyrenes (affording 2-heteroaryl indoles). Interestingly, the choice of solvent played a role in these transformations. When PhMe was replaced with tetrahydrofuran, significant amounts of *N*-hydroxyindoles and small amounts of anilines (< 8%) were formed during the cyclization reaction [49]; yields as high as 60% for the *N*-hydroxyindoles have been found at short reaction times (3 h vs. 6 h) and lower temperatures (130 °C vs. 170 °C). As suggested by results the hydroxyindole was formed as an intermediate and prior to cyclization the NO$_2$ substituent was not fully deoxygenated to nitrenoid. Indole was produced when hydroxyindole was reacted under reaction conditions. Presumably, the hydroxyindole intermediate was rapidly transformed to indole in a non-polar solvent (PhMe) whereas in a polar solvent (tetrahydrofuran) hydroxyindole was longer-lived. The complete reduction to nitrenoid cannot be ruled out as aniline by-products were isolated *albeit* in lower yields than hydroxyindoles **(Scheme 13)**. In contrast to hydroxyindoles being converted to indoles, anilines have been previously shown to not form the indole products when subjected to reductive carbonylation reaction conditions [50]. If anilines were intermediates then oxidative palladium(II) conditions would be required for a possible amino palladation/hydride elimination sequence to form the indoles.

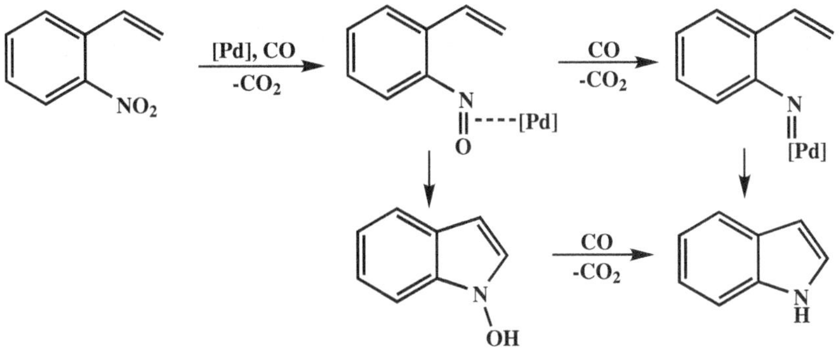

Scheme-13

To avoid the drawbacks related to need of *N*-protected iodoanilines, Djakovitch and Dufaud [51a-b] produced [Pd(PPh$_2$)$_2$]SBA-15 catalyst and compared its activity to that of [Pd(NH$_3$)$_4$]/NaY, palladium acetate and "Beller-Herrmann palladacycle" {Pd[P(o-C$_6$H$_4$CH$_3$)$_2$-(o-C$_6$H$_4$CH$_2$)(CH$_3$CO$_2$)]}$_2$. High selectivities and conversions (>89% yield) resulted in moderate to high yields in the presence of palladium catalyst (1 mol%) under standard reaction conditions (80 °C, dimethylformamide/water (4/1)) **(Scheme 14)**. The heterogeneous catalysts were more active than homogeneous ones which were deactivated by the formation of Pd black. The [Pd(PPh$_2$)$_2$]SBA-15 catalyst shown a slightly higher activity as compared to [Pd(NH$_3$)$_4$]/NaY one; however, the [Pd(PPh$_2$)$_2$]SBA-15 catalyst was reused up to five times while the [Pd(NH$_3$)$_4$]/NaY catalyst was fully deactivated after the third run. This difference was due to the negligible rate of palladium-leaching with [Pd(PPh$_2$)$_2$]SBA-15 whereas this leaching was pronounced with [Pd(NH$_3$)$_4$]/NaY. Interestingly, a further direct arylation employing [Pd(PPh$_2$)$_2$]SBA-15 catalyst was utilized for the formation of 2,3-functionalized indoles. However, the reaction was not very efficient as only 35% yield was reported after 12 d [52].

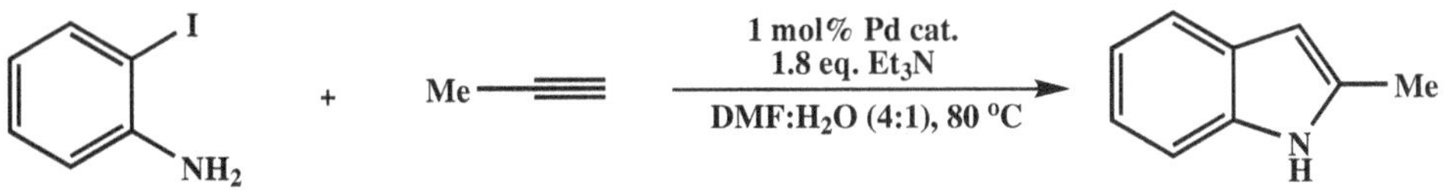

Scheme-14

The chiral *N*-heterocyclic carbene systems were designed for asymmetric catalysis during the synthesis of *N*-heterocyclic carbene ligands. This field has grown dramatically and various chiral *N*-heterocyclic carbenes were described since the first examples observed by Enders and Herrmann [53-54]. The Pd complex supported by an optically active *N*-heterocyclic carbene ligand was utilized for the formation of valuable chiral oxindoles [55-56] by amide arylation **(Scheme 15)** [57-59a, b].

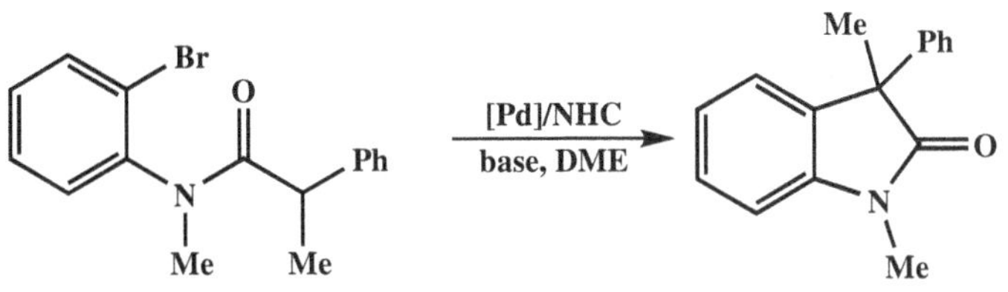

Scheme-15

The cross-coupling reactions of unactivated substrates catalyzed by metal complexes were modified *via* incorporation of an extensive library of chiral and achiral phosphine ligands. The use of phosphine ligands resulted in positive effects in terms of selectivities and turnovers in comparison to traditional industrial processes like hydrogenation. The rich field of *N*-heterocyclic carbene ligands utilized in homogeneous catalysis resulted in many limitations such as high cost of producing tertiary (especially chiral) phosphines and their degradative tendency in converting to phosphine oxides [60]. A variety of *N*-heterocyclic carbene ligands are now commercially accessible which has shown high activities in many important organic reactions when used in combination with metal pre-catalysts. *N*-heterocyclic carbene imidazolidine ligands with sterically encumbering moieties like isopropyl, mesityl, and adamantyl were utilized in palladium-catalyzed cyclization of anilides [61], amination of aryl chlorides [62], arylation with ester enolates to provide α-aryl esters [63], Sonogashira reactions of unactivated alkyl bromides [64], and the Ru-catalyzed ring-closing metathesis reaction **(Scheme 16)** [65-67].

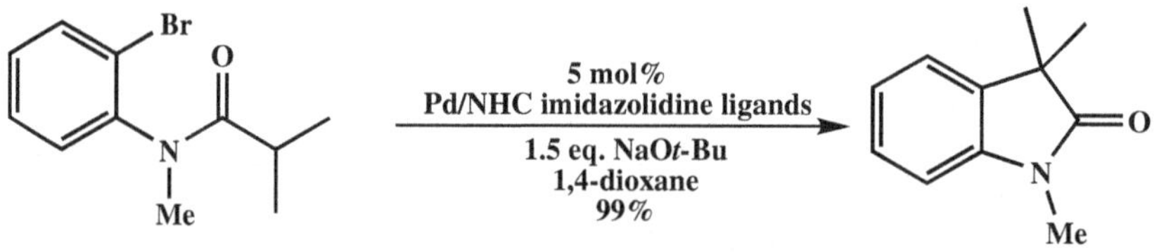

Scheme-16

The isoindole core is present in various biologically active synthetic and natural products. α-Amino(2-alkynylphenyl)methylphosphonate was produced from amine, 2-alkynyl benzaldehyde, and diethyl phosphate. Good to excellent yields of isoindol-1-ylphosphonate derivatives were obtained when α-amino(2-alkynylphenyl) methylphosphonate was reacted with PhI in catalytic amounts of DABCO (1,4-diazabicyclo[2.2.2]octane) and acetone at rt **(Scheme 17)** [68-69].

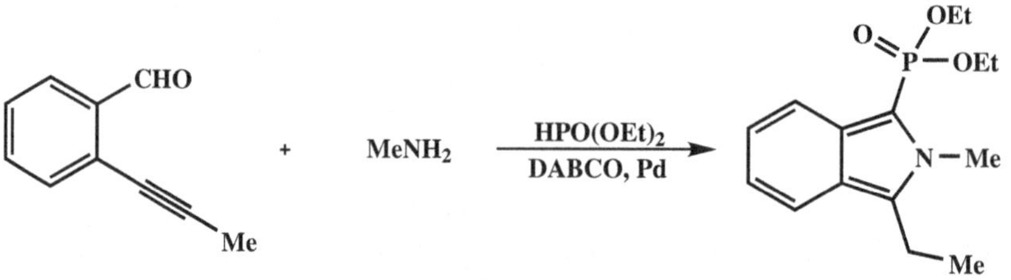

Scheme-17

The applicability of palladium-catalyzed carboamination of *N*-allylureas was explored for the preparation of imidazolidin-2-ones enantioselectively. The use of chiral ligands on metal helped in achieving the enantioselectivity in reactions. Asymmetric palladium-catalyzed insertion reactions with chiral ligands are Heck reactions as indicated by various examples in literature [70-73]. One of those examples is the Overman's enantioselective synthesis of oxindoles **(Scheme 18)**. There are less common examples of enantioselective aminopalladation. Zhu and Yang [74] provided instances of asymmetric aza-Wacker-type cyclizations in the presence of (-)-sparteine.

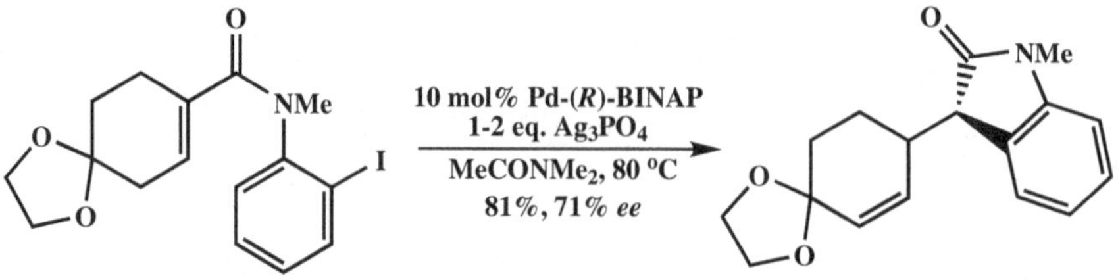

Scheme-18

The isoindolin-1-ones were generated by a sequence which involved intermolecular palladium-catalyzed carbonylative amidation followed by intramolecular Michael addition. This conversion was effective with a number of aromatic and primary aliphatic amine nucleophiles. A competitive edge was obtained with the introduction of C1 synthon CO in carbopalladation protocols. Grigg et al. [75] described a three-component reaction of primary amines, *o*-iodo cinnamic derivatives, and CO to afford 3-substituted isoindolinones in the presence of Pd catalyst. Two mechanisms were proposed. In first pathway, first a Michael addition occurred followed by oxidative addition and carbon monoxide insertion to produce an acylpalladium intermediate. The intramolecular nucleophilic attack at adjacent amine followed by reductive elimination of catalyst afforded isoindolinone. In second pathway, the acylpalladium intermediate was produced and trapped by an intermolecular attack of amine. The newly synthesized amide underwent an intramolecular addition to tethered Michael system in the presence of a base catalyst **(Scheme 19)** [76].

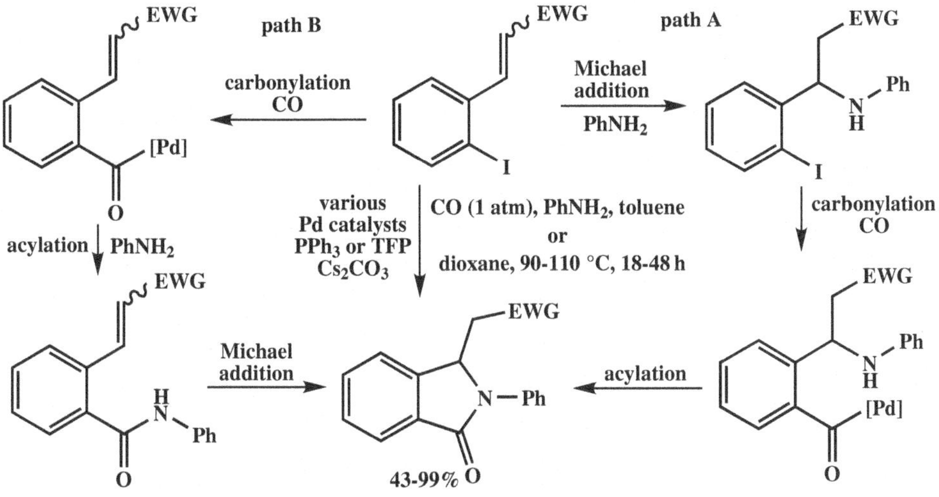

Scheme-19

Sajiki et al. [77] synthesized 2- and 2,3-substituted indoles from *N*-tosyl protected 2-iodoanilines and alkynes *via* Larock heteroannulation in the presence of palladium/carbon catalysts. Initially, the reaction was developed in lithium chloride, after that a lithium chloride-free method was reported. It afforded a method close to the one example explored by Batail and co-workers [52, 78] **(Scheme 20)**.

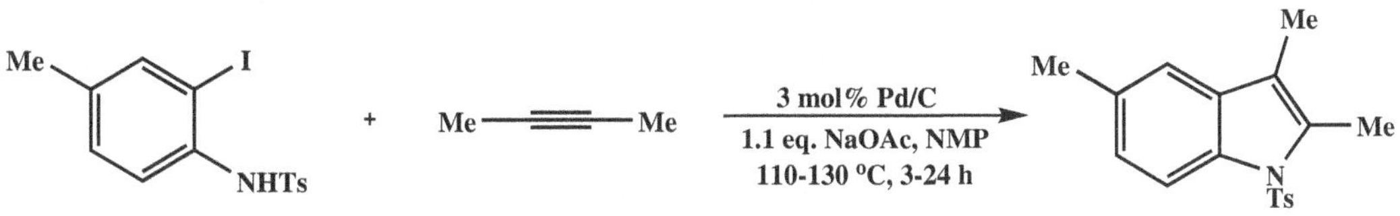

Scheme-20

Batail and co-workers [79] used a number of substituted alkynes and 2-bromoanilines in this procedure. Good to high yields (55%-95%) of indoles were afforded despite the lower reactivity of bromoaniline derivatives and it increased the versatility and efficiency of this heterogeneous process **(Scheme 21)** [80-81]. Common side reactions for this substrate (*i.e.*, amination/dimerization or multiple insertions of the substrates) were almost suppressed and good yields of targeted indoles were obtained, in spite of longer reaction times and a higher temperature (*i.e.*, 140 °C) inherent to the use of diphenylacetylene [52].

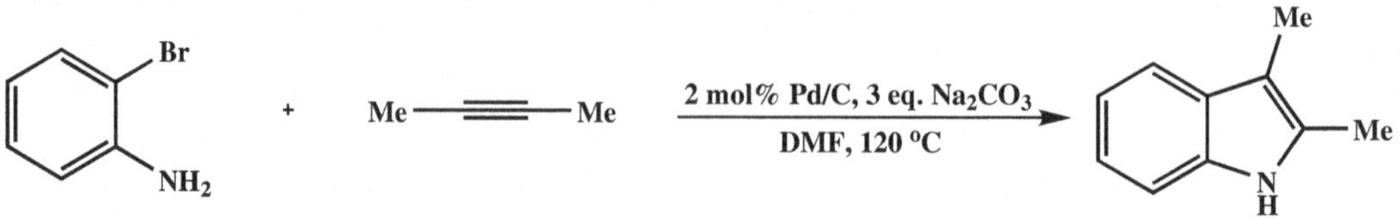

Scheme-21

In 2009, Batail and co-workers [78] carried out Larock methodology with reusable and easily separable heterogeneous Pd catalysts. Authors used easily homemade [Pd(NH$_3$)$_4$]/NaY catalyst (prepared by ion exchange of a NaY zeolite using a 0.1 M aqueous solution of [Pd(NH$_3$)$_4$]Cl$_2$) or commercially available palladium/carbon in order to develop an additive-free (*i.e.*, salt- and ligand-free) Larock indole synthesis in the presence of potentially recyclable and easily separable heterogeneous Pd catalysts. The 2,3-diphenylindole was provided in 70% yield after 14 h when 2-iodoaniline was coupled with diphenylacetylene using 2 mol% of palladium/carbon and sodium carbonate as base at 120 °C in dimethylformamide. Excellent yields of indoles were afforded when many alkynes and 2-iodoanilines were utilized **(Scheme 22)**. Higher chemical yields were obtained using homemade [Pd(NH$_3$)$_4$]/NaY catalyst, with the exception of 2-iodoaniline for which palladium/carbon exhibited a higher activity. The [Pd(NH$_3$)$_4$]/NaY or palladium/carbon catalyst was reused up to 5 and 3 times, respectively [52, 82-83].

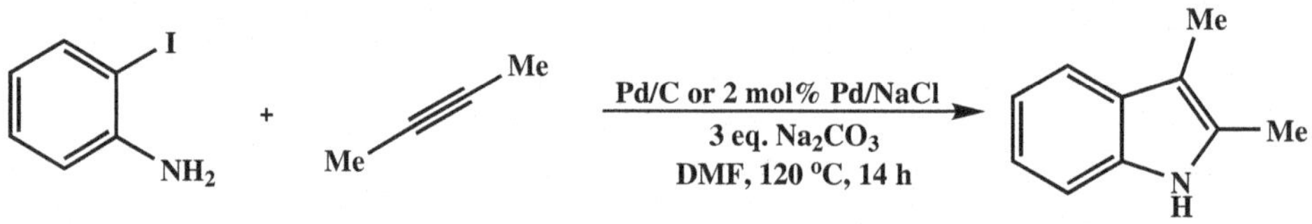

Scheme-22

Felpin et al. [84-86] described the use of aryldiazonium salts and 2-(2-nitrophenyl)acrylates for the preparation of oxindoles *via* a tandem Heck/Reduction/Cyclization (HRC) process in the presence of Pd catalyst. This protocol was developed initially using palladium/carbon catalyst and was improved by producing *in situ* catalytic material from charcoal and palladium acetate. The reaction conditions were optimized (*i.e.*, 1.2 mmol of aryldiazonium salt, 1 mmol of acrylates, 5 mol% of palladium acetate, 5 mL of methanol, 45 mg of charcoal, 15-90 min, 40 °C; then hydrogen, 24 h, 40 °C) for this Heck/Reduction/Cyclization reaction to provide good to high yields of many oxindoles **(Scheme 23)**. Interestingly, during Heck coupling (*i.e.*, HBF$_4$) the formed waste acted as a co-catalyst in further reduction-cyclization step which was beneficial to overall reaction [52].

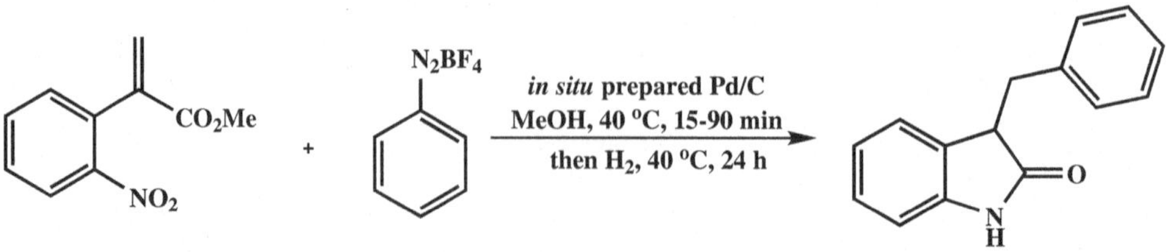

Scheme-23

An alternative approach to the synthesis of oxindoles involved ring-closing reactions, most commonly used in the formation of five-membered lactam. A number of processes that affect this ring closure have been developed, and they can be divided into two general classes. In the first, a reactive functional group (such as a nucleophilic component or a suitable leaving group) was bound directly to aromatic ring. For example, the cyclization between an aromatic amine (or a precursor thereof) and an appropriately situated carboxylic acid derivative resulted in the formation of oxindole lactam ring **(Scheme 24)** [87].

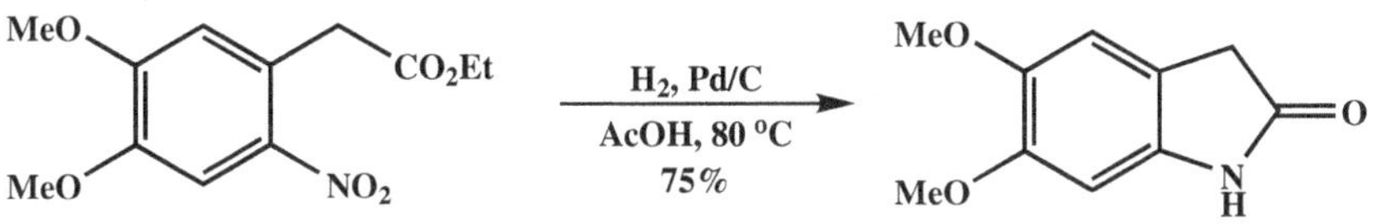

Scheme-24

Leimgruber and Batcho [88] reported the synthesis of indoles *via* reductive cyclization of nitroaromatics. This is also a very important procedure for the preparation of natural products. The Leimgruber and Batcho indole synthesis formed the indoles from *o*-NO$_2$-PhMe in two steps. Leimgruber and Batcho [88] reported an efficient method for the synthesis of indole based on the condensation of *o*-NO$_2$-PhMe with DMFDMA, subsequently the resulting *E*-*β*-dimethylamino-2-nitrostyrene was cyclized reductively **(Scheme 25)** [89].

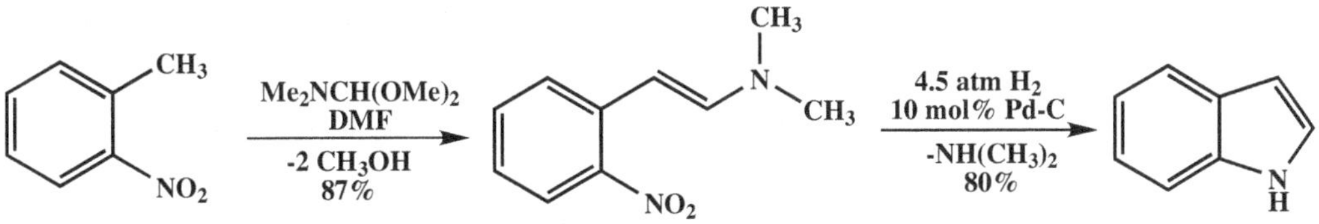

Scheme-25

Due to medicinal importance of heterocycles, the development of new methods for the formation of heterocycles catalyzed by transition metals is an active field of research [90-96]. Synthesis of such heterocycles by means of carbon-hydrogen activation followed by carbon-nitrogen bond formation was a complementary pathway to powerful Buchwald-Hartwig amination process **(Scheme 26)** [97-100].

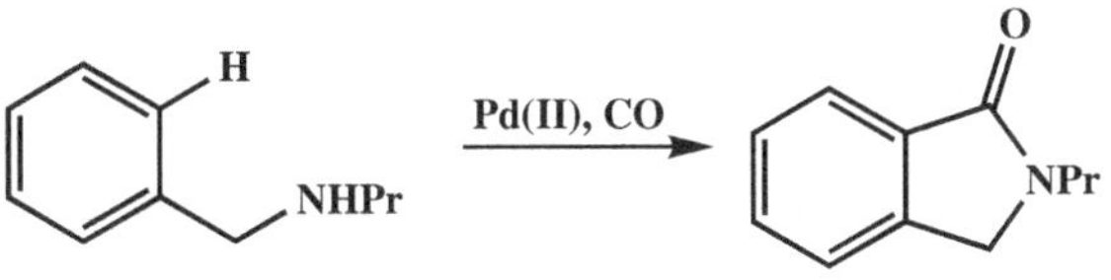

Scheme-26

Boger and co-workers [101] through 5-*exo-trig* aryl radical alkene cyclization of allylamine derivative formed a methyl 1,2,8,8a-tetrahydrocyclopropa[*c*]thieno[3,2-*e*]indol-4-one-6-carboxylate (CTI) derivatives **(Scheme 27)** and examined their biological activity. The methyl 1,2,8,8a-tetrahydrocyclopropa[*c*]thieno[3,2-*e*]indol-4-one-6-carboxylate (CTI) derivatives have a single atom change (nitrogen to sulfur) in duocarmycin SA alkylation subunit. The pyrrole NH of alkylation subunit of duocarmycin SA was replaced with a sulfur atom which maintained or slightly increased the biological activity of natural product, but not to the extent reported with MeCTI [102].

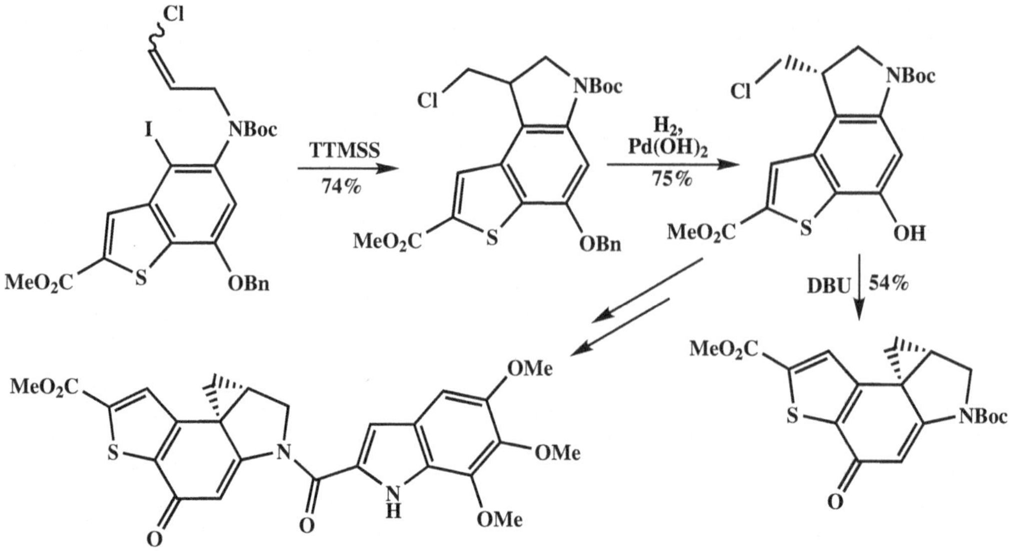

Scheme-27

Gabriele and co-workers [103] described the synthesis of 1,3-dihydroinol-2-one derivatives in good yields from the reaction of *o*-ethynylanilines with CO, MeOH, and O_2 in the presence of Pd catalyst **(Scheme 28)**. Many conversions which involved carbon monoxide insertion into a palladium-heteroatom bond were developed that resulted into the introduction of two molecules of carbon monoxide into heterocyclic compound. Gabriele [104] used this protocol for the synthesis of heterocyclic compounds like dihydroindolones. The *o*-alkynyl aniline was treated with carbon monoxide in the presence of palladium(II) catalyst in MeOH to synthesize 1,3-dihydroinol-2-one in 50% yield. The alkene was transformed to pyrrolidinone by a similar pathway [76, 105].

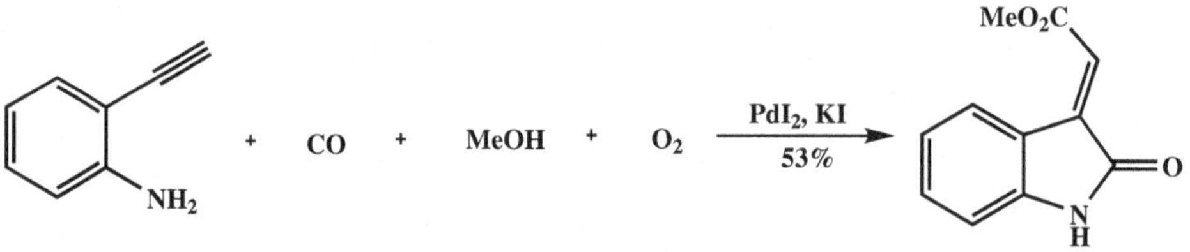

Scheme-28

A sequential intermolecular and transannular Pd-catalyzed hydroamination of cycloheptatriene synthesized biologically active azabicyclic tropene derivatives. The presence of 1-hexene favored the conversion of *N*-alkylanilines and the role of 1-hexene was highlighted although the actual role was not clear. Interestingly, under nonoxidative conditions, indol-2-acetic esters were obtained *via* 5-*exo*-*dig* cyclization **(Scheme 29)** [106-107].

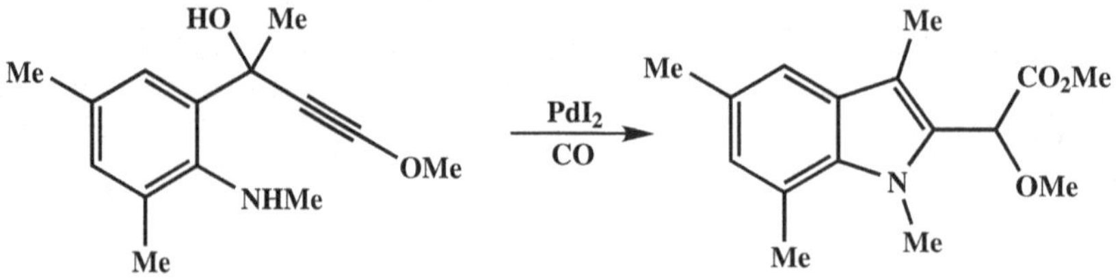

Scheme-29

Gabriele and co-workers [108] used 1-(2-aminoaryl)-2-yn-1-ols for the synthesis of indol-2-acetic esters. The alkynylmagnesium bromides were reacted with 1-(2-aminoaryl)ketones for the preparation of 1-(2-aminoaryl)-2-yn-1-ols **(Scheme 30)**. Moderate to good yields (42-88%), on the basis of starting 1-(2-aminoaryl)ketones], of indole products were obtained in methanol under 90 atm of carbon monoxide at 100 °C in the presence of potassium iodide and palladium iodide in case of 1-(2-aminoaryl)-2-yn-1-ols containing either a primary or secondary amino group and substituted with a bulky group on triple bond [29a-b].

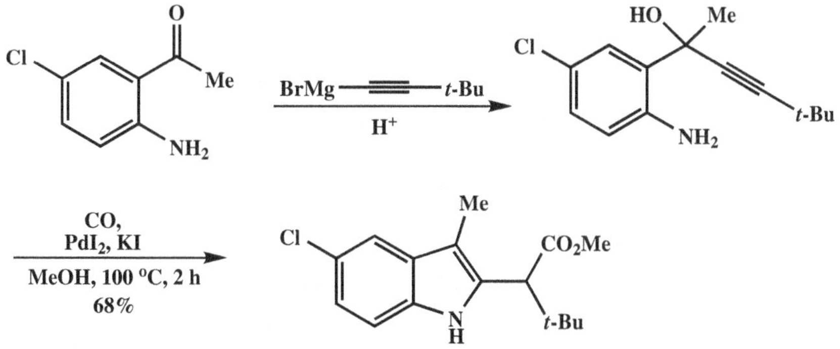

Scheme-30

Moderate yields of 2,3-disubstituted indoles were obtained *via* palladium bromide-catalyzed cyclization of *o*-alkynylphenyl *N,O*-acetals **(Scheme 31)** [29a-b, 109].

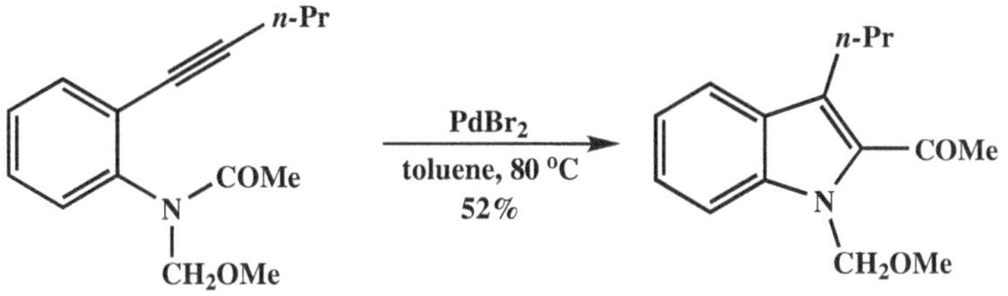

Scheme-31

This transannulation needed internal alkynes and heating at 130 °C in the presence of [Pd(PPh₃)₄] without a solvent **(Scheme 32)**. The multisubstituted indoles were obtained in good yields under reaction conditions. The reaction occurred less efficiently with solvents and other Pd catalysts. The efficiency of this reaction was influenced with the electronic nature of substituents. The electron-withdrawing groups containing triazoles reacted well. On the other hand triazoles with electron-donating groups reacted sluggishly and afforded poor yields in long reaction times. Varied regioselectivity was observed from the reactions of unsymmetrical alkynes and favored bulkier substituents at C2 of indole like the trend reported in Larock's indole synthesis. The palladium(0)-catalyzed protocol did not tolerate terminal alkynes [23, 110].

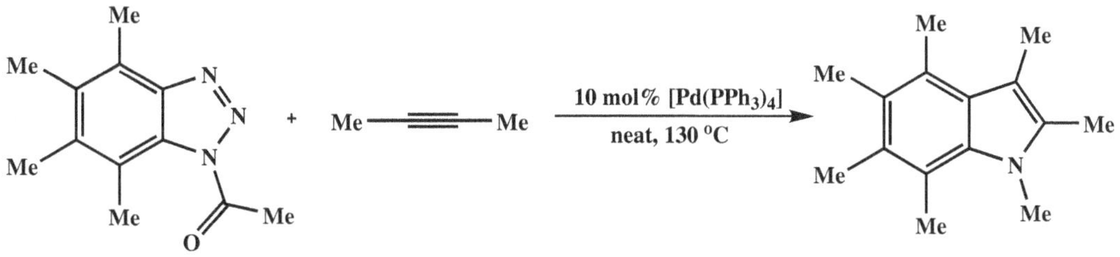

Scheme-32

This method involved the coupling of vinyl- or aryl-halides in the presence of Pd catalyst. The cyclization occurred by an initial oxidative addition of vinyl- or aryl-halides to form a Pd(II) complex with Pd(0) catalysts [110-111]. Subsequently, the reductive elimination of heterocycle-vinyl or -aryl bond occurred. A variety of polysubstituted indoles were generated by this method. For instance, Cacchi [112-113] synthesized substituted indoles in good yield by Pd(PPh$_3$)$_4$-catalyzed coupling of trifluoroacetanilides with vinyl-halides/triflates or ary-halides **(Scheme 33)** [114].

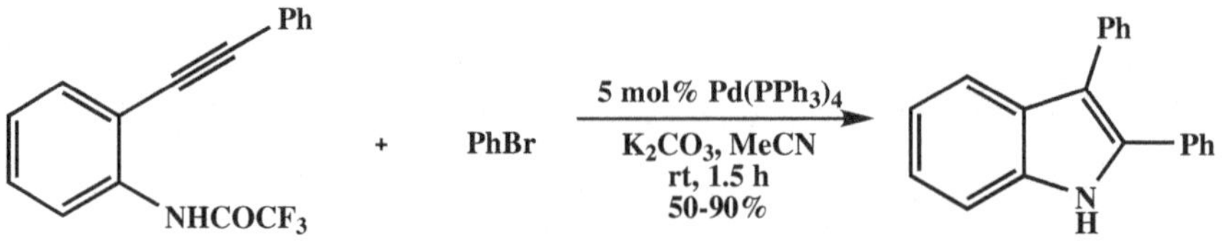

Scheme-33

Cacchi et al. [112] extended the aminopalladation-reductive elimination route to indoles. The 2-substituted 3-acyl indoles exhibited a number of therapeutic activities. The *o*-alkynyltrifluoroacetanilides were reacted with vinyl triflates and PhI in CO to provide 2-substituted 3-acyl indoles in fair to good yields. This three-component reaction gives satisfactory results with electron-rich, neutral, or slightly electron-poor vinyl triflates and PhI in the presence of Pd(PPh$_3$)$_4$ and potassium carbonate at 45 °C in acetonitrile under a balloon of CO [114-116]. The use of a higher pressure of CO and anhydrous CH$_3$CN was necessary with strongly electron-poor ArI, like ethyl *p*-iodobenzoate. Alternatively, good results were reported under a balloon of CO with Pd(dba)$_2$/P(*o*-tol)$_3$. The reaction occurred in following basic steps: (a) a σ-acylpalladium complex was formed by carbonylation of a σ-organopalladium complex produced *in situ* via oxidative addition of an organic triflate or halide to Pd(0); (b) coordination of alkyne to Pd atom of the σ-acylpalladium complex formed a π-alkyne-σ-acylpalladium complex; (c) a σ-acyl-σ-indolylpalladium complex was formed by an intramolecular nucleophilic

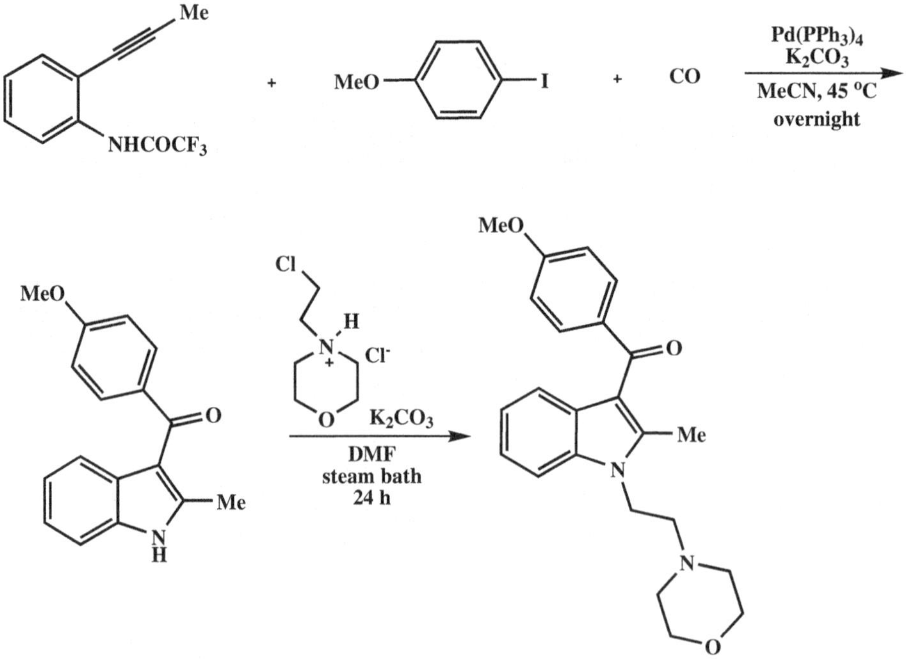

Scheme-34

attack of nitrogen on the activated C-C triple bond; (d) reductive elimination. Other mechanisms which involved the addition of σ-acylpalladium complex or carbonylation of σ-organo -σ-indolylpalladium complex to the C-C triple bond were also considered. This methodology was utilized for the preparation of pravadoline [117], an indole derivative with analgesic activity in humans **(Scheme 34)** [118-119]. The 6-aryl-11*H*-indolo[3,2-*c*]quinolines were synthesized from *o*-(*o*-aminophenylethynyl)-trifluoroacetanilide *via* a carbonylative cyclization followed by the cyclization of resulting 3-acylindoles [120]. The bis(*o*-trifluoroacetamidophenyl)-acetylene provided 12-acylindolo[1,2-*c*]quinazolines under same carbonylative cyclization conditions [29a-b, 121].

The 2-substituted 3-allylindoles were formed when *o*-alkynyltrifluoroacetanilides were reacted with allyl esters [111, 113-116]. Three basic procedures were developed by optimization studies: procedure A, *N*-allylation products were formed in a stepwise protocol *via* a Pd-catalyzed *N*-allylation (only those *N*-allyl derivatives were isolated which contain the nitrogen fragment on less substituted allyl terminus), followed by a cyclization step; procedure B, a one-pot reaction that omitted the isolation of *N*-allyl intermediates **(Scheme 35)** [29a-b].

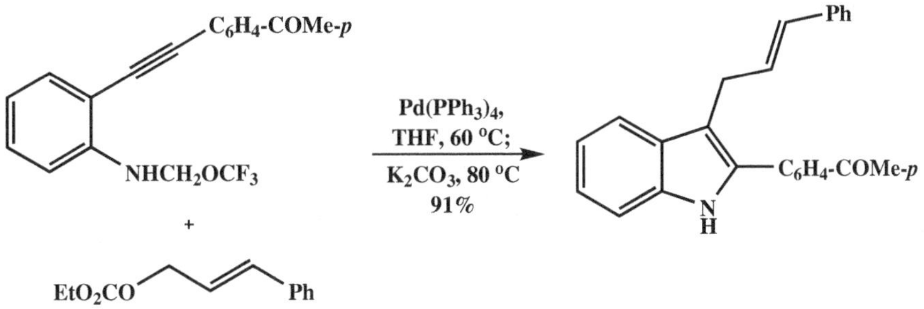

Scheme-35

Buchwald and Hartwig [122-124] reported a Pd-catalyzed coupling reaction of aryl halides with amines, and this reaction was extended to the intramolecular version to afford a number of aza-heterocycles. From the preparation of aromatic amines, the coupling of amines with aromatic halides in the presence of Pd catalyst (Buchwald-Hartwig reaction) has become a very useful protocol. Both five- and six-membered ring heterocyclic compounds were synthesized by intramolecular version of this reaction. For instance, Buchwald and co-workers [125] showed that for the synthesis of simple indulines, Pd(PPh$_3$)$_4$ was an effective catalyst **(Scheme 36)**. A variety of alkaloids were afforded by this protocol, like indazoles, indoles, benazepines, benzimidazoles, carbapenems, phenazines, carbolines, the mitomycin ring system, and polyheterocycles [126-136] and pharmacologically active natural products, like (-)-asperlicin [137-139].

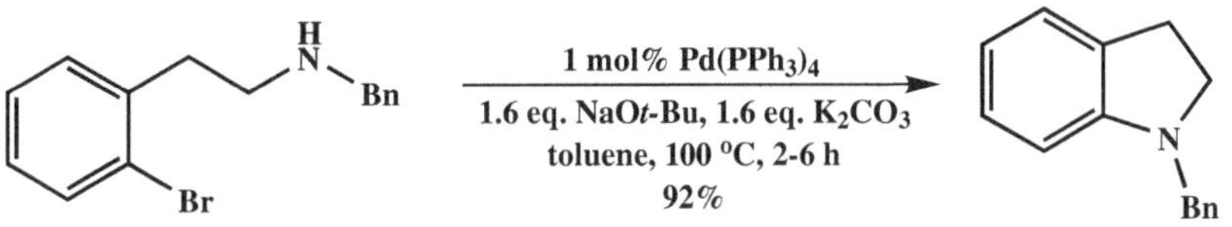

Scheme-36

Cacchi [117] synthesized libraries of three independently substituted indoles under solid-phase conditions utilizing a Wang resin **(Scheme 37)**. The alkyne precursor was obtained from Wang resin. The formed alkyne precursor was utilized for Pd-catalyzed cyclization in three steps. Interestingly, potassium carbonate was found to be optimal base for the cyclization step even though it was expected that a soluble base was required for a SPS [29a-b].

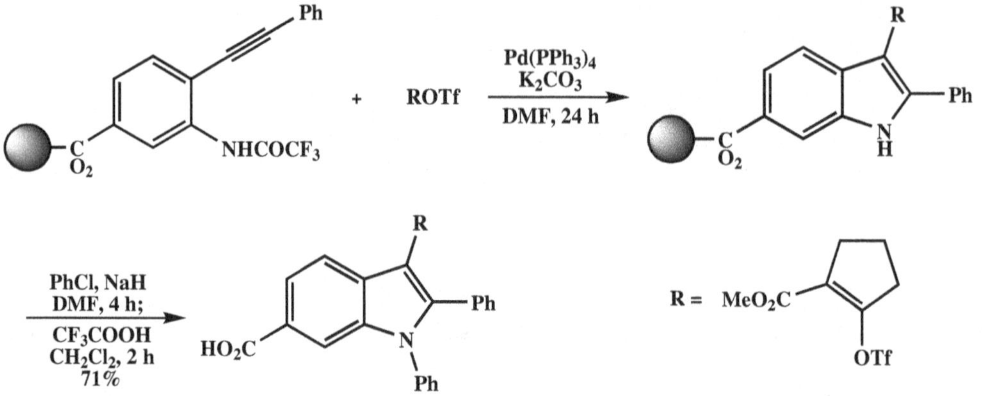

Scheme-37

During the selective synthesis of quinolones, it was reported that cyclization step for the synthesis of indoxyls was catalyzed by free phosphines. The 2-benzylideneindoxyl was formed quantitatively from 2-iodoaniline, phenyl acetylene and CO in the presence of [Pd(PPh$_3$)$_4$] catalyst. This method was further extended to a number of indoxyls, mainly observed as (*Z*)-isomer **(Scheme 38)** [52, 140].

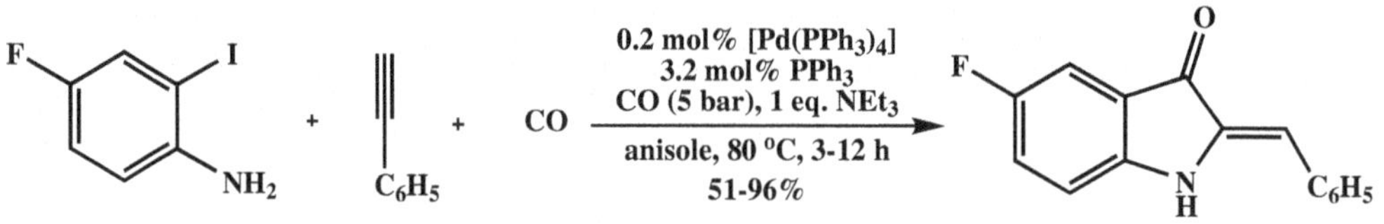

Scheme-38

The benzimide was obtained in a one-pot synthetic protocol in moderate yields when CO and nitrogen was introduced into aryl halide. The phthalimide was formed in 82% yield when 2-bromobenzoic acid was reacted in a similar way **(Scheme 39)** [141-142].

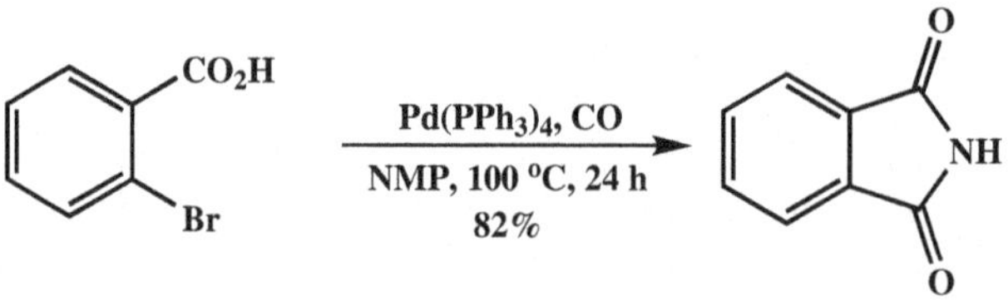

Scheme-39

The 2-alkynyltrifluoroacetanilides and arenediazonium tetrafluoroborates were reacted for the synthesis of free N-H 2,3-disubstituted indoles in the presence of Pd catalyst. The substrates tolerated a number of substituents such as bromo, nitro, chloro, keto, cyano, ether, and ester substituents **(Scheme 40)** [143].

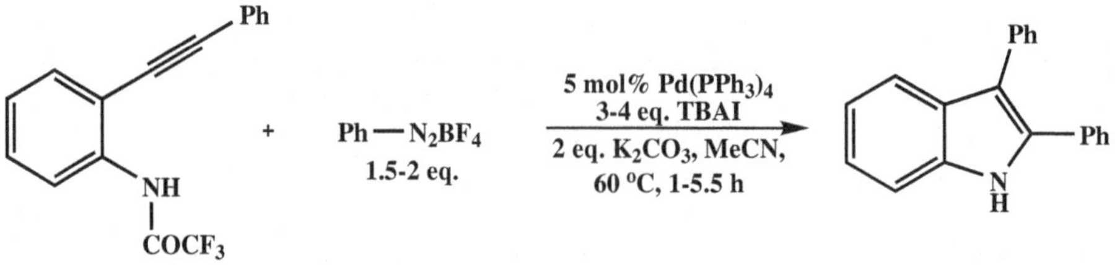

Scheme-40

The reaction occurred *via* a Pd-catalyzed denitrogenative/indolization process from *N*-aroylbenzotriazoles **(Scheme 41)**. Symmetrical alkynes provided the best results. Regioisomeric indoles were obtained from unsymmetrical alkynes. A σ-arylpalladium intermediate was produced when the diazonium functionality of a 2-iminobenzenediazonium species (produced from benzotriazole) was reacted in the presence of Pd(0). The σ-arylpalladium intermediate was in equilibrium with a four-membered palladacycle. A six-membered palladacycle was produced on subsequent carbopalladation. The indole was formed from six-membered palladacycle through reductive elimination [29a-b].

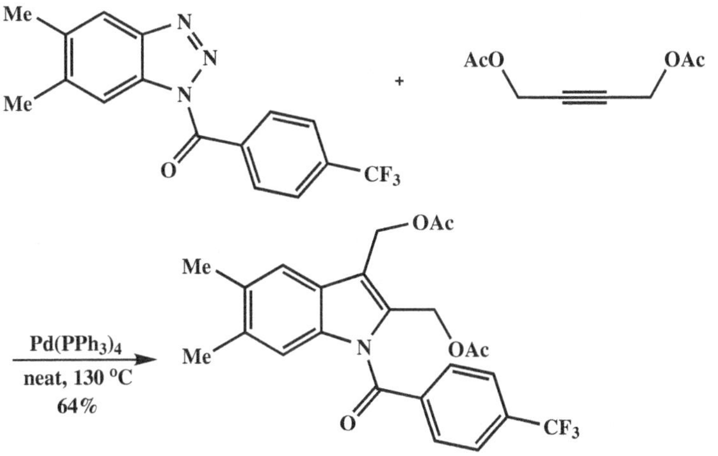

Scheme-41

Cacchi et al. [144-146] synthesized a number of 3-unsubstituted 2-substituted indoles using 3-(*o*-trifluoroacetamidoaryl)-1-propargylic esters as synthetic intermediates. Excellent yields of 2-(piperazin-1-ylmethyl)indoles were obtained when ethyl 3-(*o*-trifluoroacetamidoaryl)-1-propargylic carbonates (possessing an aryl substituent at the propargylic carbon or unsubstituted) were reacted with piperazines in the presence of Pd(PPh₃)₄ in tetrahydrofuran at 80 °C **(Scheme 42)** [147]. The indole was obtained in moderate yield only with piperazines possessing bulky substituents at the 2-position, this was due to low nucleophilicity of nitrogen derivative because of steric effects. The 2-aminomethylindoles were obtained in good to excellent yields with other secondary amines. The crucial role was played by acidity of nitrogen-hydrogen bond. The indole was produced only in trace amounts, if any, when a less acidic nitrogen-hydrogen bond possessing ethyl 3-(*o*-acetamidophenyl)-1-propargyl carbonate was treated with 4-ethylpiperazine under standard conditions [29a-b].

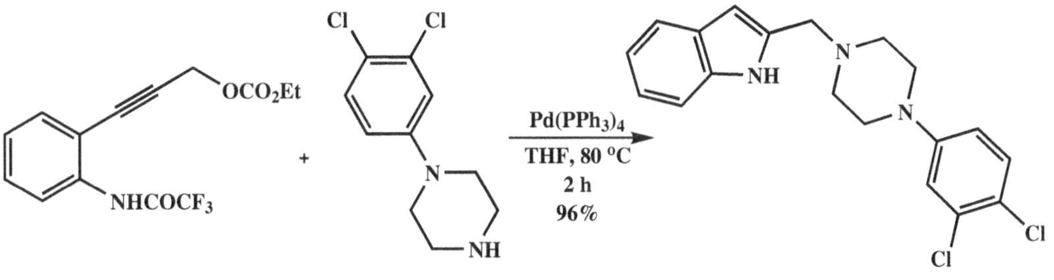

Scheme-42

The *N*-(*o*-haloaryl)enolates were utilized in the indole synthesis. The cyclization of β-(*o*-iodoanilino)carboxamides was involved here [148]. Indolines were even the main reaction products in this reaction or frequently significant side-products **(Scheme 43)** [29a-b].

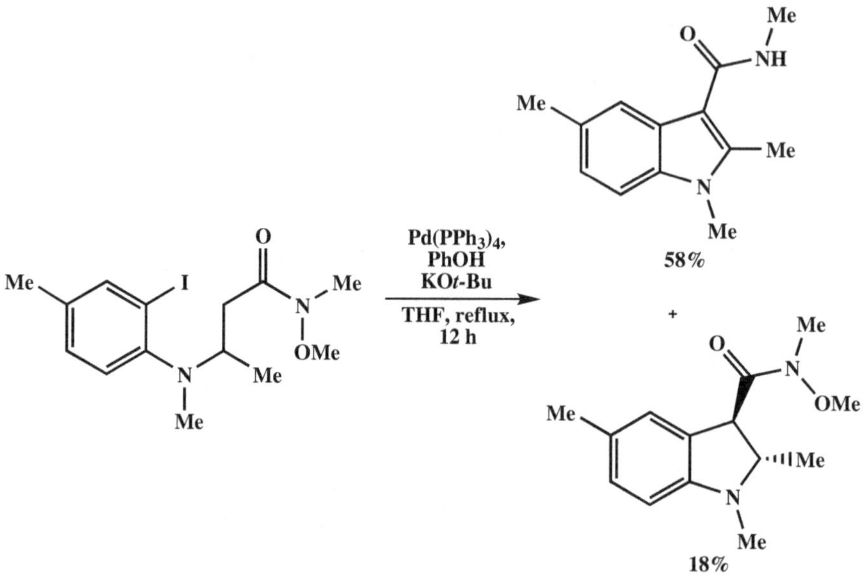

Scheme-43

The azaindoles were formed by a one-pot two-step method under dielectric heating conditions. The aminopyridines and ketones were condensed in the first step either under dielectric heating at 160-220 °C or at rt to afford intermediate enamines. Then in second step, the intramolecular Heck reactions under MWI yielded 4-,5-, 6- or 7-azaindoles in moderate to good yields **(Scheme 44)** [149].

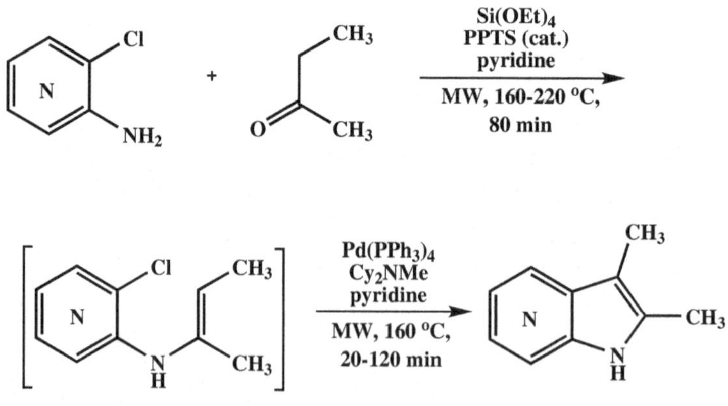

Scheme-44

The *o*-alkynyltrifluoroacetanilides were reacted with 1-haloalkynes to provide 2-substituted 3-alkynylindoles [150]. The 1-iodoalkynes did not act well in this reaction while satisfactory yields were reported with 1-bromoalkynes. Lesser yields were obtained with 1-iodoalkynes because they underwent side reactions. For instance, 1,3-diynes were obtained from 1-iodoalkynes *via* Pd-catalyzed homocoupling **(Scheme 45)** [29a-b, 118].

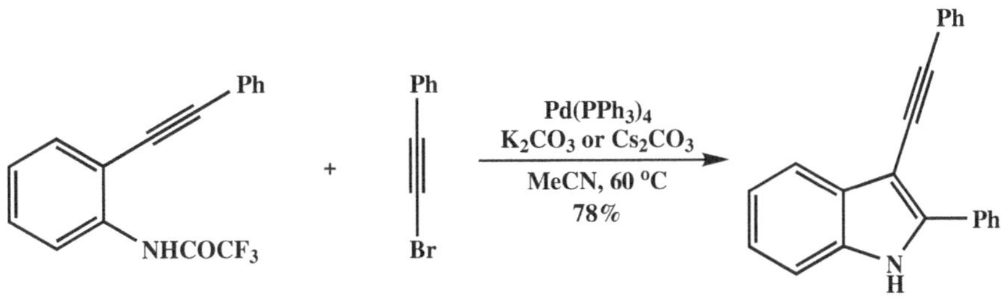

Scheme-45

A high yielding and highly diastereoselective synthesis of 2-aminomethylene indolines was reported **(Scheme 46)**. This was achieved by utilizing a reductive nitro-Mannich reaction of nitroalkenes bearing a pendant *o*-bromo-substituted aromatic ring. Reduction of β-nitroamine products to 1,2-diamines provided the substrates for selective intramolecular *N*-arylations to yield both five- and six-membered ring heterocycles. This synthesis was used to produce an array of 1,2-diamine containing fused heterocycles [151].

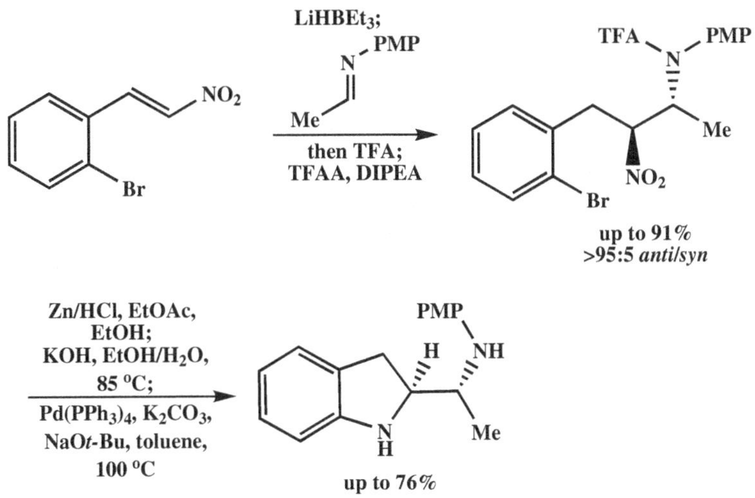

Scheme-46

Seomoon and co-workers [152] reported the allyl cross-coupling reactions using allylindium species for the synthesis of 3-vinyl indoline in the presence of palladium catalyst **(Scheme 47)**. Allylindium species were produced *in situ* by the treatment of allyl acetates with indium chloride and indium in the presence of palladium(0) catalyst [102].

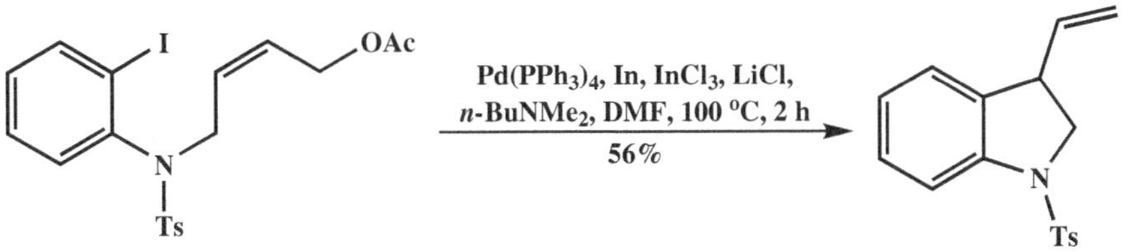

Scheme-47

Fuwa and Sasaki [153] used allenamide for the synthesis of indole-2,3-quinodimethanes *via* formation of cationic Pd π-allyl complex **(Scheme 48)**. Excellent yields of tetrahydrocarbazoles were obtained when the indole-2,3-quinodimethanes were trapped *in situ* via Diels-Alder cycloaddition with an external dienophile. Homodimers were observed through a regioselective Diels-Alder cycloaddition without an external dienophile.

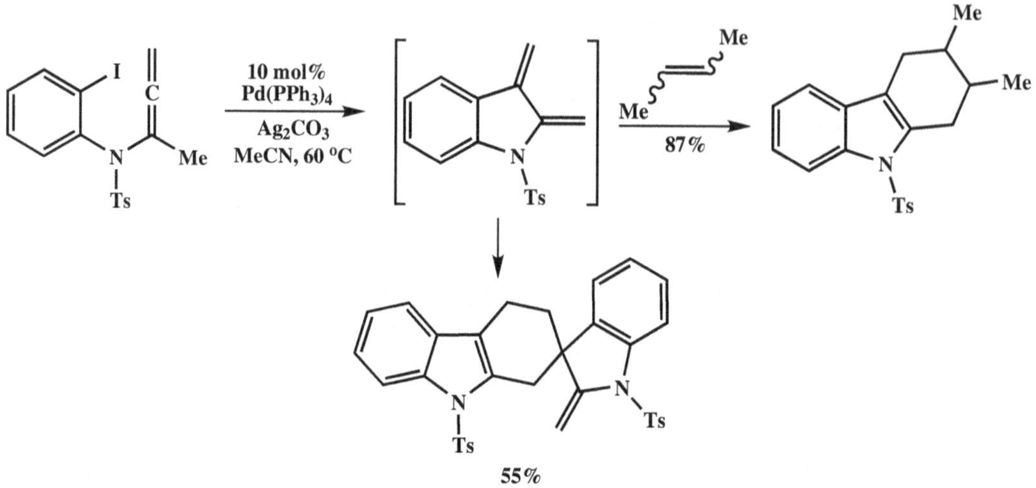

Scheme-48

A keto-carbonyl group (at the 2-position) possessing aryl halide was utilized for the preparation of lactam **(Scheme 49)**. Acylpalladium complex was produced through arylpalladium complex when the aryl halide was treated with palladium(0) under CO. The enol lactone was produced when enol part was reacted with acylpalladium complex, since the keto-carbonyl group was in equilibrium with an enol form. An isoindolinone was synthesized if the enol lactone can react with titanium-isocyanate complex [142, 154].

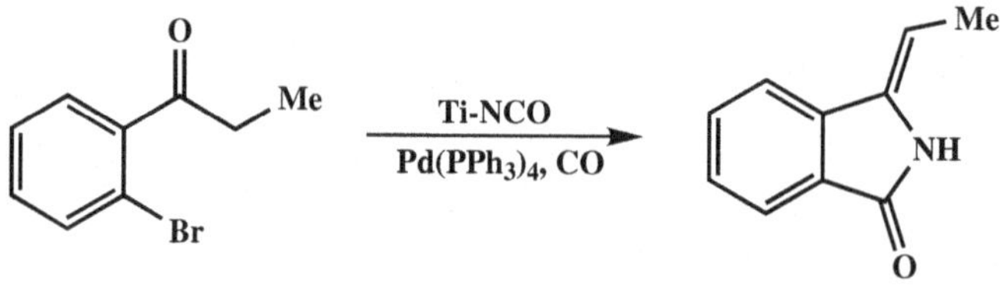

Scheme-49

The *o*-bromobutylophenone was reacted with titanium-isocyanate complex, Pd(PPh$_3$)$_4$, and potassium carbonate in the presence of *N*-methyl-2-pyrrolidone at 120 °C under CO for 24 h. The isoindolinone was formed in 70% yield. The reaction was performed in stepwise manner to understand the course of reaction. The 87% yield of enol lactone was reported when *o*-bromobutylophenone was reacted with Pd(PPh$_3$)$_4$ at 100 °C in *N*-methyl-2-pyrrolidone for 12 h under CO [155]. Then, the isoindolinone was obtained in 80% yield by reacting enol lactone with titanium-isocyanate complex at 120 °C in *N*-methyl-2-pyrrolidone for 24 h **(Scheme 50)** [142].

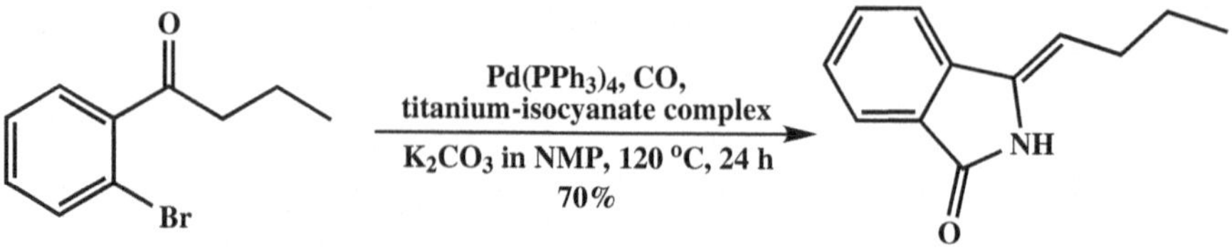

Scheme-50

The indole moiety was formed in a tandem one-pot protocol from nitriles *via* Pd-catalyzed intramolecular *N*-alkylative/*N*-arylative and *N*-arylative trappings of Blaise reaction intermediates **(Scheme 51)** [156].

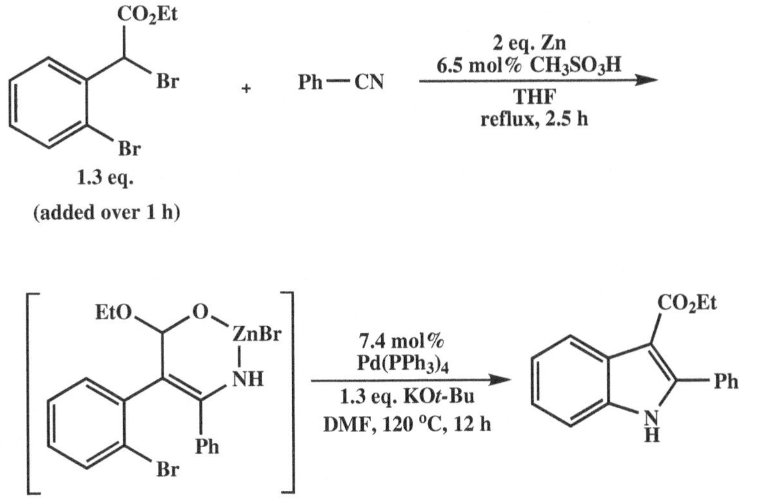

Scheme-51

The indole-thiazole moiety is possessed by many biologically significant compounds like naturally occurring BE 10988 or camalexins, an inhibitor of topoisomerase. Therefore, the synthesis of 3-thiazolyl indoles is particularly interesting. In addition, the thiazolyl group was easily transformed into a formyl group [157] for the synthesis of 2-substituted indole-3-carboxaldehydes **(Scheme 52)** [29a-b].

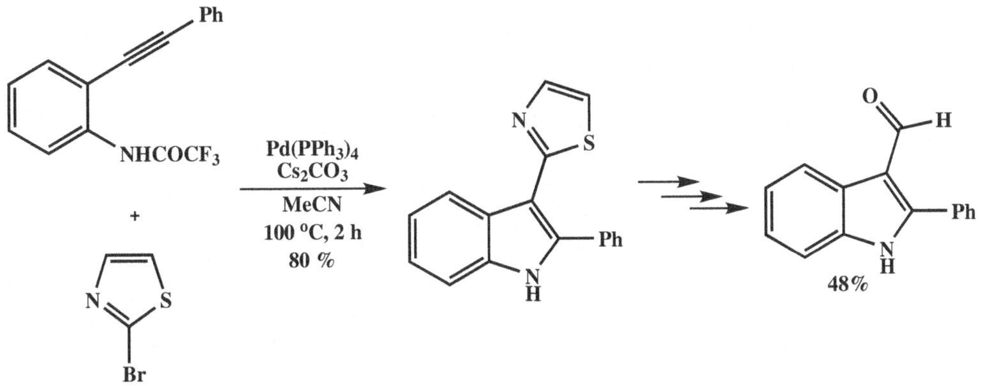

Scheme-52

Fukuyama and co-workers [158-159] synthesized 2-stannylindoles. This method provided 2-stannylindoles through cyclization of isonitriles in AIBN and TBTH and avoided the lithiation step to afford *N*-unprotected 3-substituted 2-stannylindoles. The Stille coupling with triflates and vinyl and aryl halides was best carried out *via* a one-pot method without the formation of stannyl intermediates, due to destannylation during work-up with 2-stannylindoles **(Scheme 53)** [29a-b, 160-161].

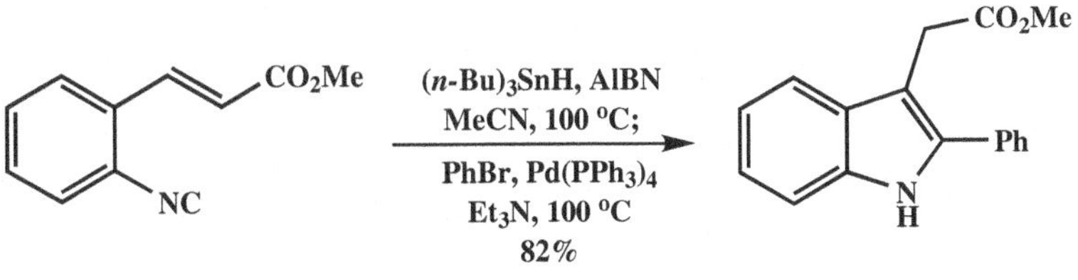

Scheme-53

The indole derivatives were produced by Larock annulation reaction. This reaction was utilized for the preparation of blue-light emitting materials [162-163] of 2,3-disubstituted pyrrolo[2,3-*b*]pyridines, 5-, 6-, and 7-azaindoles and 2,3-disubstituted indoles through an oxime-derived chloro-bridged palladacycle (not sensitive to moisture or air, thermally stable) catalyzed reaction [164], and in a traceless SPS of 2,3-disubstituted indoles and in a solid-phase preparation of trisubstituted indoles (using an amide group as a linker) (**Scheme 54**) [165-166]. Solution-phase conditions were not successful in the former case and large quantities of multiple acetylene insertion products and incomplete reactions were reported. The use of 1,1,3,3-tetramethylguanidine as base, PdCl$_2$(PPh$_3$)$_2$ as pre-catalyst, and double couplings afforded optimum yields. The reaction was also carried out using heterogeneous Pd catalysts under salt- and ligand-free conditions [29a-b, 167].

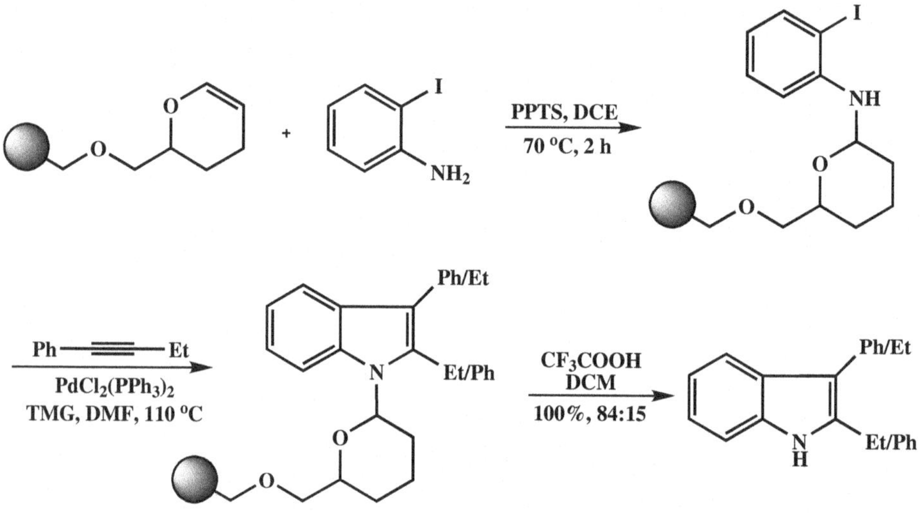

Scheme-54

The 2-carboxyindoles were synthesized through a domino carbon, nitrogen-coupling/carbonylation process (**Scheme 55**) [168]. Subsequently, 2-heteroaroyl-/aroylindoles containing a number of functional groups were afforded *via* a domino carbon, nitrogen-coupling/carbonylation/carbon, carbon-coupling process [169]. This reaction involved CO, *gem*-dibromovinylanilines, and boronic acids (**Scheme 56**). Moderate to good yields of desired indoles were obtained in dioxane. The domino reactions were carried out under carbon monoxide (12 bar) to promote the carbonylation step. Low yields of 2-aroylindoles were afforded in PhMe (solvent) at 90 °C under 1 atm of carbon monoxide along with 2-arylindoles, arising from a carbon, nitrogen-coupling/Suzuki reaction [29a-b].

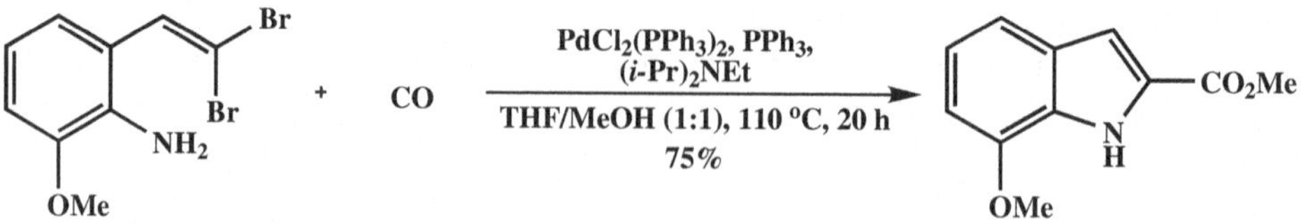

Scheme-55

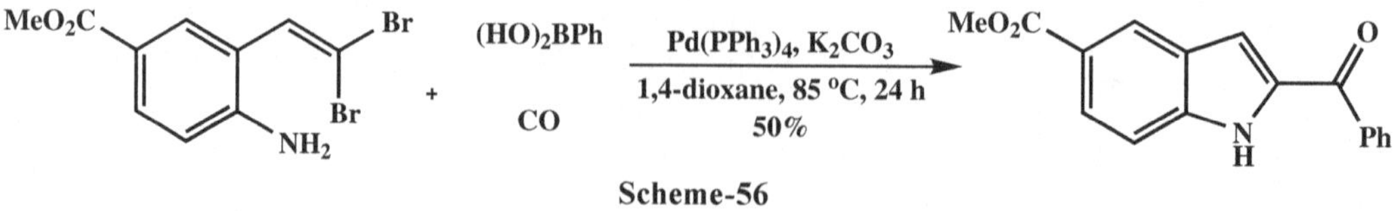

Scheme-56

Many tandem/cascade reactions which provide five-membered *N*-heterocycles involved the insertion of carbon monoxide into palladium-carbon bonds [170]. This method was applied for the synthesis of heterocyclic compounds *i.e.* preparation of isoindolinones (64% yield) through coupling of 2-bromobenzaldehyde with two eq. of a primary amine in the presence of palladium catalyst under an atmosphere of carbon monoxide [171]. Initially, an aminal was formed through reversible condensation of 2-bromobenzaldehyde with 2 eq. of amine. The acylpalladium species was produced by oxidative addition of aryl bromide to palladium(0) followed by carbon monoxide insertion, the formed acylpalladium species was captured by pendant aminal to provide the observed product. An alternative mechanism was proposed which involved an intramolecular imine insertion into the palladium-carbon bond of acylpalladium species, followed by synthesis of a palladium amido complex and carbon-nitrogen bond-forming reductive elimination **(Scheme 57)** [76, 172].

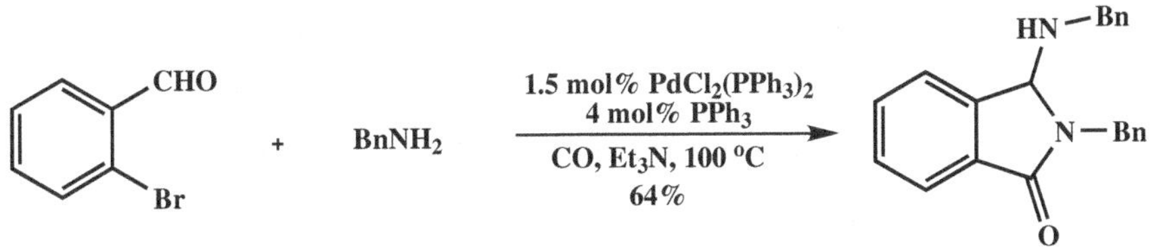

Scheme-57

The double carbonylative coupling of *o*-diiodo arenes with anilines produced the phthalimides [173]. Good yield was afforded in this transformation using a Pd/triphenylphosphine-based catalyst **(Scheme 58)** [76].

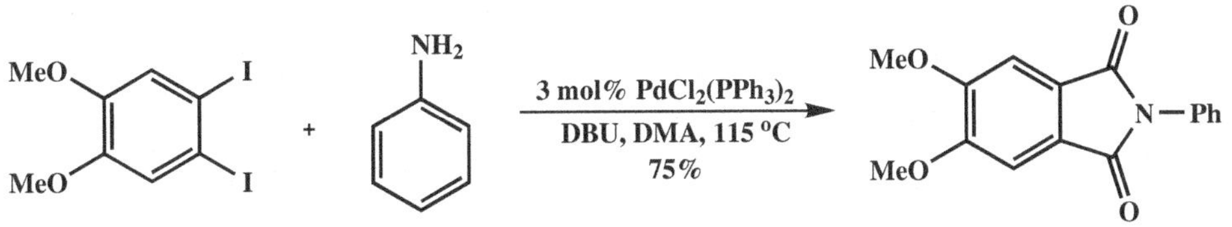

Scheme-58

Cenini's original preparation of indoles required very harsh conditions with 80 atm of carbon monoxide and reaction temperatures in excess of 200 °C. Also, this method suffered from considerable aniline by-product formation, up to 42% **(Scheme 59)**. Six yrs later, milder conditions were reported with palladium(II) catalysis. Groups of Watanabe [174-175] and Cenini [176] independently reported less harsh conditions for the cyclization of *o*-nitrostyrene substrates. With PdCl$_2$(PPh$_3$)$_2$ and a Sn(II) additive, Watanabe showed indole formation with 20 atm carbon monoxide at 100 °C. Both SnCl$_2$ and triphenylphosphine were essential to reaction as without them, little to no indole product was detected. Rather than phosphine ligands, Cenini demonstrated cyclization with a diamine ligand, TMphen, along with Pd(TMB)$_2$ at 40 atm carbon monoxide and 140 °C. The nitroarene precursors were utilized in the synthesis of aniline derivatives for indole synthesis, which was easily derivatized with alkene moiety. It was found that these nitroarenes were directly transformed into indole derivatives by this cyclization pathway. It was suggested that CO was used for the reduction of NO$_2$ group either to a nitroso or nitrene unit, which underwent cyclization with pendant unsaturated group. With the correct catalyst SnCl$_2$ was not needed, and under 1 atm of carbon monoxide atmosphere indoles were provided with good product diversity [177]. An important characteristics of this method was that halo substituted nitroarenes can be easily functionalized through Pd-catalyzed carbon-heteroatom or C-C bond forming reactions. Efficient pathways were developed by Sodenberg [178-179] for the preparation of a variety of heterocyclic compounds on the basis of this approach [180].

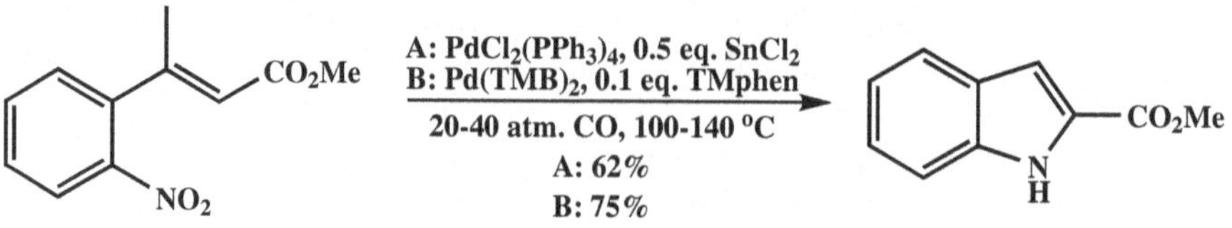

Scheme-59

Domino Heck-Michael methodology for the formation of heterocycles has not been widely reported [181-182]. Early examples of this methodology included the synthesis of pthalimidines [183] and tetrahydronapthalenes. Unfortunately these methods suffered from low yields, long reaction times and limited substrate scope. In 2005, the synthesis of isoindolinones using a domino Heck-aza-Michael reaction was reported by Khan et al. [184] **(Scheme 60)**. Although this reaction sequence allowed the synthesis of a series of isoindolinones where the amide substituent could be readily varied, attempts to use electron deficient alkenes other than acrylates (for example acrylonitrile and acrolein) failed.

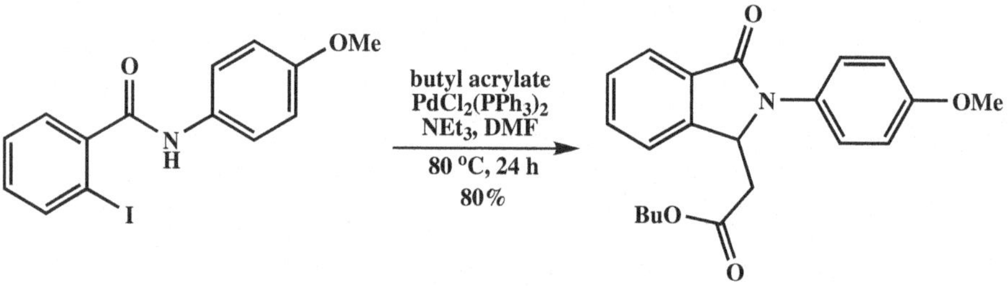

Scheme-60

Witulsky et al. [185] used *o*-halo-*N*-alkynylanilides for the synthesis of indoles. The reaction of *o*-halo-*N*-alkynylanilides with primary or secondary amines in the presence of Pd catalyst afforded 2-aminoindoles **(Scheme 61)**. For the optimization of optimal conditions, many additional bases like potassium hydroxide, 1,4-diazabicyclo[2.2.2]octane, potassium carbonate, potassium *tert*-butoxide, and cesium carbonate were tested. The most efficient bases were cesium carbonate and potassium carbonate. Tetrahydrofuran was found to be more suitable than PhMe or DMF. Higher yields were observed with PdCl$_2$(PPh$_3$)$_2$ pre-catalyst in comparison to Pd(PPh$_3$)$_4$, due to its lower phosphine content [for the success of Pd-catalyzed reactions the Pd/phosphine ratio was crucial, and the activity of actual palladium(0) catalyst was reduced at relatively high phosphine content] [29a-b].

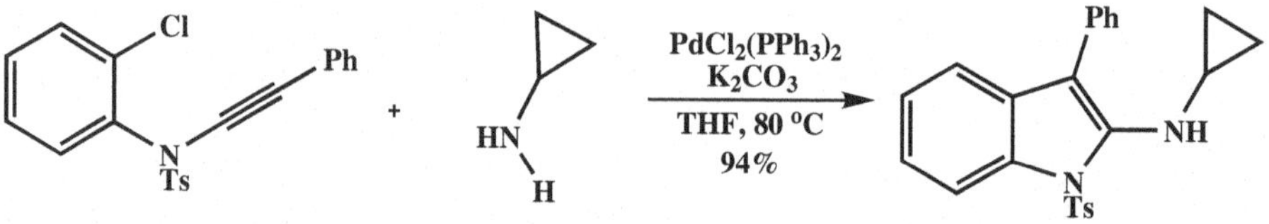

Scheme-61

In this study, several compounds were identified that combined Plm I and II inhibition in the low nanomolar range with a decent selectivity versus Cat D. Four new series with 35 novel compounds comprising different combinations of P3 and P1-side chains were produced using a sequential high-throughput protocol. The 25 compounds among 35, were formed under MW-promoted Suzuki couplings in the final step (MW increased Negishi coupling was also performed). Using sodium carbonate as a base in a DME/ethanol, cock-tail the best Suzuki couplings were obtained, yielding up to 77% of products **(Scheme 62)** [186a-b].

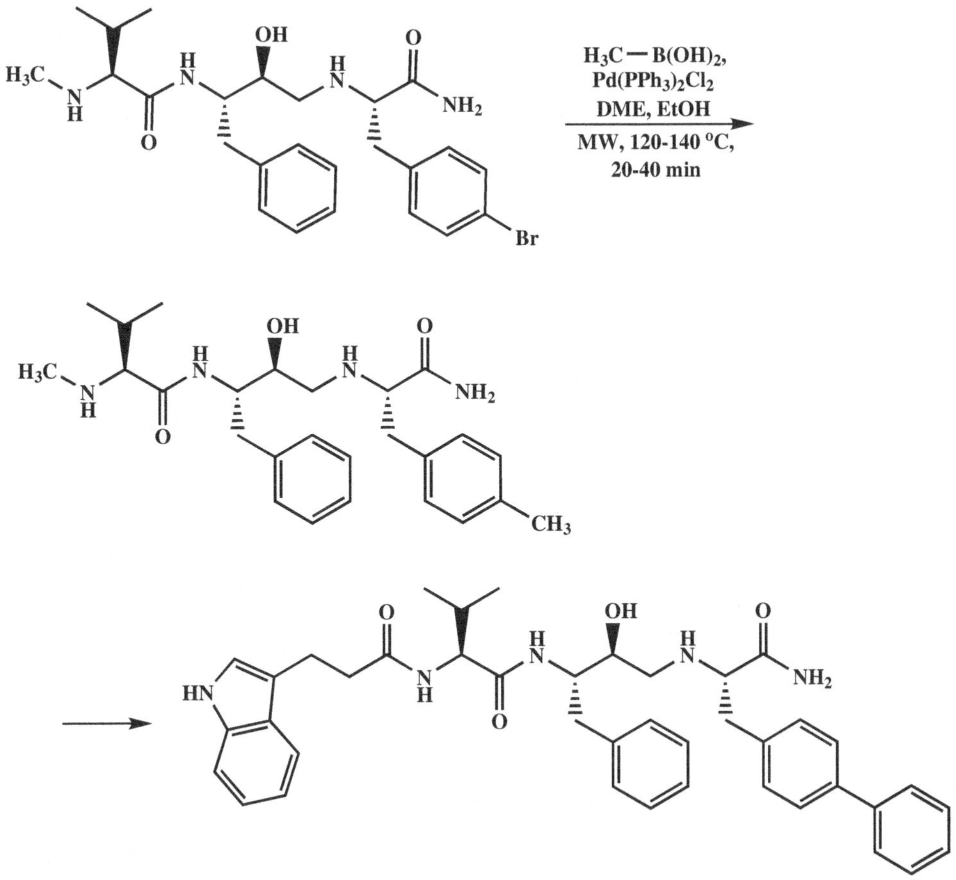

Scheme-62

In case of 3-iodo 2-amino pyridines the substituent of nitrogen atom has influenced the outcome of reaction [187]. The open coupled alkyne or indoles were provided on the basis of substituent. A mixture of compounds was obtained in the absence of substituent. With electron-donating groups only indole was formed. The open alkyne form was obtained with an electron-withdrawing group. Yum and co-workers [188] reported that internal alkynes of 3-iodo 4-amino quinolines formed substituted pyrrolo[3,2-*c*]quinolines through heteroannulation. In some cases Pd-catalyzed annulation of ketones and 2-haloanilines has been observed **(Scheme 63)** [39, 189].

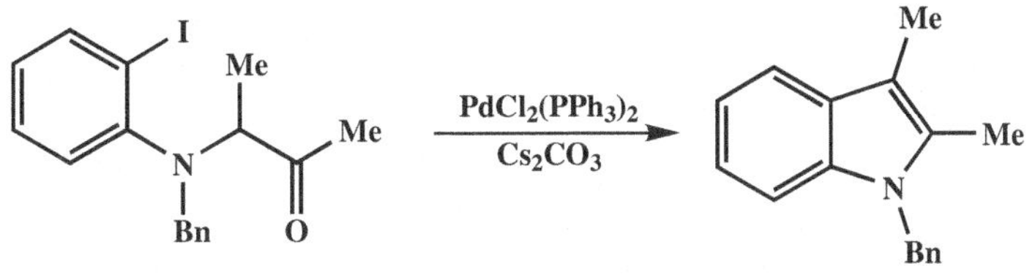

Scheme-63

Kasahara and co-workers [190] first reported the direct synthesis of indoles from *o*-nitrostyrenes substrates in the presence of Pd catalyst. The *o*-nitrostyrenes and in some cases significant amounts of indole products were isolated upon Heck reactions of *o*-bromonitrobenzenes with ethylene in the presence of Pd(OAc)$_2$. For instance, a mixture of indole (22% yield) and *o*-nitrostyrene (43% yield) was obtained from *o*-bromonitrobenzene. In this reaction *o*-nitrostyrenes (produced through Heck reaction) were reduced to o-vinylanilines by hydridopalladium species (formed in Heck reaction), followed by a palladium(II)-catalyzed cyclization. Subsequently, Watanabe and co-workers [174-175] reported the synthesis of indoles in moderate to good yields through reductive N-heteroannulation with CO, $PdCl_2(PPh_3)_2$, and $SnCl_2$ (Sn/Pd = 10:1). Other additives like cupric chloride, $SnCl_4$, $BF_3.3Et_2O$, and ferric chloride were ineffective (Scheme 64) [29a-b].

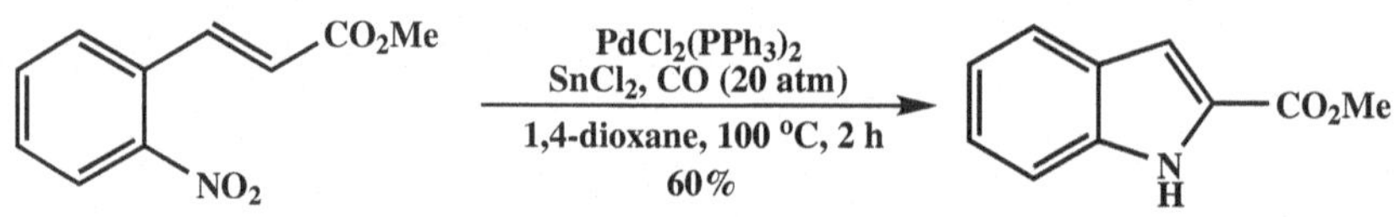

Scheme-64

This reaction was explored for the synthesis of indoles [191]. For instance, in 1985 Taylor and McKillop [37] described the synthesis of indoles when o-alkynyl substituted anilines underwent cyclization in palladium chloride catalysts (Scheme 65). This reaction occurred through initial coordination of palladium chloride to alkyne for cyclization, followed by subsequent protonation of Pd-C bond to reform the active Pd(II) catalyst and to produce the product.

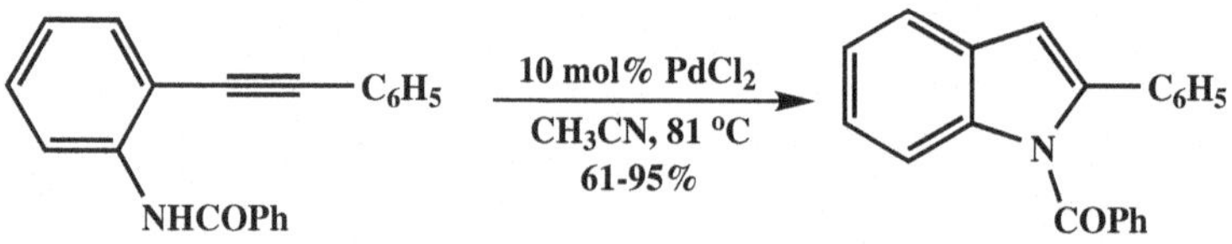

Scheme-65

The (Z)-didehydrophenylalanine derivatives via an intramolecular Pd-catalyzed cyclization provided N-aryl indole-2-carboxylates (Scheme 66) [192]. The process was expanded to the formation of N-acylindoles starting from (Z)-N-acyldidehydroamino acid derivatives [29a-b].

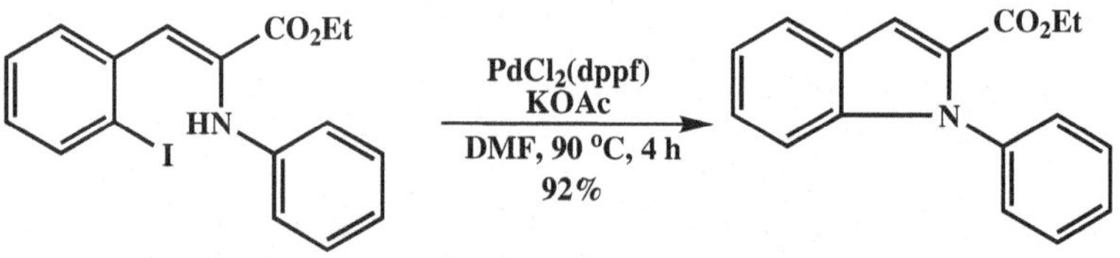

Scheme-66

An allylative cyclization of o-alkynyl-N-methoxycarbonylanilides was described by Utimoto and co-workers [38] (Scheme 67). The nitrogen nucleophile played an important role in the cyclization reaction. Unsatisfactory results were observed with acetamido group and unprotected amino group. The reaction occurred under mild conditions with N-methoxycarbonylanilides and proceeded via regioselective attack of σ-indolylpalladium intermediate on γ-position of

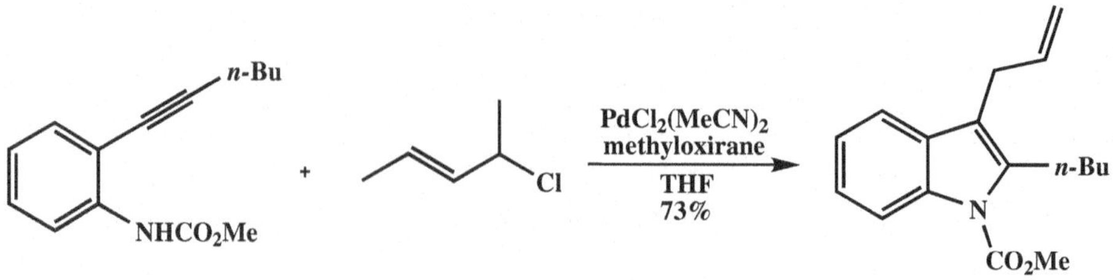

Scheme-67

allyl chorides. In some cases lack of olefin geometry was reported. To obtain the best results excess amounts of allyl chloride (10:1 allyl chloride: alkyne) were required. The competitive protonation, which led to 3-unsubstituted 2-substituted indoles, was prevented with the use of an oxirane (typically methyl oxirane) as proton scavenger. For instance, 20-35% of protonated product and about 30% of allylated product were obtained when allylative cyclization of *o*-(hexyn-1-yl)-acetanilide was carried out omitting methyl oxirane. Even under best conditions different amounts of 3-unsubstituted 2-substituted indoles were reported. The starting material was recovered upon using proton sponge and AcOK instead of methyl oxirane [29a-b].

Dai and co-workers [193] reported a transition metal, SPOS and MW mediated cyclization of 2-alkynylanilides to indoles in the presence of either palladium(II) or copper(II) catalyst **(Scheme 68)**. Following standard solid-phase organic synthesis procedures the required alkynylanilide precursor was produced on Rink resin. Under conventional thermal conditions the desired cyclization step was extremely sluggish and only partial ring closure was reported (4-5 h, 80 °C). In contrast, indole was provided in 94% purity and 75% yield after cleavage upon dielectric heating with microwaves at 160 °C for 10 min in the presence of 20 mol% of [PdCl$_2$(MeCN)$_2$] in tetrahydrofuran. Alternatively, the desired indoles were also afforded in similar purities and yields with cuprous iodide mediated reaction. No decomposition of resin occurred even at 200 °C. For all three steps of synthesis (<140 °C, <15 min) and final cleavage reaction, open-vessel MW technology was used at rt. Under MW conditions (as compared to conventional heating) higher yields of final products were reported in much shorter times [29a-b].

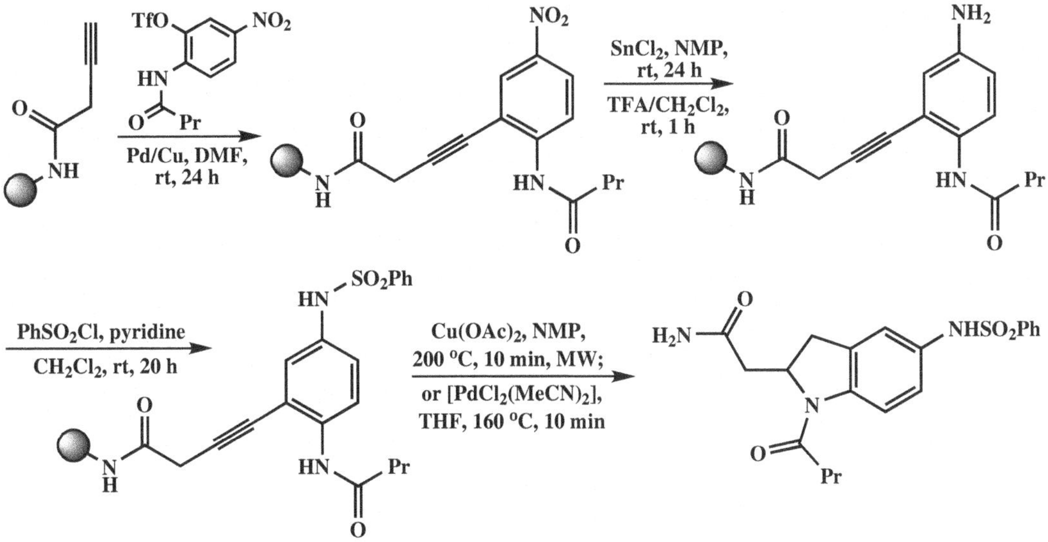

Scheme-68

Since aromatic amines were much less basic than aliphatic ones, these substances were readily cyclized to indole derivatives without *N*-functionalization **(Scheme 69)** [194].

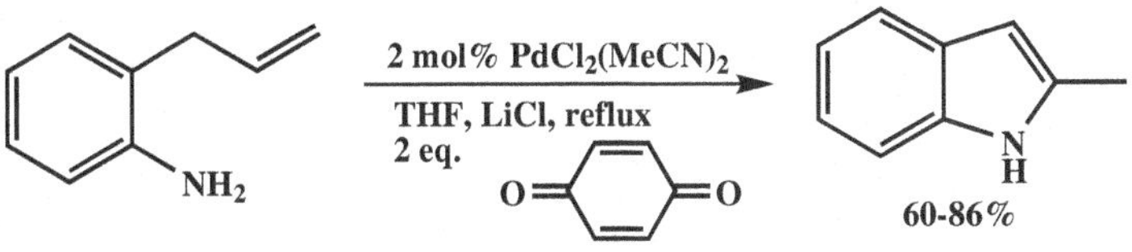

Scheme-69

A variety of aromatic heterocyclic compounds were synthesized by oxidative cyclization of alkenes. Hegedus et al. [195] used *o*-vinylaniline for the synthesis of indole in the presence of Pd catalyst **(Scheme 70)**. Stille coupling of 2-haloaniline derivatives with vinylstannanes produced 2-vinyl-*N*-tosyl-aniline substrates through Pd catalysis, followed by oxidative cyclization for the transformation of 2-vinyl-*N*-tosyl-aniline into indole [196]. Remarkably, under stoichiometric conditions no cyclization of same substrate was reported. Subsequently, the method was employed for the cyclization of *o*-vinyl-*N*-tosylanilines [197-199], *o*-vinylacetanilides [200-204], *o*-vinylanilines, and *o*-vinyl-*N*-alkylanilines [205]. Indoles were generated from 2-allylaniline derivatives in the presence of PdCl$_2$(MeCN)$_2$ or palladium chloride and stoichiometric amount of BQ (benzoquinone) as re-oxidant [206-207]. The degree of substitution determined several changes in cyclization reaction. The 2-methylquinoline was formed exclusively by cyclization of 2-crotylaniline under standard conditions, whereas in the presence of excess amounts of lithium chloride the sole product was 2-ethylindole. Harrington and Hegedus [208] reported better results in coupling reactions with electron-poor nitrogen of sulfonamides or amides [29a-b, 100, 209].

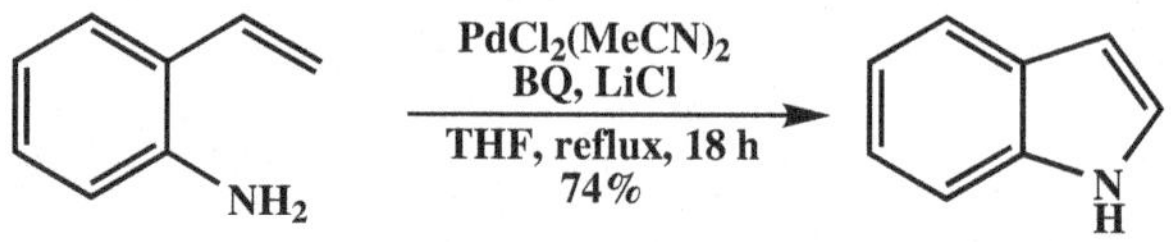

Scheme-70

3-Silyloxyindoles were formed upon intramolecular cyclization of 2-(1-silyloxyallyl)-anilines. 3-Alkoxyindoles were obtained by removal of protecting group and trapping of hydroxyl anion with alkyl halides [210]. This reaction was rarely used for the synthesis of indoles. The formation of 3-alkoxyindoles comprised one of the few examples **(Scheme 71)** [29a-b, 100].

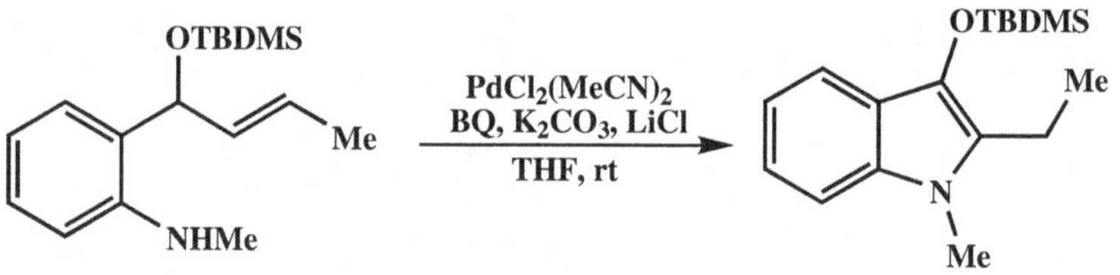

Scheme-71

The indoloquinone was generated by cyclization of allyl-substituted aminobenzoquinone **(Scheme 72)** [100, 211].

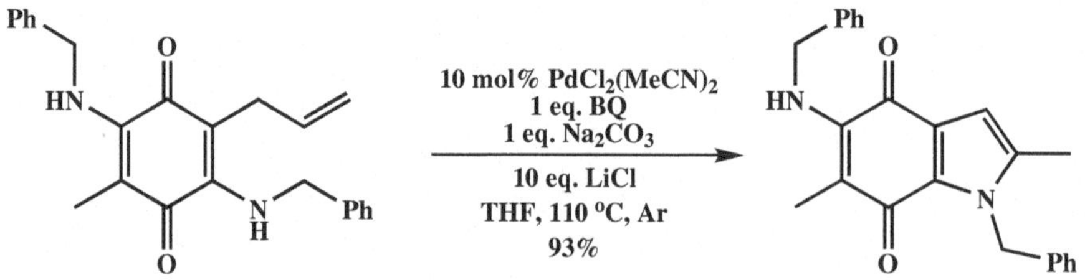

Scheme-72

The isocyanides can also be used in this transannulation reaction [212]. The isocyanide incorporated products were afforded in excellent yields when 1,2,3-benzotriazinone underwent smooth transannulation with isocyanides in the presence of a phosphine ligand and a Pd catalyst **(Scheme 73)**. All substrates exhibited excellent reactivity, with the exception of *N*-alkyl-substituted triazinones, to afford products in almost quantitative yields. The reaction was also quite general with respect to isocyanides, as benzyl, aryl, cyclohexyl, and even aliphatic isocyanides were competent in this reaction for giving high yields of transannulation products [23].

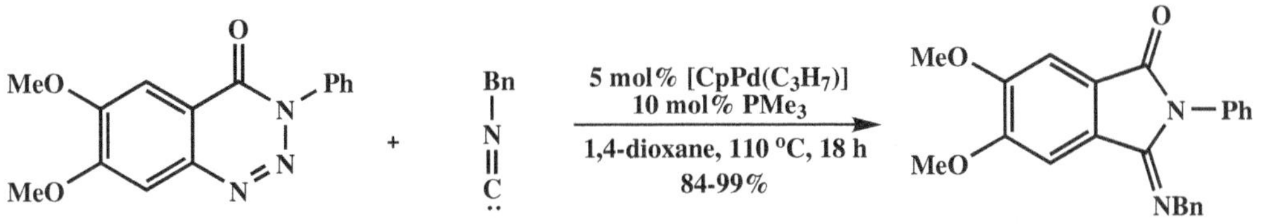

Scheme-73

Lin and Kazmaier [213] performed intramolecular Stille couplings for the transformation of substituted vinylstannanes into indoles derivatives **(Scheme 74)** [102].

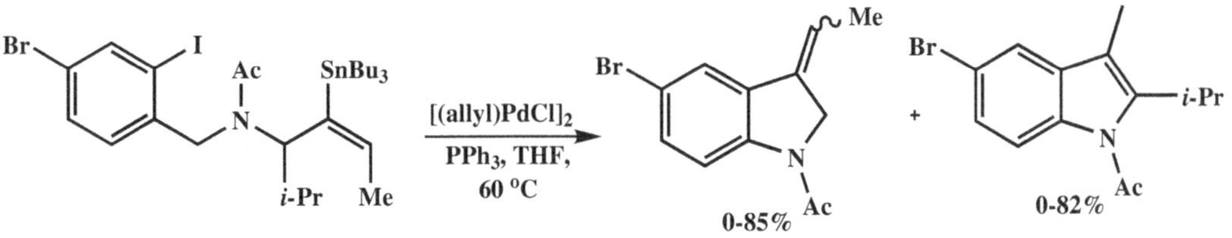

Scheme-74

The *N*-aminoindole and indazole product were produced in 56% and 31% yields after 1 h under standard conditions employing 5 mol% of palladium. Attempts to bias the product ratio by altering the solvent, base, or additives (cupric chloride or silver carbonate) were not successful. With additional substrates other *N*-aminoindoles were produced in moderate yields. In cross-coupling reactions the use of hydrazine as a nitrogen-source was associated with difficulties and this conversion represented a significant contribution towards the establishment of direct routes to hydrazine-possessing heterocyclic compounds **(Scheme 75)** [214-218].

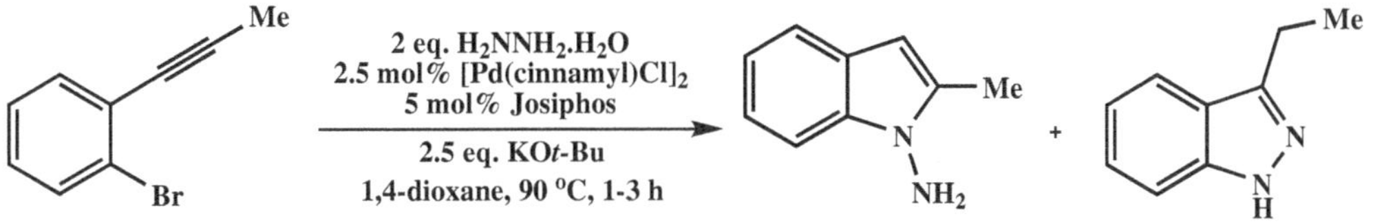

Scheme-75

Active ligands were investigated for palladium-catalyzed amination reactions in order to develop a more effective catalytic protocol. The indole product was obtained in 89% GC yield with Josiphos (CyPFtBu) ligand, whereas ligands [219-225] like *S*-Phos (2-dicyclohexylphosphino-2′,6′-dimethoxybiphenyl), *t*-Bu-DavePhos, P*t*-Bu$_3$, X-Phos, Q-Phos, DiPPF, IPr, TrippyPhos, and CataCXium ligands afforded poor results. For amine cross-coupling, including NH$_3$, Josiphos was found to be a highly effective ligand as discovered by Hartwig et al. [24-28]. In the presence of Josiphos ligand standard reaction conditions were varied to demonstrate the significance of potassium *tert*-butoxide [226-229]. The desired product was formed in lower yield using a lower catalyst loading (0.5 mol% of [Pd(cinnamyl)Cl]$_2$). Aryl tosylates or chlorides were not suitable substrates. The highest yield of indoles was reported with [Pd(cinnamyl)Cl]$_2$, other palladium catalysts such as Pd[P(*o*-tolyl)$_3$]$_2$ or Pd(dba)$_2$ were also used. Initially the reaction of 1-bromo-2-(phenylethynyl)-benzene with primary amines was reported in the presence of Pd/L1 (2.5 mol% each) catalyst mixtures to afford indoles through carbon-nitrogen cross-coupling/cyclization processes [230-233]. The Pd precursor based on [Pd(cinnamyl)Cl]$_2$/Mor-DalPhos catalyst system [9] was utilized, and for comparative studies parallel reactions were performed with *p*-isomer of OTips-DalPhos, as well as IPr, DavePhos, and Mor-DalPhos **(Scheme 76)** [217, 234].

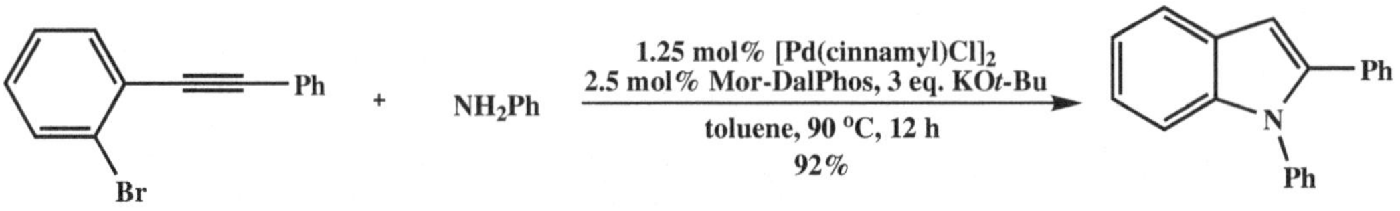

Scheme-76

The development of a Pd-catalyzed route to 2*H*-isoindoles was initiated by reacting activated oxime with a base in the presence of Pd. The cyclization of oxime was investigated because the activated oxime was a mixture of oxime isomers, which have been reported to be active in Pd-catalyzed aza-Heck reactions [235-236], and the pentafluorobenzoyl activated oxime was previously proposed to undergo oxidative addition to Pd [237-238]. The potassium hexamethyldisilazide (KHMDS) was selected as a base because its use has been reported in Pd-catalyzed enolate cross-coupling reactions [239]. The mechanism for this transformation included initial oxidative addition of Pd into N-O bond of protected oxime, followed by enolate attack on Pd center **(Scheme 77)**. Reductive elimination and then tautomerization would provide desired isoindole derivative.

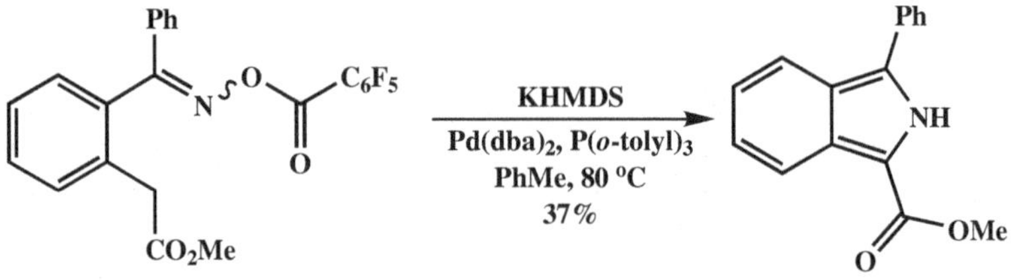

Scheme-77

Larock and others generated indole derivatives *via* intramolecular carbon-heteroatom bond formation [240-242]. The coupling of *o*-halo substituted anilines with internal alkynes was involved in this reaction. While the reaction was similar to Pd-catalyzed preparation of indoles through the formation of *o*-alkynylanilines, this conversion utilized internal alkynes, which cannot synthesize these intermediates. This reaction occurred similar to C-N bond forming reactions **(Scheme 78)**. Initially, the intermediate was produced by oxidative addition of aryl halide. While this intermediate cannot undergo cyclization with pendant *o*-amino group, alkyne insertion can occur to form Pd intermediate, which can now undergo C-N bond formation through palladation of NH bond, followed by reductive elimination [39].

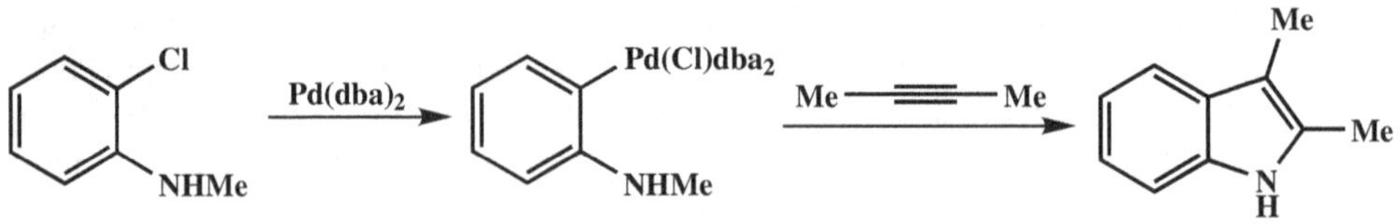

Scheme-78

New reaction conditions were developed which do not require dimethylsulphoxide solvent and only molecular O_2 was used as a co-oxidant [243]. The Pd catalysts supported by NHC or pyridine as ligands were utilized. Under similar reaction conditions, Stoltz [244-245] transformed the amide into lactam. The stereochemistry of aminopalladation step depends on reaction conditions, and both *syn-* and *anti*-aminopalladation pathways were possible in oxidative amination reactions **(Scheme 79)** [76, 99, 246-247].

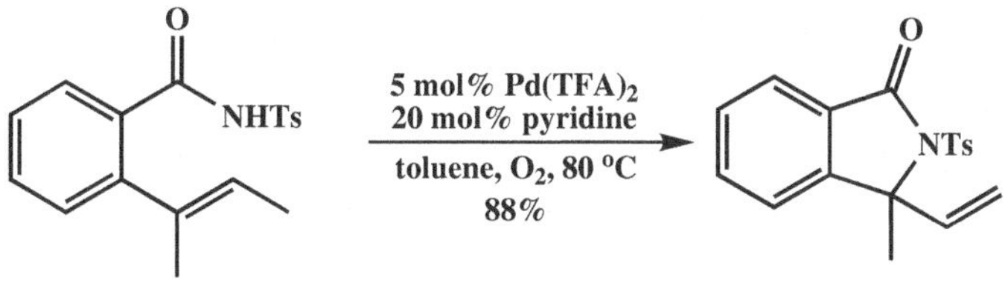

Scheme-79

Akermark, Backvall, Zetterberg, and Hegedus [248-255] reported that aminopalladation reactions occurred by the reaction of palladium-alkene complexes with amine nucleophiles to form carbon-nitrogen bonds. Molecular O_2 was used as a sole oxidant in palladium-catalyzed intermolecular oxidative amination of alkenes. With the initial applications of vinyl arenes the reaction was extended to unactivated alkyl olefins. Stahl et al. [99] reported that for the intramolecular oxidative amination of alkenes with molecular O_2 (as oxidant) the *N*-heterocyclic carbene-coordinated palladium complexes were effective catalysts **(Scheme 80)**. For the related intramolecular oxidative amination of alkenes, IMes was also ligand of choice. The reaction was not limited to aromatic-tethered substrates. The reaction outcome was improved with the use of carboxylic acids as co-catalysts. The acid was reacted with Pd(0) species to produce Pd(II)-hydride derivatives, less prone to aggregation into inactive palladium black. This conversion occurred *via* a *cis*-aminopalladation. However, *trans*-aminopalladation was also possible and depending on the reaction conditions, catalyst and substrate, this strategy become major protocol. The *trans*-aminopalladation was promoted in the presence of NHC [256-257].

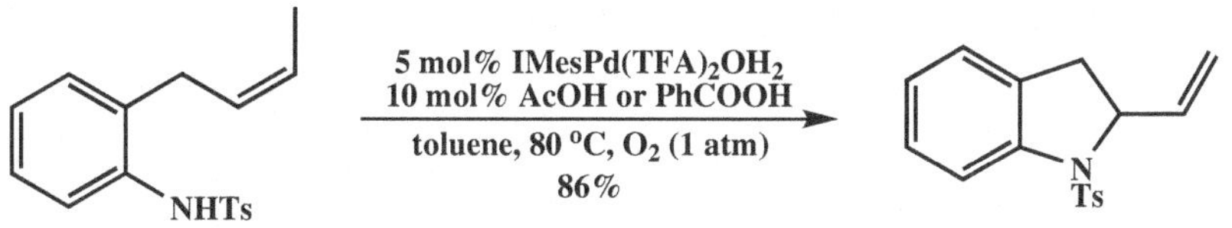

Scheme-80

Niwa and co-workers [258] explained the synthesis of pyridylethyl-substituted dihydroindole with the transfer of 2-pyridylmethyl from 2-(2-pyridyl)ethanol derivative to *N*-allyl-2-chloroaniline in the presence of palladium catalyst by chelation-assisted cleavage of unstrained sp^3-sp^3 bonds **(Scheme 81)** [102].

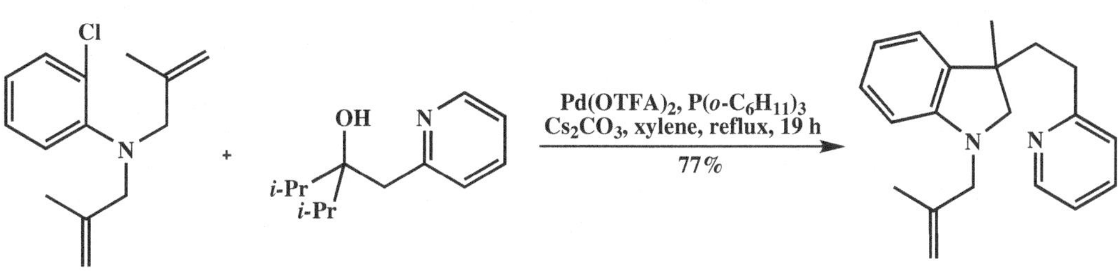

Scheme-81

Yum et al. [259] described the preparation of 2-substituted indoles in the presence of palladium using [palladium(II)]/NaY (formed by calcination of [Pd(NH$_3$)$_4$]/NaY). While efficient, as shown by moderate to high isolated yields (*i.e.*, 40%-80%), this protocol needed *N*-acetyl *o*-iodoanilide and Cs$_2$CO$_3$ (base) in lithium chloride to achieve competitive transformations **(Scheme 82)** [52].

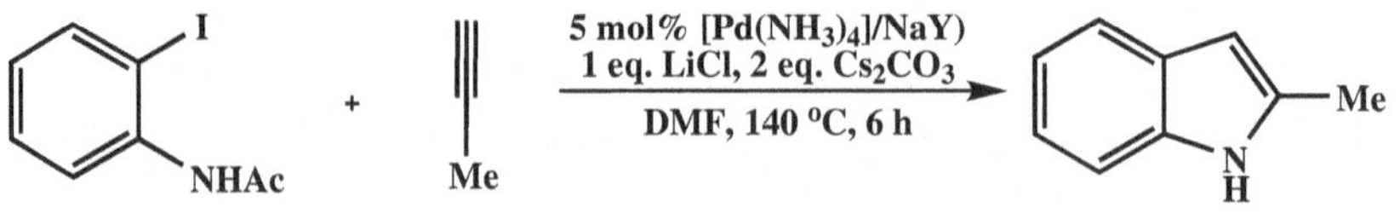

Scheme-82

Kamijo and Yamamoto [260-261] utilized *o*-(alkynyl)phenylisocyanates for the synthesis of 2-substituted indoles **(Scheme 83)**. Reactions were performed with Na_2PdCl_4, but other palladium(II) catalysts, like $PdCl_2(MeCN)_2$ and palladium chloride also exhibited similar catalytic activities. Among other transition metals, platinum(II) and gold(III) showed catalytic activity to synthesize the indole products. Interestingly, an argon atmosphere was not necessary. Even in the presence of O_2, the catalytic activity was found to be high for a few hr. The catalyst activated the alkynes for subsequent cyclization and accelerated the addition of alcohols to isocyanate group. For the synthesis of 2-phenyl indole (72% yield) from phenylacetylene *via* a domino Sonogashira coupling-intramolecular heteroannulation, the Pd on activated carbon was an selective and active single catalyst [262]. No coupling intermediate was formed which indicated that heteroannulation was rapid under reaction conditions (1 mol% of cuprous iodide, 1 mol% of palladium/carbon, 6 h, 120 °C). The catalyst was deactivated strongly during the first run and a palladium/carbon catalyst with an average activity of ca. 20% was observed. The terminal alkynes and *o*-iodoanilides were reacted in a one-pot domino sequence for the preparation of 2-aryl- and 2-alkyl-substituted indoles in the presence of 10% palladium/carbon in H_2O [263]. The reaction was conducted in 2-aminoethanol, triphenylphosphine and cuprous iodide as the co-catalyst system at 80 °C. With *N*-mesylanilides (producing *N*-mesylindoles) the highest yields were observed, whereas good yields were not reported when *o*-iodotrifluoroacetanilides were used. A variety of 2,5-disubstituted indoles were obtained under almost identical conditions in H_2O [29a-b].

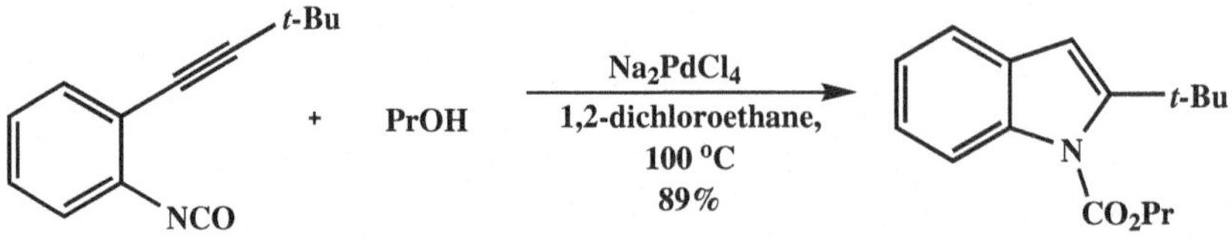

Scheme-83

The substituted 2-chloroanilines were reacted directly with acyclic or cyclic ketones by this mild, broadly applicable, simple, and efficient protocol for the preparation of polyfunctionalized indoles. In addition to these protocols, carbon-heteroatom bond formation was also coupled with these Heck cyclizations. Other straightforward protocol to couple carbon-heteroatom bond formation with Heck cyclization was through enamine production. For instance, enamines for subsequent Heck cyclization were produced by the reaction of enolizable ketones or aldehydes with 2-haloanilines. Nazare [264] reacted *o*-chloroanilines with enolizable ketones to form indoles **(Scheme 84)**. The reaction occurred in good yields with a number of unsymmetrical and symmetrical ketones and afforded only one enamine isomer, and was applied to many substituted indoles. Zhu [265] has shown that enolizable aldehydes were also utilized in this cyclization. This method was applied for the introduction of a range of aryl, alkyl, or functionalized units into 3-indole position, many of which were not easily available through other routes. A range of electron-poor and electron-rich cyclic and acyclic ketones and *o*-chloroanilines possessing functional moieties such as free acids and amides as well as *N*-alkylated anilines were transformed into indoles [29a-b].

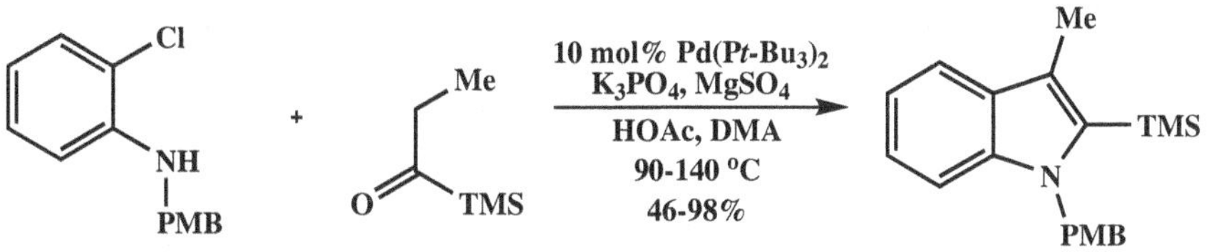

Scheme-84

A bromovinylic fragment possessing (at nitrogen atom) phenolic carbamates were utilized for the synthesis of indole carbamates [266]. Optimum yields were observed with Herrmann's catalyst. Mixtures of indole derivatives were obtained by cyclization both at the *para* and at the *ortho* position. One of the cyclizable positions was blocked with a substituent or using a symmetrical phenol to avoid the issue of *ortho* versus *para* selectivity **Scheme 85** [29a-b].

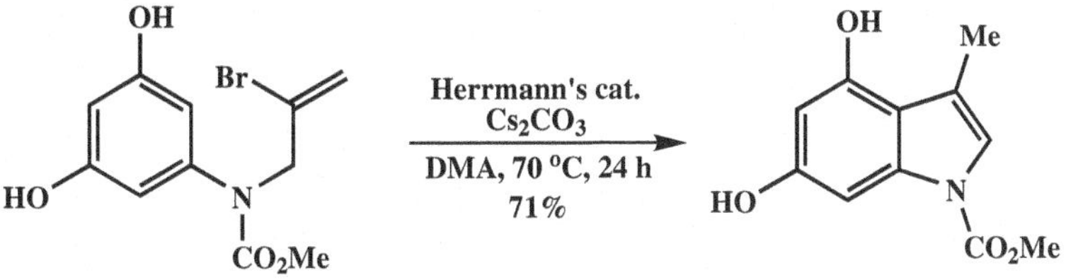

Scheme-85

Efforts were attempted to use lower amounts of Pd because lower catalyst loading increased the uptake of this methodology [267]. Good results were reported using 2 mol% of 1,10-phenanthroline (phen) and 1 mol% of palladium acetate at 80 °C under a 15 psi carbon monoxide atmosphere in dimethylformamide for 16 h. Under same conditions 2.0 mol% of TMP (3,4,7,8-tetramethyl-1,10-phenanthroline) and 1.0 mol% of $Pd(O_2CCF_3)_2$ or 0.7 mol% of TMP and 0.1 mol% of $Pd(O_2CCF_3)_2$ were also effective. A novel class of KDR kinase inhibitors was generated under former conditions **(Scheme 86)** [29a-b, 268].

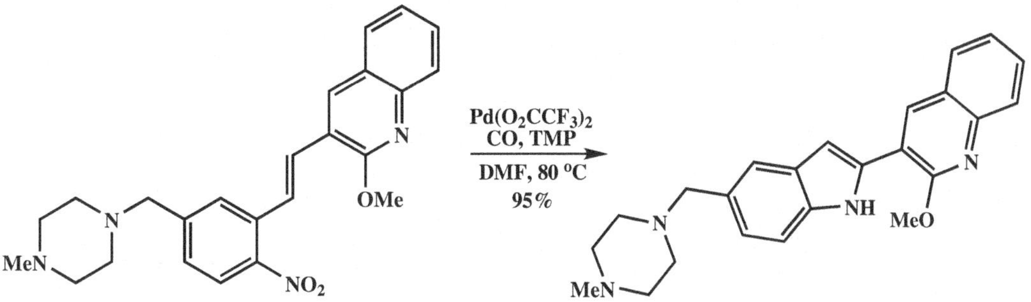

Scheme-86

REFERENCES

[1]   (a) N. Kaur. 2015. Role of microwaves in the synthesis of fused five-membered heterocycles with three *N*-heteroatoms. Synth. Commun. 45: 403-431.
      (b) N. Kaur. 2015. Recent impact of microwave-assisted synthesis on benzo derivatives of five-membered *N*-heterocycles. Synth. Commun. 45: 539-568.
      (c) N. Kaur and D. Kishore. 2014. Microwave-assisted synthesis of seven- and higher-membered *N*-heterocycles. Synth. Commun. 44: 2577-2614.
      (d) N. Kaur and D. Kishore. 2014. Microwave-assisted synthesis of six-membered *S*-heterocycles. Synth. Commun. 44: 2615-2644.

(e) N. Kaur and D. Kishore. 2014. Microwave-assisted synthesis of seven- and higher-membered *O*-heterocycles. Synth. Commun. 44: 2739-2755.

[2]   K. Kubo, Y. Kohara, E. Imamiya, Y. Sugiura, Y. Inada, Y. Furukawa, K. Nishikawa and T. Naka. 1993. Nonpeptide angiotensin II receptor antagonists. Synthesis and biological activity of benzimidazolecarboxylic acids. J. Med. Chem. 36: 2182-2195.

[3]   A. Chimirri, S. Grasso, A.M. Monforte, P. Monforte and M. Zappala. 1991. Anti-HIV agents II. Synthesis and *in vitro* anti-HIV activity of novel 1*H*,3*H*-thiazolo[3,4-*a*]benzimidazoles. Farmaco 46: 925-933.

[4]   J. Benavidesm, H. Schoemaker, C. Dana, Y. Claustre, M. Delahaye, M. Prouteau, P. Manoury, J. Allen, B. Scatton, S.Z. Langer and S. Arbilla. 1995. *In vivo* and *in vitro* interaction of the novel selective histamine H1 receptor antagonist mizolastine with H1 receptors in the rodent. F Arzneim. 45: 551-558.

[5]   K. Ishihara, T. Ichikawa, Y. Komuro, S. Ohara and K. Hotta. 1994. Effect on gastric mucus of the proton pump inhibitor leminoprazole and its cytoprotective action against ethanol-induced gastric injury in rats. F Arzneim. Drug Res. 44: 827-830.

[6]   V. Sharma, P. Kumar and D. Pathak. 2010. Biological importance of the indole nucleus in recent years: a comprehensive review. J. Heterocycl. Chem. 47: 491-502.

[7]   W. Gul and M.T. Hamann. 2005. Indole alkaloid marine natural products: an established source of cancer drug leads with considerable promise for the control of parasitic, neurological and other diseases. Life Sci. 78: 442-453.

[8]   M. Somei, F. Yamada, T. Kurauchi, Y. Nagahama, M. Hasegawa, K. Yamada, S. Teranishi, H. Sato and C. Kaneko. 2001. The chemistry of indoles. CIII. Simple syntheses of serotonin, *N*-methylserotonin, bufotenine, 5-methoxy-*N*-methyltryptamine, bufobutanoic acid, *N*-(indol-3-yl) methyl-5-methoxy-*N*-methyltryptamine, and lespedamine based on 1-hydroxyindole chemistry. Chem. Pharm. Bull. 49: 87-96.

[9]   F.E. Chen and J. Huang. 2005. Reserpine: a challenge for total synthesis of natural products. Chem. Rev. 105: 4671-4706.

[10]   M. Kale and K. Patwardhan. 2013. Synthesis of heterocyclic scaffolds with anti-hyperlipidemic potential: a review. Der Pharma Chemica 5: 213-222.

[11]   S. Antoniotti, E. Genin, V. Michelet and J.-P. Genet. 2005. Highly efficient access to strained bicyclic ketals *via* gold-catalyzed cycloisomerization of bis-homopropargylic diols. J. Am. Chem. Soc. 127: 9976-9977.

[12]   L.-P. Liu and G.B. Hammond. 2009. Highly efficient and tunable synthesis of dioxabicyclo[4.2.1] ketals and tetrahydropyrans *via* gold-catalyzed cycloisomerization of 2-alkynyl-1,5-diols. Org. Lett. 11: 5090-5092.

[13]   B. Liu and J.K. De Brabander. 2006. Metal-catalyzed regioselective oxy-functionalization of internal alkynes: an entry into ketones, acetals, and spiroketals. Org. Lett. 8: 4907-4910.

[14]   B. Alcaide, P. Almendros and J.M. Alonso. 2011. Gold-catalyzed cyclizations of alkynol-based compounds: synthesis of natural products and derivatives. Molecules 16: 7815-7843.

[15]   L.-Z. Dai and M. Shi. 2009. Gold(I) catalysis: selective synthesis of six- or seven-membered heterocycles from epoxy alkynes. Eur. J. Org. Chem. 19: 3129-3133.

[16]   Z. Shi and C. He. 2004. An Au-catalyzed cyclialkylation of electron-rich arenes with epoxides to prepare 3-chromanols. J. Am. Chem. Soc. 126: 5965-5964.

[17]   R. Grigg and V. Sridharan. 1994. Spirocycles *via* palladium-catalyzed cascade cyclization-carbonylation-anion capture processes. Tetrahedron Lett. 34: 7471-7474.

[18]   Akanksha and D. Maiti. 2012. Microwave-assisted palladium mediated decarbonylation reaction: synthesis of eulatachromene. Green Chem. 14: 2314-2320.

[19]   R. Grigg, B. Putnikovic and C. Urch. 1996. Palladium catalyzed ter- and tetra-molecular queuing processes. One-pot routes to 3-spiro-2-oxindoles and 3-spiro-2(3*H*)-benzofuranones. Tetrahedron Lett. 37: 695-698.

[20]   R. Grigg and V. Sridharan. 1998. Heterocycles *via* Pd catalyzed molecular queuing processes. Relay switches and the maximization of molecular complexity. Pure Appl. Chem. 70: 1047-1057.

[21]   I. Nakamura, T. Nemoto, N. Shiraiwa and M. Terada. 2009. Palladium-catalyzed indolization of *N*-aroylbenzotriazoles with disubstituted alkynes. Org. Lett. 11: 1055-1058.

[22] S. Mehta and R.C. Larock. 2010. Iodine/palladium approaches to the synthesis of polyheterocyclic compounds. J. Org. Chem. 75: 1652-1658.

[23] B. Chattopadhyay and V. Gevorgyan. 2012. Transition-metal-catalyzed denitrogenative transannulation: converting triazoles into other heterocyclic systems. Angew. Chem. Int. Ed. 51: 862-872.

[24] J.F. Hartwig. 1997. Palladium-catalyzed amination of aryl halides: mechanism and rational catalyst design. Synlett 4: 329-340.

[25] D. Baranano, G. Mann and J.F. Hartwig. 1997. Nickel and palladium-catalyzed cross-couplings that form carbon-heteroatom and carbon-element bonds. Curr. Org. Chem. 1: 287-305.

[26] J.F. Hartwig. 1998. Carbon-heteroatom bond-forming reductive eliminations of amines, ethers, and sulfides. Acc. Chem. Res. 31: 852-860.

[27] J.F. Hartwig. 1998. Filtering algorithm for noise reduction in phase-map images with 2π phase jumps. Angew. Chem. Int. Ed. 37: 2046-2050.

[28] J.F. Hartwig. 1999. Approaches to catalyst discovery. New carbon-heteroatom and carbon-carbon bond formation. Pure Appl. Chem. 71: 1417-1423.

[29] (a) S. Cacchi and G. Fabrizi. 2011. Palladium-catalyzed reactions. Chem. Rev. 111: 215-283.
(b) S. Cacchi and G. Fabrizi. 2005. Synthesis and functionalization of indoles through palladium-catalyzed reactions. Chem. Rev. 105: 2873-2920.

[30] R.C. Larock, E.K. Yum, M.J. Doty and K.K.C. Sham. 1996. Synthesis of aromatic heterocycles *via* palladium-catalyzed annulation of internal alkynes. J. Org. Chem. 60: 3270-3271.

[31] E.J. Latham and S.P. Stanfoth. 1996. Synthesis of indoles and quinolones by sequential Wittig and Heck reactions. Chem. Commun. 19: 2253-2254.

[32] E.J. Latham and S.P. Stanfoth. 1997. Synthesis of indoles and quinolones by sequential Wittig and Heck reactions. J. Chem. Soc. Perkin Trans. 1 14: 2059-2064.

[33] H. Alper and N. Hamel. 1987. Regiospecific synthesis of α-methylene-β-lactams by a homogeneous palladium catalyzed ring expansion-carbonylation reaction. Tetrahedron Lett. 28: 3237-3240.

[34] T. Sakamoto, T. Nagano, Y. Kondo and H. Yamanaka. 1990. Palladium-catalyzed cyclization of β-(2-halophenyl)amino substituted α,β-unsaturated ketones and esters to 2,3-disubstituted indoles. Synthesis 3: 215-218.

[35] J. Barluenga and C. Valdes. 2005. Palladium catalyzed alkenyl amination: from enamines to heterocyclic synthesis. Chem. Commun. 39: 4891-4901.

[36] Y. Tan and J.F. Hartwig. 2010. Palladium-catalyzed amination of aromatic C-H bonds with oxime esters. J. Am. Chem. Soc. 132: 3676-3677.

[37] E.C. Taylor, A.H. Katz, H. Salgado-Zamora and A. McKillop. 1985. Thallium in organic synthesis. A convenient synthesis of 2-phenylindoles from anilides. Tetrahedron Lett. 26: 5963-5966.

[38] K. Iritani, S. Matsubara and K. Utimoto. 1988. Palladium catalyzed reaction of 2-alkynylanilines with allyl chlorides. Formation of 3-allylindoles. Tetrahedron Lett. 29: 1799-1802.

[39] G. Kirsch, S. Hesse and A. Comel. 2004. Synthesis of five- and six-membered heterocycles through palladium-catalyzed reactions. Curr. Org. Synth. 1: 47-63.

[40] A. Fayol, Y.-Q. Fang and M. Lautens. 2006. Synthesis of 2-vinylic indoles and derivatives *via* a Pd-catalyzed tandem coupling reaction. Org. Lett. 8: 4203-4206.

[41] Y.-Q. Fang and M. Lautens. 2008. A highly selective tandem cross-coupling of *gem*-dihaloolefins for a modular, efficient synthesis of highly functionalized indoles. J. Org. Chem. 73: 538-549.

[42] S.C. Bryan and M. Lautens. 2008. Silver-promoted domino Pd-catalyzed amination/direct arylation: access to polycyclic heteroaromatics. Org. Lett. 10: 4633-4636.

[43] L.T. Kaspar and L. Ackermann. 2005. Three-component indole synthesis using *o*-dihaloarenes. Tetrahedron 61: 11311-11316.

[44] X.-H. Duan, X.-Y. Li, L.-N. Guo, M.-C. Liao, W.-M. Liu and Y.-M. Liang. 2005. Palladium-catalyzed one-pot synthesis of highly substituted furans by a three-component annulation reaction. J. Org. Chem. 70: 6980-6983.

[45] M. Syamala. 2009. Recent progress in three-component reactions: an update. Org. Prep. Proced. Int. 41: 1-68.

[46]   R.S. Colemen and W. Chen. 2001. A convergent approach to the mitomycin ring system. Org. Lett. 3: 1141-1144.

[47]   S. Cenini, E. Bettettini, M. Fedele and S. Tollari. 1996. Intramolecular amination catalyzed by ruthenium and palladium. Synthesis of 2-acyl indoles and 2-aryl quinolines by carbonylation of 2-nitrochalcones. J. Mol. Catal. A: Chem. 111: 37-41.

[48]   S. Tollari, S. Cenini, A. Rossi and G. Palmisano. 1998. Synthesis of 2-hetaryl substituted indoles *via* palladium-catalyzed reductive *N*-heterocyclization. J. Mol. Catal. A: Chem. 135: 241-248.

[49]   S. Tollari, A. Penoni and S. Cenini. 2000. The unprecedented detection of the intermediate formation of *N*-hydroxy derivatives during the carbonylation of 2'-nitrochalcones and 2-nitrostyrenes catalyzed by palladium. J. Mol. Catal. A: Chem. 152: 47-54.

[50]   F. Ragaini, P. Sportiello and S. Cenini. 1999. Investigation of the possible role of arylamine formation in the *o*-substituted nitroarenes reductive cyclization reactions to afford heterocycles. J. Organomet. Chem. 577: 283-291.

[51]   (a) L. Djakovitch, V. Dufaud and R. Zaidi. 2006. Heterogeneous palladium catalysts applied to the synthesis of 2- and 2,3-functionalized indoles. Adv. Synth. Catal. 348: 715-724.
        (b) N. Batail, M. Genelot, V. Dufaud, L. Joucla and L. Djakovitch. 2011. Palladium based innovative catalytic procedures: designing new homogeneous and heterogeneous catalysts for the synthesis and functionalization of *N*-containing heteroaromatic compounds. Catal. Today 173: 2-14.

[52]   L. Djakovitch, N. Batail and M. Genelot. 2011. Recent advances in the synthesis of *N*-containing heteroaromatics *via* heterogeneously transition metal catalyzed cross-coupling reactions. Molecules 16: 5241-5267.

[53]   D. Enders and H. Gielen. 2001. Synthesis of chiral triazolinylidene and imidazolinylidene transition metal complexes and first application in asymmetric catalysis. J. Organomet. Chem. 617: 70-80.

[54]   W.A. Herrmann, L.J. Goossen, C. Kocher and G.R.J. Artus. 1996. Chiral heterocylic carbenes in asymmetric homogeneous catalysis. Angew. Chem. Int. Ed. Engl. 35: 2805-2807.

[55]   K.C. Nicolaou, J.L. Hao, M.V. Reddy, P.B. Rao, G. Rassias, S.A. Snyder, X.H. Huang, D.Y.K. Chen, W.E. Brenzovich, N. Giuseppone, P. Giannakakou and A. O'Brate. 2004. Chemistry and biology of diazonamide A: second total synthesis and biological investigations. J. Am. Chem. Soc. 126: 12897-12906.

[56]   C. Marti and E.M. Carreira. 2003. Construction of spiro[pyrrolidine-3,3'-oxindoles] - recent applications to the synthesis of oxindole alkaloids. Eur. J. Org. Chem. 12: 2209-2219.

[57]   F. Glorius, G. Altenhoff, R. Goddard and C. Lehmann. 2002. Oxazolines as chiral building blocks for imidazolium salts and *N*-heterocyclic carbene ligands. Chem. Commun. 22: 2704-2705.

[58]   T. Arao, K. Kondo and T. Aoyama. 2006. Asymmetric construction of quaternary carbon stereocenter by Pd-catalyzed intramolecular α-arylation. Chem. Pharm. Bull. 54: 1743-1744.

[59]   (a) T. Arao, K. Sato, K. Kondo and T. Aoyama. 2006. Function of an *N*-heterocyclic carbene ligand based on concept of chiral mimetic. Chem. Pharm. Bull. 54: 1576-1581.
        (b) J.A. Mata and M. Poyatos. 2011. Recent developments in the applications of palladium complexes bearing *N*-heterocyclic carbene ligands. Curr. Org. Chem. 15: 3309-3324.

[60]   W.A. Herrmann. 2002. *N*-Heterocyclic carbenes: a new concept in organometallic catalysis. Angew. Chem. Int. Ed. 41: 1290-1309.

[61]   S. Lee and J.F. Hartwig. 2001. Improved catalysts for the palladium-catalyzed synthesis of oxindoles by amide α-arylation. Rate acceleration, use of aryl chloride substrates, and a new carbene ligand for asymmetric transformations. J. Org. Chem. 66: 3402-3415.

[62]   S.R. Stauffer, S. Lee, J.P. Stambuli, S.I. Hauck and J.F. Hartwig. 2000. High turnover number and rapid, room-temperature amination of chloroarenes using saturated carbene ligands. Org. Lett. 2: 1423-1426.

[63]   M. Jørgensen, S. Lee, X. Liu, J.P. Wolkowski and J.F. Hartwig. 2002. Efficient synthesis of α-aryl esters by room-temperature palladium-catalyzed coupling of aryl halides with ester enolates. J. Am. Chem. Soc. 124: 12557-12565.

[64]   M. Eckhardt and G.C. Fu. 2003. The first applications of carbene ligands in cross-couplings of alkyl electrophiles: Sonogashira reactions of unactivated alkyl bromides and iodides. J. Am. Chem. Soc. 125: 13642-13643.

[65] A. Fürstner, O.R. Thiel, L. Ackermann, H.-J. Schanz and S.P. Nolan. 2000. Ruthenium carbene complexes with *N,N'*-bis(mesityl)imidazol-2-ylidene ligands: RCM catalysts of extended scope. J. Org. Chem. 65: 2204-2207.

[66] R.R. Schrock, J.S. Murdzek, G.C. Bazan, J. Robbins, M. DiMare and M. O'Regan. 1990. Synthesis of molybdenum imido alkylidene complexes and some reactions involving acyclic olefins. J. Am. Chem. Soc. 112: 3875-3886.

[67] B.M. Trost and G. Dong. 2010 Total synthesis of bryostatin 16 using a Pd-catalyzed diyne coupling as macrocyclization method and synthesis of C20-*epi*-bryostatin 7 as a potent anti-cancer agent. J. Am. Chem. Soc. 132: 16403-16416.

[68] Q. Ding, B. Wanga and J. Wu. 2007. Synthesis of isoindol-1-ylphosphonate derivatives *via* Pd(0)-catalyzed reaction of α-amino (2-alkynylphenyl) methylphosphonate with aryl iodide. Tetrahedron Lett. 48: 8599-8602.

[69] B. Baghernejad. 2010. 1,4-Diazabicyclo[2.2.2]octane (DABCO) as a useful catalyst in organic synthesis. Eur. J. Chem. 1: 54-60.

[70] L.F. Tietze, H. Ila and H.P. Bell. 2004. Enantioselective palladium-catalyzed transformations. Chem. Rev. 104: 3453-3516.

[71] A.B. Dounay and L.E. Overman. 2003. The asymmetric intramolecular Heck reaction in natural product total synthesis. Chem. Rev. 103: 2945-2964.

[72] C. Bolm, J.P. Hildebrand, K. Muniz and N. Hermanns. 2001. Catalyzed asymmetric arylation reactions. Angew. Chem. Int. Ed. 40: 3284-3308.

[73] S.F. Kirsch and L.E. Overman. 2005. Catalytic asymmetric intramolecular aminopalladation: improved palladium(II) catalysts. J. Org. Chem. 70: 2859-2861.

[74] N.-Y. Zhu and D. Yang. 2007. Catalytic asymmetric diamination of conjugated dienes and triene. J. Am. Chem. Soc. 129: 11688-11689.

[75] X. Gai, R. Grigg, T. Khamnaen, S. Rajviroongit, V. Sridharan, L. Zhang, S. Collard and A. Keep. 2003. Synthesis of 3-substituted isoindolin-1-ones *via* a palladium-catalyzed 3-component carbonylation/amination/Michael addition process. Tetrahedron Lett. 44: 7441-7443.

[76] D.M. D'Souza and T.J.J. Muller. 2007. Multi-component syntheses of heterocycles by transition-metal catalysis. Chem. Soc. Rev. 36: 1095-1108.

[77] Y. Monguchi, S. Mori, S. Aoyagi, A. Tsutsui, T. Maegawa and H. Sajiki. 2010. Palladium on carbon-catalyzed synthesis of 2- and 2,3-substituted indoles under heterogeneous conditions. Org. Biol. Chem. 8: 3338-3342.

[78] N. Batail, A. Bendjeriou, T. Lomberget, R. Barret, V. Dufaud and L. Djakovitch. 2009. First heterogeneous ligand- and salt-free Larock indole synthesis. Adv. Synth. Catal. 351: 2055-2062.

[79] N. Batail, V. Dufaud and L. Djakovitch. 2011. Larock heteroannulation of 2-bromoanilines with internal alkynes *via* ligand and salt free Pd/C catalyzed reaction. Tetrahedron Lett. 52: 1916-1918.

[80] M. Shen, G. Li, B.Z. Lu, A. Hossain, F. Roschangar, V. Farina and C.H. Senanayake. 2004. The first regioselective palladium-catalyzed indolization of 2-bromo- or 2-chloroanilines with internal alkynes: a new approach to 2,3-disubstituted indoles. Org. Lett. 6: 4129-4132.

[81] X. Cui, J. Li, Y. Fu, L. Liu and Q.-X. Guo. 2008. Regioselective Pd-catalyzed indolization of 2-bromoanilines with internal alkynes using phosphine-free ligands. Tetrahedron Lett. 49: 3458-3462.

[82] L. Djakovitch and K. Koehler. 1999. Heterogeneously catalyzed Heck reaction using palladium modified zeolites. J. Mol. Catal. A: Chem. 142: 275-284.

[83] L. Djakovitch and K. Koehler. 2001. Heck reaction catalyzed by Pd-modified zeolites. J. Am. Chem. Soc. 123: 5990-5999.

[84] F.-X. Felpin, O. Ibarguren, L. Nassar-Hardy and E. Fouquet. 2009. Synthesis of oxindoles by tandem Heck-reduction-cyclization (HRC) from a single bifunctional, *in situ* generated Pd/C catalyst. J. Org. Chem. 74: 1349-1352.

[85] F.-X. Felpin, K. Miqueu, J.-M. Sotiropoulos, E. Fouquet, O. Ibarguren and J. Laudien 2010. Room temperature, ligand- and base-free Heck reactions of aryl diazonium salts at low palladium loading: sustainable preparation of substituted stilbene derivatives. Chem. Eur. J. 16: 5191-5204.

[86] O. Ibarguren, C. Zakri, E. Fouquet and F.-X. Felpin. 2009. Heterogeneous palladium multi-task catalyst for sequential Heck-reduction-cyclization (HRC) reactions: influence of the support. Tetrahedron Lett. 50: 5071-5074.

[87] G.N. Walker. 1955. Synthesis of 5,6-dimethoxyindoles and 5,6-dimethoxyoxindoles. A new synthesis of indoles. J. Am. Chem. Soc. 77: 3844-3850.

[88] W. Leimgruber, A.D. Batcho and F. Schenker. 1965. The structure of anthramycin. J. Am. Chem. Soc. 87: 5793-5795.

[89] E. Srisook and D.Y. Chi. 2004. The syntheses of 3-substituted 4-(pyridin-2-ylthio)indoles *via* Leimgruber-Batcho indole synthesis. Bull. Korean Chem. Soc. 25: 895-899.

[90] K.R. Roesch and R.C. Larock. 1998. Synthesis of isoquinolines and pyridines *via* palladium-catalyzed iminoannulation of internal acetylenes. J. Org. Chem. 63: 5306-5307.

[91] A.M. Kearney and C.D. Vanderwal. 2006. Synthesis of nitrogen heterocycles by the ring opening of pyridinium salts. Angew. Chem. 118: 7967-7970; Angew. Chem. Int. Ed. 45: 7803-7806.

[92] I.V. Seregin, V. Ryabova and V. Gevorgyan. 2007. Direct palladium-catalyzed alkynylation of *N*-fused heterocycles. J. Am. Chem. Soc. 129: 7742-7743.

[93] S. Chuprakov and V. Gevogyan. 2007. Regiodivergent metal-catalyzed rearrangement of 3-iminocyclopropenes into *N*-fused heterocycles. Org. Lett. 9: 4463-4466.

[94] X.-Y. Liu, P. Ding, J.-S. Huang and C.-M. Che. 2007. Synthesis of substituted 1,2-dihydroquinolines and quinolines from aromatic amines and alkynes by gold(I)-catalyzed tandem hydroamination-hydroarylation under microwave-assisted conditions. Org. Lett. 9: 2645-2648.

[95] T. Pei, C.-Y. Chen, P.G. Dormer and I.W. Davies. 2008. Expanding the [1,2]-aryl migration to the synthesis of substituted indoles. Angew. Chem. Int. Ed. 120: 4299-4301; 47: 4231-4233.

[96] D.L. Boger and J.S. Panek. 1984. Palladium (O) mediated β-carboline synthesis: preparation of the CDE ring system of lavendamycin. Tetrahedron Lett. 25: 3175-3178.

[97] B. Yin, X. Zhang, X. Zhang, H. Peng, W. Zhou, B. Liu and H. Jiang. 2015. Access to polysubstituted indoles or benzothiophenes *via* palladium-catalyzed cross-coupling of furfural tosylhydrazones with 2-iodoanilines or 2-iodothiophenols. Chem. Commun. 51: 6126-6129.

[98] J.-J. Li, T.-S. Mei and J.-Q. Yu. 2008. Synthesis of indolines and tetrahydroisoquinolines from arylethylamines by PdII-catalyzed C-H activation reactions. Angew. Chem. 120: 6552-6555.

[99] M.M. Rogers, J.E. Wendlandt, I.A. Guzei and S.S. Stahl. 2006. Aerobic intramolecular oxidative amination of alkenes catalyzed by NHC-coordinated palladium complexes. Org. Lett. 8: 2257-2260.

[100] E.M. Beccalli, G. Broggini, M. Martinelli and S. Sottocornola. 2007. C-C, C-O, C-N Bond formation on sp^2 carbon by Pd(II)-catalyzed reactions involving oxidant agents. Chem. Rev. 107: 5318-5365.

[101] K.S. MacMillan, J.P. Lajiness, C.L. Cara, R. Romagnoli, W.M. Robertson, I. Hwang, P.G. Baraldi and D.L. Boger. 2009. Synthesis and evaluation of a thio analogue of duocarmycin SA. Bioorg. Med. Chem. Lett. 19: 6962-6965.

[102] S. Nag and S. Batra. 2011. Applications of allylamines for the syntheses of aza-heterocycles. Tetrahedron 67: 8959-9061.

[103] B. Gabriele, G. Salerno, L. Veltri, M. Costa and C. Massera. 2001. Stereoselective synthesis of (*E*)-3-(methoxycarbonyl)methylene-1,3-dihydroindol-2-ones by palladium-catalyzed oxidative carbonylation of 2-ethynylanilines. Eur. J. Org. Chem. 24: 4607-4613.

[104] B. Gabriele, G. Salerno, A. Fazio and F.B. Campana. 2002. Unprecedented carbon dioxide effect on a Pd-catalyzed oxidative carbonylation reaction: a new synthesis of pyrrole-2-acetic esters. Chem. Commun. 13: 1408-1409.

[105] T. Mizutani, Y. Ukaji and K. Inomata. 2003. Palladium-catalyzed carbonylation of homoallylic amine derivatives in the presence of a copper co-catalyst. Bull. Chem. Soc. Jpn. 76: 1251-1256.

[106] S. Anguille, J. Brunet, N.C. Chu, O. Diallo, C. Pages and S. Vincendeau. 2006. Platinum catalyzed formation of quinolines from anilines. Aliphatic α-C-H activation of alkylamines and aromatic *ortho*-C-H activation of anilines. Organometallics 25: 2943-2948.

[107] B. Gabriele, R. Mancuso, G. Salerno, G. Ruffolo and P. Plastina. 2007. Novel and convenient synthesis of substituted quinolines by copper- or palladium-catalyzed cyclodehydration of 1-(2-aminoaryl)-2-yn-1-ols. J. Org. Chem. 72: 6873-6877.

[108] B. Gabriele, R. Mancuso, G. Salerno, E. Elvira Lupinacci, G. Ruffolo and M. Costa. 2008. Versatile synthesis of quinoline-3-carboxylic esters and indol-2-acetic esters by palladium-catalyzed carbonylation of 1-(2-aminoaryl)-2-yn-1-ols. J. Org. Chem. 73: 4971-4977.

[109] I. Nakamura, Y. Mizushima, U. Yamagishi and Y. Yamamoto. 2007. Synthesis of 2,3-disubstituted benzofurans and indoles by π-Lewis acidic transition metal-catalyzed cyclization of *o*-alkynylphenyl *O,O*- and *N,O*-acetals. Tetrahedron 63: 8670-8676.

[110] T. Miura, M. Yamauchi and M. Murakami. 2008. Synthesis of 1(2*H*)-isoquinolones by the nickel-catalyzed denitrogenative alkyne insertion of 1,2,3-benzotriazin-4(3*H*)-ones. Org. Lett. 10: 3085-3088.

[111] M. Edin and S. Grivas. 2001. On the preparation of 1,2,5-selenadiazolo [3,4-*e*]indole and its [3,4-*f*] and [3,4-*g*] isomers through the Batcho-Leimgruber indole synthesis. ARKIVOC (i): 144-153.

[112] S. Cacchi, G. Fabrizi and A. Goggiamani. 2006. 2,3-Disubstituted indoles through the palladium-catalyzed reaction of aryl chlorides with *o*-alkynyltrifluoroacetanilides. Adv. Synth. Catal. 348: 1301-1305.

[113] S. Cacchi, G. Fabrizi, F. Marinelli, L. Moro and P. Pace. 1997. 2-Unsubstituted 3-arylindoles through the palladium-catalyzed reaction of 2-ethynyltrifluoroacetanilide with aryl iodides. Synlett 12: 1363-1366.

[114] P.S. Baran and E.J. Corey. 2002. A short synthetic route to (+)-austamide, (+)-deoxyisoaustamide, and (+)-hydratoaustamide from a common precursor by a novel palladium-mediated indole-dihydroindoloazocine cyclization. J. Am. Chem. Soc. 124: 7904-7905.

[115] A. Arcadi, S. Cacchi, A. Cassetta, G. Fabrizi and L.M. Parisi. 2001. Indole[1,2-*c*]quinazolines by palladium-catalyzed cyclization of bis(*o*-trifluoroacetamidophenyl) acetylene with aryl and vinyl halides or triflates. Synlett 10: 1605-1607.

[116] S. Cacchi, G. Fabrizi and L.M. Parisi. 2004. Preparation of indoles from *o*-alkynyltrifluoroacetanilides through the aminopalladation-reductive elimination process. Synthesis 11: 1889-1894.

[117] A. Arcadi, S. Cacchi, V. Carnicelli and F. Marinelli. 1994. 2-Substituted-3-acylindoles through the palladium-catalyzed carbonylative cyclization of 2-alkynyltrifluoroacetanilides with aryl halides and vinyl triflates. Tetrahedron 50: 437-452.

[118] S.V. Damle, D. Semoon and P.H. Lee. 2003. Palladium-catalyzed homocoupling reaction of 1-iodoalkynes: a simple and efficient synthesis of symmetrical 1,3-diynes. J. Org. Chem. 68: 7085-7087.

[119] B.L. Flynn, E. Hamel and M.K. Jung. 2002. One-pot synthesis of benzo[*b*]furan and indole inhibitors of tubulin polymerization. J. Med. Chem. 45: 2670-2673.

[120] S. Cacchi, G. Fabrizi, P. Pace and F. Marinelli. 1999. 6-Aryl-11*H*-indolo[3,2-*c*]quinolines through the palladium-catalyzed carbonylative cyclization of *o*-(*o*-aminophenyl)trifluoroacetanilide with aryl iodides. Synlett 5: 620-622.

[121] G. Battistuzzi, S. Cacchi, G. Fabrizi, F. Marinelli and L.M. Parisi. 2002. 12-Acylindolo[1,2-*c*] quinazolines by palladium-catalyzed cyclocarbonylation of *o*-alkynyltrifluoroacetanilides. Org. Lett. 4: 1355-1358.

[122] J.P. Wolfe, R.A. Rennels and S.L. Buchwald. 1996. Intramolecular palladium-catalyzed aryl amination and aryl amidation. Tetrahedron 52: 7525-7546.

[123] B.H. Yang and S.L. Buchwald. 1999. Palladium-catalyzed amination of aryl halides and sulfonates. J. Organomet. Chem. 576: 125-146.

[124] T. Hama and J.F. Hartwig. 2008. α-Arylation of esters catalyzed by the Pd(I) dimer {[P(*t*-Bu)₃] PdBr}₂. Org. Lett. 10: 1545-1548.

[125] A.S. Guram, R.A. Rennels and S.L. Buchwald. 1995. A simple catalytic method for the conversion of aryl bromides to arylamines. Angew. Chem. Int. Ed. Engl. 34: 1348-1350.

[126] J. Louie and J.F. Hartwig. 1995. Palladium-catalyzed synthesis of arylamines from aryl halides. Mechanistic studies lead to coupling in the absence of tin reagents. Tetrahedron Lett. 36: 3609-3612.

[127] R. Omar-Amrani, A. Thomas, E. Brenner, R. Schneider and Y. Fort. 2003. Efficient nickel-mediated intramolecular amination of aryl chlorides. Org. Lett. 5: 2311-2314.

[128] J.J. Song and N.K. Yee. 2000. A novel synthesis of 2-aryl-2*H*-indazoles *via* a palladium-catalyzed intramolecular amination reaction. Org. Lett. 2: 519-521.

[129] J.J. Song and N.K. Yee. 2001. Synthesis of 1-aryl-1*H*-indazoles *via* the palladium-catalyzed cyclization of *N*-aryl-*N'*-(*o*-bromobenzyl)hydrazines and [*N*-aryl-*N'*-(*o*-bromobenzyl)-hydrazinato-*N'*]-triphenylphosphonium bromides. Tetrahedron Lett. 42: 2937-2940.

[130] C.T. Brain and S.A. Brunton. 2002. An intramolecular palladium-catalyzed aryl amination reaction to produce benzimidazoles. Tetrahedron Lett. 43: 1893-1895.

[131] C.T. Brain and J.T. Steer. 2003. An improved procedure for the synthesis of benzimidazoles, using palladium-catalyzed aryl-amination chemistry. J. Org. Chem. 68: 6814-6816.

[132] M. Catellani, C. Catucci, G. Celentano and R. Ferraccioli. 2001. Palladium-catalyzed synthesis of enantiopure 1,2,4,5-tetrahydro-1,4-benzodiazepin-3-(3*H*)-one derivatives. Synlett 6: 803-805.

[133] B.J. Margolis, J.J. Swidorski and B.N. Rogers. 2003. An efficient assembly of heterobenzazepine ring systems utilizing an intramolecular palladium-catalyzed cycloamination. J. Org. Chem. 68: 644-647.

[134] T. Emoto, N. Kubosaki, Y. Yamagiwa and T. Kamikawa. 2000. A new route to phenazines. Tetrahedron Lett. 41: 355-358.

[135] Y. Kozawa and M. Mori. 2002. Synthesis of 3-alkoxycarbonyl-1*β*-methylcarbapenem using palladium-catalyzed amidation of vinyl halide. Tetrahedron Lett. 43: 111-114.

[136] G. Cuny, M. Bois-Choussy and J. Zhu. 2003. One-pot synthesis of polyheterocycles by a palladium-catalyzed intramolecular *N*-arylation/C-H activation/aryl-aryl bond-forming domino process. Angew. Chem. Int. Ed. 42: 4774-4777.

[137] F. He, B.M. Foxman and B.B. Snider. 1998. Total syntheses of (-)-asperlicin and (-)-asperlicin C. J. Am. Chem. Soc. 120: 6417-6418.

[138] X. Luo, E. Chenard, P. Martens, Y.-X. Cheng and M.J. Tomaszewshi. 2010. Practical synthesis of quinoxalinones *via* palladium-catalyzed intramolecular *N*-arylations. Org. Lett. 12: 3574-3577.

[139] G.S. Lemen and J.P. Wolfe. 2011. Cascade intramolecular *N*-arylation/intermolecular carboamination reactions for the construction of tricyclic heterocycles. Org. Lett. 13: 3218-3221.

[140] M. Genelot, A. Bendjeriou, V. Dufaud and L. Djakovitch. 2009. Optimized procedures for the one-pot selective syntheses of indoxyls and 4-quinolones by a carbonylative Sonogashira/cyclization sequence. Appl. Catal. A: Gen. 369: 125-132.

[141] R.C. Larock and D. Yue. 2002. Synthesis of 2,3-disubstituted benzo[*b*]thiophenes *via* palladium-catalyzed coupling and electrophilic cyclization of terminal acetylenes. J. Org. Chem. 67: 1905-1909.

[142] M. Mori. 2009. Synthesis of nitrogen heterocycles utilizing molecular nitrogen as a nitrogen source and attempt to use air instead of nitrogen gas. Heterocycles 78: 281-318.

[143] S. Cacchi, G. Fabrizi, A. Goggiamani, A. Perboni, P. Stabile and A. Sferrazza. 2010. 2,3-Disubstituted indoles *via* palladium-catalyzed reaction of 2-alkynyltrifluoroacetanilides with arenediazonium tetrafluoroborates. Org. Lett. 12: 3279-3281.

[144] I. Ambrogio, S. Cacchi, G. Fabrizi and A. Prastaro. 2009. 3-(*o*-Trifluoroacetamidoaryl)-1-propargylic esters: common intermediates for the palladium-catalyzed synthesis of 2-aminomethyl-, 2-vinylic, and 2-alkylindoles. Tetrahedron 65: 8916-8929.

[145] I. Ambrogio, S. Cacchi and G. Fabrizi. 2007. 2-Alkylindoles *via* palladium-catalyzed reductive cyclization of ethyl 3-(*o*-trifluoroacetamidophenyl)-1-propargyl carbonates. Tetrahedron Lett. 48: 7721-7725.

[146] S. Cacchi, G. Fabrizi and E. Filisti. 2009. Palladium-catalyzed synthesis of free-NH indole 2-acetamides and derivatives from ethyl 3-(*o*-trifluoroacetamidoaryl)-1-propargylic carbonates. Synlett 11: 1817-1821.

[147] I. Ambrogio, S. Cacchi and G. Fabrizi. 2006. Palladium-catalyzed synthesis of 2-(aminomethyl) indoles from ethyl 3-(*o*-trifluoroacetamidophenyl)-1-propargyl carbonate. Org. Lett. 8: 2083-2086.

[148] D. Sole and O. Serrano. 2008. Intramolecular Pd(0)-catalyzed reactions of *β*-(2-iodoanilino carboxamides: enolate arylation and nucleophilic substitution at the carboxamide group. J. Org. Chem. 73: 9372-9378.

[149] N. Lachance, M. April and M.-A. Joly. 2005. Rapid and efficient microwave-assisted synthesis of 4-, 5-, 6- and 7-azaindoles. Synthesis 15: 2571-2577.

[150] A. Arcadi, S. Cacchi, G. Fabrizi, F. Marinelli and L.M. Parisi. 2005. Palladium-catalyzed reaction of *o*-alkynyltrifluoroacetanilides with 1-bromoalkynes. An approach to 2-substituted 3-alkynylindoles and 2-substituted 3-acylindoles. J. Org. Chem. 70: 6213-6217.

[151] T. Fukuyama, A.A. Laird and L.M. Hotchkiss. 1985. *p*-Anisyl group: a versatile protecting group for primary alcohols. Tetrahedron Lett. 26: 6291-6292.

[152] D. Seomoon, K. Lee, H. Kim and P.H. Lee. 2007. Inter- and intramolecular palladium-catalyzed allyl cross-coupling reactions using allylindium generated *in situ* from allyl acetates, indium, and indium trichloride. Chem. Eur. J. 13: 5197-5206.

[153] H. Fuwa, T. Tako, M. Ebine and M. Sasaki. 2008. A new method for the generation of indole-2,3-quinodimethanes from allenamides. Chem. Lett. 37: 904-905.

[154] M. Mori, Y. Uozumi and M. Shibasaki. 1990. Incorporation of molecular nitrogen into organic compounds III. Reaction of titanium-nitrogen complexes with acid halides and acid anhydrides. J. Organomet. Chem. 395: 255-267.

[155] Y. Uozumi, E. Mori, M. Mori and M. Shibasaki. 1990. Incorporation of molecular nitrogen into organic compounds: IV. Novel lactam synthesis by nitrogenation of enol lactones. J. Organomet. Chem. 399: 93-102.

[156] J.H. Kim and S.-G. Lee. 2011. Palladium-catalyzed intramolecular trapping of the Blaise reaction intermediate for tandem one-pot synthesis of indole derivatives. Org. Lett. 13: 1350-1353.

[157] A. Dondoni, A. Marra and D. Perrone. 1993. Efficacious modification of the procedure for the aldehyde release from 2-substituted thiazoles. J. Org. Chem. 58: 275-277.

[158] T. Fukuyama, X. Chen and G. Peng. 1994. A novel tin-mediated indole synthesis. J. Am. Chem. Soc. 116: 3127-3128.

[159] Y. Kobayashi and T. Fukuyama. 1998. Development of a novel indole synthesis and its application to natural products synthesis. J. Heterocycl. Chem. 35: 1043-1056.

[160] J.C. Torres, R.A. Pilli, M.D. Vargas, F.A. Violante, S.J. Garden and A.C. Pinto. 2002. Synthesis of 1-ferrocenyl-2-aryl(heteroaryl)acetylenes and 2-ferrocenylindole derivatives *via* the Sonogashira-Heck-Cassar reaction. Tetrahedron 58: 4487-4492.

[161] T. Kalai, M. Balog, J. Jeko, W.L. Hubbell and K. Hideg. 2002. Palladium-catalyzed coupling reactions of paramagnetic vinyl halides. Synthesis 16: 2365-2372.

[162] J.R. Hwu, Y.C. Hsu, T. Josephrajan and S.-C. Tsay. 2009. Fine tuning of blue photoluminescence from indolesfor device fabrication. J. Mater. Chem. 19: 3084-3090.

[163] F. Ujjainwalla and D. Warner. 1998. Synthesis of 5-, 6- and 7-azaindoles *via* palladium-catalyzed heteroannulation of internal alkynes. Tetrahedron Lett. 39: 5355-5358.

[164] D.A. Alonso, C. Najera and M.C. Pacheco. 2002. Oxime-derived palladium complexes as very efficient catalysts for the Heck-Mizoroki reaction. Adv. Synth. Catal. 344: 172-183.

[165] T. Nishikawa, K. Wada and M. Isobe. 2002. Synthesis of novel α-C-glycosylamino acids and reverse regioselectivity in Larock's heteroannulation for the synthesis of the indole nucleus. Biosci. Biotechnol. Biochem. 66: 2273-2278.

[166] H.-C. Zhang, K.K. Brumfield and B.E. Maryanoff. 1997. Synthesis of trisubstituted indoles on the solid phase *via* palladium-mediated heteroannulation of internal alkynes. Tetrahedron Lett. 38: 2439-2442.

[167] A.L. Smith, G.I. Stevenson, C.J. Swain and J.L. Castro. 1998. Traceless solid phase synthesis of 2,3-disubstituted indoles. Tetrahedron Lett. 39: 8317-8320.

[168] T.O. Viera, L.A. Meaney, Y.-L. Shi and H. Alper. 2008. Tandem palladium-catalyzed N,C-coupling/carbonylation sequence for the synthesis of 2-carboxyindoles. Org. Lett. 10: 4899-4901.

[169] M. Arthuis, R. Pontikis and J.-C. Florent. 2009. Palladium-catalyzed domino C,N-coupling/carbonylation/Suzuki coupling reaction: an efficient synthesis of 2-aroyl-/heteroaroylindoles. Org. Lett. 11: 4608-4611.

[170] C.S. Cho, D.Y. Chu, D.Y. Lee, S.C. Shim, T.J. Kim, W.T. Lim and N.H. Heo. 1997. Palladium-catalyzed diastereoselective synthesis of isoindolinones. Synth. Commun. 27: 4141-4158.

[171] C.S. Cho, L.H. Jiang, D.Y. Lee, S.C. Shim, H.S. Lee and S.-D. Cho. 1997. Palladium-catalyzed synthesis of 3-(alkylamino)isoindolin-1-ones by carbonylative cyclization of 2-bromobenzaldehyde with primary amines. J. Heterocycl. Chem. 34: 1371-1374.

[172] C.S. Cho, H.S. Shim, H.-J. Choi, T.-J. Kim and S.C. Shim. 2002. Palladium-catalyzed convenient synthesis of 3-methyleneisoindolin-1-ones. Synth. Commun. 32: 1821-1827.

[173] R.J. Perry and S.R. Turner. 1991. Preparation of *N*-substituted phthalimides by the palladium-catalyzed carbonylation and coupling of *o*-dihalo aromatics and primary amines. J. Org. Chem. 56: 6573-6579.

[174] M. Akazome, T. Kondo and Y. Watanabe. 1992. Novel synthesis of indoles *via* palladium-catalyzed reductive *N*-heterocyclization of *o*-nitrostyrene derivatives. Chem. Lett. 5: 769-772.

[175] M. Akazome, T. Kondo and Y. Watanabe. 1994. Palladium complex-catalyzed reductive *N*-heterocyclization of nitroarenes: novel synthesis of indole and 2*H*-indazole derivatives. J. Org. Chem. 59: 3375-3380.

[176] S. Tollari, S. Cenini, C. Crotti and E. Gianella. 1994. Synthesis of heterocycles *via* palladium-catalyzed carbonylation of *o*-substituted organic nitro compounds in relatively mild conditions. J. Mol. Catal. 87: 203-214.

[177] A. Deagostino, V. Farina, C. Prandi, C. Zavattaro and P. Venturello. 2006. New metal-catalyzed synthesis of quinoline and chromene skeletons. Eur. J. Org. Chem. 15: 3451-3456.

[178] B.C. Söderberg and J.A. Shriver. 1997. Palladium-catalyzed synthesis of indoles by reductive *N*-heteroannulation of 2-nitrostyrenes. J. Org. Chem. 62: 5838-5845.

[179] B.C. Söderberg, A.C. Chisnell, S.N. O'Neil and J.A. Shriver. 1999. Synthesis of indoles isolated from *Tricholoma* species. J. Org. Chem. 64: 9731-9734.

[180] B.C. Soderberg, S.R. Banini, M.R. Turner, A.R. Minter and A.K. Arrington. 2008. Palladium-catalyzed synthesis of 3-indolecarboxylic acid derivatives. Synthesis 6: 903-912.

[181] G. Dyker and P. Grundt 1996. Annulated ring-systems by domino-Heck-aldol-condensation and domino Heck-Michael-addition processes. Tetrahedron Lett. 37: 619-622.

[182] A. Rolfe, K. Young and P.R. Hanson. 2008. Domino Heck-Aza-Michael reactions: a one-pot, sequential three-component approach to 1,1-dioxido-1,2-benzisothiazoline-3-acetic acid. Eur. J. Org. Chem. 31: 5254-5262.

[183] N. Barr, J.P. Bartley, P.W. Clark, P. Dunstan and S.F. Dyke. 1986. Palladium-assisted organic reactions. Simple syntheses of 2,3-disubstituted phthalimidines. J. Organomet. Chem. 302: 117-126.

[184] M.W. Khan and A.F.G. Masud Reza. 2005. Palladium mediated synthesis of isoindolinones and isoquinolinones. Tetrahedron 61: 11204-11210.

[185] B. Witulski, C. Alayrac and L. Tevzadze-Saeftel. 2003. Palladium-catalyzed synthesis of 2-aminoindoles by a heteroanulation reaction. Angew. Chem. Int. Ed. 42: 4257-4260.

[186] (a) D. Noteberg, W. Schaal, E. Hamelink, L. Vrang and M. Larhed. 2003. High-speed optimization of inhibitors of the malarial proteases plasmepsin I and II. J. Comb. Chem. 5: 456-464.
      (b) M. Larhed, J. Wannberg and A. Hallberg. 2007. Controlled microwave heating as an enabling technology: expedient synthesis of protease inhibitors in perspective. QSAR & Comb. Sci. 26: 51-68.

[187] S.S. Park, J.-K. Choi, E.K. Yum and D.-C. Ha. 1998. A facile synthesis of 2,3-disubstituted pyrrolo[2,3-*b*]pyridines *via* palladium-catalyzed heteroannulation with internal alkynes. Tetrahedron Lett. 39: 627-630.

[188] S.K. Kang, S.S. Park, S.S. Kim, J.-K. Choi and E.K. Yum. 1999. Synthesis of 1,2,3-trisubstituted pyrrolo[3,2-*c*]quinolines *via* palladium-catalyzed heteroannulation with internal alkynes. Tetrahedron Lett. 40: 4379-4382.

[189] D. Sole, L. Vallverdu, E. Peidro and J. Bonjoch. 2001. Palladium-catalyzed intramolecular annulation of 2-haloanilines and ketones: enolate arylation vs. nucleophilic addition to the carbonyl group. Chem. Commun. 18: 1888-1889.

[190] A. Kasahara, T. Izumi, S. Murakami, K. Miyamoto and T. Hino. 1989. A regiocontrolled synthesis of substituted indoles by palladium-catalyzed coupling of 2-bromonitrobenzenes and 2-bromoacetanilides. J. Heterocycl. Chem. 26: 1405-1413.

[191] F. Alonso, I.P. Beletskaya and M. Yus. 2004. Transition-metal-catalyzed addition of heteroatom-hydrogen bonds to alkynes. Chem. Rev. 104: 3079-3160.

[192] J.A. Brown. 2000. Synthesis of *N*-aryl indole-2-carboxylates *via* an intramolecular palladium-catalyzed annulation of didehydrophenylalanine derivatives. Tetrahedron Lett. 41: 1623-1626.

[193] W.-M. Dai, D.-S. Guo, L.-P. Sun and X.-H. Huang. 2003. Microwave-assisted solid-phase organic synthesis (MASPOS) as a key step for an indole library construction. Org. Lett. 5: 2919-2922.

[194] E.M. Beccalli, G. Broggini, M. Martinelli and G. Paladino. 2005. Pd-catalyzed intramolecular cyclization of pyrrolo-2-carboxamides: regiodivergent routes to pyrrolo-pyrazines and pyrrolo-pyridines. Tetrahedron 61: 1077-1082.

[195] L.S. Hegedus, G.F. Allen, J.J. Bozell and E.L. Waterman. 1978. Palladium-assisted intramolecular amination of olefins. Synthesis of nitrogen heterocycles. J. Am. Chem. Soc. 100: 5800-5807.

[196] M.E. Krolski, A.F. Renaldo, D.E. Rudisill and J.K. Stille. 1988. Palladium-catalyzed coupling of 2-bromoanilines with vinylstannanes. A regiocontrolled synthesis of substituted indoles. J. Org. Chem. 53: 1170-1176.

[197] W.C. Frank, Y.C. Kim and R.F. Heck. 1978. Palladium-catalyzed vinylic substitution reactions with heterocyclic bromides. J. Org. Chem. 43: 2947-2949.

[198] P.J. Harrington, L.S. Hegedus and K.F. McDaniel. 1987. Palladium-catalyzed reactions in the synthesis of 3- and 4-substituted indoles. Total synthesis of the *N*-acetyl methyl ester of (+)-clavicipitic acids. J. Am. Chem. Soc. 109: 4335-4338.

[199] D.R. Adams, M.A.J. Duncton, J.R.A. Roffey and J. Spencer. 2002. Preparation of 6-chloro-5-fluoroindole *via* the use of palladium and copper-mediated heterocyclizations. Tetrahedron Lett. 43: 7581-7583.

[200] T. Sato, S. Ishida, H. Ishibashi and M. Ikeda. 1991. Regiochemistry of radical cyclizations (6-*exo*/7-*endo* and 7-*exo*/8-*endo*) of *N*-(*o*-alkenylphenyl)-2,2-dichloroacetamides. Chem. Soc. Perkin Trans. 1 22: 353-359.

[201] S. Hibino and E. Sugino. 1987. A facile and alternative synthesis of quinoline nucleus using thermal cyclization of 2-azahexatriene system generated from 2-alkenyl-acylaniline with POCl$_3$. Heterocycles 26: 1883-1889.

[202] M.K. Coooper and D.W. Yaniuk. 1981. Preparation and characterization of chelating monoolefin-aniline ligands and their platinum(II) complexes. J. Organomet. Chem. 221: 231-247.

[203] C. Subramanyam, M. Noguchi and S.M. Weinreb. 1989. An approach to amphimedine and related marine alkaloids utilizing an intramolecular Kondrat'eva pyridine synthesis. J. Org. Chem. 54: 5580-5585.

[204] J.E. Plevyak and R.F. Heck. 1978. Palladium-catalyzed arylation of ethylene. J. Org. Chem. 43: 2454-2456.

[205] M. Yamaguchi, M. Arisawa and M. Hirama. 1998. *o*-Vinylation reaction of anilines. Chem. Commun. 13: 1399-1400.

[206] N. Kaur. 2018. Ruthenium catalysis in six-membered *O*-heterocycles synthesis. Synth. Commun. 48: 1551-1587.

[207] C.C. Scarborough, A. Bergant, G.T. Sazama, I.A. Guzei, L.C. Spencer and S.S. Stahl. 2009. Synthesis of PdII complexes bearing an enantiomerically-resolved seven-membered *N*-heterocyclic carbene ligands and initial studies of their use in asymmetric Wacker-type oxidative cyclization reactions. Tetrahedron 65: 5084-5092.

[208] P.J. Harrington and L.S. Hegedus. 1984. Palladium-catalyzed reactions in the synthesis of 3- and 4-substituted indoles. Approaches to ergot alkaloids. J. Org. Chem. 49: 2657-2662.

[209] J. Siu, I.R. Baxendale and S.V. Ley. 2004. Microwave assisted Leimgruber-Batcho reaction for the preparation of indoles, azaindoles and pyrroylquinolines. Org. Biomol. Chem. 2: 160-167.

[210] M. Gowan, A.S. Caille and C.K. Lau. 1997. Synthesis of 3-alkoxyindoles *via* palladium-catalyzed intramolecular cyclization of *N*-alkyl *o*-siloxyallylanilines. Synlett 11: 1312-1314.

[211] P.R. Weider, L.S. Hegedus, H. Asada and V. D'Andreq. 1985. Oxidative cyclization of unsaturated aminoquinones. Synthesis of quinolinoquinones. Palladium-catalyzed synthesis of pyrroloindoloquinones. J. Org. Chem. 50: 4276-4281.

[212] T. Miura, Y. Nishida, M. Morimoto, M. Yamauchi and M. Murakami. 2011. Palladium-catalyzed denitrogenation reaction of 1,2,3-benzotriazin-4(3*H*)-ones incorporating isocyanides. Org. Lett. 13: 1429-1431.

[213] H. Lin and U. Kazmaier. 2009. Molybdenum-catalyzed α-hydrostannations of propargylamines as the key step in the synthesis of *N*-heterocycles. Eur. J. Org. Chem. 8: 1221-1227.

[214] N. Halland, M. Nazare, O. Rkyek, J. Alonso, M. Urmann and A. Lindenschmidt. 2009. A general and mild palladium-catalyzed domino reaction for the synthesis of 2*H*-indazoles. Angew. Chem. Int. Ed. 48: 6879-6882.

[215] N. Halland, M. Nazare, J. Alonso, O. R'kyek and A. Lindenschmidt. 2011. A general and mild domino approach to substituted 1-aminoindoles. Chem. Commun. 47: 1042-1044.

[216] R. Martin, R.M. Rivero and S.L. Buchwald. 2006. Domino Cu-catalyzed C-N coupling/hydro-amidation: a highly efficient synthesis of nitrogen heterocycles. Angew. Chem. Int. Ed. 45: 7079-7082.

[217] P.G. Alsabeh, R.J. Lundgren, L.E. Longobardi and M. Stradiotto. 2011. Palladium-catalyzed synthesis of indoles *via* ammonia cross-coupling-alkyne cyclization. Chem. Commun. 47: 6936-6938.

[218] C.J. Ball and M.C. Willis. 2013. Cascade palladium- and copper-catalyzed aromatic heterocycle synthesis: the emergence of general precursors. Eur. J. Org. Chem. 3: 425-441.

[219] A. Salim, H. Haitham and Y. Maher. 2008. Palladium-based chemotherapeutic agents: routes toward complexes with good anti-tumor activity. Cancer Therapy 6: 1-10.

[220] J.L. Klinkenberg and J.F. Hartwig. 2010. Slow reductive elimination from arylpalladium parent amido complexes. J. Am. Chem. Soc. 132: 11830-11833.

[221] G.D. Vo and J.F. Hartwig. 2009. Palladium-catalyzed coupling of ammonia with aryl chlorides, bromides, iodides, and sulfonates: a general method for the preparation of primary arylamines. J. Am. Chem. Soc. 131: 11049-11061.

[222] Q. Shen and J.F. Hartwig. 2006. Palladium-catalyzed coupling of ammonia and lithium amide with aryl halides. J. Am. Chem. Soc. 128: 10028-10029.

[223] D.S. Surry and S.L. Buchwald. 2007. Selective palladium-catalyzed arylation of ammonia: synthesis of anilines as well as symmetrical and unsymmetrical di- and triarylamines. J. Am. Chem. Soc. 129: 10354-10355.

[224] T. Schulz, C. Torborg, S. Enthaler, B. Schaffner, A. Dumrath, A. Spannenberg, H. Neumann, A. Borner and M. Beller. 2009. A general palladium-catalyzed amination of aryl halides with ammonia. Chem. Eur. J. 15: 4528-4533.

[225] R.J. Lundgren, B.D. Peters, P.G. Alsabeh and M. Stradiotto. 2010. A P,N-ligand for palladium-catalyzed ammonia arylation: coupling of deactivated aryl chlorides, chemoselective arylations, and room temperature reactions. Angew. Chem. Int. Ed. 49: 4071-4074.

[226] E. Avaro and J.F. Hartwig. 2009. Resting state and elementary steps of the coupling of aryl halides with thiols catalyzed by alkylbisphosphine complexes of palladium. J. Am. Chem. Soc. 131: 7858-7868.

[227] Q. Shen and J.F. Hartwig. 2008. [(CyPF-*t*-Bu)PdCl$_2$]: an air-stable, one-component, highly efficient catalyst for amination of heteroaryl and aryl halides. Org. Lett. 10: 4109-4112.

[228] M.A. Fernandez-Rodriguez, Q. Shen and J.F. Hartwig. 2006. Highly efficient and functional group tolerant catalysts for the palladium-catalyzed coupling of aryl chlorides with thiols. Chem. Eur. J. 12: 7782-7796.

[229] Q. Shen, S. Shekhar, J.P. Stambuli and J.F. Hartwig. 2005. Highly reactive, general, and long-lived catalysts for coupling heteroaryl and aryl chlorides with primary nitrogen nucleophiles. Angew. Chem. Int. Ed. 44: 1371-1375.

[230] R.J. Lundgren and M. Stradiotto. 2010. Palladium-catalyzed cross-coupling of aryl chlorides and tosylates with hydrazine. Angew. Chem. Int. Ed. 49: 8686-8690.

[231] K.D. Hesp, R.J. Lundgren and M. Stradiotto. 2011. Palladium-catalyzed mono-α-arylation of acetone with aryl halides and tosylates. J. Am. Chem. Soc. 133: 5194-5197.

[232] D.S. Surry and S.L. Buchwald. 2011. Dialkylbiaryl phosphines in Pd-catalyzed amination: a user's guide. Chem. Sci. 2: 27-50.

[233] J.F. Hartwig. 2008. Evolution of a fourth generation catalyst for the amination and thioetherification of aryl halides. Acc. Chem. Res. 41: 1534-1544.

[234] C.B. Lavery, R. McDonald and M. Stradiotto. 2012. Efficient palladium-catalyzed synthesis of substituted indoles employing a new (silanyloxyphenyl)phosphine ligand. Chem. Commun. 48: 7277-7279.

[235] K. Narasaka and M. Kitamura. 2005. Amination with oximes. Eur. J. Org. Chem. 21: 4505-4519.

[236] M. Kitamura and K. Narasaka. 2002. Synthesis of aza-heterocycles from oximes by amino-Heck reaction. Chem. Rec. 2: 268-277.

[237] H. Tsutsui and K. Narasaka. 1999. Synthesis of pyrrole derivatives by the Heck-type cyclization of γ,δ-unsaturated ketone *O*-(pentafluorobenzoyl)oximes. Chem. Lett. 1: 45-46.

[238] N. Kaur. 2018. Green synthesis of three to five-membered *O*-heterocycles using ionic liquids. Synth. Commun. 48: 1588-1613.

[239] D.A. Culkin and J.F. Hartwig. 2003. Palladium-catalyzed α-arylation of carbonyl compounds and nitriles. Acc. Chem. Res. 36: 234-245.

[240] M. Rubin, A.W. Sromek and V. Gevorgyan. 2003. New advances in selected transition metal-catalyzed annulations. Synlett 15: 2265-2291.

[241] D. Conreaux, D. Bouyssi, N. Monteiro and C. Balme. 2006. Palladium-catalyzed bicyclization processes in the one step construction of heteropolycyclic ring systems. Cur. Org. Chem. 10: 1325-1340.

[242] A. Banerjee, S.K. Santra, S.K. Rout and B.K. Patel. 2013. A ligand free copper(II) catalyst is as effective as a ligand assisted Pd(II) catalyst towards intramolecular C-S bond formation *via* C-H functionalization. Tetrahedron 69: 9096-9104.

[243] S.S. Stahl. 2004. Palladium oxidase catalysis: selective oxidation of organic chemicals by direct dioxygen-coupled turnover. Angew. Chem. Int. Ed. 43: 3400-3420.

[244] R.M. Trend, Y.K. Ramthohul and B.M. Stoltz. 2005. Oxidative cyclizations in a nonpolar solvent using molecular oxygen and studies on the stereochemistry of oxypalladation. J. Am. Chem. Soc. 127: 17778-17788.

[245] R.M. Trend, Y.K. Ramthohul, E.M. Ferreira and B.M. Stoltz. 2003. Palladium-catalyzed oxidative Wacker cyclizations in nonpolar organic solvents with molecular oxygen: a stepping stone to asymmetric aerobic cyclizations. Angew. Chem. Int. Ed. 42: 2892-2895.

[246] S.R. Fix, J.L. Brice and S.S. Stahl 2002. Efficient intramolecular oxidative amination of olefins through direct dioxygen-coupled palladium catalysis. Angew. Chem. Int. Ed. 41: 164-166.

[247] G. Liu and S.S. Stahl. 2007. Two-faced reactivity of alkenes: *cis*- versus *trans*-aminopalladation in aerobic Pd-catalyzed intramolecular aza-Wacker reactions. J. Am. Chem. Soc. 129: 6328-6335.

[248] B. Akermark, J.E. Backvall, K. Siiralah, K. Sjoberg and K. Zetterberg. 1974. The steric course of the palladium promoted amination of simple olefins. Tetrahedron Lett. 15: 1363-1366.

[249] B. Akermark, J.E. Backvall, L.S. Hegedus, K. Zetterberg, K. Siirala-Hansen and K. Sjoberg. 1974. Palladium-promoted addition of amines to isolated double bonds. J. Organomet. Chem. 72: 127-138.

[250] B. Akermark and J.E. Backvall. 1975. Competitive palladium-promoted amination of butenes. Tetrahedron Lett. 16: 819-822.

[251] L.S. Hegedus, G.F. Allen and E.L. Waterman. 1976. Palladium assisted intramolecular amination of olefins. A new synthesis of indoles. J. Am. Chem. Soc. 98: 2674-2676.

[252] J.E. Backvall. 1978. Stereospecific palladium-promoted vicinal diamination of olefins. Tetrahedron Lett. 19: 163-166.

[253] J.E. Backvall and E.E. Bjorkman. 1980. Stereospecific palladium-promoted oxyamination of alkenes. J. Org. Chem. 45: 2893-2898.

[254] J.E. Backvall, E.E. Bjorkman and S.E. Bystrom. 1982. Palladium-promoted asymmetric oxyamination of alkenes application to the synthesis of optically active aryloxypropanolamines. Tetrahedron Lett. 23: 943-946.

[255] L.S. Hegedus, B. Akermark, K. Zetterberg and L.F. Olsson. 1984. Palladium-assisted amination of olefins. A mechanistic study. J. Am. Chem. Soc. 106: 7122-7126.

[256] Z. Shi, C. Zhang, C. Tanga and N. Jiao. 2012. Recent advances in transition-metal catalyzed reactions using molecular oxygen as the oxidant. Chem. Soc. Rev. 41: 3381-3430.

[257] S. Diez-Gonzalez, N. Marion and S.P. Nolan. 2009. *N*-Heterocyclic carbenes in late transition metal catalysis. Chem. Rev. 109: 3612-3676.

[258] T. Niwa, H. Yorimitsu and K. Oshima. 2007. Palladium-catalyzed 2-pyridylmethyl transfer from 2-(2-pyridyl)ethanol derivatives to organic halides by chelation-assisted cleavage of unstrained $C(sp^3)$-$C(sp^3)$ bonds. Angew. Chem. Int. Ed. 46: 2643-2645.

[259] K.B. Hong, C.W. Lee and E.K. Yum. 2004. Synthesis of 2-substituted indoles by palladium-catalyzed heteroannulation with Pd-NaY zeolite catalysts. Tetrahedron Lett. 45: 693-697.

[260] S. Kamijo and Y. Yamamoto. 2002. A new Pd(0)-Cu(I) bimetallic catalyst for the synthesis of indoles from isocyanates and allyl carbonates. Angew. Chem. Int. Ed. 41: 3230-3233.

[261] S. Kamijo and Y. Yamamoto. 2003. A bimetallic catalyst and dual role catalyst: synthesis of N-(alkoxycarbonyl)indoles from 2-(alkynyl)phenylisocyanates. J. Org. Chem. 68: 4764-4771.

[262] M. Gruber, S. Chouzier, K. Koehler and L. Djakovitch. 2004. Palladium on activated carbon: a valuable heterogeneous catalyst for one-pot multi-step synthesis. Appl. Catal. A 265: 161-169.

[263] M. Pal, V. Subramanian, V.R. Batchu and I. Dager. 2004. Synthesis of 2-substituted indoles *via* Pd/C-catalyzed reaction in water. Synlett 11: 1965-1969.

[264] M. Nazare, C. Schneider, A. Lindenschmidt and D.W. Will. 2004. A flexible, palladium-catalyzed indole and azaindole synthesis by direct annulation of chloroanilines and chloroaminopyridines with ketones. Angew. Chem. Int. Ed. 43: 4526-4528.

[265] J. Jia and J. Zhu. 2006. Palladium-catalyzed, modular synthesis of highly functionalized indoles and tryptophans by direct annulation of substituted *o*-haloanilines and aldehydes. J. Org. Chem. 71: 7826-7834.

[266] D.D. Hennnings, S. Iwasa and V.H. Rawal. 1997. Anion-accelerated palladium-mediated intramolecular cyclizations: synthesis of benzofurans, indoles, and a benzopyran. Tetrahedron Lett. 38: 6379-6382.

[267] I.W. Davies, J.H. Smitrovich, R. Sidler, C. Qu, V. Gresham and C. Bazaral. 2005. A highly active catalyst for the reductive cyclization of *o*-nitrostyrenes under mild conditions. Tetrahedron 61: 6425-6437.

[268] J.T. Kuethe, A. Wong, C. Qu, J. Smitrovich, I.W. Davies and D.L. Hughes. 2005. Synthesis of 5-substituted-1*H*-indol-2-yl-1*H*-quinolin-2-ones: a novel class of KDR kinase inhibitors. J. Org. Chem. 70: 2555-2567.

CHAPTER 3

Five-Membered Fused N-Heterocycles

3.1 Introduction

For more than a century, heterocyclic compounds are the largest classical divisions of organic chemistry with industrial and biological importance. Numerous biologically active agrochemicals, pharmaceuticals, additives and modifiers applied in industrial applications such as information storage, cosmetics reprography, and plastics are heterocycles in nature. One striking structural feature of heterocyclic compounds lies in their ability to manifest substituents around a core scaffold in defined three dimensional representations [1a-c]. Heterocycles have contributed to the understanding of life processes as well as to industrial and biological development. By the end of second millennium among 20 million chemical compounds identified, more than two-thirds at partially or fully aromatic and approximately half are heterocyclic compounds. The presence of heterocyclic compounds in organic compounds of interest in biology, electronics, pharmacology, optics, and material sciences is very well known [2-8].

Although various protocols have been developed, their functional group tolerance and substrate scope are often limited. In recent yrs, for the synthesis of heterocycles many new protocols have been developed which involved palladium-catalyzed carbon-nitrogen bond-forming reactions. These reactions tolerate a number of functional groups, occur under mild conditions, and proceed with high stereoselectivity. The utilization of palladium allows highly convergent multi-component coupling approaches, which form many bonds and/or stereocenters in one-pot protocol. This chapter describes the preparation of fused five-membered nitrogen heterocycles through palladium assisted reactions [9-16].

3.2 Palladium assisted synthesis of five-membered N-heterocycles fused with other heterocycles

3.3 Synthesis of five-membered heterocycles fused with aromatics

Beller and Tse [17], and Sanford [18] independently transformed 1,6-enynes into bicyclo-[3.1.0] hexanes by cyclopropanation at a palladium(IV) center **(Scheme 1)** and thus shown the power of higher-oxidation-state Pd catalysis for carbon-carbon bond-forming reactions which was not possible through conventional palladium(II) catalysis. Yin and Liu [19] synthesized chloro-substituted lactones by a related conversion under aerobic conditions in the presence of LiCl (large excess) in CH_3COOH. In this case, the opposite relative configuration of products pointed towards a direct reductive elimination from within the coordination sphere of palladium(IV) catalyst [20].

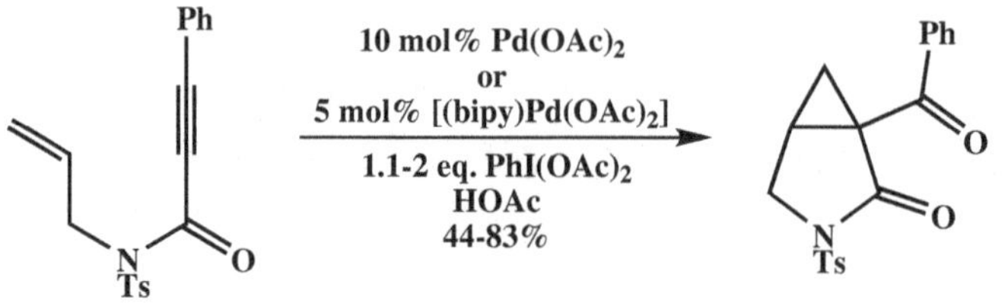

Scheme-1

Oxidative addition of Pd(0) to vinyl triflate followed by stereospecific 5-*exo-trig* cyclization, anion exchange and reductive elimination proceeded in excellent yield. Boronic acids due to their stability, ease of availability, and diverse structures, form a valuable substrate for cyclization-anion capture protocol. Allenylpalladium(II) was produced by a biscyclization which involved the formation of three new bonds using Tsuji's [21] efficient and simple protocol **(Scheme 2)** [22].

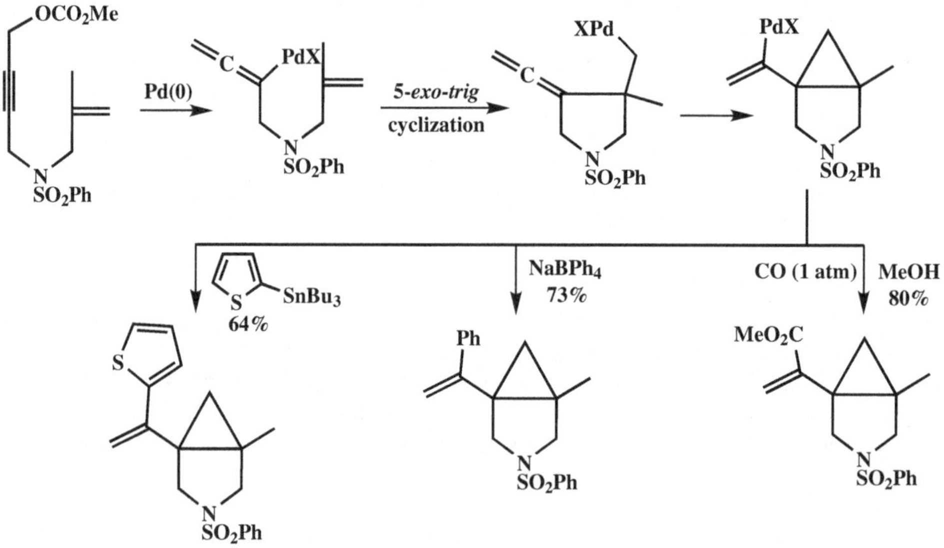

Scheme-2

Grigg and co-workers [23] observed the synthesis of vinylic Pd intermediate. The 2-bicyclic propenoate was prepared by the reaction of *N*-(2-methylallyl)-*N*-(4-methoxycarbonyloxy-2-butynyl)benzenesulfonamide in the presence of palladium catalyst and carbon monoxide in methanol through the formation of vinylic Pd intermediate. However, the Heck-type of carbopalladation-β-H elimination had not been observed **(Scheme 3)** [24].

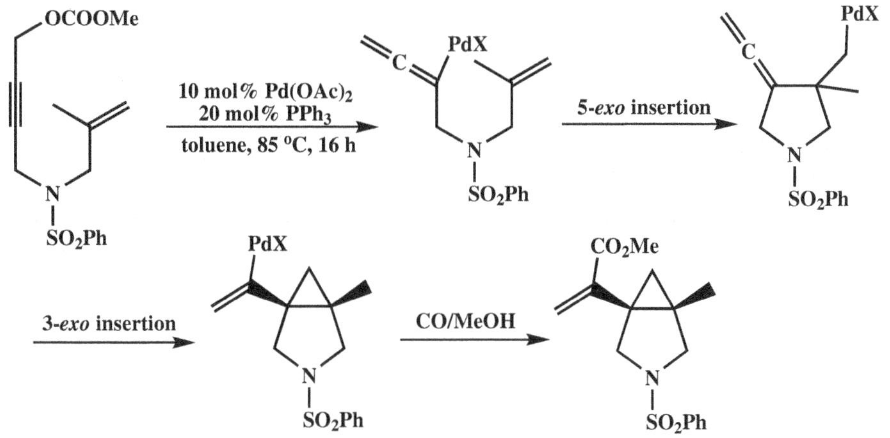

Scheme-3

Mascarenas and co-workers [25] prepared bicyclic aza-heterocyclic compounds by palladium-catalyzed intramolecular [4+3]-cycloaddition of *N*-tethered alkylidenecyclopropane with dienes **(Scheme 4)**. The utilization of a phosphorous ligand C-20 afforded the best results in this reaction [26].

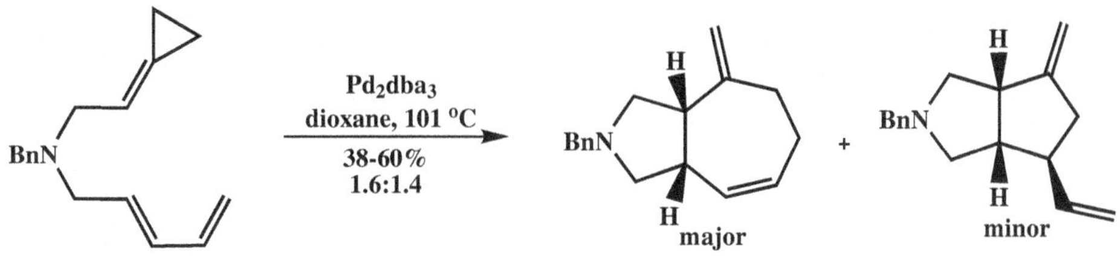

Scheme-4

Initial Heck-type carbopalladation of an alkene with an alkenyl halide, followed by rearrangement of resulting alkylpalladium species through reversible β-hydride elimination processes were involved in the synthesis of allylpalladium complex intermediate during the synthesis of heterocyclic compounds [27-28]. The olefinic amides were utilized in the preparation of lactams employing this pathway [29]. In addition, the pyrrolidine was synthesized in an intramolecular fashion **(Scheme 5)** [30-31].

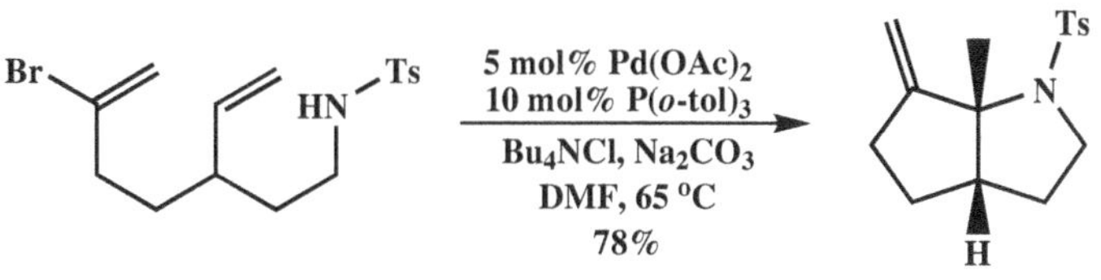

Scheme-5

The aminoalkenes underwent intramolecular amidation reactions. The aminoalkenes were first transformed into *p*-toluenesulfonamides which were cyclized to *N*-tosylated cyclic enamines **(Scheme 6)** [32]. In general, more difficulties were encountered during the synthesis of six-membered rings as compared to five-membered rings [33].

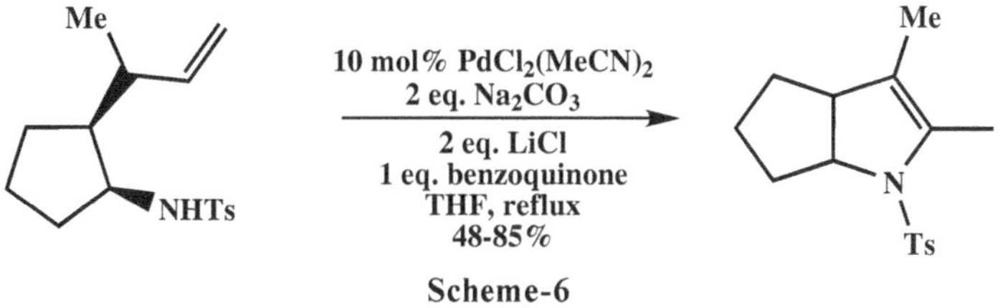

Scheme-6

Recent direct evidence for intermolecular palladium-mediated *syn*-aminopalladations of ethylene and 1-octene has been put forth by Hartwig et al. [34]. Stahl and Liu [35] have also shown that oxidative, intramolecular *anti*- or *syn*-aminopalladations both were possible depending on the nature of catalyst employed. For example, a catalyst composed of palladium acetate/ dimethylsulphoxide/oxygen yielded only *anti*-aminopalladation product whereas a palladium acetate/pyridine/oxygen catalyst system afforded *syn*-aminopalladation products **(Scheme 7)**.

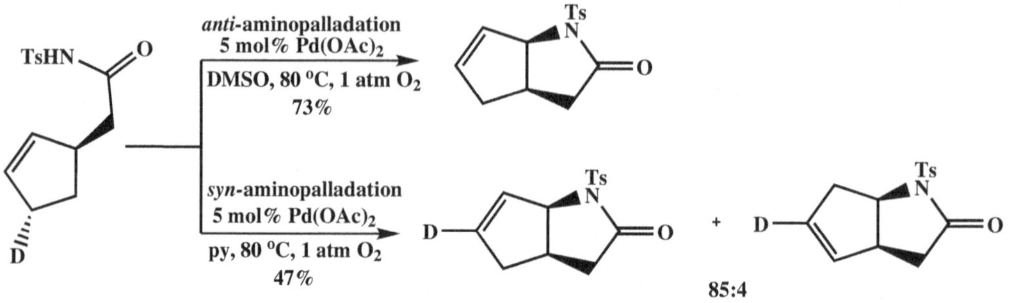

Scheme-7

A wide range of fused-heterocyclic systems were synthesized from alkene moiety of the appropriately substituted allylamine by intramolecular [3+2]-cycloaddition reactions. Mascarenas and co-workers [36] synthesized cyclopenta[*c*]pyrrol-4(5*H*)-ones with three stereocenters from *N*-tethered alk-5-enylidenecyclopropanes *via* palladium-catalyzed intramolecular [3+2]-cycloaddition reactions **(Scheme 8)** [26].

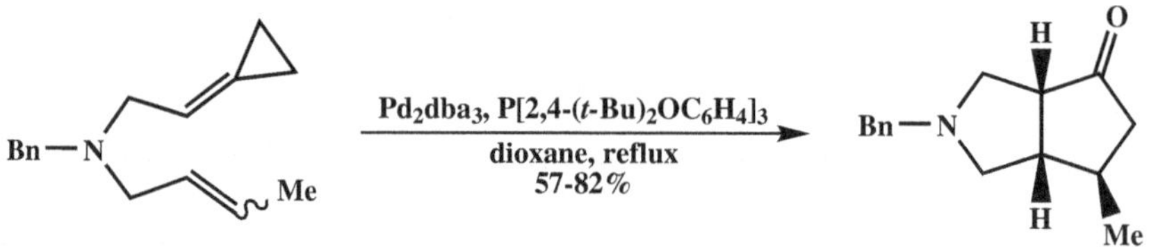

Scheme-8

Arai and co-workers [37] described the dicyanative cyclization of 1,6-dienynes to form the aza-heterocyclic systems by *syn*- and *anti*-cyanopalladation through the formation of three carbon-carbon bonds in a single operation **(Scheme 9)** [26].

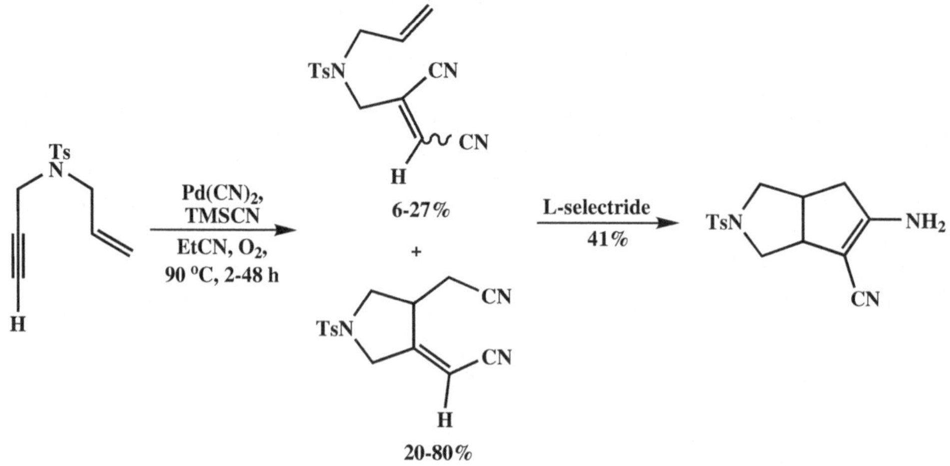

Scheme-9

Palladium-catalyzed carboamination of alkenes has also become a useful method for the synthesis of a broad array of nitrogen-containing heterocycles [38]. In addition to pyrrolidines being an interesting class of medicinally-relevant compounds [39], this carboamination method was demonstrated to involve a novel, intramolecular *syn*-aminopalladation step. In 2005, Wolfe and Ney [40a] illustrated that carboamination of *γ-N*-arylaminoalkene substrate gave products derived from *syn*-addition of nitrogen and aryl group across the pendant alkene **(Scheme 10)**.

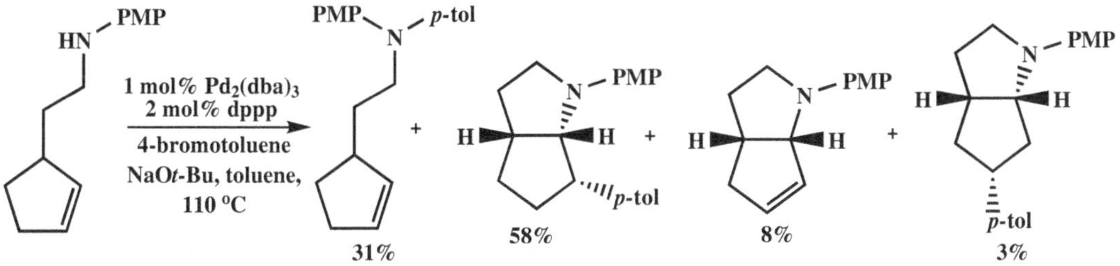

Scheme-10

Moderate to good yield of target products with excellent diastereoselectivity was afforded upon selective coupling of starting compound with 4-Br-PhMe in the presence of phosphine ligand **(Scheme 11)**. The *N-p*-methoxyphenyl group was replaced with *N-p*-cyanophenyl group for the improvement of selectivity of this regioisomer. Good yield of a number of *N*-aryl-5- and 6-aryl azabicyclo[3.3.0]octane derivatives was obtained in subsequent experiments [38, 40b].

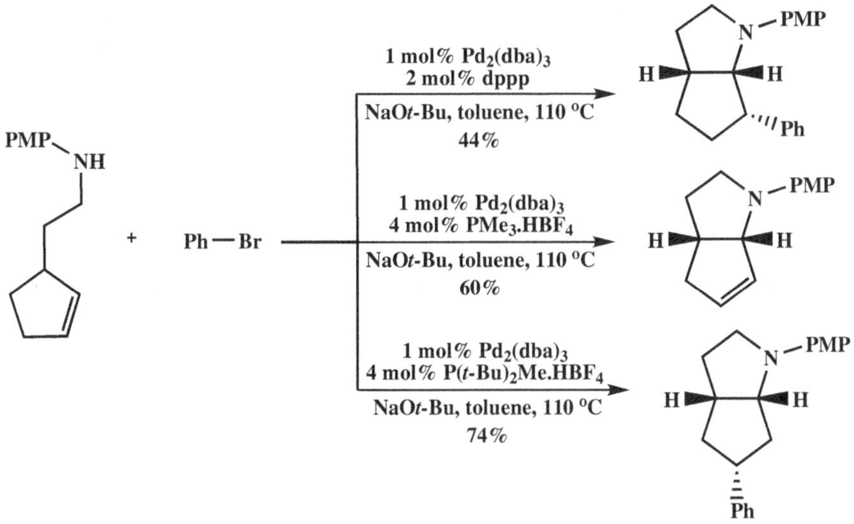

Scheme-11

Unsuccessful carboamination reactions of acyclic internal alkenes in the presence of palladium catalyst were reported, when the conversions of *N*-protected cyclopent-2-enyl ethylamine derivatives were conducted. A mixture of four products was obtained when *N*-(4-methoxyphenyl) protected substrate was reacted with 4-bromobiphenyl in Pd₂(dba)₃/P(*o*-tol)₃ catalyst and sodium *tert*-butoxide. The expected product was only afforded in moderate yield *via syn*-addition across the alkene when Boc-protected substrate was reacted with 4-bromobiphenyl and sodium *tert*-butoxide in the presence of palladium catalyst [41]. However, the coupling of Boc-protected substrate with 4-bromobiphenyl synthesized benzocyclobutene rather than pyrrolidine when dioxane solvent and cesium carbonate base were used **(Scheme 12)** [42-44]. The pyrrolidine-synthesizing reactions are mechanistically similar to THF-forming reactions in so far as both the conversions involved *syn*-insertion of an alkene into palladium-heteroatom bond of intermediate palladium(aryl)(amido) or palladium(aryl) (alkoxide) complexes. The palladium-nitrogen bond-forming step was reversible, and the position of equilibrium presumably was related to both the strength of base and the acidity of NH proton [45-46]. In addition, the alkene insertion step may be reversible [47], and both the position of this equilibrium and the rate of insertion depend on nucleophilicity, basicity, and/or leaving group ability of amino group, as well as the steric encumbrance of both the complex and the alkene produced after aminopalladation [38, 48-51].

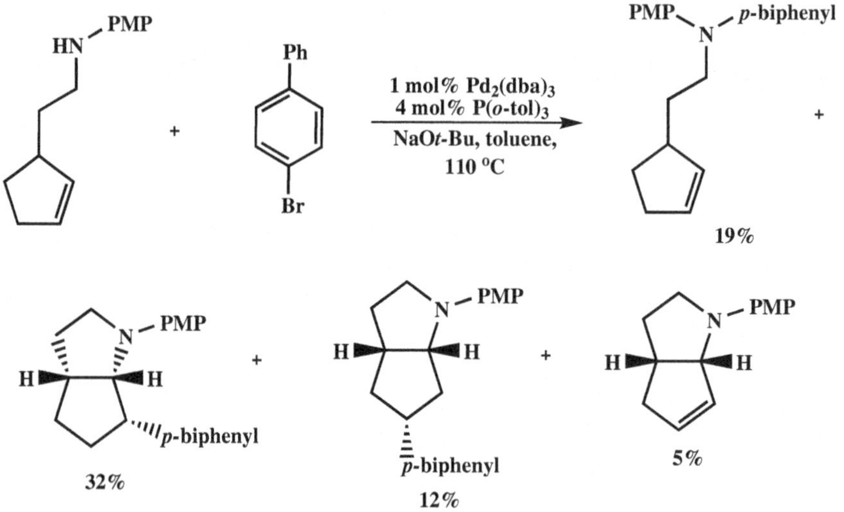

Scheme-12

Wolfe group [52-53] demonstrated the palladium-catalyzed carboamination of γ-(*N*-arylamino) alkenes and γ-(*N*-Boc-amino)alkenes to afford substituted pyrrolidines. The carboamination of an internal cyclic alkene to afford the bicyclic pyrrolidine proceeded with high diastereoselectivity **(Scheme 13)**.

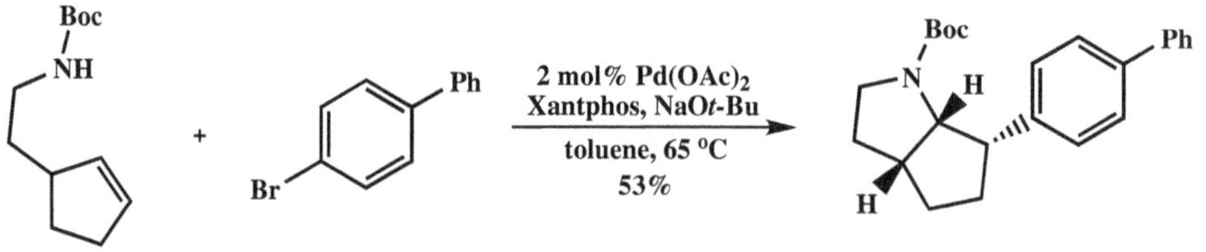

Scheme-13

Jeong and co-workers [54] synthesized bicyclopentenones in high yields by a tandem allylic alkylation/Pauson-Khand reaction of the propargylic amines with carbon monoxide and allyl acetate in a mixture of Rh and Pd catalysts **(Scheme 14)**. The enyne was prepared by allylation of propargylic amines with allyl acetate in the presence of Pd catalyst. The formed enyne underwent Pauson-Khand reaction with carbon monoxide and Rh catalyst.

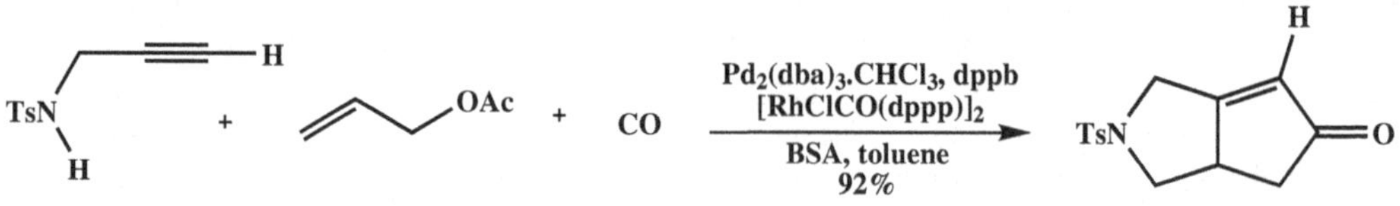

Scheme-14

Nucleophilic attack on palladium(II)-complexed alkenes was one of the most efficient organometallic process to generate valuable organic compounds. A prominent example was Wacker process, an industrial method for the preparation of acetaldehyde from ethylene. The pioneering work of Hegedus showed that nitrogen nucleophiles too can be used as reactants in such transformations. In case of cyclopentylamine derivatives, both the starting amine and the product were good ligands for Pd, though when suitably derivatized in order to decrease their basicity, such transformations can be performed in a catalytic fashion (**Scheme 15**) [55-57].

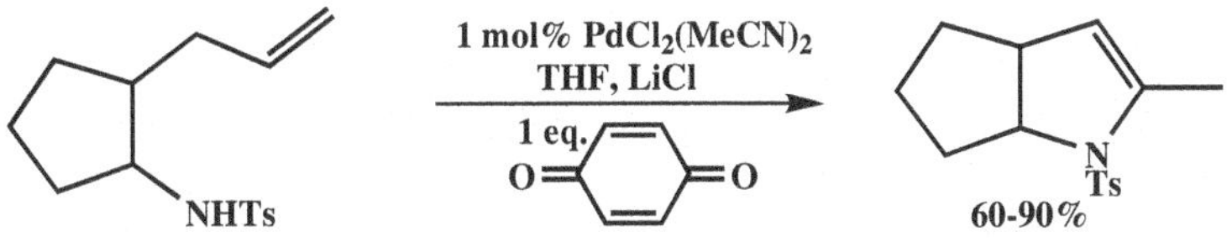

Scheme-15

An allylic nitrogen possessing heterocyclic compounds were synthesized by cyclization of cyclic olefinic *N*-tosylamines (**Scheme 16**) [58]. To avoid the other re-oxidants, the reaction was performed under an O_2 atmosphere in dimethylsulphoxide. The mechanism proposed the use of palladium acetate/oxygen/dimethylsulphoxide catalytic oxidation system which demonstrated that the turnover limiting step of catalytic cycle was reoxidation of Pd by molecular O_2. The catalytic efficiency in oxidative amination reactions was increased with the use of pyridine or other imine donor ligands. The palladium acetate/pyridine (1:2) catalytic system acted well in a number of solvents ranging from non-polar to polar, and to achieve efficient dioxygen-coupled turnover the need for a co-catalyst was obviated.

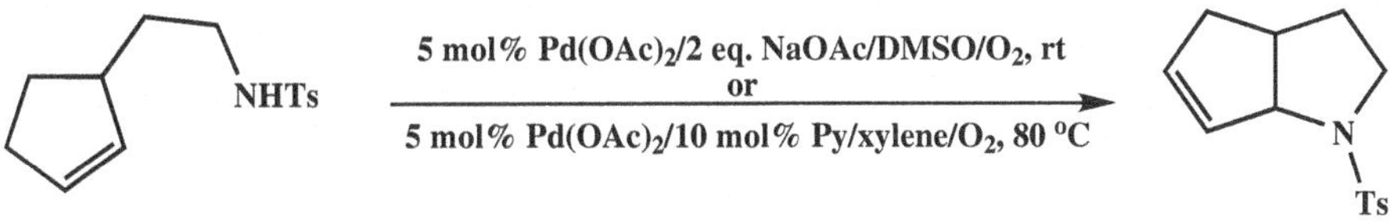

Scheme-16

In 1978, Hegedus [59] synthesized dihydropyrrole and indoles derivatives by palladium-catalyzed oxidative amination reactions of alkenes. Although with catalytic amounts of Pd these reactions occurred in good yield but a stoichiometric amount of a co-oxidant, including cupric chloride or benzoquinone, was needed to facilitate catalyst turnover. Through a loss of HX, a palladium(0) complex was formed from Pd(H)X intermediate. Subsequently, the palladium(0) complex was re-oxidized to palladium(II) with O_2 in dimethylsulphoxide. This protocol was used for the synthesis of bicyclic pyrrolidines and indolines containing carbamate or sulfonyl protecting groups (**Scheme 17**) [60].

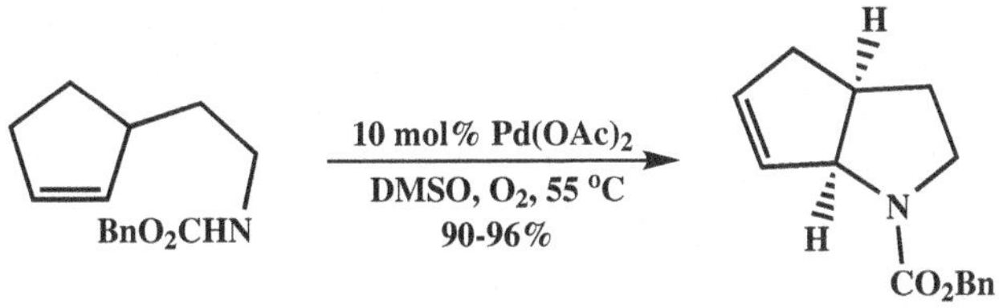

Scheme-17

The reaction of *N*-cyclohexenyl derivative was investigated (**Scheme 18**). The tetracyclic compound was formed as a single isomer upon exposure of *N*-cyclohexenyl derivative under standard cyclization conditions. NMR analysis, including COSY and NOE, experiments were performed to confirm the structure of tetracyclic compound. The complex heterocyclic compounds were prepared utilizing this tandem cyclization as a novel protocol [61].

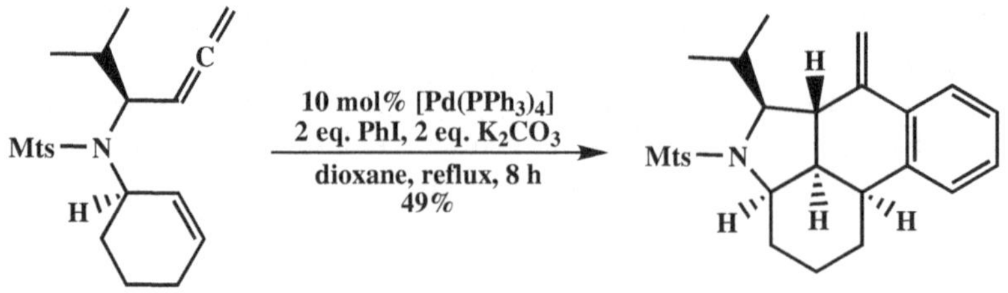

Scheme-18

The desired tandem cyclization was promoted with inhibition of β-hydride elimination. The β-hydride elimination was suppressed and allowed another carbopalladation step upon replacement of β-hydrogen atom with an alkyl group. However, the reactivity of allenene was decreased with the incorporation of a methyl group at 2'-position, and 2'-methylated allenene afforded the desired tricyclic product after 36 h in just 5% yield **(Scheme 19)** [61].

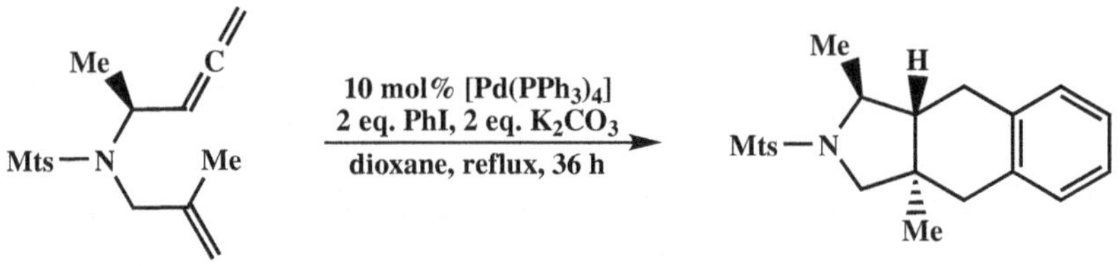

Scheme-19

The pyrrole derivatives were synthesized by nitrogen-Heck-type reaction. The pyrroles were prepared smoothly upon cyclization of many α,β-unsaturated ketone oximes having substituted terminal methylene groups **(Scheme 20)** [62].

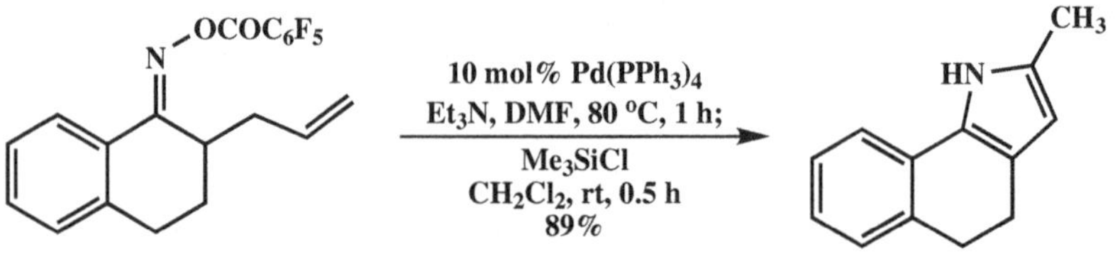

Scheme-20

The l-azaazulenes were formed in good yields from oximes by Pd-catalyzed amino-Heck reaction and subsequent treatment with manganese(IV) oxide **(Scheme 21)** [63-64]. Cyclic amines like azaazulene, aza-spiro compound, indoles and imidazoles, other than isoquinolines and pyrroles, were produced when many unsaturated open tafluorobenzoyloximes were reacted with a palladium(0) catalyst by an intramolecular amino-Heck reaction [65-66]. The aza-azulenes were also generated by this straightforward protocol *via* Pd-catalyzed cyclization. The cycloheptatrienylmethyl ketone *O*-pentafluorobenzoyloximes were treated with Pd catalyst and TEA and were successively oxidized with manganese(IV) oxide to afford 1-aza-azulenes [67].

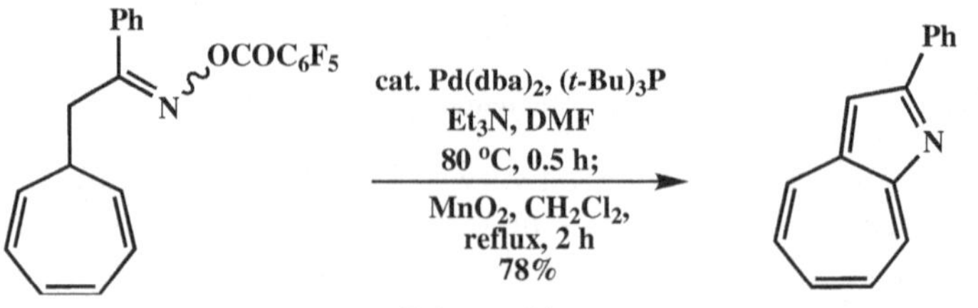

Scheme-21

Mascarenas and co-workers [68] used alkynes, alkylidenecyclopropanes, and alkenes for a palladium-catalyzed multi-component intramolecular [3+2+2]-cycloaddition reaction to provide *N*-possessing tricyclic systems with complete diastereoselectivities and moderate to excellent chemoselectivities **(Scheme 22)**. In addition, minor yields of another bicyclic product were obtained [26].

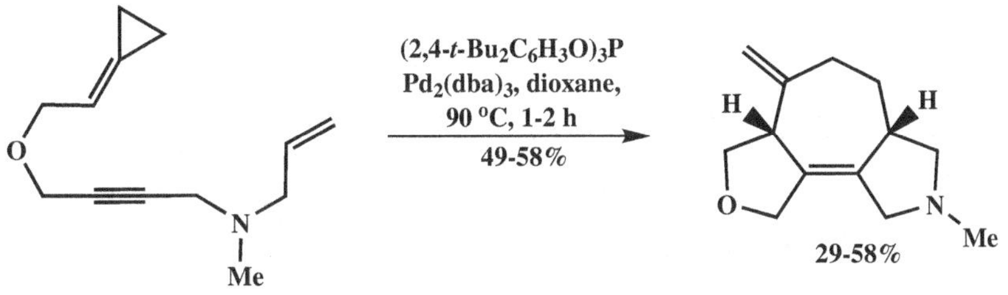

$(2,4\text{-}t\text{-}Bu_2C_6H_3O)_3P$
$Pd_2(dba)_3$, dioxane,
90 °C, 1-2 h
49-58%

29-58%

Scheme-22

3.4 Synthesis of five-membered heterocycles fused with four-membered heterocycles

The D2-carbapenems were produced by aminocyclization of allene-substituted β-lactams in the presence of metal salt catalyst (Au-, Pt-, and Pd-based catalysts) **(Scheme 23)** [69-75].

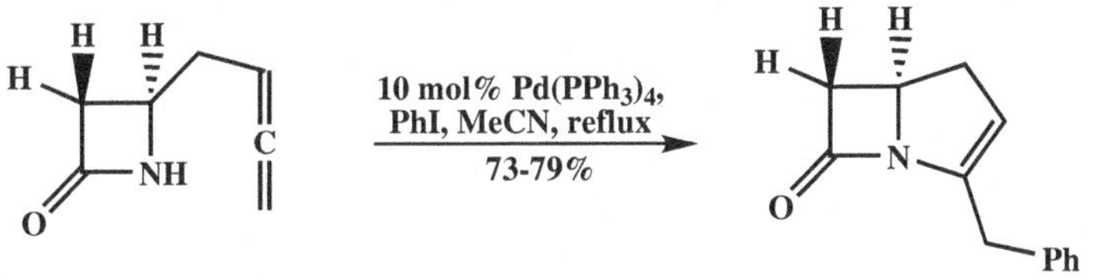

10 mol% $Pd(PPh_3)_4$,
PhI, MeCN, reflux
73-79%

Scheme-23

The salinosporamide A was prepared as shown in **Scheme 24**. The amide was synthesized by cyclization of chiral propargyl alcohol in the presence of $In(OTf)_3$ catalyst [76]. Marshall [77] reported the transformation of propargyl alcohol into the mesylate, which was then reacted with (*tert*-butyldimethylsilyloxy)acetaldehyde through allenylzinc species to provide alkyne as a 90:10 mixture of epimers. Alkyne provided diol upon elimination of PMB (*p*-methoxybenzyl) group, selective acetylation [78], and desilylation. The carboxylic acid was formed when diol was exposed to HIO_4 and CrO_3 [79] in aqueous acetone. The formed carboxylic acid was then condensed with dimethyl 2-(4-methoxybenzylamino)malonate [80] through the formation of acid chloride. During the purification by column chromatography on silica gel, amide was partially cyclized to afford an inseparable 72:28 mixture. The amide was completely transformed into acetate to provide quantitative yield when this mixture was treated with a catalytic amount of $In(OTf)_3$ at reflux in PhMe. There was no significant loss of enantiomeric purity of substrate in this process. Under mild lipase-catalyzed reaction conditions, the acetoxy group was hydrolyzed to afford an alcohol as acetate was very labile under basic conditions, then the formed alcohol was oxidized to aldehyde. Aldehyde was subjected to acetal-mediated cationic cyclization for the assembly of C3 quaternary center. The selenium derivative was obtained upon treating aldehyde with $AgBF_4$ and phenylselenenyl bromide in benzyl alcohol, selenium derivative underwent radical deselenenylation to provide deselenium derivative. There was an excellent discrimination of geminal esters upon reduction of deselenium derivative with sodium borohydride, and aldehyde was formed as sole product after oxidation with DMP (Dess-Martin periodinane). A single stereoisomer was generated when aldehyde was reacted with cyclohex-2-enylzinc chloride. Removal of PMB (*p*-methoxybenzyl) group provided product, which was subjected to reductive ring-opening with cyclic acetal to give known intermediate. Finally, the dealkylative cleavage of methyl ester was promoted with $(Me_2AlTeMe)_2$, then β-lactonization and chlorination of intermediate furnished (-)-salinosporamide A [81].

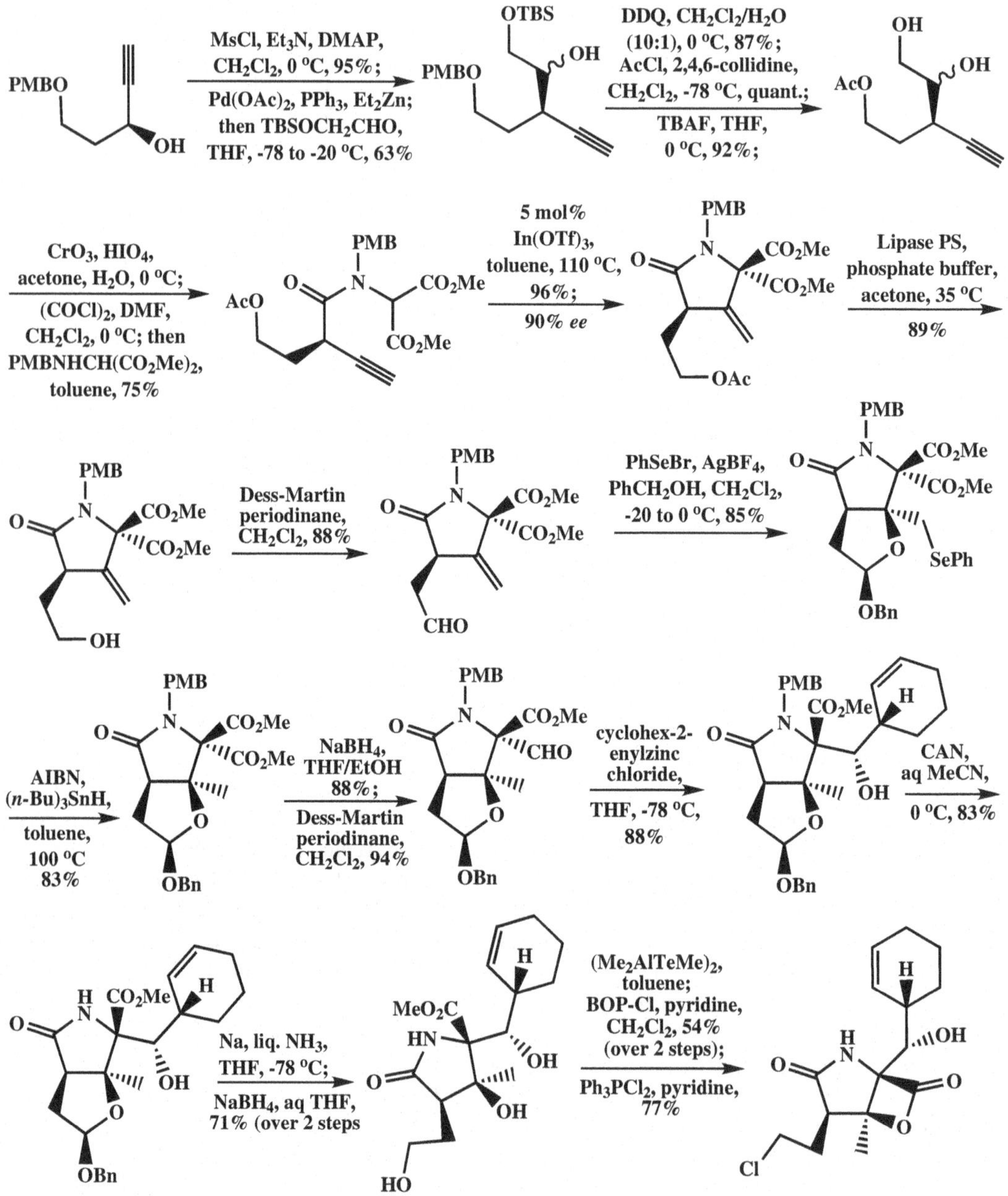

Scheme-24

3.5 Synthesis of five-membered heterocycles fused with five-membered heterocycles

The tandem 1,4-additions which involved the formation of two carbon-nitrogen bonds occurred with amides of alkadienoic acids. The length of tether between amide group and conjugated unsaturation was varied for the production of pyrrolizidine **(Scheme 25)** [82].

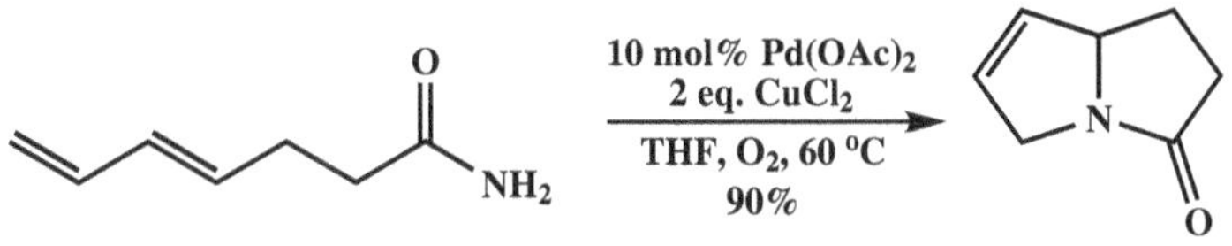

Scheme-25

Indolizidines and pyrrolizidines are alkaloid derivatives with useful biological activity. The indolizidines and pyrrolizidines were synthesized from nitro-diketones having two carbonyl groups. The addition of nitro-ketone to vinyl ketone afforded nitro-diketone in the presence of Bu₃P **(Scheme 26)** [83]. A mixture of stereoisomeric pyrrolizidines was obtained, whose diastereomeric composition depends on the reducing system, upon reduction of nitro-diketone [84].

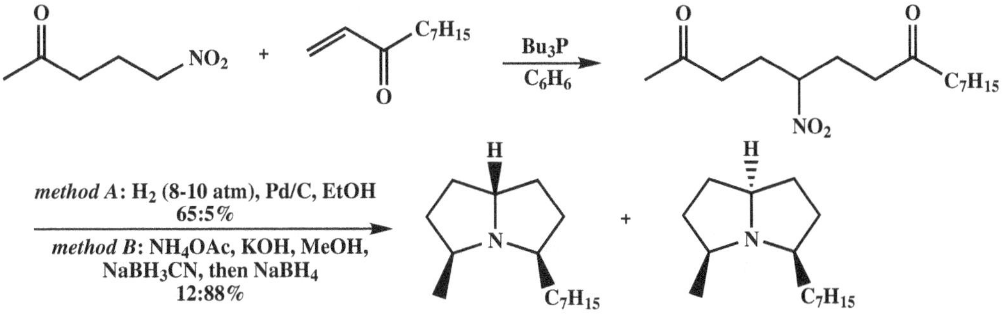

Scheme-26

The mitosenes (a large class of anti-neoplastic and anti-biotic pyrroloindoloquinones) were synthesized from bis(allylamino)benzoquinone *via* tandem oxidative cyclization/olefin insertion reaction in the presence of PdCl₂(MeCN)₂/benzoquinone catalytic system **(Scheme 27)** [85]. The reaction proceeded *via* primary alkylpalladium intermediate through sequential elimination/ addition of a hydridopalladium species [33].

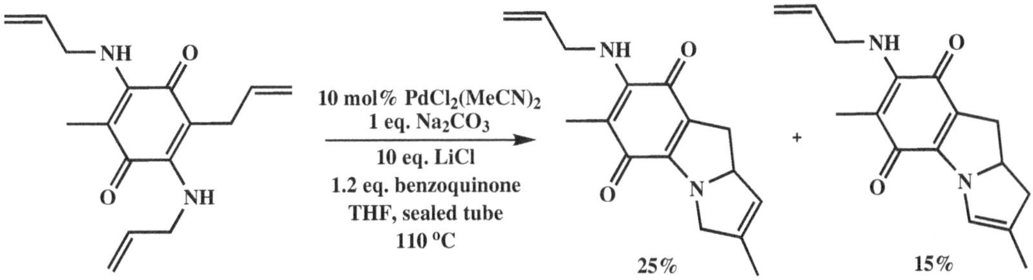

Scheme-27

The synthesis of pyrrolizidines could be achieved in a two-step procedure from 1,2-oxazines. In the first step hydrogenolysis of different substituted 1,2-oxazines with hydrogen/Pd on charcoal led to pyrrolizidinone derivatives. Subsequent treatment of pyrrolizidinone derivatives with borane dimethylsulfide complex at rt furnished expected pyrrolizines in good yields **(Scheme 28)** [86-90].

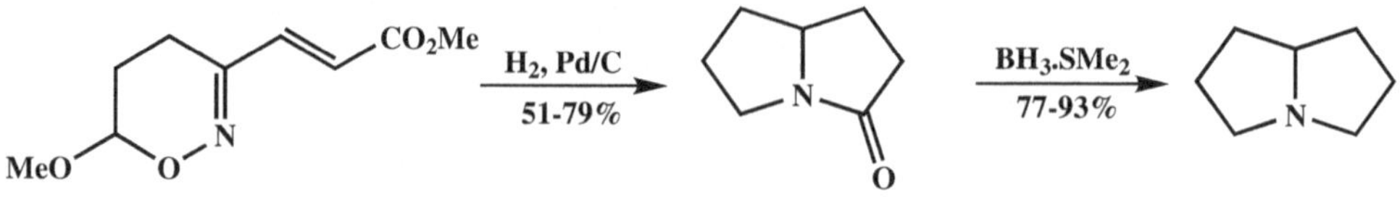

Scheme-28

The desymmetrization of cyclic *meso*-2-methyl-2-propargyl-1,3-cyclohexane-diols and 1,3-diones was accomplished in the presence of palladium(II)-complex containing chiral bis(oxazoline) ligands by first asymmetric variant of a palladium-catalyzed alkoxylation-methoxycarbonylation. The asymmetric palladium(II)-catalyzed cyclization of allylanilines and allylphenols was carried out using chiral bis(oxazolines) based on a biphenyl or binaphthyl backbone. The asymmetric cyclization of aminoalkenes, alkenyl alcohols, and alkenoic acids was performed with spiro bis(isoxazolines). Dohanosova and co-workers [91] described the asymmetric intramolecular amido and alkoxylactonization of amino alcohols and alkene-1,3-diols employing palladium acetate-{2,20-methylenebis[(4R,5S)-4,5-diphenyl-2-oxazoline] and palladium acetate-{(R,S)-indabox}, respectively **(Scheme 29)**.

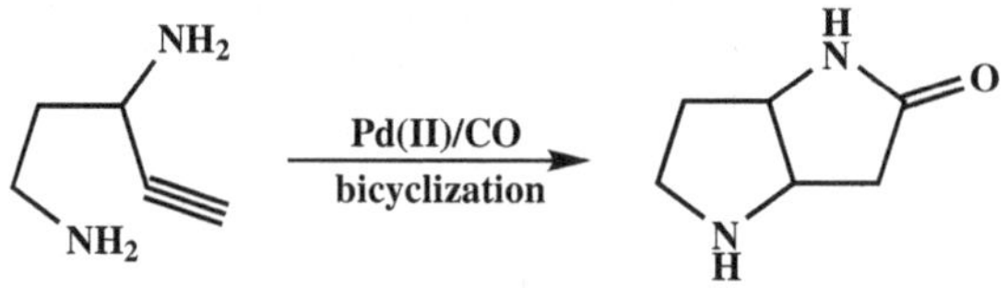

Scheme-29

The exact mechanism of this transformation was the subject of much debate, although many reports proposed a palladium(II)/palladium(IV) catalytic pathway under these oxidizing conditions. For example, Muniz [92] reported the intramolecular diamination of olefins under similar conditions to those for diacetoxylation **(Scheme 30)**. An initial intramolecular aminopalladation of olefin provided Pd-C-species, which then underwent nucleophilic substitution by other amine to give diaminated product. Muniz proposed that Pd-C-species was oxidized to palladium(IV) species under these highly oxidizing conditions prior to substitution by second amine. This suggestion was supported by the observation that no diaminated product was observed in a stoichiometric example in the absence of iodobenzene diacetate.

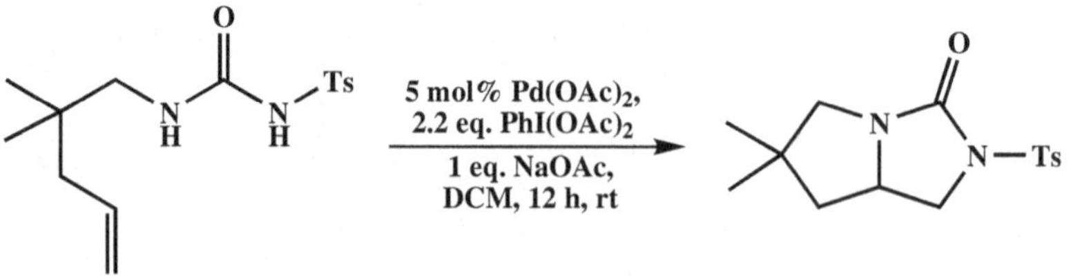

Scheme-30

A catalytic diamination of alkenes was conducted using Pd(IV) catalysis [92]. Initially, the intramolecular vicinal alkene oxidation occurred in the presence of robust tosyl ureas (nitrogen source). The most effective oxidants were hypervalent iodine oxidants, like iodobenzene diacetate. This method was utilized for the preparation of a number of five- and six-membered-ring annelation products of cyclic ureas. The example of diastereoselective alkene diamination is shown in **Scheme 31**. There was a *syn* aminopalladation followed by *anti* alkyl-nitrogen bond formation from a palladium(IV) intermediate. This mechanism was also proposed for related aminoacetoxylation reactions reported by Liu and Stahl [35]. The theoretical calculations have confirmed the involvement of a palladium(IV) catalyst state resulting from the oxidation of *s*-alkyl Pd intermediate produced by aminopalladation [20, 93-95].

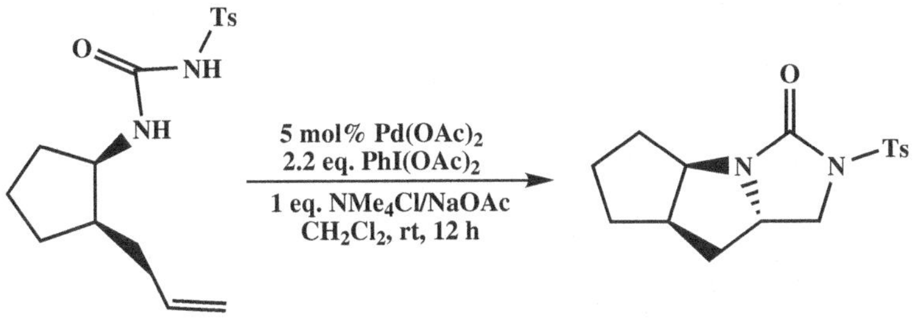

Scheme-31

Three different protocols, involving palladium-catalyzed alkene diamination reactions, were developed for the formation of five-membered cyclic ureas. The heteropalladation proceeded in a *syn*- rather than *anti*-fashion, and the reductive elimination occurred with intramolecular formation of a carbon-nitrogen bond rather than intermolecular formation of a carbon-oxygen bond. The bisindolines **(Scheme 32)** [96-98] and bicyclic guanidines **(Scheme 33)** [99-100] were produced by alkene diamination reactions.

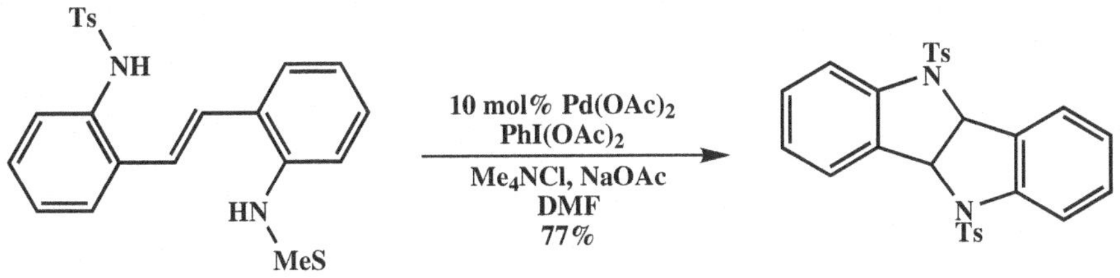

Scheme-32

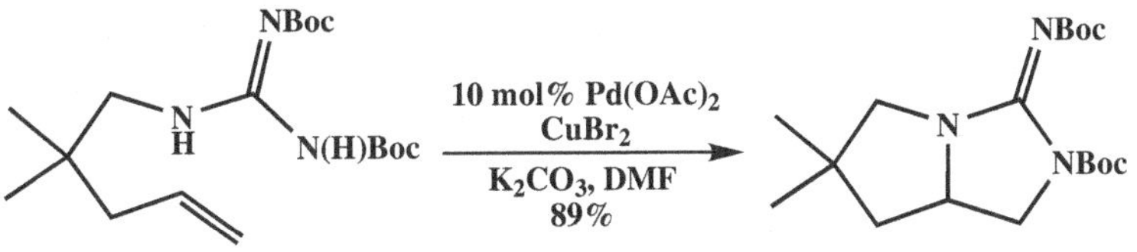

Scheme-33

In addition, intramolecular aminopalladation process has been demonstrated as a preferred route for the synthesis of valuable nitrogen heterocycles. For example, intramolecular alkene diamination **(Scheme 34)**, chloroamination, [101] and hetero-Heck-type transformations [102] have appeared in literature for the synthesis of a plethora of valuable nitrogen-containing structures [95].

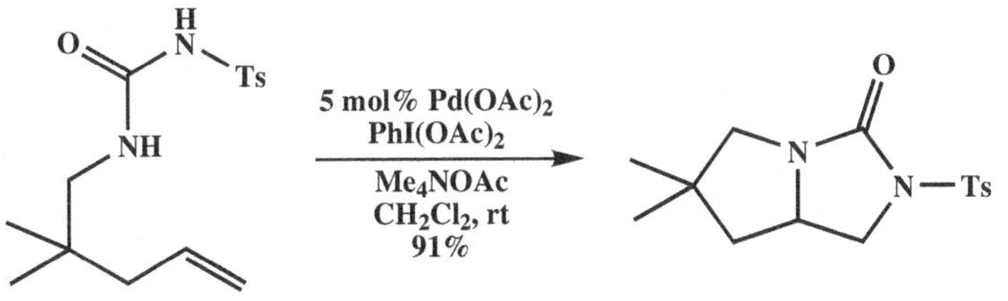

Scheme-34

Fused bis(heterocycles) were prepared by alkene aminopalladation/carbonylation [103]. This pathway was utilized for the synthesis of 1,4-iminoglycitols, and Geissman-Waiss lactone. The Geissman-Waiss lactone was employed as a key intermediate for the construction of necine bases. Lactones were provided upon aminocarbonylation of *N*-(3-hydroxy-4-pentenyl)-substituted carbamates, tosylamides, and ureas with palladium chloride/cupric chloride in acetic acid **(Scheme 35)** [33, 104-105].

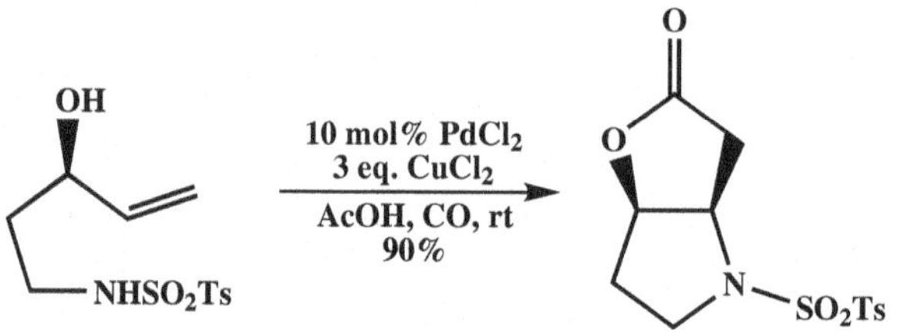

Scheme-35

3.6   Synthesis of five-membered heterocycles fused with six-membered heterocycles

A number of KDR kinase inhibitors were synthesized by this method. The intramolecular amination preceded the intermolecular Suzuki coupling although no reaction intermediates were detected [106]. The modular nature of this method makes it particularly effective for such preparations. A variety of analogues were synthesized rapidly by simple variation of Suzuki coupling partner [107]. Same group extended this chemistry to show that thiophene- and pyridine-derived substrates could be employed **(Scheme 36)** [108]. A variety of 5-, 6- and 7-azaindoles, as well as thienopyrroles, were prepared in good yields from *gem*-dichloro substrates under reaction conditions almost identical to those employed for parent indole. The *N*-protecting groups were utilized to modify the parent system to achieve high yields. Preparation of regioisomeric 4-azaindoles was more challenging and needed *N*-oxide substrates [109].

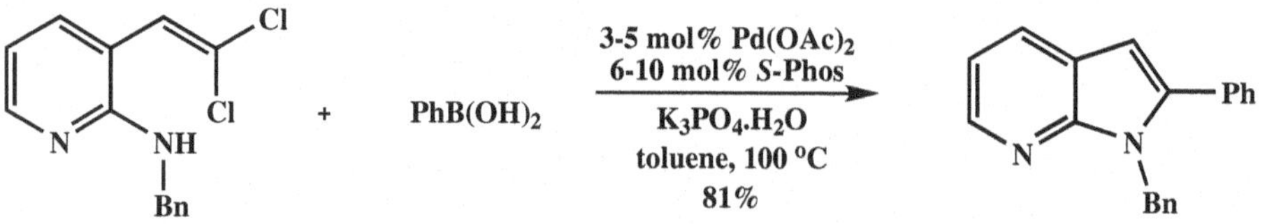

Scheme-36

Berteina-Raboin and co-workers [110] synthesized indole skeleton of new melatoninergic analogs under solid-phase in association with MWI. This combined use speeded up the reactions. Bedeschi and co-workers [111] reported the reaction of resin-bound *o*-iodoaniline (ester linkage) and a terminal alkyne for the production of 2-subtituted indoles. Five-, six- and seven-azaindoles were obtained in low to good yields (5-78%) (depending upon the substituents present on alkyne) from *o*-iodoaminopyridines *via* Pd-catalyzed heteroannulation employing trimethylsilylalkynes [112]. The 7-azaindoles were synthesized as shown in **Scheme 37** [113].

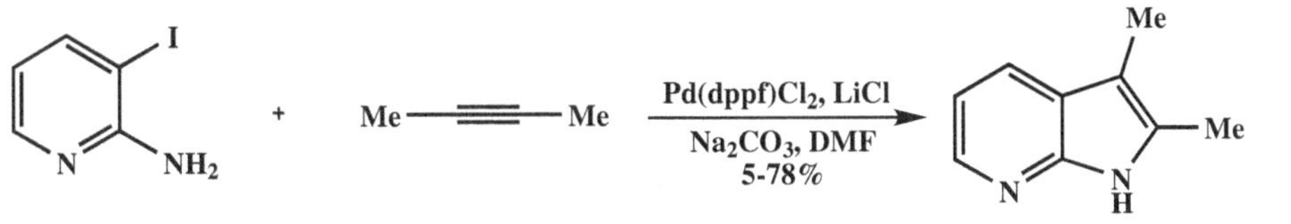

Scheme-37

The 3-(arylmethylene)isoindolin-1-ones were prepared from ynamines in two palladium(0)-catalyzed steps, a Heck and a Suzuki-Miyaura reaction. Heck reaction was general as ynamines were converted into 3-(arylmethylene)isoindolin-1-ones in good yields **(Scheme 38)** [114-115]. The efficient stereoselective synthesis of (*E*)-cyclic enamines, particularly (*E*)-3-(arymethylene) isoindolin-1-ones, was carried out from ynamines using a HSM cascade reaction in the presence of palladium(0) catalyst [116].

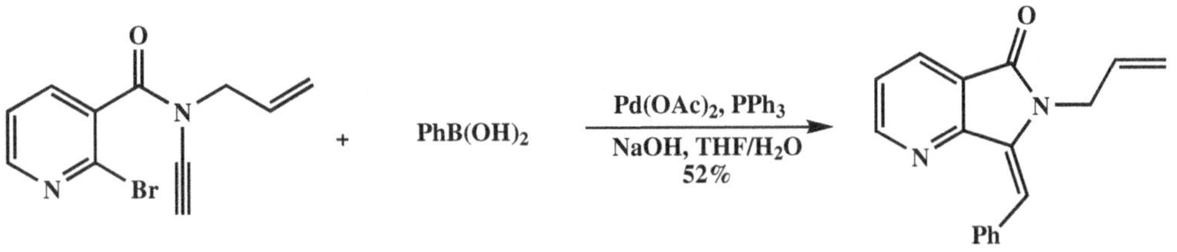

Scheme-38

Wipf and Maciejewski [117] observed the formation of epoxide tethered to substituted aminopyridine from allyl carbamate. The 3,3-disubstituted azaindoline was produced from epoxide in the presence of manganese metal- and titanocene dichloride-promoted radical annulation **(Scheme 39)** [26].

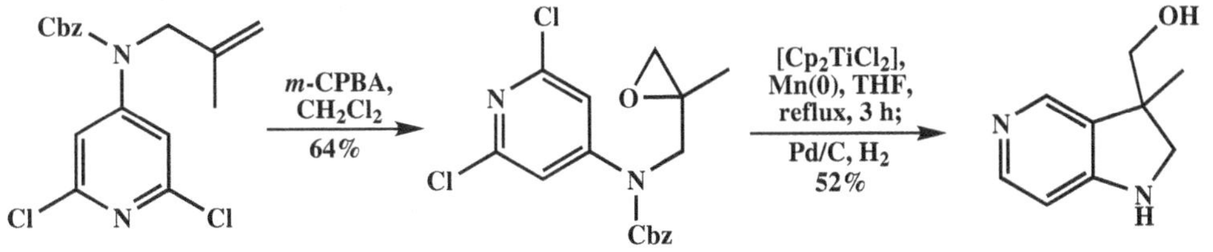

Scheme-39

The reaction of substituted 2-chloroanilines with acyclic or cyclic ketones was reported for the direct preparation of polyfunctionalized indoles by this simple, broad, mild, new, and efficient protocol **(Scheme 40)** [118].

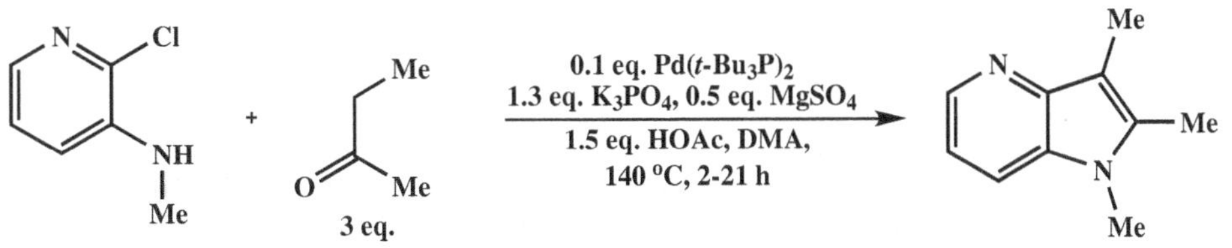

Scheme-40

Grimaud et al. [119] employed allylamine as amine component in Ugi reaction for the formation of indoles by Ugi-Smiles reaction coupled with Heck cyclization **(Scheme 41)** [26].

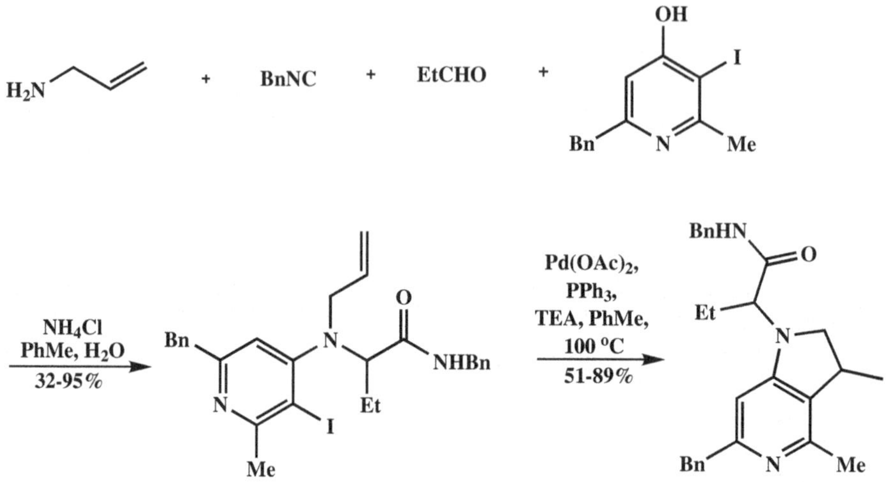

Scheme-41

Jorgensen et al. [120] transformed the primary allylamines into aza-indoles by this novel one-flask approach, through sequential aryl amination and Heck cyclization reactions with single catalyst **(Scheme 42)** [26].

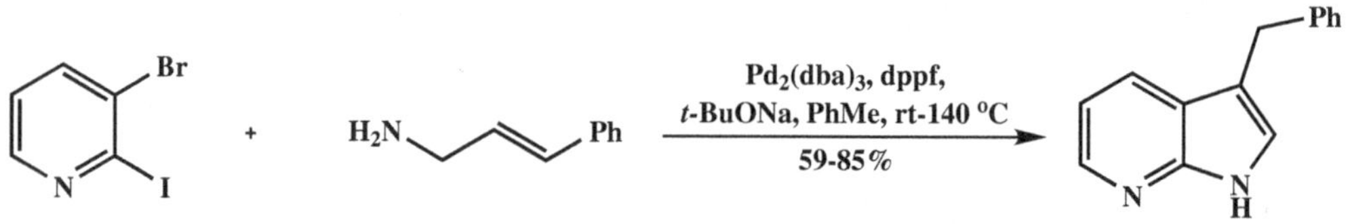

Scheme-42

The 2-(1-hydroxyallyl)-3-aminopyridines were utilized for the preparation of 1*H*-pyrrolo[3,2-*b*] pyridines **(Scheme 43)** [121]. The final products were obtained by protection of hydroxyl group with *tert*-butyldimethylsilyl group followed by treatment with palladium(II)/benzoquinone.

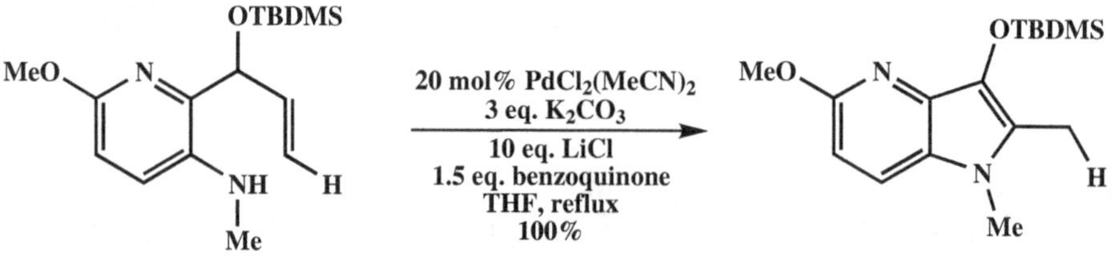

Scheme-43

The indolizidine skeletons were synthesized efficiently by cycloisomerization of alkynyl *N*-acyl enamines with Pd catalyst [122]. The quinolizidines were prepared through iminium ion species by cationic cyclization of alkynyl *N*-acyl enamines in HCO_2H. On the other hand, good to excellent yields of indolizidines were obtained when alkynyl *N*-acyl enamines were reacted in the presence of a ligand such as *N,N*-bis-(benzylidene)ethylene-diamine (BBEDA) or PPh₃, palladium catalyst like palladium acetate and Pd₂(dba)₃ in CH₃COOH. The palladium acetate exerted an excellent control on the stereochemistry of newly forming exocyclic double bond (afforded only one stereoisomer) and *N,N*-bis-(benzylidene)ethylene-diamine was a better ligand than PPh₃ **(Scheme 44)** [123].

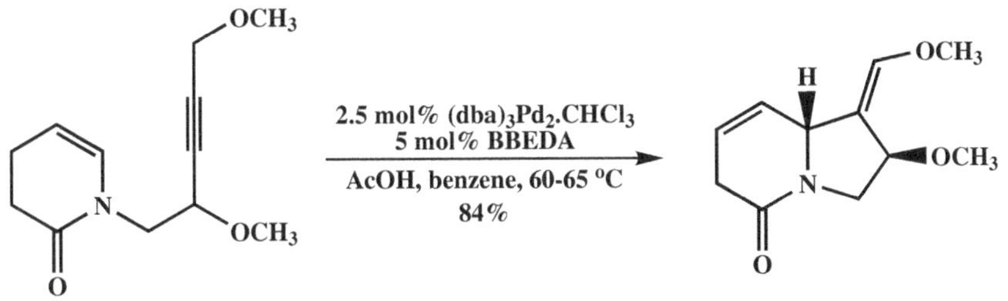

Scheme-44

The development of reactions which employed easily accessible substrates to afford the densely substituted pyrroloheterocycles is in high demand [124]. These protocols were general with respect to heterocyclic core but these were limited to the preparation of 1,2- or 1,3-disubstituted indolizines, while either the C-3 or C-2 position remained unfunctionalized. By using stoichiometric amounts of iodine [125] followed by cross-coupling steps, this drawback was mitigated. The 1,2,3-trisubstituted *N*-fused heterocyclic compounds were formed in good to excellent yields by a palladium-catalyzed two-component arylation/cyclization cascade protocol [126]. The indolizine was formed when Ph-Pd-X species underwent carbopalladation of propargylic moiety with subsequent 5-*endo-dig* cyclization. The readily available propargyl-possessing pyridine was subjected to Pd-catalyzed arylation/cyclization reaction. The indolizine was synthesized in 49% yield using iodobenzene as electrophilic component. The substitution of dimethylformamide with other solvents was not successful. The reaction yields were improved significantly employing different ammonium and lithium salts. The replacement of base from triethylamine to potassium carbonate was also beneficial **(Scheme 45)** [127-128].

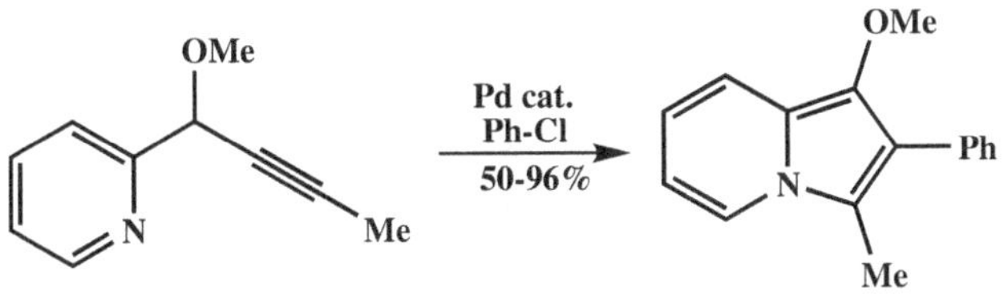

Scheme-45

This method was applied for the preparation of functionalized indolizidine derivatives from iodoalkane **(Scheme 46)** [129]. Spirooxindoles served as key intermediates for the synthesis of (-)-physostigmine, (-)-eptazocine, halenaquinol [130] and indolizidine alkaloids [123, 131-132].

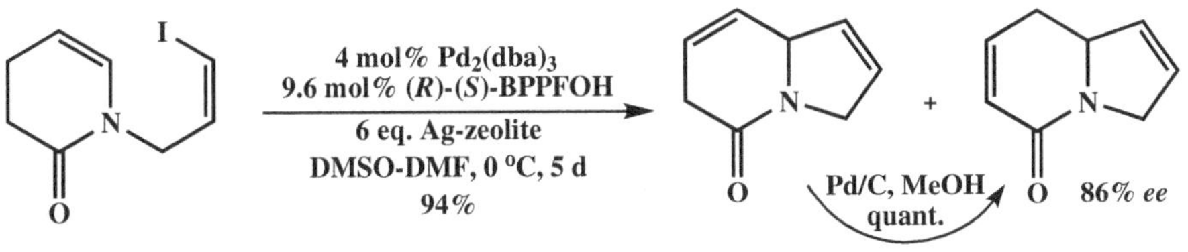

Scheme-46

2-Nitro-ketones underwent conjugate additions under milder conditions as compared to nitroalkanes due to the enhanced acidity of C-2 hydrogen atom. An adduct was formed when 2-nitrocyclohexanone was reacted with unsaturated ketone in triphenylphosphine **(Scheme 47)** [133]. In adduct the cyclohexanone moiety suffered a fast base-catalyzed retro-Claisen ring-opening and provided open-chain NO_2 derivative which was reduced chemoselectively to afford *cis*-pyrrolidine. The *cis*-pyrrolidine was a central intermediate for the preparation of indolizidine alkaloid monomorine I, a trail pheromone of Pharaoh Ant, and other similar biologically active substances [84, 134].

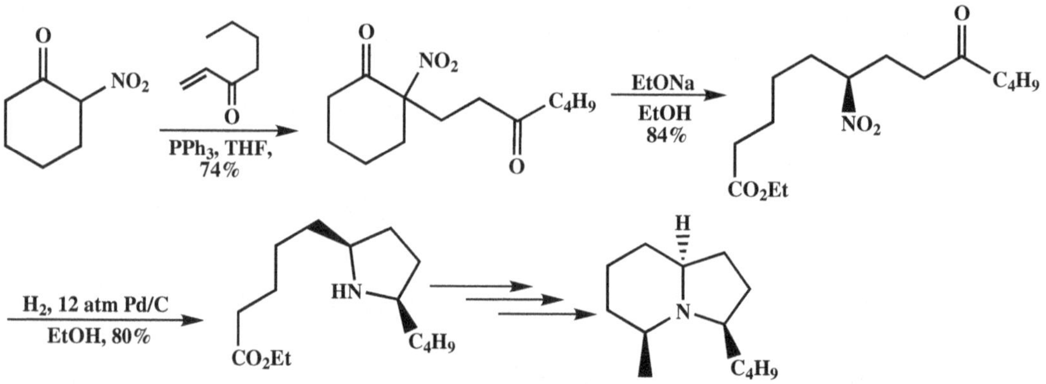

Scheme-47

The use of propargylic phenylethers was investigated in this conversion **(Scheme 48)**. In this process the bromobenzenes worked equally well. The indolizine was formed in 73% yield by cascade cyclization of propargylic silylether. This Pd-catalyzed arylation/cyclization reaction occurred upon coordination of triple bond of an alkyne with PhPdX which triggered the 5-*endo-dig* cyclization by nucleophilic attack of pyridyl nitrogen and afforded zwitterionic adduct. The zwitterionic adduct underwent deprotonation/tautomerization and subsequent reductive elimination to afford the product [135-137].

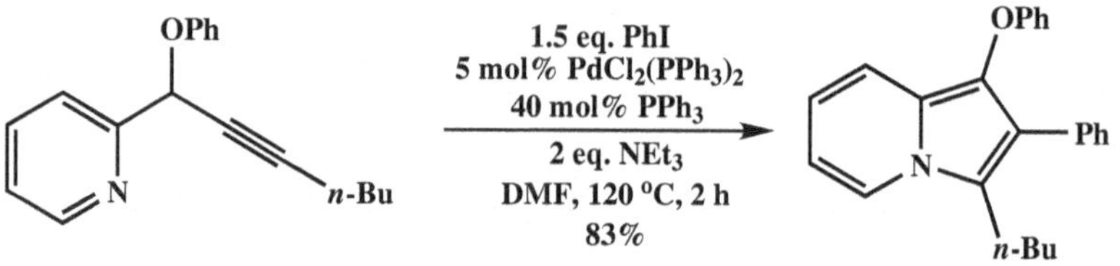

Scheme-48

Cycloaddition reaction represented an attractive approach for accessing azabicyclic frameworks, as several bonds and stereocenters can be generated in a single step during ring formation. For example, the synthesis of functionalized indolizidine **(Scheme 49)** was achieved through intermolecular [3+2] nitrone cycloaddition reactions of a dienophile with either nitrone substrates [138].

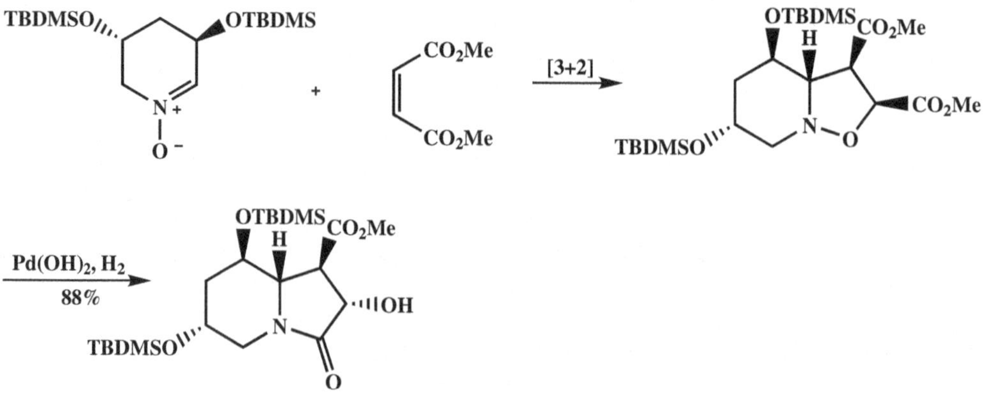

Scheme-49

The absolute stereochemistry of product was determined during carbon-nitrogen bond forming step. However, the palladium/Siphos-PE system was different from bidentate phosphine ligands (*e.g.*, dpe-phos or 1,4-bis(diphenylphosphino)butane) used for the synthesis of racemic pyrrolidines [40a-b, 52, 139]. As shown in **Scheme 50**, coupling of deuterated substrate and bromobenzene provided pyrrolidine product, which resulted from suprafacial addition of alkene into palladium-nitrogen and suggested that both asymmetric and nonasymmetric variants of carboamination reaction proceeded through similar pathways. The stereochemistry of pyrrolidine was established by conversion to known compound [140].

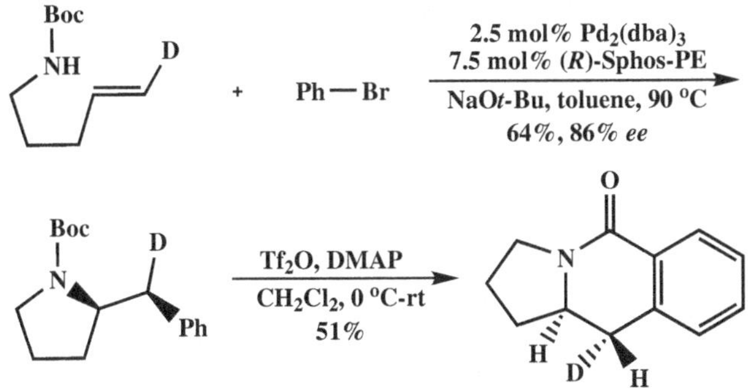

Scheme-50

Several different solvents, such as dimethylformamide, acetonitrile, 1,4-dioxane and tetrahydrofuran, have been employed in Heck reaction as they were able to weakly coordinate with Pd complex, increasing its stability [141]. Dimethylsulphoxide, benzene and PhMe have also been used in controlling both the regioselectivity and stereoselectivity in a number of processes [142-143]. The importance of solvent choice in enantioselective Pd-catalyzed transformations was demonstrated by Sulikowski and co-workers [144] where the use of tetrahydrofuran afforded indolizidine, however when the reaction was carried out in dimethylformamide, the desired asymmetric enamide was major product **(Scheme 51)**.

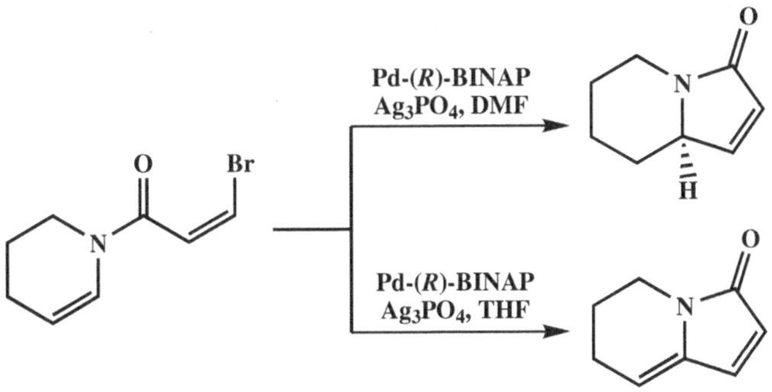

Scheme-51

The Pd-catalyzed carbonylative cyclization/arylation was an efficient method for the construction of densely substituted 2-aroylindolizines. The conversion occurred *via* 5-*endo-dig* cyclization of 2-propargylpyridine triggered by an aroyl palladium complex to afford good to excellent yields of diversely substituted 2-aroylindolizines **(Scheme 52)** [145].

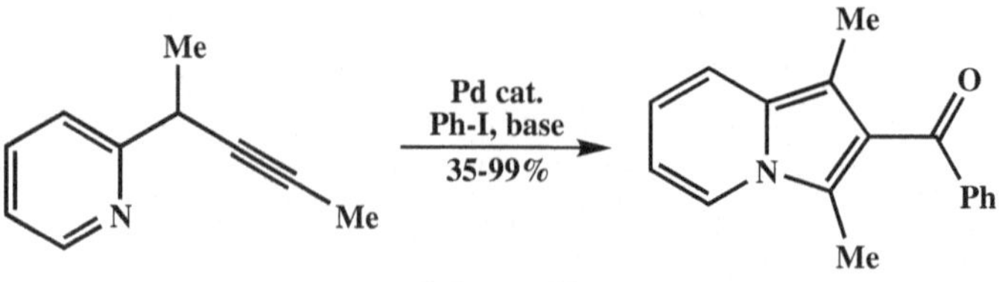

Scheme-52

A number of *N*-fused pyrroloheterocycles were synthesized by an efficient two-component arylation/cyclization cascade protocol in the presence of Pd catalyst. This conversion occurred through the coupling of aryl halides with propargylic ethers or esters with Pd catalyst followed by 5-*endo-dig* cyclization to provide highly functionalized pyrroloheterocycles in good to excellent yield **(Scheme 53)** [146-150].

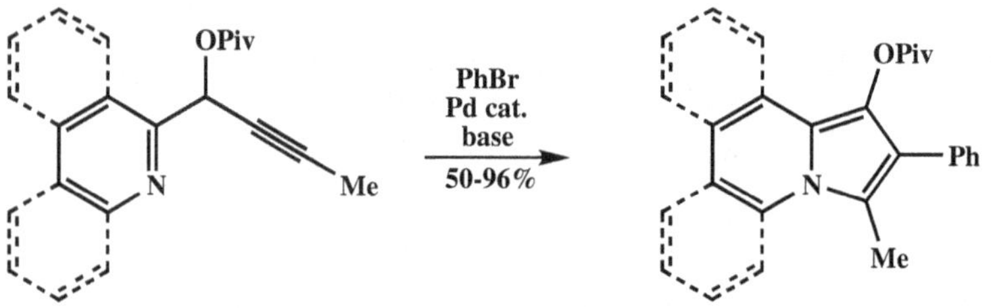

Scheme-53

The phenanthroindolizidine alkaloid tylophorine possess anti-viral and anti-tumor activities [151-154]. The preparation of tylophorine was carried out to establish the absolute configuration of pyrrolidine products and demonstrated the applicability of enantioselective carboamination reaction **(Scheme 54)**. For the synthesis of (±)-tylophorine an analogous route was developed by Herr [155]. The aryl bromide was synthesized in four steps, and then the aryl bromide was coupled with starting substrate in the presence of palladium/Siphos-PE system to provide 88% *ee* and 69% yield. The de-protection of Boc protecting group followed by treatment with refluxing formalin resulted in the transformation of intermediate into tylophorine in two steps [40a-b].

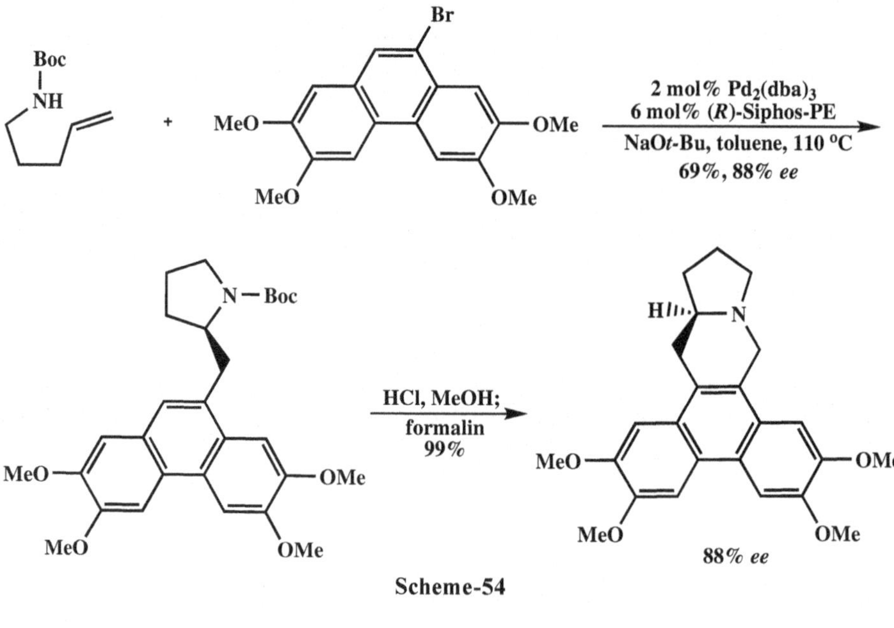

Scheme-54

Muller et al. [156] described a three-component coupling-[3+2] sequence in which alkynone was formed and after that 1-(2-oxoethyl)pyridinium bromides were added to reaction mixture for the construction of pyridinium ylides which reacted as allyl type 1,3-dipoles after oxidative aromatization to afford highly fluorescent indolizines **(Scheme 55)**. The indolizines were formed in 41-59% yield at rt after 14 h when (hetero)aroyl chlorides were reacted with terminal alkynes under Sonogashira coupling reaction conditions in a mixture of TEA and tetrahydrofuran and then adding 1-(2-oxoethyl)pyridinium bromides after 2 h at ambient temperature [84]. A cross-coupling and a sequential cycloaddition were combined to afford a variety of indolizines. The 7-(pyridin-4-yl)-substituted compounds displayed pronounced fluorescence and in their protonated form they showed even strong daylight fluorescence. The fluorescence sensitivity of protonation as well as its reversibility in weakly acidic media render 7-(pyridin-4-yl)indolizines ideal candidates for studying p*H*-alternating cellular processes and p*H*-dependent and for fluorescence labeling [157-159].

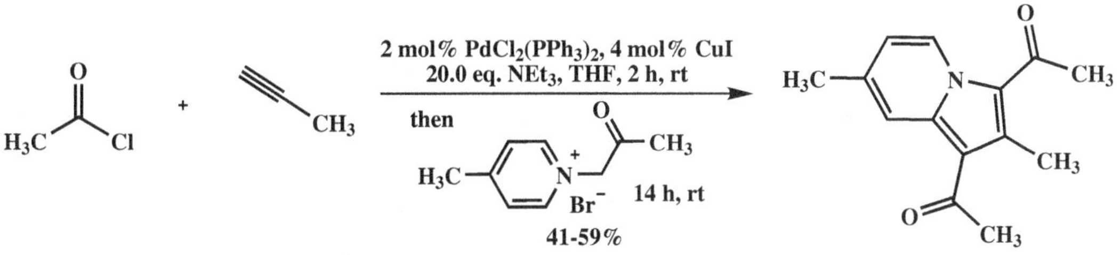

Scheme-55

The lepadiformine and cylindricine alkaloids contain a tricyclic pyrroloquinoline derivative. Tanner and co-workers [160] synthesized tricyclic pyrroloquinoline derivative in a single operation through a transannular Mannich reaction which involved a macrocyclic diketoamine. The macrocyclic diketoamine was formed from *N*-Boc-allylamine as depicted in **Scheme 56** [26].

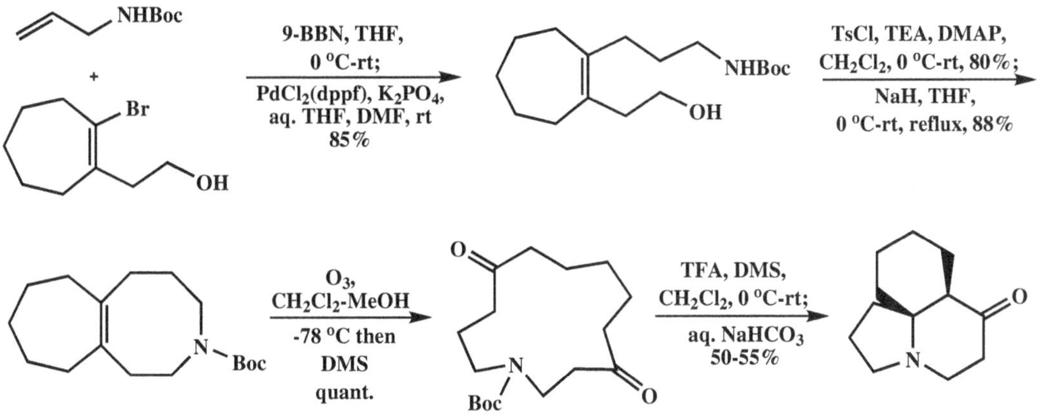

Scheme-56

The 2-substituted indoles were synthesized from functionalized 2-alkynylanilines. The heterocyclic core of marine alkaloid hinckdentine A was also synthesized by this base mediated reaction. The reaction was successfully conducted under solid-phase conditions. The indole was prepared on solid-phase as shown in **Scheme 57** [161].

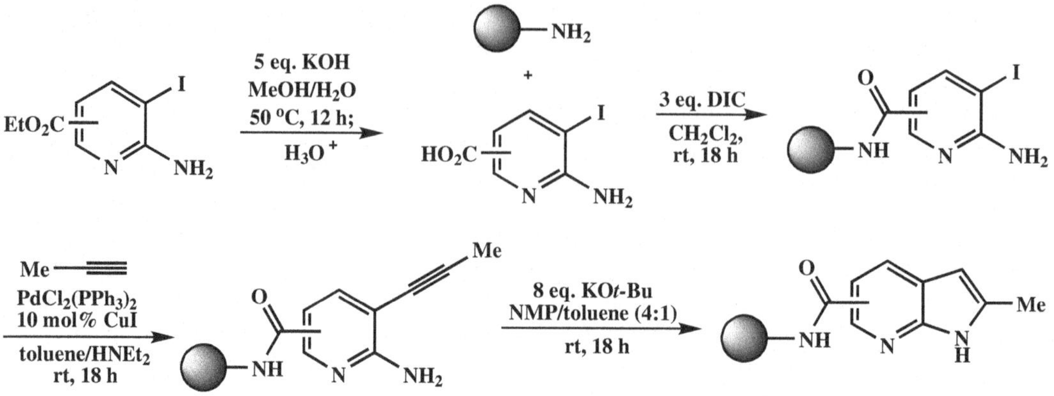

Scheme-57

The isocryptolepine was produced by a coupling in which two tethered pyridine moieties were utilized as model compounds **(Scheme 58)** [162]. The direct arylation with pyridyl chloride proceeded in 52% yield.

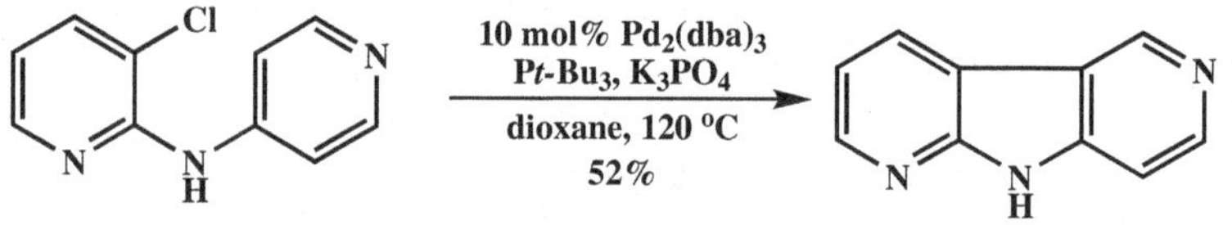

Scheme-58

Comins [163-165] synthesized camptothecin in final step *via* an intramolecular Pd-catalyzed cyclization **(Scheme 59)**. Subsequently, this strategy was employed in the preparation of camptothecin analogue [166] and also for the formation of many homocamptothecin analogues [167-168].

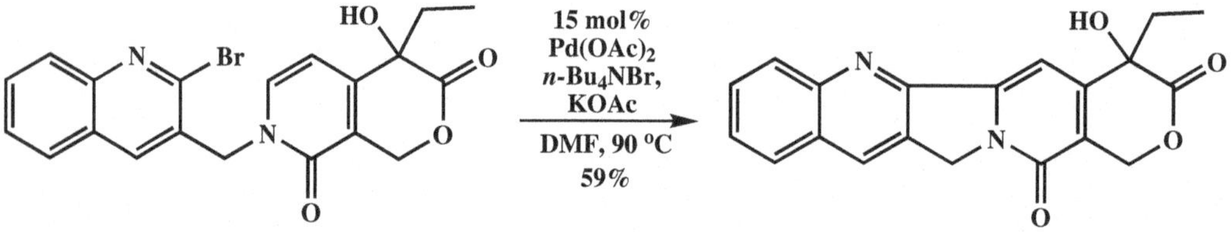

Scheme-59

Wani and Wall [169] in 1966 discovered camptothecin which acts as a cytotoxic pentacyclic quinoline alkaloid and screened natural products for anti-cancer activity. The stem and bark of *Camptotheca acuminata* (tree native to China) contain natural product. CPT possessed anti-cancer activity which stabilized and targeted the covalent binary complex produced between topoisomerase I and DNA during DNA relaxation, leading to aptosis [170-172]. Medicinal and synthetic chemists have developed many methods for the preparation of camptothecin and many derivatives because of their promising bioactivity [173-174]. Methods for the synthesis of CPT have some limitations such as long steps and difficult operations which render these syntheses impractical for large scale synthesis. The preparation of multiple carbon-carbon bonds in one operation was attractive pathway for the synthesis of complex molecular architectures. Yao and co-workers [175] developed an efficient and very short cascade pathway for this class of alkaloids and analogues. The tetracyclic A/B/C/D ring core of CPT-family alkaloids was synthesized in high yield in the presence of a mild Hendrickson-reagent which involved an imidate formation, an intramolecular aza-Diels-Alder reaction, and an eliminative aromatization. The camptothecin was synthesized from chloropyridine **(Scheme 60)** which was carbonylated under carbon monoxide atmosphere to produce methyl ester in 97% yield. The *N*-propargyl pyridone was obtained in 67% yield upon selective *O*-demethylation of methyl ester with iodotrimethylsilane, followed by *N*-propargylation of resulting pyridone with potassium carbonate, propargyl bromide, lithium bromide, and TBAB in PhMe. The key amide precursor (90% overall) was provided upon transformation of methyl ester into acyl chloride, followed by coupling with aniline. The advanced intermediate possessing A/B/C/D-ring core of CPT was formed in 96% yield when amide was treated with reagent (1.5 eq. Tf_2O and 3 eq. triphenylphosphine oxide and manganese(IV) oxide) at rt. The camptothecin was provided in 95% *ee* and 83% yield through a highly enantioselective Sharpless asymmetric dihydroxylation and an iodine/calcium carbonate-based hemiacetal oxidation [176].

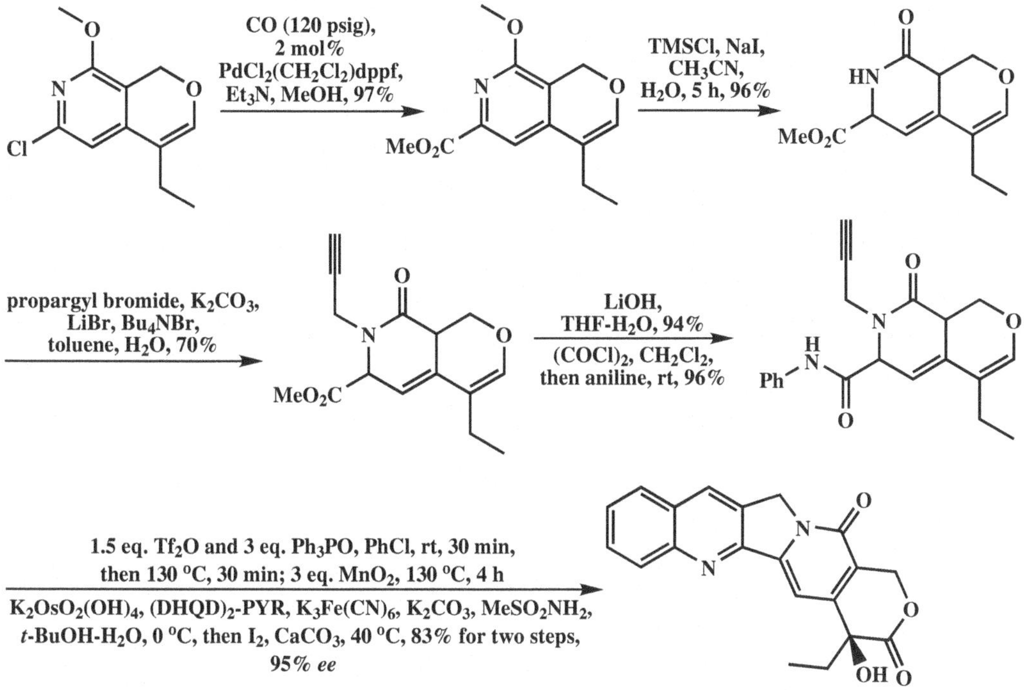

Scheme-60

Comins's [177] approach for the construction of camptothecin was also applied for the preparation of many natural products such as luotonin A and B, mappicine, and rutaecarpine [178-180]. A camptothecin-like alkaloid, 22-hydroxyacuminatine was also synthesized employing this similar pathway. The cyclization occurred to afford desired 22-hydroxyacuminatine in 96% yield **(Scheme 61)** [181-190].

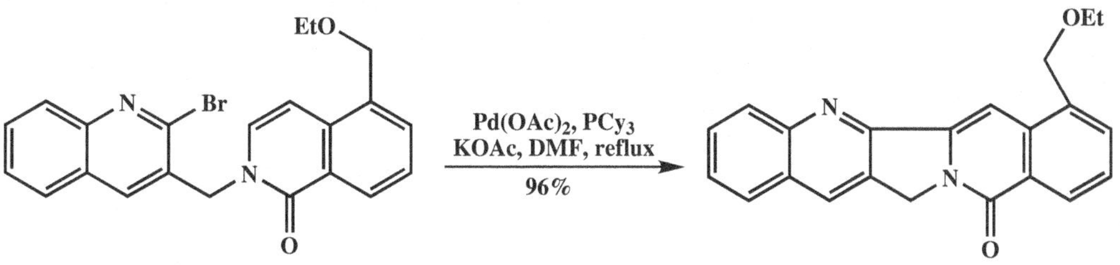

Scheme-61

Sasai et al. [191] have reported a highly enantioselective aminocarbonylation reaction for the synthesis of bicyclic β-amino acid. A catalyst system of $[Pd(MeCN)_4](BF_4)_2$ and spiro bisisoxazoline ligand were effective for the conversion of starting compound into piperazine derivative in 89% yield and 88% *ee* **(Scheme 62)**. The authors proposed a mechanism that involved coordination of alkene and nucleophilic attack to generate alkylpalladium complex. Carbon monoxide insertion provided acylpalladium intermediate, in which ring closure *via* nucleophilic trapping of acylpalladium intermediate by tethered tosylamide yielded piperazine derivative and palladium(0), which was reoxidized by benzoquinone to regenerate the palladium(II) catalyst. However, the reaction required low temperatures and long reaction times (7 d), there was potential for other spiro bisisoxazoline ligands to be employed as effective ligands for enantioselective oxidative cyclization reactions.

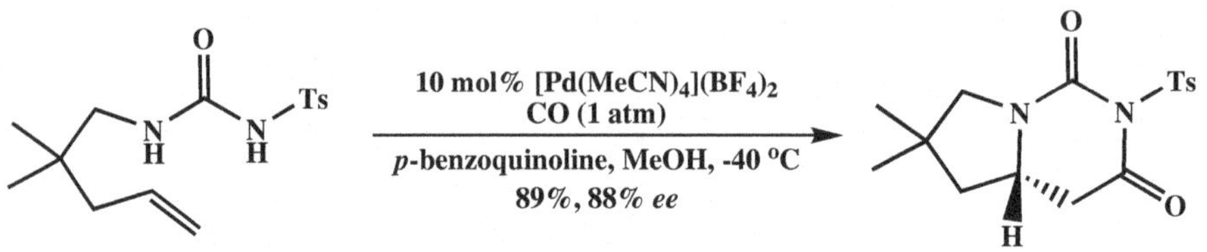

Scheme-62

Carbon monoxide insertion into intermediate aminopalladium adducts provided an intriguing entry to functionalized nitrogen heterocycles. Tamaru [192-194] has shown that *N*-tosyl protected alkene substrate cyclized to afford pyrrolidine, with reaction proceeding through a nucleophilic attack of heteroatom onto palladium-activated olefin **(Scheme 63)**. Upon nucleophilic attack and loss of hydrogen chloride, insertion of carbon monoxide occurred into palladium-carbon bond to afford intermediate, which upon methanolysis afforded pyrrolidine. It was important to note that heteroatom and metal add *anti* across the olefin, which has important consequences with regard to the mechanism of reaction. This reaction was very useful for the synthesis of pyrrolidines but was limited to the preparation of molecules bearing an ester group in Cl′ position [195-197].

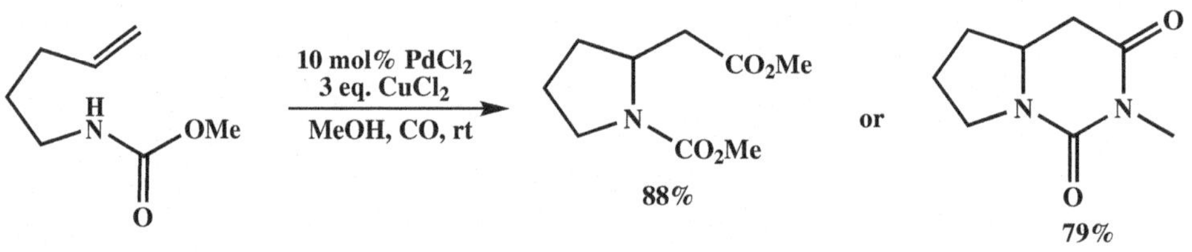

Scheme-63

The bis-alkynylpyrimidines underwent double cycloisomerization-reduction for the synthesis of tricyclic alkaloids. The dibromopyrimidines through regioselective sequential Sonogashira coupling produced bis-alkynylpyrimidines. The tricyclic heteroaromatic cores were formed from bis-alkynylpyrimidines *via* copper(I) assisted double cycloisomerization reaction. The highly diastereoselective total synthesis of (±)-tetraponerine T6 and its analogues was carried out by hydrogenation of bis-pyrrolopyrimidines with PtO$_2$ catalyst in acidic media, followed by reduction with lithium aluminium hydride **(Scheme 64)** [198].

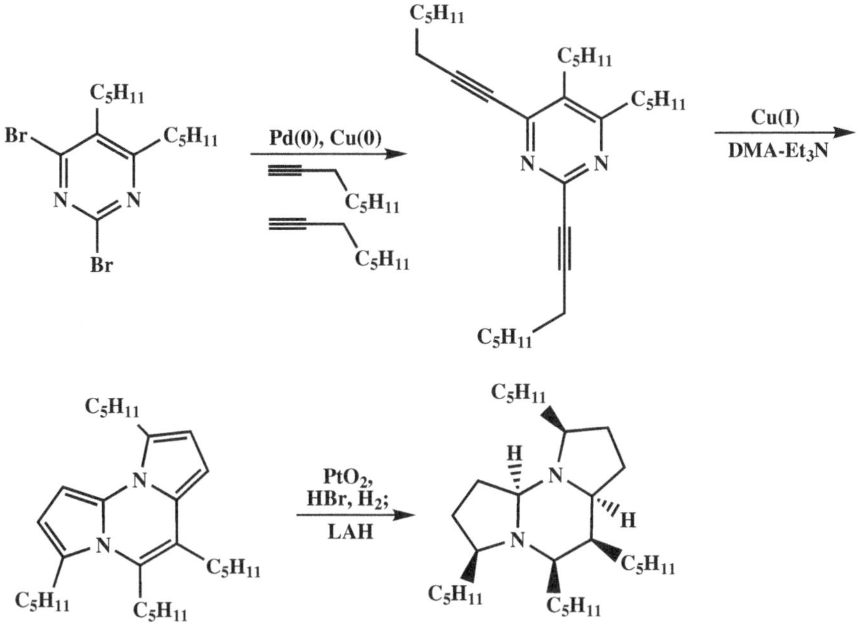

Scheme-64

The *N*-heterocycles (-)-spirotryprostatin B was constructed by Heck reactions of dienes [199]. As depicted in **Scheme 65**, the complex pentacycle was obtained by intramolecular Heck reaction of starting substrate. After the cleavage of SEM ([2-(trimethylsilyl)ethoxy]methyl acetal) protecting group, the complex pentacycle was transformed into natural product.

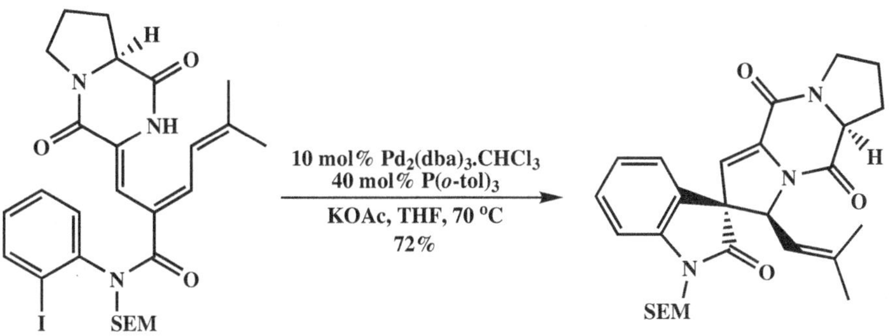

Scheme-65

The 14-azacamptothecin was successfully produced but no asymmetric induction occurred under Sharpless asymmetric dihydroxylation conditions, providing only racemic product. Same result was observed when chiral ligands like (DHQD)$_2$-PHAL (3-dehydroquinate dehydratase 1,4-phthalazinediyl) were employed. During AD reaction, coordination of osmium with chiral ligand was disrupted by two proximal nitrogen atoms (*N*-1 and *N*-14) in the rigid cyclic enol ether. The enantioselective dihydroxylation was also performed to afford the oxygenated stereogenic center in 94% *ee* **(Scheme 66)**. Because of poor regioselectivity obtained in *N*- and *O*-propargylation step, it was decided to conduct a palladium-catalyzed rearrangement of *O*-allyl to *N*-allyl derivative and to synthesize the *N*- and *O*-allyl mixture. The rearrangement proceeded successfully to afford a remarkable yield (100%) of *N*-allyl amide. Previously, allyl amides were not used in aza-Diels-Alder cascade reaction as designed earlier with alkyne tethers.

The pentacyclic intermediate was obtained in 89% yield when allyl amide was treated with 1.5 eq. of Tf$_2$O and 3 eq. of triphenylphosphine oxide at 0 °C, followed by oxidation with freshly prepared manganese(IV) oxide. This conversion represented the application of Hendrickson reagent in which an allyl group underwent a highly efficient aza-Diels-Alder cascade reaction. The enantioselective preparation was completed to afford (*S*)-14-azacamptothecin in >99% *ee* and 95% yield by deacetylation of pentacyclic intermediate with concentrated hydrogen chloride in ethanol [176].

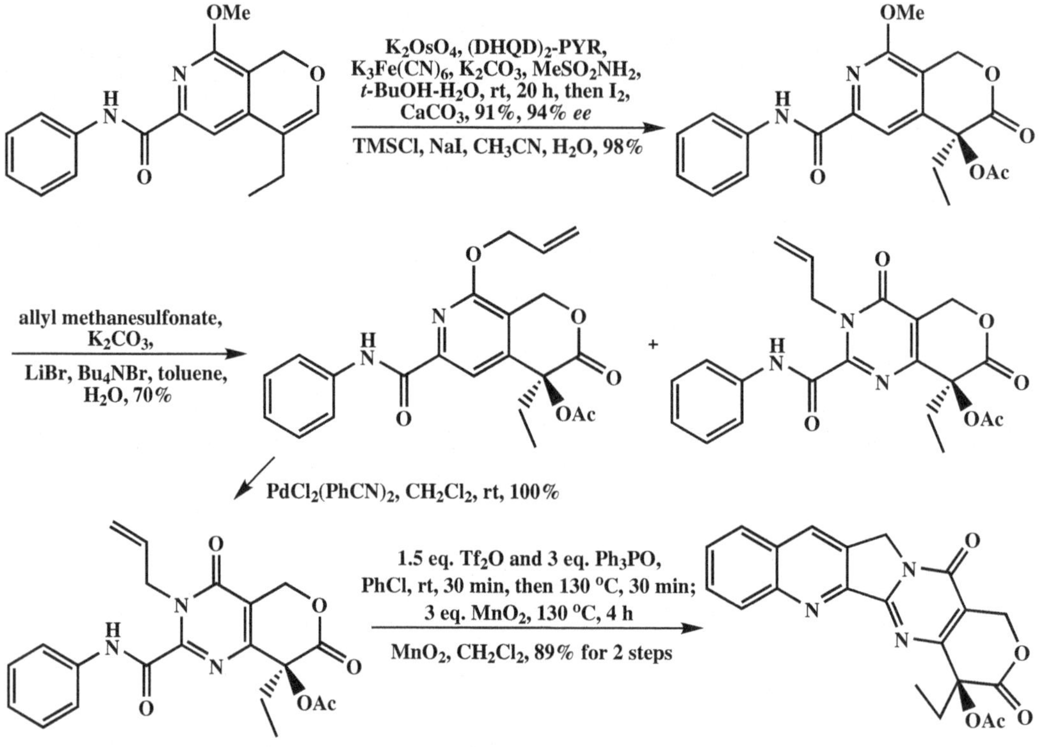

Scheme-66

In combination with MW heating many reaction steps proceeded in a one-pot synthetic protocol and increased the throughput. One-pot and sequential three-step Sonogashira coupling-heteroannulation occurred smoothly and Hopkins and Collar [200] utilized MWI for de-protection process **(Scheme 67)**.

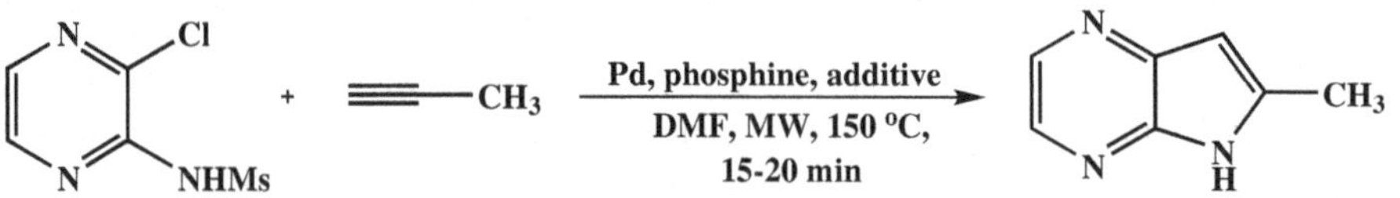

Scheme-67

This protocol was expanded for the preparation of münchnone, which was inert toward imines in the absence of P(*o*-tolyl)$_3$ [201]. There were some drawbacks brought on by the complex series of reactions occurring during catalysis. This method was utilized for the synthesis of pyrroles where each of the five substituents can be varied by modulation of three substrates and independently controlled. As shown in **Scheme 68**, this protocol was important for the introduction of further levels of product complexity into pyrrole product in minimum steps. This class of multicyclic pyrroles is useful as retinoic acid regulators and potential therapeutics [202]. An aldehyde, amine, alkyne, and acid chloride were reacted in three steps for the preparation of pyrroles. The three basic building blocks were coupled through Pd catalysis for the formation of heterocyclic compounds with high atom economy and facile diversity [203].

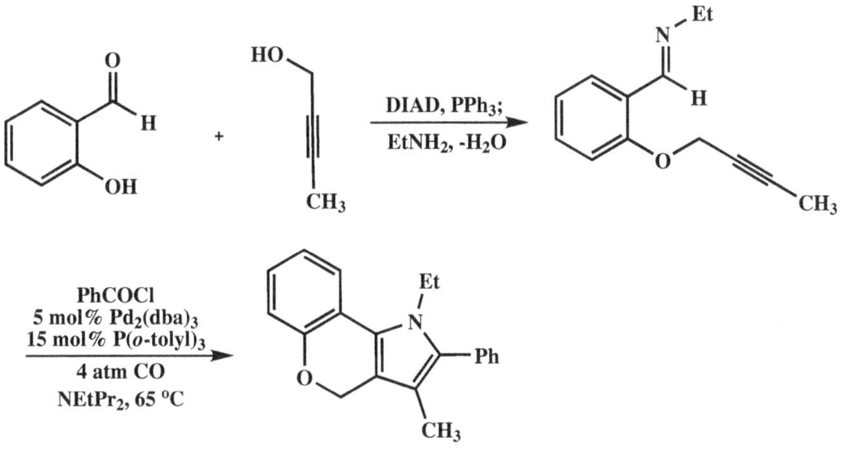

Scheme-68

3.7 Synthesis of five-membered heterocycles fused with seven- and higher-membered heterocycles

The phenyliodine(III) bis(trifluoroacetate)-mediated ring closure of *N*-(3-aminopropyl) alkynamides provided functionalized 5-aryl-2-pyrrolidinones, which underwent ring closure to afford the corresponding perhydropyrrolodiazepines. The method was then readily adapted for the preparation of isomeric pyrrolobenzodiazepines **(Scheme 69)** [204].

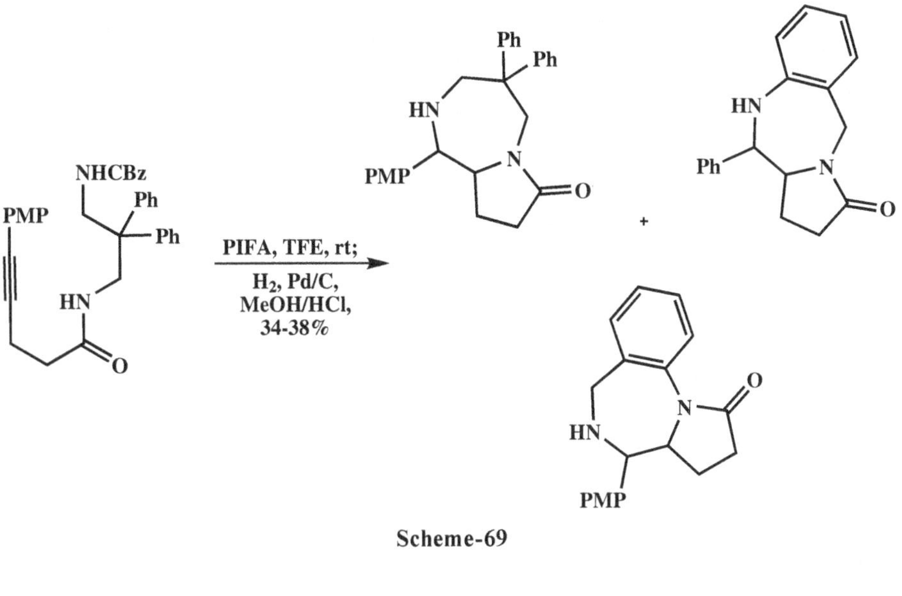

Scheme-69

Winkler and co-workers [205] utilized allyl carbamate in intramolecular nucleophilic displacement of tosylprotected hydroxyl group with amide in the presence of sodium hydride for the preparation of tricyclic ketones. The *N*-alloc-protected eight-membered intermediate was formed from allyl carbamate. The tricyclic ketones were formed upon de-protection of alloc group and then intrmolecular cyclization of 3-butyne-2-one in the presence of ultraviolet light **(Scheme 70)**. The manazamine A, a marine natural product was produced from tricyclic ketones [26].

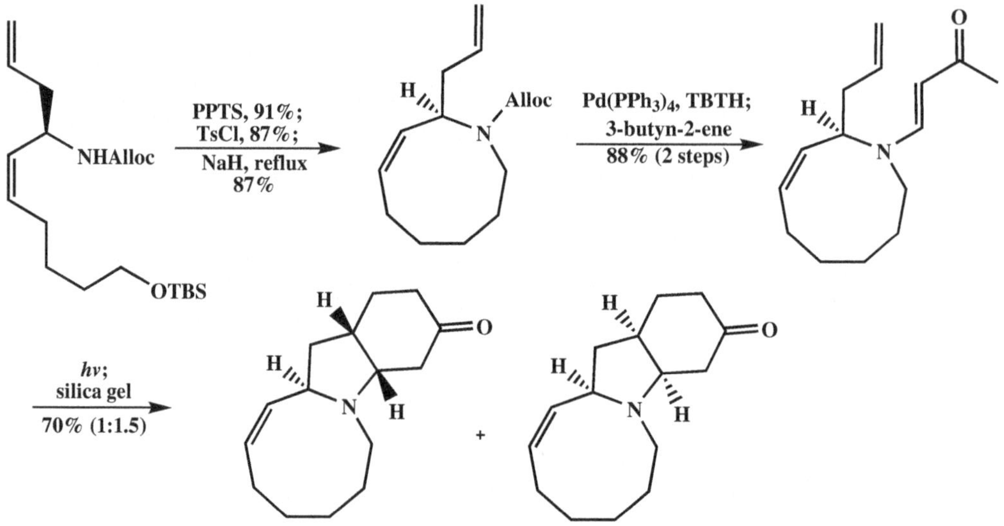

Scheme-70

REFERENCES

[1]   (a) J.A.R. Salvador, R.M.A. Pinto and S.M. Silvestreb. 2009. Recent advances of bismuth(III) salts in organic chemistry: application to the synthesis of heterocycles of pharmaceutical interest. Curr. Org. Synth. 6: 426-470.

        (b) N. Kaur. 2018. Photochemical mediated reactions in five-membered *O*-heterocycles synthesis. Synth. Commun. 48: 2119-2149.

        (c) N. Kaur. 2018. Solid-phase synthesis of sulfur-containing heterocycles. J. Sulfur Chem. 39: 544-577.

[2]   G.S. Singh and Z.Y. Desta. 2012. Isatins as privileged molecules in design and synthesis of spiro-fused cyclic frameworks. Chem. Rev. 112: 6104-6155.

[3]   N. Krause, V. Belting, C. Deutsch, J. Erdsack, H.-T. Fan, B. Gockel, A. Hoffmann-Röder, N. Morita and F. Volz. 2008. Golden opportunities in catalysis. Pure Appl. Chem. 80: 1063-1069.

[4]   A. Das, S.M.A. Sohel and R.-S. Liu. 2010. Carbo- and heterocyclization of oxygen- and nitrogen-containing electrophiles by platinum, gold, silver and copper species. Org. Biomol. Chem. 8: 960-979.

[5]   J.-M. Weibel, A. Blanc and P. Pale. 2008. Ag-Mediated reactions: coupling and heterocyclization reactions. Chem. Rev. 108: 3149-3173

[6]   J.-J. Li, T.-S. Mei and J.-Q. Yu. 2008. Synthesis of indolines and tetrahydroisoquinolines from arylethylamines by PdII-catalyzed C-H activation reactions. Angew. Chem. 120: 6552-6555.

[7]   R.K. Friedman, K.M. Oberg, D.M. Dalton and T. Rovis. 2010. Phosphoramidite-rhodium complexes as catalysts for the asymmetric [2+2+2] cycloaddition of alkenyl isocyanates and alkynes. Pure Appl. Chem. 82: 1353-1364.

[8]   N. Krause, Ö. Aksin-Artok, V. Breker, C. Deutsch, B. Gockel, M. Poonoth, Y. Sawama, Y. Sawama, T. Sun and C. Winter. 2010. Combined coinage metal catalysis for the synthesis of bioactive molecules. Pure Appl. Chem. 82: 1529-1536.

[9] A. Padwa, D.M. Danca, J.D. Ginn and S.M. Lynch. 2001. Application of the tandem thionium/*N*-acyliminium ion cascade toward heterocyclic synthesis. J. Braz. Chem. Soc. 12: 571-585.

[10] D.-H. Zhang, Z. Zhang and M. Shi. 2012. Transition metal-catalyzed carbocyclization of nitrogen and oxygen-tethered 1,n-enynes and diynes: synthesis of five- or six-membered heterocyclic compounds. Chem. Commun. 48: 10271-10279

[11] B. Montaignac, V. Östlund, M.R. Vitale, V.R. Vidal and V. Michelet. 2012. Copper(I)-amine metallo-organocatalyzed synthesis of carbo- and heterocyclic systems. Org. Biomol. Chem. 10: 2300-2306.

[12] A. Fürstner and G. Seidel. 1995. Palladium-catalyzed arylation of polar organometallics mediated by 9-methoxy-9-borabicyclo 3.3.1 nonane - Suzuki reactions of extended scope. Tetrahedron 51: 11165-11176.

[13] A. Mori, T. Kondo, T. Kato and Y. Nishihara. 2001. Palladium-catalyzed cross-coupling polycondensation of bisalkynes with dihaloarenes activated by tetrabutylammonium hydroxide or silver(I) oxide. Chem. Lett. 30: 286-287.

[14] Y. Bai, J. Zeng, J. Ma, B.K. Gorityala and X.-W. Liu. 2010. Quick access to drug like heterocycles: facile silver-catalyzed one-pot multicomponent synthesis of aminoindolizines. J. Comb. Chem. 12: 696-699.

[15] A. Minatti and K. Muniz. 2007. Intramolecular aminopalladation of alkenes as a key step to pyrrolidines and related heterocycles. Chem. Soc. Rev. 36: 1142-1152.

[16] G. Balme, E. Bossharth and N. Monteiro. 2003. Pd-Assisted multicomponent synthesis of heterocycles. Eur. J. Org. Chem. 21: 4101-4111.

[17] X. Tong, M. Beller and M.K. Tse. 2007. A palladium-catalyzed cyclization-oxidation sequence: synthesis of bicyclo[3.1.0]hexanes and evidence for S_N2 C-O bond formation. J. Am. Chem. Soc. 129: 4906-4907.

[18] L.L. Welbes, T.W. Lyons, K.A. Cychosz and M.S. Sanford. 2007. Synthesis of cyclopropanes *via* Pd(II/IV)-catalyzed reactions of enynes. J. Am. Chem. Soc. 129: 5836-5837.

[19] G. Yin and G. Liu. 2008. Palladium-catalyzed oxidative cyclization of enynes with hydrogen peroxide as the oxidant. Angew. Chem. Int. Ed. 47: 5442-5445.

[20] K. Muniz. 2009. High-oxidation-state palladium catalysis: new reactivity for organic synthesis. Angew. Chem. Int. Ed. 48: 2-14.

[21] J. Tsuji and T. Mandai. 1995. Palladium-catalyzed reactions of propargylic compounds in organic synthesis. Angew. Chem. Int. Ed Engl. 34: 2589-2612.

[22] R. Grigg and V. Sridharan. 1998. Heterocycles *via* Pd catalyzed molecular queuing processes. Relay switches and the maximization of molecular complexity. Pure Appl. Chem. 70: 1047-1057.

[23] R. Grigg, R. Rasul, J. Redpath and D. Wilson. 1996. Palladium catalyzed cascade bis-cyclisation-anion capture processes proceeding *via* allenyl-palladium(II) starter species. 1-vinyl-3-azabicyclo[3.1.0] hexanes. Tetrahedron Lett. 37: 4609-4612.

[24] S. Ma. 2006. Transition-metal-catalyzed reactions of allenes. Pure Appl. Chem. 78: 197-208.

[25] M. Gulias, J. Duran, F. Lopez, L. Castedo and J.L. Mascarenas. 2007. Palladium-catalyzed [4+3] intra-molecular cycloaddition of alkylidenecyclopropanes and dienes. J. Am. Chem. Soc. 129: 11026-11027.

[26] S. Nag and S. Batra. 2011. Applications of allylamines for the syntheses of aza-heterocycles. Tetrahedron 67: 8959-9061.

[27] R.C. Larock, P. Pace, H. Yang, C. Russell, S. Cacchi and G. Fabrizi. 1998. Synthesis of nitrogen heterocycles *via* Pd-catalyzed cross-coupling of *o*-alkenyl anilides with vinylic halides and triflates. Tetrahedron 54: 9961-9980.

[28] R.C. Larock, H. Yang, S.M. Weinreb and R.J. Herr. 1994. Synthesis of pyrrolidines and piperidines *via* palladium-catalyzed coupling of vinylic halides and olefinic sulfonamides. J. Org. Chem. 59: 4172-4178.

[29] P. Pinho, A.J. Minnaard and B.L. Feringa. 2003. The tandem Heck-allylic substitution reaction: a novel route to lactams. Org. Lett. 5: 259-261.

[30] G.D. Harris, R.J. Herr and S.M. Weinreb. 1992. A palladium-mediated approach to construction of nitrogen heterocycles. J. Org. Chem. 57: 2528-2530.

[31] G.D. Harris, R.J. Herr and S.M. Weinreb. 1993. Synthesis of bicyclic nitrogen compounds *via* tandem intramolecular Heck cyclizations and subsequent trapping of intermediate π-allylpalladium complexes. J. Org. Chem. 58: 5452-5464.

[32] L.S. Hegedus and J.M. McKearin. 1982. Palladium-catalyzed cyclization of Ω-olefinic tosamides. Synthesis of nonaromatic nitrogen heterocycles. J. Am. Chem. Soc. 104: 2444-2451.

[33] E.M. Beccalli, G. Broggini, M. Martinelli and S. Sottocornola. 2007. C-C, C-O, C-N Bond formation on sp^2 carbon by Pd(II)-catalyzed reactions involving oxidant agents. Chem. Rev. 107: 5318-5365.

[34] P.S. Hanley, D. Markovic and J.F. Hartwig. 2010. Intermolecular insertion of ethylene and octene into a palladium-amide bond. Spectroscopic evidence for an ethylene amido intermediate. J. Am. Chem. Soc. 132: 6302-6303.

[35] G. Liu and S.S. Stahl. 2007. Two-faced reactivity of alkenes: *cis*- versus *trans*-aminopalladation in aerobic Pd-catalyzed intramolecular aza-Wacker reactions. J. Am. Chem. Soc. 129: 6328-6335.

[36] M. Gulias, R. Garcia, A. Delgado, L. Castedo and J.L. Mascarenas. 2006. Palladium-catalyzed [3+2] intramolecular cycloaddition of alk-5-enylidenecyclopropanes. J. Am. Chem. Soc. 128: 384-385.

[37] S. Arai, T. Sato, Y. Koike, M. Hayashi and A. Nishida. 2009. Palladium-catalyzed cyanation of carbon-carbon triple bonds under aerobic conditions. Angew. Chem. Int. Ed. 48: 4528-4531.

[38] J.P. Wolfe. 2008. Stereoselective synthesis of saturated heterocycles *via* Pd-catalyzed alkene carboetherification and carboamination reactions. Synlett 19: 2913-2937.

[39] D. O'Hagan. 2000. Pyrrole, pyrrolidine, pyridine, piperidine and tropane alkaloids. Nat. Prod. Rep. 17: 435-446.

[40] (a) J. Ney and J.P. Wolfe. 2005. Selective synthesis of 5- or 6-aryl octahydrocyclopenta[*b*]pyrroles from a common precursor through control of competing pathways in a Pd-catalyzed reaction. J. Am. Chem. Soc. 127: 8644-8651.

(b) D.N. Mai and J.P. Wolfe. 2010. Asymmetric palladium-catalyzed carboamination reactions for the synthesis of enantiomerically enriched 2-(arylmethyl)- and 2-(alkenylmethyl)pyrrolidines. J. Am. Chem. Soc. 132: 12157-12159.

[41] M. Beaudoin and J.P. Wolfe. 2007. Palladium-catalyzed synthesis of cyclopentane-fused benzocyclobutenes *via* tandem directed carbopalladation/C-H bond functionalization. Org. Lett. 9: 3073-3075.

[42] M. Catellani, G.P. Chiusoli and S. Ricotti. 1985. A new palladium-catalyzed synthesis of 1,2,3,4,4a,8b-hexahydro-1,4-methanobiphenylenes and 2-phenylbicyclo[2.2.1]hept-2-enes. J. Organomet. Chem. 296: C11- C15.

[43] M. Catellani, G.P. Chiusoli, S. Ricotti and F. Sabini. 1985. Palladium-catalyzed C-C bond formation involving aromatic C-H activation. IV. New synthetic applications of insertion reactions coupled with intramolecular aromatic substitution. Gazz. Chim. Ital. 115: 685-689.

[44] M. Catellani and L. Ferioli. 1996. An improved synthesis of 1,4-*cis*, *exo*-hexa- or tetrahydromethano- or -ethanobiphenylene derivatives catalyzed by palladium complexes. Synthesis 6: 769-772.

[45] C. Meyers, B.U.W. Maes, K.T.J. Loones, G. Bal, G.L.F. Lemiere and R.A. Dommisse. 2004. Study of a new rate increasing "base effect" in the palladium-catalyzed amination of aryl iodides. J. Org. Chem. 69: 6010-6017.

[46] M.S. Driver and J.F. Hartwig. 1997. Energetics and mechanism of alkylamine N-H bond cleavage by palladium hydroxides: N-H activation by unusual acid-base chemistry. Organometallics 16: 5706-5715.

[47] U. Hacksell and G.D. Daves. 1983. Apparent *syn* elimination of palladium oxide from a β-hydroxy organopalladium intermediate. Organometallics 2: 772-775.

[48] G. Zhu and X. Lu. 1995. Reactivity and stereochemistry of β-heteroatom elimination. A detailed study through a palladium-catalyzed cyclization reaction model. Organometallics 14: 4899-4904.

[49] H. Zhao, A. Ariafard and Z. Lin. 2006. β-Heteroatom versus β-hydrogen elimination: a theoretical study. Organometallics 25: 812-819.

[50] J.E. Ney, M.B. Hay, Q. Yang and J.P. Wolfe. 2005. Synthesis of *N*-aryl-2-allyl pyrrolidines *via* palladium-catalyzed carboamination reactions of γ-(*N*-arylamino)alkenes with vinyl bromides. Adv. Synth. Catal. 347: 1614-1620.

[51] J.P. Wolfe. 2006. Stereoselective synthesis of saturated heterocycles *via* Pd-catalyzed alkene carboetherification and carboamination reactions. Synlett 4: 571-582.

[52] J.E. Ney and J.P. Wolfe. 2004. Palladium-catalyzed synthesis of *N*-aryl pyrrolidines from γ-(*N*-arylamino) alkenes: evidence for chemoselective alkene insertion into Pd-N bonds. Angew. Chem. Int. Ed. 43: 3605-3608.

[53] M.B. Bertrand and J.P. Wolfe. 2006. A concise stereoselective synthesis of preussin, 3-*epi*-preussin, and analogs. Org Lett. 8: 2353-2356.

[54] N. Jeong, S.D. Seo and J.Y. Shin. 2000. One-pot preparation of bicyclopentenones from propargyl malonates (and propargylsulfonamides) and allylic acetates by a tandem action of catalysts. J. Am. Chem. Soc. 122: 10220-10221.

[55] M. Kimura, H. Harayama, S. Tanaka and Y. Tamaru. 1994. Palladium(II) catalyzed 5-*endo*-trigonal cyclization of 2-hydroxybut-3-enylamines: synthesis of five-membered nitrogen heterocycles. J. Chem. Soc. Chem. Commun. 26: 2531-2533.

[56] R.C. Larock, T.R. Hightower, L.A. Hasvold and K.P. Peterson. 1996. Palladium(II)-catalyzed cyclization of olefinic tosylamides. J. Org. Chem. 61: 3584-3585.

[57] S.R. Fix, J.L. Brice and S.S. Stahl 2002. Efficient intramolecular oxidative amination of olefins through direct dioxygen-coupled palladium catalysis. Angew. Chem. Int. Ed. 41: 164-166.

[58] M. Ronn, J.-E. Backvall and P.G. Andersson. 1995. Palladium(II)-catalyzed cyclization using molecular oxygen as reoxidant. Tetrahedron Lett. 36: 7749-7752.

[59] L.S. Hegedus, G.F. Allen, J.J. Bozell and E.L. Waterman. 1978. Palladium-assisted intramolecular amination of olefins. Synthesis of nitrogen heterocycles. J. Am. Chem. Soc. 100: 5800-5807.

[60] J. Barreiro, E. Pezanha and C. Fraga. 1998. Studies on diastereoselective synthesis of 3-vinyl 5-carbomethoxy-2-oxabicyclo[3.3.0]octane derivatives employing palladium(II) oxidative cyclization. Heterocycles 48: 2621-2630.

[61] H. Ohno, K. Miyamura, Y. Takeoka and T. Tanaka. 2003. Palladium(0)-catalyzed tandem cyclization of allenenes. Angew. Chem. Int. Ed. 42: 2647-2650.

[62] K. Narasaka. 2002. Metal-assisted amination with oxime derivatives. Pure Appl. Chem. 74: 143-149.

[63] M. Kitamura, S. Zaman and K. Narasaka. 2001. Synthesis of spiro imines from oximes by palladium-catalyzed cascade reaction. Synlett 974-976.

[64] S. Zaman, M. Kitamura and K. Narasaka. 2003. Synthesis of polycyclic imines by palladium-catalyzed domino cyclization of di- and trienyl ketone *O*-pentafluorobenzoyloximes. Bull. Chem. Soc. Jpn. 76: 1055-1062.

[65] M. Kitamura, S. Chiba, O. Saku and K. Narasaka. 2002. Palladium-catalyzed synthesis of 1-azaazulenes from cycloheptatrienylmethyl ketone *O*-pentafluorobenzoyl oximes. Chem. Lett. 31: 606-607.

[66] S. Chiba, M. Kitamura, O. Saku and K. Narasaka. 2004. Synthesis of 1-azaazulenes from cycloheptatrienylmethyl ketone *O*-pentafluorobenzoyloximes by palladium-catalyzed cyclization. Bull. Chem. Soc. Jpn. 77: 785-796.

[67] A.A. Aly, A.B. Brown, T.I. El-Emary, A.M.M. Ewas and M. Ramadane. 2009. Hydrazinecarbothioamide group in the synthesis of heterocycles. ARKIVOC (i): 150-197.

[68] G. Bhargava, B. Trillo, M. Araya, F. Lopez, L. Castedo and J.L. Mascarenas. 2010. Palladium-catalyzed [3+2+2] cycloaddition of enynylidenecyclopropanes: efficient construction of fused 5-7-5 tricyclic systems. Chem. Commun. 46: 270-272.

[69] P.H. Lee, H. Kim, K. Lee, M. Kim, K. Noh, H. Kim and D. Seomoon. 2005. The indium-mediated selective introduction of allenyl and propargyl groups at the C4-position of 2-azetidinones and the AuCl₃-catalyzed cyclization of 4-allenyl-2-azetidinones. Angew. Chem. 117: 1874-1877.

[70] B. Jiang and H. Tian. 2007. Synthesis of 4-allenyl and 4-proparyl-2-azetidinone *via* Zn-mediated Barbier-type reaction and Pt-catalyzed intramolecular amidation to carbapenem skeletons. Tetrahedron Lett. 48: 7942-7945.

[71] W.F.J. Karstens, F.P.J.T. Rutjes and H. Hiemstra. 1997. Palladium-catalyzed coupling/cyclization reactions of allene-substituted lactams. Tetrahedron Lett. 38: 6275-6278.

[72] B. Alcaide and P. Almendros. 2011. Allenyl-β-lactams: versatile scaffolds for the synthesis of heterocycles. Chem. Rec. 11: 311-330.

[73] Y. Kozawa and M. Mori. 2001. Construction of a carbapenam skeleton using palladium-catalyzed cyclization. Tetrahedron Lett. 42: 4869-4873.

[74] Y. Kozawa and M. Mori. 2002. Synthesis of different ring-size heterocycles from the same propargyl alcohol derivative by ligand effect on Pd(0). Tetrahedron Lett. 43: 1499-1502.

[75] Y. Kozawa and M. Mori. 2003. Novel synthesis of carbapenam by intramolecular attack of lactam nitrogen toward η^1-allenyl and η^3-propargylpalladium complex. J. Org. Chem. 68: 8068-8074.

[76] Y. Kiyotsuka, J. Igarashi and Y. Kobayashi. 2002. A study toward a total synthesis of fostriecin. Tetrahedron Lett. 43: 2725-2729.

[77] J.A. Marshall. 2007. Chiral allylic and allenic metal reagents for organic synthesis. J. Org. Chem. 72: 8153-8166.

[78] K. Ishihara, H. Kurihara and H. Yamamoto. 1993. An extremely simple, convenient, and selective method for acetylating primary alcohols in the presence of secondary alcohols. J. Org. Chem. 58: 3791-3793.

[79] M.A. Kinsella, V.J. Kalish and S.M. Weinreb. 1990. Approaches to the total synthesis of the anti-tumor anti-biotic echinosporin. J. Org. Chem. 55: 105-111.

[80] S. Husinec, I. Juranic, A. Llobera and A.E.A. Porter. 1988. Bis(methoxycarbonyl)carbene insertion into N-H bonds: a facile route to *N*-substituted aminomalonic esters. Synthesis 9: 721-723.

[81] K. Takahashi, M. Midori, K. Kawano, J. Ishihara and S. Hatakeyama. 2008. Entry to heterocycles based on indium-catalyzed Conia-ene reactions: asymmetric synthesis of (-)-salinosporamide A. Angew. Chem. Int. Ed. 47: 6244-6246.

[82] P.G. Andersson and J.-E. Backvall. 1992. Palladium-catalyzed tandem cyclization of 4,6- and 5,7-diene amides. A new route toward the pyrrolizidine and indolizidine alkaloids. J. Am. Chem. Soc. 114: 8696-8698.

[83] M. Vavrecka, A. Janowitz and M. Hesse. 1991. Transformation of 4-nitroalkane-1,7-diones into pyrrolizidines. Tetrahedron Lett. 32: 5543-5546.

[84] R. Ballini and M. Petrini. 2009. Nitroalkanes as key building blocks for the synthesis of heterocyclic derivatives. ARKIVOC (ix): 195-223.

[85] P.R. Weider, L.S. Hegedus, H. Asada and V. D'Andreq. 1985. Oxidative cyclization of unsaturated aminoquinones. Synthesis of quinolinoquinones. Palladium-catalyzed synthesis of pyrroloindolo-quinones. J. Org. Chem. 50: 4276-4281.

[86] P.G. Tsoungas. 2002. Synthesis of 1,2-oxazines and their *N*-oxides. Heterocycles 57: 1149-1178.

[87] R. Zimmer, M. Hoffmann and H.-U. Reissig. 1992. Model studies of the reduction of 3-phenyl-6*H*-1,2-oxazines, chemo- and stereoselectivity: synthesis of amino alcohols, amino acids, and related compounds. Chem. Ber. 125: 2243-2248.

[88] J. Angermann, K. Homann, H.-U. Reissig and R. Zimmer. 1995. Synthesis and *cis*-dihydroxylation of 6*H*-1,2-oxazines: synthesis of dihydroxyprolinols. Synlett 10: 1014-1016.

[89] A.A. Tishkov, H.-U. Reissig and S.L. Ioffe. 2002. Preparation of cyclic and bicyclic β-amino acids derivatives from methyl 6-ethoxy-5,6-dihydro-4*H*-1,2-oxazine-4-carboxylate. Synlett 6: 863-866.

[90] R. Zimmer, M. Collas, M. Roth and H.-U. Reissig. 1992. 6-Siloxy-substituted 5,6-dihydro-4*H*-1,2-oxazines as key building blocks for natural products. Liebigs Ann. Chem. 7: 709-714.

[91] J. Dohanosova, A. Lasikova, M. Toffano, T. Gracza and G. Vo-Thanh. 2012. Kinetic resolution of pent-4-ene-1,3-diol by Pd(II)-catalyzed oxycarbonylation in ionic liquids. New J. Chem. 36: 1744-1750.

[92] J. Streuff, C.H. Hvelmann, M. Nieger and K. Muniz. 2005. Palladium(II)-catalyzed intramolecular diamination of unfunctionalized alkenes. J. Am. Chem. Soc. 127: 14586-14587.

[93] H. Yu, Y. Fao, Q. Guo and Z. Lin. 2009. Theoretical investigations on mechanisms of Pd(OAc)$_2$ catalyzed intramolecular diaminations in the presence of bases and oxidants. Organometallics 28: 4507-4512.

[94] G. Liu and S.S. Stahl. 2006. Highly regioselective Pd-catalyzed intermolecular aminoacetoxylation of alkenes and evidence for *cis*-aminopalladation and S_N2 C-O bond formation. J. Am. Chem. Soc. 128: 7179-7181.

[95] K. Muniz, C.H. Hoevelmann and J. Streuff. 2008. Oxidative diamination of alkenes with ureas as nitrogen sources: mechanistic pathways in the presence of a high oxidation state palladium catalyst. J. Am. Chem. Soc. 130: 763-773.

[96] K. Muniz. 2007. Advancing palladium-catalyzed C-N bond formation: bisindoline construction from successive amide transfer to internal alkenes. J. Am. Chem. Soc. 129: 14542-14543.

[97] C.H. Hovelmann, J. Streuff, L. Brelot and K. Muniz. 2008. Direct synthesis of bicyclic guanidines through unprecedented palladium(II) catalyzed diamination with copper chloride as oxidant. Chem. Commun. 20: 2334-2336.

[98] K. Muniz, C.H. Hovelmann, J. Streuff and E. Campoz-Gomez. 2008. First palladium- and nickel-catalyzed oxidative diamination of alkenes: cyclic urea, sulfamide, and guanidine building blocks. Pure Appl. Chem. 80: 1089-1096.

[99] K. Muniz, C.H. Hovelmann, E. Campos-Gomez, J. Barluenga, J.M. Gonzalez, J. Streuff and M. Nieger. 2008. Intramolecular diamination of alkenes with palladium(II)/copper(II) bromide and IPy$_2$BF$_4$: the role of halogenated intermediates. Chem. Asian J. 3: 776-788.

[100] K. Muniz, J. Streuff, P. Chavez and C.H. Hovelmann. 2008. Synthesis of diamino carboxylic esters by palladium-catalyzed oxidative intramolecular diamination of acrylates. Chem. Asian J. 3: 1248-1255.

[101] J. Helaja and R. Gottlich. 2002. A new catalytic hetero-Heck type reaction. Chem. Commun. 7: 720-721.

[102] H. Tsutsui and K. Narasaka. 1999. Synthesis of pyrrole derivatives by the Heck-type cyclization of γ,δ-unsaturated ketone O-(pentafluorobenzoyl)oximes. Chem. Lett. 1: 45-46.

[103] Y. Tamaru, T. Kobayashi, S.I. Kawamura, H. Ochiai and Z.-I. Yoshida. 1985. Stereoselective intramolecular aminocarbonylation of 3-hydroxypent-4-enylamides catalyzed by palladium. Tetrahedron Lett. 26: 4479-4482.

[104] W. Hummer, E. Dubois, T. Gracza and V. Jager. 1997. Halocyclization and palladium(II)-catalyzed amidocarbonylation of unsaturated aminopolyols - synthesis of 1,4-iminoglycitols as potential glycosidase inhibitors. Synthesis 6: 634-642.

[105] H. Takahata, Y. Banba and T. Momose. 1991. The shortest synthesis of optically active Geissman-Waiss lactone, a key synthetic intermediate for necine bases. Tetrahedron: Asymmetry 2: 445-448.

[106] Y.Q. Fang, R. Karisch and M. Lautens. 2007. Efficient syntheses of KDR kinase inhibitors using a Pd-catalyzed tandem C-N/Suzuki coupling as the key step. J. Org. Chem. 72: 1341-1346.

[107] Y.-Q. Fang and M. Lautens. 2008. A highly selective tandem cross-coupling of *gem*-dihaloolefins for a modular, efficient synthesis of highly functionalized indoles. J. Org. Chem. 73: 538-549.

[108] Y.Q. Fang, J. Yuen and M. Lautens. 2007. A general modular method of azaindole and thienopyrrole synthesis *via* Pd-catalyzed tandem couplings of *gem*-dichloroolefins. J. Org. Chem. 72: 5152-5160.

[109] C.J. Ball and M.C. Willis. 2013. Cascade palladium- and copper-catalyzed aromatic heterocycle synthesis: the emergence of general precursors. Eur. J. Org. Chem. 3: 425-441.

[110] A. Fînaru, A. Berthault, T. Besson, G. Guillaumet and S. Berteina-Raboin. 2002. Microwave-assisted solid-phase synthesis of 5-carboxamido-*N*-acetyltryptamine derivatives. Org. Lett. 4: 2613-2615.

[111] M.C. Fagnola, I. Candiani, G. Visentin, W. Cabri, F. Zarini, N. Mongelli and A. Bedeschi. 1997. Solid-phase synthesis of indoles using the palladium-catalyzed coupling of alkynes with iodoaniline derivatives. Tetrahedron Lett. 38: 2307-2310.

[112] F. Ujjainwalla and D. Warner. 1998. Synthesis of 5-, 6- and 7-azaindoles *via* palladium-catalyzed heteroannulation of internal alkynes. Tetrahedron Lett. 39: 5355-5358.

[113] G. Kirsch, S. Hesse and A. Comel. 2004. Synthesis of five- and six-membered heterocycles through palladium-catalyzed reactions. Curr. Org. Synth. 1: 47-63.

[114] S. Couty, B. Liegault, C. Meyer and J. Cossy. 2004. Heck-Suzuki-Miyaura domino reactions involving ynamides. An efficient access to 3-(arylmethylene)isoindolinones. Org. Lett. 6: 2511-2514.

[115] S. Couty, B. Liegault, C. Meyer and J. Cossy. 2006. Synthesis of 3-(arylmethylene)isoindolin-1-ones from ynamides by Heck-Suzuki-Miyaura domino reactions. Application to the synthesis of lennoxamine. Tetrahedron Lett. 62: 3882-3895.

[116] J. Cossy. 2010. Efficient cyclization routes to substituted heterocyclic compounds mediated by transition metal catalysts. Pure Appl. Chem. 82: 1365-1373.

[117] P. Wipf and J.P. Maciejewski. 2008. Titanocene(III)-catalyzed formation of indolines and azaindolines. Org. Lett. 10: 4383-4386.

[118] M. Nazare, C. Schneider, A. Lindenschmidt and D.W. Will. 2004. A flexible, palladium-catalyzed indole and azaindole synthesis by direct annulation of chloroanilines and chloroaminopyridines with ketones. Angew. Chem. Int. Ed. 43: 4526-4528.

[119] L. El Kaim, M. Gizzi and L. Grimaud. 2008. New MCR-Heck-isomerization cascade toward indoles. Org. Lett. 10: 3417-3419.

[120] T. Jensen, H. Pedersen, B. Bang-Andersen, R. Madsen and M. Jorgensen. 2008. Palladium-catalyzed aryl amination-Heck cyclization cascade: a one-flask approach to 3-substituted indoles. Angew. Chem. Int. Ed. 47: 888-890.

[121] P. Zakrzewski, M. Gowan, L.A. Trimble and C.K. Lau. 1999. o-Hydroxyalkylation of aminopyridines: a novel approach to heterocycles. Synthesis 11: 1893-1902.

[122] B.M. Trost and C. Pedregal. 1992. Palladium-catalyzed cycloisomerization of alkynyl N-acyl enamines. J. Am. Chem. Soc. 114: 7292-7294.

[123] I. Ojima, M. Tzamarioudaki, Z. Li and R.J. Donovan. 1996. Transition metal-catalyzed carbocyclizations in organic synthesis. Chem. Rev. 96: 635-662.

[124] A.R. Hardin and R. Sarpong. 2007. Electronic effects in the Pt-catalyzed cycloisomerization of propargylic esters: synthesis of 2,3-disubstituted indolizines as a mechanistic probe. Org. Lett. 9: 4547-4550.

[125] B. Yan, Y. Zhou, H. Zhang, J. Chen and Y. Liu. 2007. Highly efficient synthesis of functionalized indolizines and indolizinones by copper-calayzed cycloisomerization of propargylic pyridines. J. Org. Chem. 72: 7783-7786.

[126] I. Kim and K. Kim. 2010. Expeditious synthesis of highly substituted indolizinones via a palladium-catalyzed domino sequence. Org. Lett. 12: 2500-2503.

[127] M. Lautens, J.-F. Paquin, S. Piguel and M. Dahlmann. 2001. Palladium-catalyzed sequential alkylation-alkenylation reactions and their application to the synthesis of fused aromatic rings. J. Org. Chem. 66: 8127-8134.

[128] M.B. Bertrand, M.L. Leathen and J.P. Wolfe. 2007. Mild conditions for the synthesis of functionalized pyrrolidines via Pd-catalyzed carboamination reactions. Org. Lett. 9: 457-460.

[129] Y. Sato, S. Nukui, M. Sodeoka and M. Shibasaki. 1994. Asymmetric Heck reaction of alkenyl iodides in the presence of silver salts. Catalytic asymmetric synthesis of decalin and functionalized indolizidine derivatives. Tetrahedron 50: 371-382.

[130] S. Nukui, M. Sodeoka and M. Shibasaki. 1993. Catalytic asymmetric synthesis of a functionalized indolizidine derivative. A useful intermediate suitable for the synthesis of various glycosidase inhibitors. Tetrahedron Lett. 34: 4965-4968.

[131] M. Shibasaki and M. Sodeoka. 1994. Asymmetric Heck reaction: catalytic asymmetric syntheses of bioactive molecules. J. Synth. Org. Chem. Jpn. 52: 956-967.

[132] M.A. Alvarez-Corral, M. Munoz-Dorado and I. Rodriguez-Garcia. 2008. Silver-mediated synthesis of heterocycles. Chem. Rev. 108: 3174-3198.

[133] M. Vavrecka and M. Hesse. 1991. Synthese von Monomorin I, einem Spurpheromon der Pharao-Ameise (Monomorium pharaonis). Helv. Chim. Acta 74: 438-444.

[134] W. Francke, F. Schroder, F. Walter, V. Sinnwell, H. Baumann and M. Kaib. 1995. New alkaloids from ants: identification and synthesis of (3R,5S,9R)-3-butyl-5-(1-oxopropyl)indolizidine and (3R,5R,9R)-3-butyl-5-(1-oxopropyl)indolizidine, constituents of the poison gland secretion in *Myrmicaria eumenoides* (Hymenoptera, Formicidae). Liebig's Ann. Chem. 6: 965-977.

[135] G. Zeni and R.C. Larock. 2004. Synthesis of heterocycles via palladium π-olefin and π-alkyne chemistry. Chem. Rev. 104: 2285-2310.

[136] S. Cacchi and G. Fabrizi. 2005. Synthesis and functionalization of indoles through palladium-catalyzed reactions. Chem. Rev. 105: 2873-2920.

[137] G. Zeni and R.C. Larock. 2006. Synthesis of heterocycles *via* palladium-catalyzed oxidative addition. Chem. Rev. 106: 4644-4680.

[138] A. Brandi, F. Cardona, S. Cicchi, F.M. Cordero and A. Goti. 2009. Stereocontrolled cyclic nitrone cycloaddition strategy for the synthesis of pyrrolizidine and indolizidine alkaloids. Chem. Eur. J. 15: 7808-7821.

[139] M.B. Bertrand and J.P. Wolfe. 2005. Carbamoylimidazolium and thiocarbamoylimidazolium salts: novel reagents for the synthesis of ureas, thioureas, carbamates, thiocarbamates and amides. Tetrahedron 61: 6447-6459.

[140] M.B. Bertrand, J.D. Neukom and J.P. Wolfe. 2008. Mild conditions for Pd-catalyzed carboamination of *N*-protected hex-4-enylamines and 1-, 3-, and 4-substituted pent-4-enylamines. Scope, limitations, and mechanism of pyrrolidine formation. J. Org. Chem. 73: 8851-8860.

[141] T. Gerfaud, L. Neuville and J. Zhu. 2009. Palladium-catalyzed annulation of acyloximes with arynes (or alkynes): synthesis of phenanthridines and isoquinolines. Angew. Chem. Int. Ed. 48: 572-577.

[142] P.R. Halfpenny, D.C. Horwell, J. Hughes, J.C. Hunter and D.C. Rees. 1990. Highly selective kappa-opioid analgesics. Synthesis and structure-activity relationships of novel *N*-[2-(1-pyrrolidinyl)-4- or -5-substituted-cyclohexyl]arylacetamide derivatives. J. Med. Chem. 33: 286-291.

[143] L.F. Tietze, H. Ila and H.P. Bell. 2004. Enantioselective palladium-catalyzed transformations. Chem. Rev. 104: 3453-3516.

[144] K. Kiewel, M. Tallant and G.A. Sulikowski. 2001. Asymmetric Heck cyclization route to indolizidine and azaazulene alkaloids: synthesis of (+)-5-epiindolizidine 167B and indolizidine 223AB. Tetrahedron Lett. 42: 6621-6623.

[145] Z. Li, D. Chernyak and V. Gevorgyan. 2012. Palladium-catalyzed carbonylative cyclization/arylation cascade for 2-aroylindolizine synthesis. Org. Lett. 14: 6056-6059.

[146] D. Chernyak, C. Skontos and V. Gevorgyan. 2010. Two-component approach toward fully-substituted *N*-fused pyrrole ring. Org. Lett. 12: 3242-3245.

[147] S. Hanessian, G. McNaughton-Smith, H.-G. Lombart and W.D. Lubell. 1997. Design and synthesis of conformationally constrained amino acids as versatile scaffolds and peptide mimetics. Tetrahedron 53: 12789-12854.

[148] A. Furstner and J.W.J. Kennedy. 2006. Total syntheses of the *Tylophora* alkaloids cryptopleurine, (-)-antofine, (-)-tylophorine, and (-)-ficuseptine C. Chem. Eur. J. 12: 7398-7410.

[149] R.G. Vaswani and A.R. Chamberlin. 2008. Stereocontrolled total synthesis of (-)-kaitocephalin. J. Org. Chem. 73: 1661-1681.

[150] G. Evano, N. Blanchard and M. Toumi. 2008. Copper-mediated coupling reactions and their applications in natural products and designed biomolecules synthesis. Chem. Rev. 108: 3054-3131.

[151] Z. Li, Z. Jin and R. Huang. 2001. Isolation, total synthesis and biological activity of phenanthro-indolizidine and phenanthroquinolizidine alkaloids. Synthesis 16: 2365-2378.

[152] W. Zeng and S.R. Chemler. 2008. Total synthesis of (*S*)-(+)-tylophorine *via* enantioselective intramolecular alkene carboamination. J. Org. Chem. 73: 6045-6047.

[153] A. McIver, D.D. Young and A. Dieters. 2008. A general approach to triphenylenes and azatriphenylenes: total synthesis of dehydrotylophorine and tylophorine. Chem. Commun. 39: 4750-4752.

[154] Z. Wang, Z. Li, K. Wang and Q. Wang. 2010. Efficient and chirally specific synthesis of phenanthro-indolizidine alkaloids by Parham-type cycloacylation. Eur. J. Org. Chem. 2: 292-299.

[155] L.M. Rossiter, M.L. Slater, R.E. Gissert, S.A. Sakwa and R.J. Herr. 2009. A concise palladium-catalyzed carboamination route to (+/-)-tylophorine. J. Org. Chem. 74: 9554-9557.

[156] A.V. Rotaru, I.D. Druta, T. Oeser and T.J.J. Muller. 2005. A novel coupling 1,3-dipolar cycloaddition sequence as a three-component approach to highly fluorescent indolizines. Helv. Chim. Acta 88: 1798-1812.

[157] D.M. D'Souza and T.J.J. Muller. 2007. Multi-component syntheses of heterocycles by transition-metal catalysis. Chem. Soc. Rev. 36: 1095-1108.

[158] K. Shimizu, M. Takimoto and M. Mori. 2003. Novel synthesis of heterocycles having a functionalized carbon center *via* nickel-mediated carboxylation: total synthesis of erythrocarine. Org. Lett. 5: 2323-2325.

[159] K.C. Majumdar, S. Muhuri, R.U. Islam and B. Chattopadhyay. 2009. Synthesis of five- and six-membered heterocyclic compounds by the application of the metathesis reactions. Heterocycles 78: 1109-1169.

[160] P. Vital, M. Hosseini, M.S. Shanmugham, C.H. Gotfredsen, P. Harris and D. Tanner. 2009. Polycyclic alkaloids *via* transannular Mannich reactions. Chem. Commun. 14: 1888-1890.

[161] C. Koradin, W. Dohle, A.L. Rodriguez, B. Schmid and P. Knochel. 2003. Synthesis of polyfunctional indoles and related heterocycles mediated by cesium and potassium bases. Tetrahedron 59: 1571-1587.

[162] T.H.M. Jonckers, B.U.W. Maes, G.L.F. Lemiere, G. Rombouts, L. Pieters, A. Haemers and R.A. Dommisse. 2003. Synthesis of isocryptolepine *via* a Pd-catalyzed 'amination-arylation' approach. Synlett 5: 615-618.

[163] D.L. Comins, M.F. Baevsky and H. Hong. 1992. A 10-step, asymmetric synthesis of (*S*)-camptothecin. J. Am. Chem. Soc. 114: 10971-10972.

[164] D.L. Comins, H. Hong, J.K. Saha and G. Jianhua. 1994. A six-step synthesis of (+)-camptothecin. J. Org. Chem. 59: 5120-5121.

[165] D.L. Comins and J.M. Nolan. 2001. A practical six-step synthesis of (*S*)-camptothecin. Org. Lett. 3: 4255-4257.

[166] F.G. Fang, D.D. Bankston, E.M. Huie, M.R. Johnson, M.-C. Kang, C.S. LeHoullier, G.C. Lewis, T.C. Lovelace, M.W. Lowery, D.L. McDougald, C.A. Meerholz, J.J. Partridge, M.J. Sharp and S. Xie. 1997. Convergent catalytic asymmetric-synthesis of camptothecin analog GI147211C. Tetrahedron 53: 10953-10970.

[167] O. Lavergne, D. Demarquay, C. Bailly, C. Lanco, A. Rolland, M. Huchet, H. Coulomb, N. Muller, N. Baroggi, J. Camara, C. Breton, E. Manginot, J.-B. Cazaux and D.C.H. Bigg. 2000. Topoisomerase I-mediated anti-proliferative activity of enantiomerically pure fluorinated homocamptothecins. J. Med. Chem. 43: 2285-2289.

[168] O. Lavergne, L. Lesueur-Ginot, F. Pla Rodas, P.G. Kasprzyk, J. Pommier, D. Demarquay, G. Prevost, G. Ulibarri, A. Rolland, A.-M. Schiano-Liberatore, J. Harnett, D. Pons, J. Camara and D.C.H. Bigg. 1998. Homocamptothecins: synthesis and anti-tumor activity of novel E-ring-modified camptothecin analogues. J. Med. Chem. 41: 5410-5419.

[169] M.E. Wall, M.C. Wani, C.E. Cook, K.H. Palmer, A.T. McPhail and G.A. Sim. 1966. Plant anti-tumor agents. I. The isolation and structure of camptothecin, a novel alkaloidal leukemia and tumor inhibitor from *Camptotheca acuminata*. J. Am. Chem. Soc. 88: 3888-3890.

[170] Y.H. Hsiang, R. Hertzberg, S.M. Hecht and L.F. Liu. 1985. Camptothecin induces protein-linked DNA breaks *via* mammalian DNA topoisomerase I. J. Biol. Chem. 260: 14873-14878.

[171] K.W. Kohn and Y. Pommier. 2000. Molecular and biological determinants of the cytotoxic actions of camptothecins. Perspective for the development of new topoisomerase I inhibitors. Ann. N.Y. Acad. Sci. 922: 11-26.

[172] B.L. Staker, K. Hjerrild, M.D. Feese, C.A. Behnke, A.B. Burgin and L. Stewart. 2002. The mechanism of topoisomerase I poisoning by a camptothecin analog. Proc. Natl. Acad. Sci. 99: 15387-15392.

[173] W. Du. 2003. Towards new anti-cancer drugs: a decade of advances in synthesis of camptothecins and related alkaloids. Tetrahedron 59: 8649-8687.

[174] C.R. Hutchinson. 1981. Camptothecin: chemistry, biogenesis, and medicinal chemistry. Tetrahedron 37: 1047-1065.

[175] H.-B. Zhou, G.-S. Liu and Z.-J. Yao. 2007. Highly efficient and mild cascade reactions triggered by bis(triphenyl)oxodiphosphonium trifluoromethanesulfonate and a concise total synthesis of camptothecin. Org. Lett. 9: 2003-2006.

[176] Z. Moussa. 2012. The Hendrickson 'POP' reagent and analogues thereof: synthesis, structure, and application in organic synthesis. ARKIVOC (i): 432-490.

[177] D.L. Comins and J.K. Saha. 1996. Concise synthesis of mappicine ketone and (±)-mappicine. J. Org. Chem. 61: 9623-9624.

[178] T. Harayama, Y. Morikami, A. Hori, H. Nishioka, H. Abe and Y. Takeuchi. 2004. Concise synthesis of 11*H*-indolizino[1,2-*b*]quinolin-9-one by an aryl-aryl coupling reaction using Pd reagent. Heterocycles 62: 803-806.

[179] T. Harayama, Y. Morikami, Y. Shigeta, H. Abe and Y. Takeuchi. 2003. A convenient synthesis of luotonins A and B. Synlett 6: 847-848.

[180] T. Harayama, A. Hori, G. Serban, Y. Morikami, T. Matsumoto, H. Abe and Y. Takeuchi. 2004. Concise synthesis of quinazoline alkaloids, luotonins A and B, and rutaecarpine. Tetrahedron 60: 10645-10649.

[181] Z. Ma and D.Y.W. Lee. 2004. Total synthesis of the cytotoxic alkaloid 22-hydroxyacuminatine. Tetrahedron Lett. 45: 6721-6723.

[182] D.P. Curran and W. Du. 2002. Palladium-promoted cascade reactions of isonitriles and 6-iodo-*N*-propargylpyridones: synthesis of mappicines, camptothecins, and homocamptothecins. Org. Lett. 4: 3215-3218.

[183] S. Cacchi. 1999. Heterocycles *via* cyclization of alkynes promoted by organopalladium complexes. J. Organomet. Chem. 576: 42-64.

[184] R. Grigg and V. Sridharan. 1999. Palladium catalyzed cascade cyclization-anion capture, relay switches and molecular queues. J. Organomet. Chem. 576: 65-87.

[185] R.C. Larock. 1999. Palladium-catalyzed annulations. J. Organomet. Chem. 576: 111-124.

[186] F. Zeng and H. Alper. 2011. Palladium-catalyzed domino C-S coupling/carbonylation reactions: an efficient synthesis of 2-carbonylbenzo[*b*]thiophene derivatives. Org. Lett. 13: 2868-2871.

[187] J. Garcia-Fortanet and S.L. Buchwald. 2008. Asymmetric palladium-catalyzed intramolecular α-arylation of aldehydes. Angew. Chem. Int. Ed. 47: 8108-8111.

[188] B.D. Chapsal and I. Ojima. 2005. Total synthesis of enantiopure (+)-γ-lycorane using highly efficient Pd-catalyzed asymmetric allylic alkylation. Org. Lett. 8: 1395-1398.

[189] B.D. Chapsal and I. Ojima. 2006. Catalytic asymmetric transformations with fine-tunable biphenol-based monodentate ligands. Tetrahedron: Asymmetry 17: 642-657.

[190] M. Sodeoka and Y. Hamashima. 2008. Synthesis of optically active heterocyclic compounds using Pd-catalyzed asymmetric reactions as a key step. Pure Appl. Chem. 80: 763-776.

[191] T. Tsujihara, T. Shinohara, K. Takenaka, S. Takizawa, K. Onitsuka, M. Hatanaka and H. Sasai. 2009. Enantioselective intramolecular oxidative aminocarbonylation of alkenylureas catalyzed by palladium-spiro bis(isoxazoline) complexes. J. Org. Chem. 74: 9274-9279.

[192] Y. Tamaru, M. Hojo, H. Higashimura and Z.-I. Yoshida. 1988. Urea as the most reactive and versatile nitrogen nucleophile for the palladium(2+)-catalyzed cyclization of unsaturated amines. J. Am. Chem. Soc. 110: 3994-4002.

[193] H. Harayama, A. Abe, T. Sakado, M. Kimura, K. Fugami, S. Tanaka and Y. Tamaru. 1997. Palladium(II)-catalyzed intramolecular aminocarbonylation of *endo*-carbamates under Wacker-type conditions. J. Org. Chem. 62: 2113-2122.

[194] Y. Tamaru, H. Tanigawa, S. Itoh, M. Kimura, S. Tanaka, K. Fugami, T. Sekiyama and Z. Yoshida. 1992. Palladium(II)-catalyzed oxidative aminocarbonylation of unsaturated carbamates. Tetrahedron Lett. 33: 631-634.

[195] Y. Tamaru and Z. Yoshida. 1987. Heterocyclic synthesis by the use of the oxidizing potential of palladium(II). J. Organomet. Chem. 334: 213-223.

[196] Y. Tamaru and M. Kimura. 1997. C-N bond formation reactions *via* transition metal catalysis. Synlett 7: 749-757.

[197] S. Tanimori, H. Kashiwagi, T. Nishimura and M. Kirihata. 2010. A general and practical access to chiral quinoxalinones with low copper-catalyst loading. Adv. Synth. Catal. 352: 2531-2537.

[198] J.T. Kim, J. Butt and V. Gevorgyan. 2004. Highly diastereoselective approach toward (+/-)-tetraponerine T6 and analogues *via* the double cycloisomerization-reduction of bis-alkynylpyrimidines. J. Org. Chem. 69: 5638-5645.

[199] L.E. Overman and M.D. Rosen. 2000. Total synthesis of (-)-spirotryprostatin B and three stereoisomers. Angew. Chem. Int. Ed. 39: 4596-4599.

[200] C.R. Hopkins and N. Collar. 2004. An improved method for the synthesis of 6-substituted-5*H*-pyrrolo[2,3-*b*]pyrazines *via* palladium-catalyzed heteroannulation using microwave heating. Tetrahedron Lett. 45: 8631-8633.

[201] R. Dhawan, R.D. Dghaym and B.A. Arndtsen. 2003. The development of a catalytic synthesis of münchnones: a simple four-component coupling approach to α-amino acid derivatives. J. Am. Chem. Soc. 125: 1474-1475.

[202] H. Yoshimura, M. Nagai, S. Hibi, K. Kikuchi, S. Abe, T. Hida, S. Higashi, I. Hishinuma and T. Yamanaka. 1995. A novel type of retinoic acid receptor antagonist: synthesis and structure-activity relationships of heterocyclic ring-containing benzoic acid derivatives. J. Med. Chem. 38: 3163-3173.

[203] R. Dhawan and B.A. Arndtsen. 2004. Palladium-catalyzed multicomponent coupling of alkynes, imines, and acid chlorides: a direct and modular approach to pyrrole synthesis. J. Am. Chem. Soc. 126: 468-469.

[204] L.M. Pardo, I. Tellitu and E. Dominguez. 2010. A versatile PIFA-mediated approach to structurally diverse pyrrolo (benzo) diazepines from linear alkynylamides. Tetrahedron 66: 5811-5818.

[205] J.D. Winkler, A.T. Londregan and M.T. Hamann. 2006. Anti-malarial activity of a new family of analogues of manzamine A. Org. Lett. 8: 2591-2594.

CHAPTER 4

Five-Membered N,N-Heterocycles

4.1 Introduction

Pyrazolones are present in drugs in view of their pharmacological importance. For example, pyrazolones exhibit anti-fungal, anti-microbial, anti-bacterial, anti-mycobacterial, anti-tumor, anti-platelet, anti-inflammatory, anti-depressant, gastric secretion stimulatory, and anti-filarial activities. Pyrazolones also work as substrates for pigments, dyes, chelating agents, and pesticides [1-3]. These compounds are also inhibitors of CDK2 with good activity against a number of human tumour cell lines, cannabinoid type-1 (CB1) receptor antagonists, and inhibitors of tissue-nonspecific alkaline phosphatase (TNAP). In pesticide chemistry, they emerged as fungicides, insecticides, and herbicides. Pyrazole moiety is the core structure of a wide range of biologically active compounds, such as blockbuster drugs like celecoxib and sildenafil (viagra). Celecoxib exhibits anti-arthritic and analgesic activities and is a powerful COX-2 inhibitor whereas sildenafil (viagra) is a FDA approved drug used to treat erectile dysfunction. Difenamizole is a drug with anti-inflammatory, analgesic, and anti-pyretic properties [4-5].

The imidazole ring is present in many natural products such as histamine, purine, nucleic acid and histidine. The pharmacological activities of imidazole related drugs have encouraged the medicinal chemists to produce a number of chemotherapeutic agents [6].

Benzimidazole is a significant heterocycle due to its pharmacological activities and synthetic utility. The benzimidazole exhibits different biological properties such as anti-helmintic, anti-fungal, anti-histaminic, anti-HIV, cardio tonic, anti-ulcer, neuroleptic and anti-hypertensive. Extensive pharmacological and biochemical studies have confirmed that benzimidazoles are effective against many strains of microorganisms and have an important place as chemotherapeutic agents. The pharmacological importance of benzimidazoles is because of its close relationship with structure of purines. The role of purines in biological system was established and it is found that 5,6-dimethyl-1-(α-D-ribofuranosyl) benzimidazole is an integral constituent of structure of Vitamin B12 [7-16].

4.2 Palladium assisted synthesis of five-membered heterocycles with two nitrogen atoms

4.3 Palladium assisted synthesis of five-membered 1,2-*N,N*-heterocycles

Substituted pyrazoles were synthesized regioselectively in one-pot strategy due to electronic and pharmacological properties of pyrazoles, specially fluorophores, and the increased quest for tailor-made functional π-electron systems by diversity-oriented strategies. The diversity-oriented rapid synthetic protocol to fine tunable fluorophores (with fluorescence quantum yields up to 0.78) are of considerable interest for the development of tailor-made emitters in OLED applications and fluorescence labeling of surfaces, biomolecules or mesoporous materials. For more than a century, pyrazoles were synthesized from hydrazines and alkynones by Michael addition [17-18]. Despite of few cases [19], the regioselective synthesis of *N*-substituted pyrazoles by alkynone strategy has remained unexplored. Hydrazines and CH_3COOH were reacted in same reaction vessel after the formation of alkynones. By dielectric heating under MW for 10 min at 150 °C in MeOH, the pyrazoles were obtained in good to excellent yields **(Scheme 1)**. Three types of hydrazines such as methyl hydrazine, hydrazine, and aryl hydrazines were used in this reaction. In every case only one of the two possible regioisomers was preferentially produced depending on the nature of hydrazine substituent. Other regioisomers were formed in traces only (regioselectivity >98:2) [20a-b].

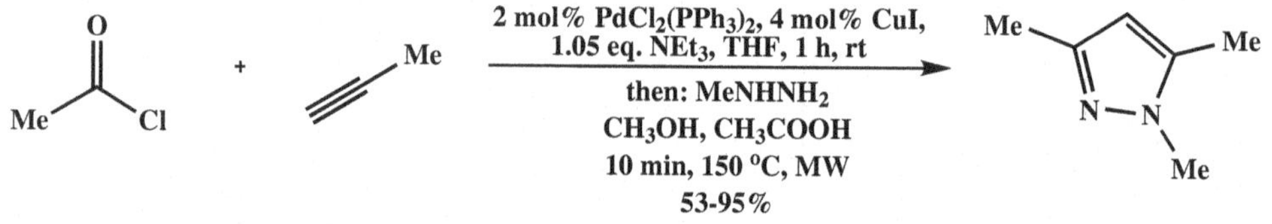

Scheme-1

Many *N*-heterocycles were synthesized when nitrogen-centred nucleophiles were reacted with α,β-unsaturated ketones (produced *in situ* by palladium-catalyzed Sonogashira cross-coupling). For example, Muller et al. [21] reacted acid chlorides, terminal alkynes, and hydrazines by a three-component pathway for the synthesis of 3,5-bis(hetero)aromatic pyrazoles. Traditional methods involved the cyclocondensation of hydrazine derivatives with 1,3-disubstituted three-carbon units (*i.e.* alkynones and α,β-unsaturated ketones). An interesting means of overcoming the poor commercial availability was *in situ* formation of 1,3-disubstituted three-carbon units. Several terminal alkynes and (hetero)aryl acid chlorides were heated in the presence of triethylamine, $PdCl_2(PPh_3)_2$, and cuprous iodide in tetrahydrofuran. A number of pyrazoles were synthesized under MW heating when ynones were treated *in situ* with diversely substituted hydrazine derivatives **(Scheme 2)**. In this cycloaddition, depending on the hydrazine derivatives one of the two possible regioisomers was obtained preferentially, *N*-aryl- and *N*-alkylhydrazines afforded opposite regioselectivities [22-23].

Mori et al. [24] reported carbonylative coupling of terminal alkynes with aryl (and heteroaryl) halides for the synthesis of α,β-alkynyl ketone derivatives as pyrazole precursors. A four-component domino approach of many terminal alkynes, organic halides, hydrazines, and CO was developed at rt. All components were mixed at very beginning of the reaction, under ambient pressure of carbon monoxide in the presence of 1 mol% of $PdCl_2(PPh_3)_2$ in aqueous tetrahydrofuran. This reaction was limited to *N*-methylhydrazine and simple hydrazine **(Scheme 3)**. The intermediacy of α,β-alkynyl ketones was not confirmed (thin layer chromatography). In addition, their reaction with hydrazines was ineffective in the absence or presence of Pd catalyst in present solvent. If α,β-alkynyl ketones were produced, they react immediately with hydrazine to synthesize pyrazole by a specific fast one-pot method [23].

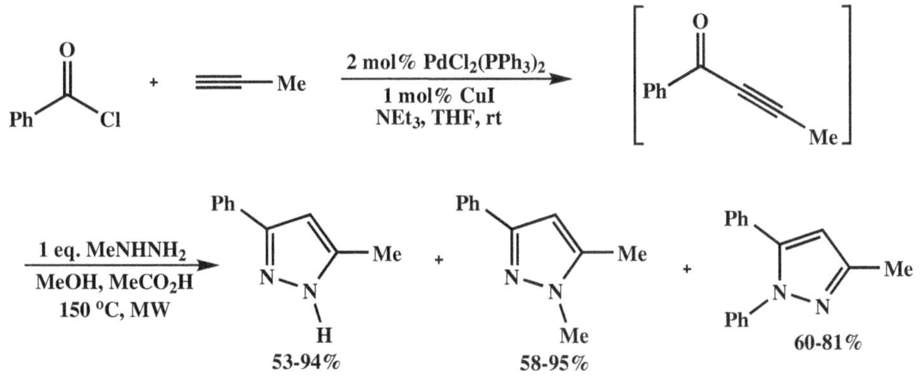

Scheme-2

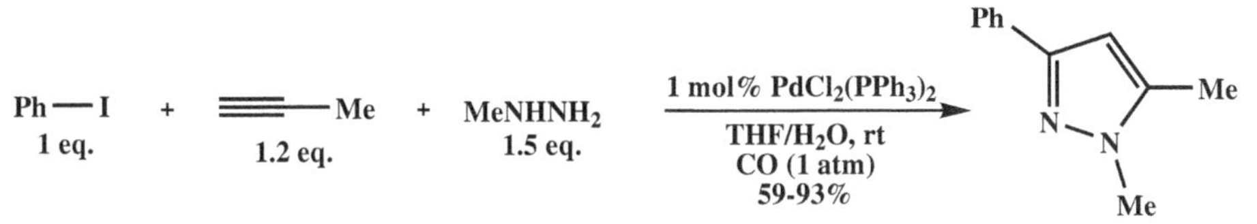

Scheme-3

Stonehouse et al. [25] utilized *in situ* produced imidazole to synthesize pyrazines. Here, carbonylative coupling of terminal alkynes with vinyl- or aryl-halides for the synthesis of imidazole was coupled with hydrazine addition **(Scheme 4)** [26].

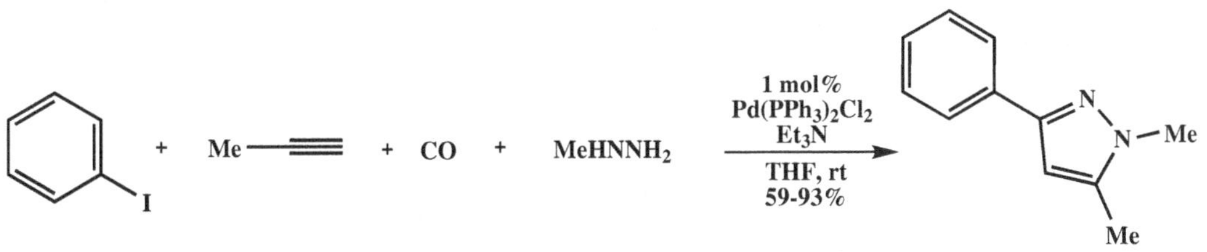

Scheme-4

A wide range of agrochemical and pharmaceutical products contain substituted pyrazoles. The core of many drugs like zometapine [27] or sildenafil [28] is formed by pyrazoles. Chalcones and hydrazines were reacted to form 1,3,5-trisubstituted pyrazoles in the presence of palladium/ carbon/K-10 bifunctional catalyst [29a-b]. The catalyst was a mechanical mixture of commercially available K-10 montmorillonite and palladium/carbon. The condensation of chalcones with hydrazines and cyclization occurred in the reaction. K-10 catalyzed these two steps. Good to excellent yields (80-98%) of 1,3,5-trisubstituted pyrazoles were obtained in the presence of palladium/carbon which ensured high rates in aromatization step **(Scheme 5)**.

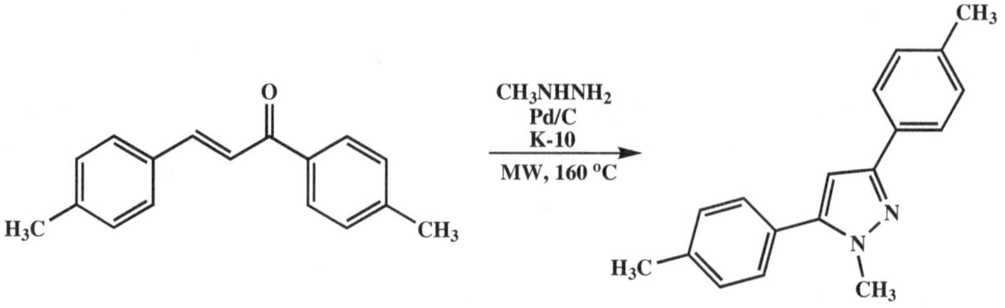

Scheme-5

This protocol was used for the generation of a large number of *N*-heterocycles such as imidazolidin-2-ones [30], and isoxazolidines [31-34]. The *cis*- and *trans*-3,5-disubstituted pyrazolidines were formed in high stereoselectivity and the absence or presence of *N*-1 protecting group controlled product stereochemistry [35]. For instance, the *trans*-disubstituted product was formed when starting substrate (R = Boc) was reacted with 4-bromophenyl in the presence of Pd catalyst and sodium *tert*-butoxide, whereas when starting compound (R = H) was treated under similar reaction conditions the *cis*-disubstituted product was obtained (**Scheme 6-7**).

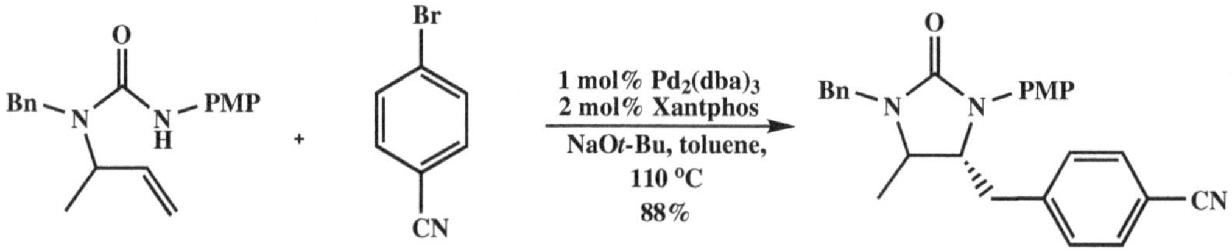

Scheme-6

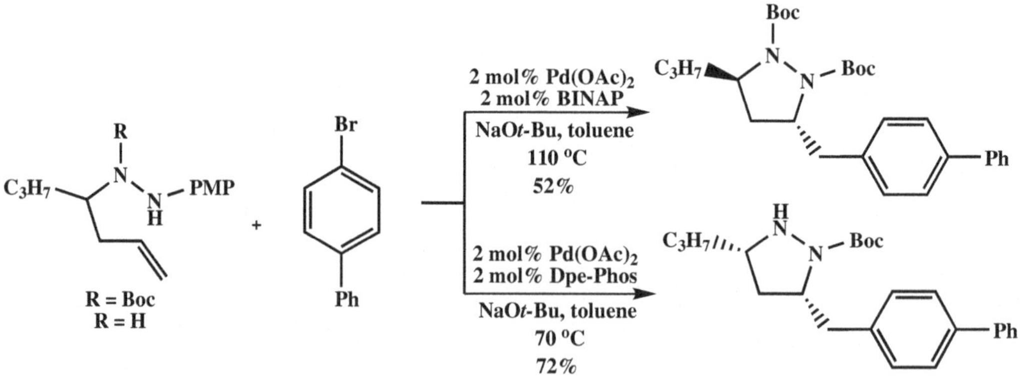

Scheme-7

4.4   Palladium assisted synthesis of five-membered 1,3-*N*,*N*-heterocycles

The good "combinatorial" capability of fluorous technology has demonstrated its great potential in this area [36a-b]. Perfluorosulfonates were valuable fluorous synthons. The perfluorooctanesulfonyl tag played three roles in multistep synthesis: 1) as a fluorous tag to facilitate intermediate purification; 2) as a protecting agent for hydroxyl group; and 3) as an activating group to promote the coupling reaction. Cyclic and acyclic amide compounds were synthesized as shown in **Scheme 8**. The reductive amination reactions of fluorous benzaldehydes were carried out. The substituted hydantoin rings were formed when amines were reacted with isocyanates. The biaryl products were synthesized from purified F-sulfonates *via* Pd-catalyzed cross-coupling reactions [37].

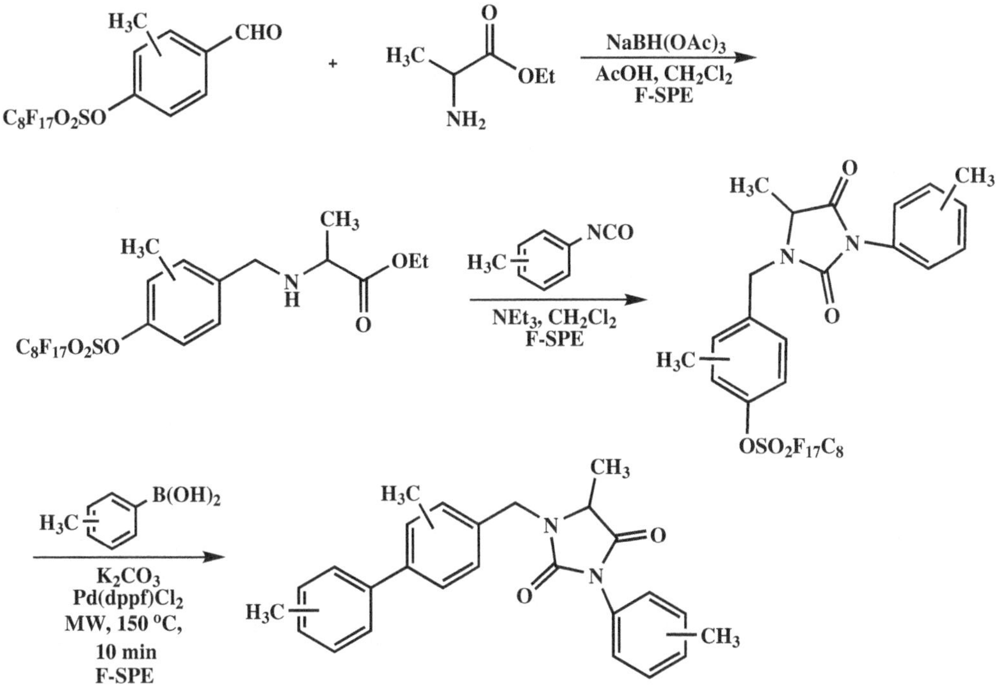

Scheme-8

Suzuki coupling of boronic acids with aryl halides was enabled under MW activation without solvent in the presence of Pd catalyst (**Scheme 9**). A number of boronic acids and chloro-, bromo-, and iodoaryls provided biaryls with fast rate of reaction in 10 min [38].

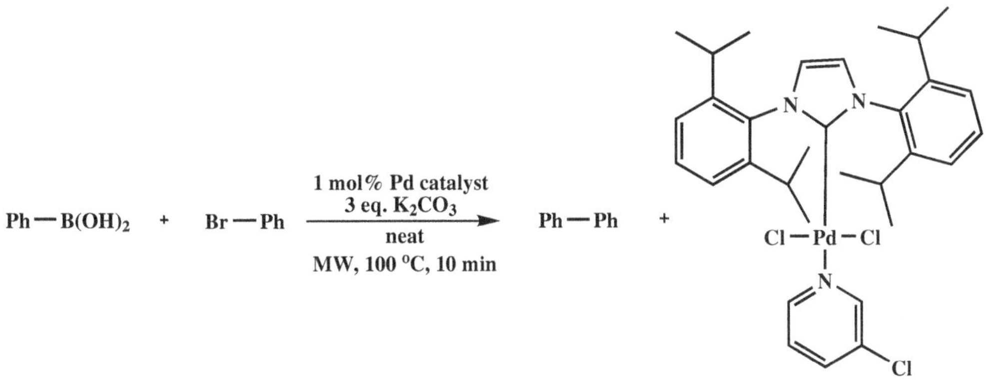

Scheme-9

An intramolecular amino-Heck reaction produced cyclic amines like azaazulene, aza-spiro compound, indoles and imidazoles, other than isoquinolines and pyrroles, in which many unsaturated open tafluorobenzoyloximes reacted with a palladium(0) catalyst (**Scheme 10**) [39-43].

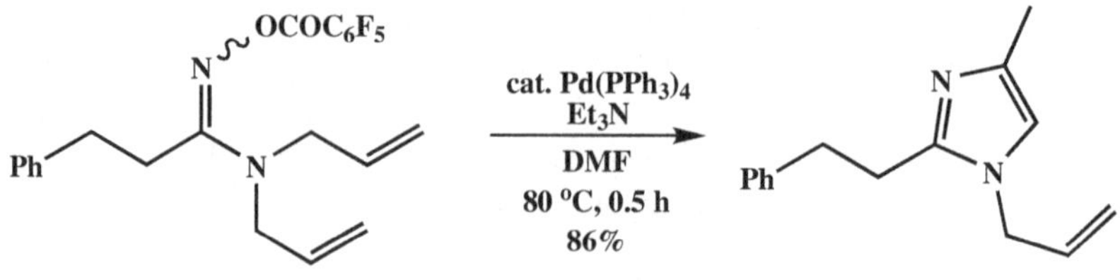

Scheme-10

Imidazolines are possessed by many biologically active compounds. The imidazolines substituted with carboxylate group have attracted the attention as potent cell sensitizers and as peptide bond isoteres for cancer treatment [44]. The simple substrates such as CO and imines coupled for the preparation of imidazolines. However, low yield (40%) of heterocycle was obtained, and the reaction occurred in a multistep manner that was stoichiometric in Pd complex. Despite these problems, the mechanism can be in sighted so that this reaction can be made an efficient pathway **(Scheme 11)** [45-46].

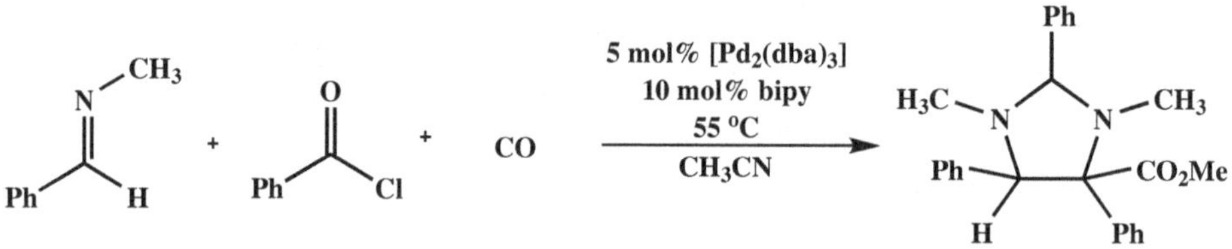

Scheme-11

Imidazole derivative acts as a potent p38 MAP kinase inhibitor. Siamaki and Arndtsen [47] synthesized this imidazole derivative regioselectively in one-step through palladium-catalyzed coupling of acid chloride and imines **(Scheme 12)**. This compound was used for the synthesis of new anti-inflammatory agents [48]. Two distinct imines were simultaneously coupled into imidazole core in this reaction. This occurred from inability of *N*-tosyl imines to form the iminium salts, but instead underwent a more fast 1,3-dipolar addition. As such, imidazoles were formed with selective variation of every substituent about the heterocyclic core and with high regiocontrol. Here, sterically encumbered phosphanes like P(*o*-tolyl)$_3$ provoked a 7 times fast oxidative addition of imine to acid chloride and carbon monoxide leading to 1,3-dipole. To prevent the side reactions with iminium ion, preformation of 1,3-dipole was required in reactive dipolarophiles. The trisubstituted imidazoles were formed when münchnones were reacted with *N*-tosyl imines [49-50]. The concurrent synthesis of *N*-(*a*-sulfonyl alkyl)amides was avoided in the presence of lithium chloride and P(*o*-tolyl)$_3$ at lower reaction temperatures [46].

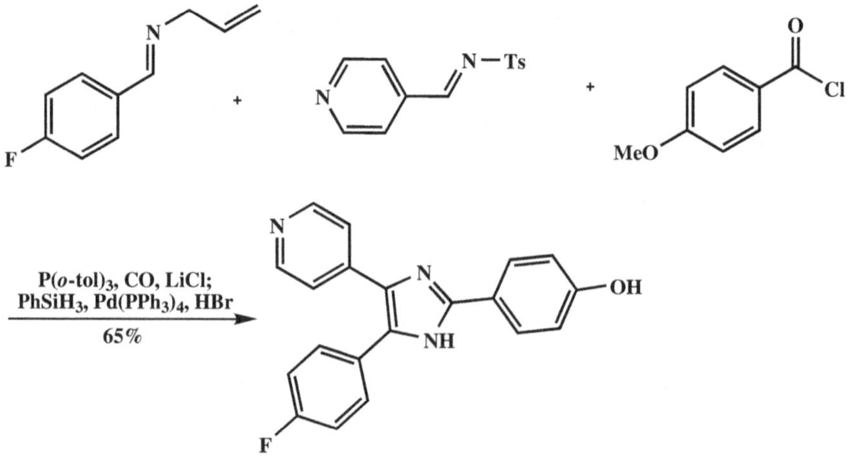

Scheme-12

Ketocarbamates were formed *via* carbonylative coupling reaction under 1 atmosphere of CO by replacing acid chloride with a chloroformate [51]. Many imines and chloroformates participated in this reaction, stannanes being limited to benzyl, aryl, or ethyl ones. The transmetallation step occurred in fast rates when vinylstannane was utilized, subsequently carbon monoxide insertion provided substituted carbamates. Postcyclization led to imidazolones, with elimination of chloroformate substituent after the removal of solvents in vacuo, with the addition of 15 eq. of NH$_4$OAc and CH$_3$COOH to crude mixture **(Scheme 13)**. Acid chlorides activated the imines toward cross-coupling with organostannanes [52-54], their utilization led to imidazolines under carbonylative conditions. The cyclization of carbonylated Pd intermediate synthesized 1,3-oxazolium-5-olate, followed by 1,3-dipolar cycloaddition of an imine [55]. The carbonylative cross-coupling product was formed in quantitative yield upon replacing acid chloride with chloroformate at ambient temperature [56]. Since transition metal catalyst was involved in these C-C bond-forming reactions, they incorporated further levels of molecular complexity. For instance, the iminium salt oxidative addition was combined with carbonylation, followed by a Stille-like coupling, to afford amido ketones. This was a relatively rare four-component cross-coupling reaction for the synthesis of final product from chloroformate, imine, CO and arylstannane. This was used to design a one-pot route for the synthesis of imidazolones from five separate units: acid chloride, an imine, arylstannane, CO, and NH$_3$ [23, 46].

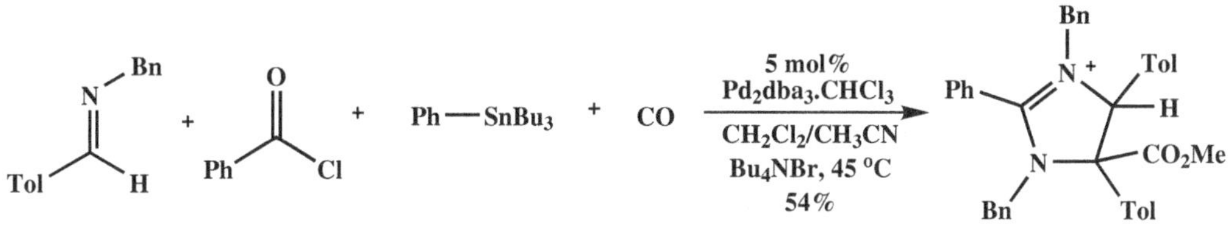

Scheme-13

The precursor(s) were built with the desired substituents prior to cyclization. The synthesis of highly substituted imidazolines occurred in multiple steps which complicated its synthesis as well as product diversification. An alternative was to synthesize polysubstituted heterocyclic compounds like imidazolines directly from multiple, available building blocks. The coupling of acid chlorides, imines, and carbon monoxide in the presence of Pd catalyst produced imidazolinium carboxylates **(Scheme 14)**. This method utilized either easily synthesized (imines, from aldehydes and amines) or available (PhCOCl and CO) building blocks and avoided the requirement of complex substrates for cyclization [57-63, 132].

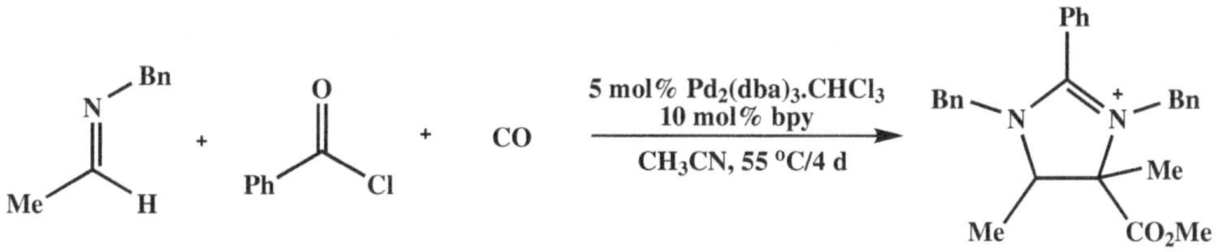

Scheme-14

With a large panel of framework accessible from cyclohexyl to an alkyl, the ligand backbone was changed easily. Due to the availability of various benzaldehydes the left arm was highly tuneable. Along with this blocking part was derived from aryl bromide derivatives. A three-step pathway was followed for the production of ligands **(Scheme 15)** [64].

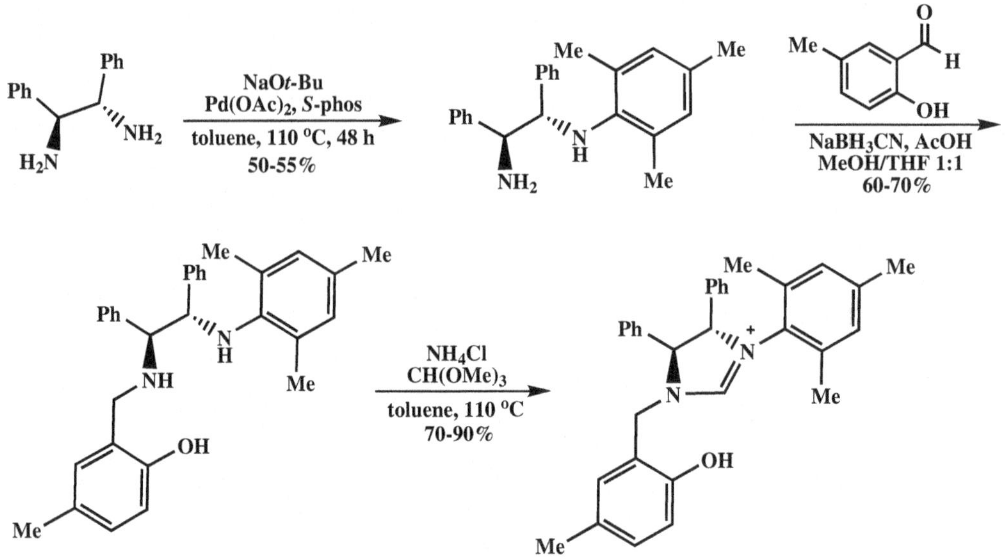

Scheme-15

The addition of Tol(H)C.NR (Tol. *p*-C$_6$H$_4$CH$_3$) and 1 atm carbon monoxide to complex led to palladium-chelated amide complex [65]. The oxidative addition of acyliminium salt to [Pd$_2$(dba)$_3$] CHCl$_3$ in the presence of 2,2′-bipyridine formed Pd complex in 92% yield [66-70]. In contrast to the behavior of palladium-chelated amide complex, the reaction of Pd complex with 1 atm carbon monoxide in CD$_3$CN led to the slow disappearance of starting materials over the course of 5 d at 55 °C. Surprisingly, however, product isolation yields carboxylate-substituted imidazoline in 35% yield. Carboxylate-substituted imidazolines are biologically relevant heterocycles, formally incorporating an amino acid residue into heterocyclic core [10±12]. Thus, the generation of imidazolines from Pd complex suggested that imine and carbon monoxide have been coupled into a peptide unit, followed by subsequent reactions. To determine the origin of imidazolines, and to optimize its synthesis, the mechanism of transformation was examined. This presumably arises from insertion of 13CO into Pd complex to form the Pd-bound amino acid derivative **(Scheme 16)**.

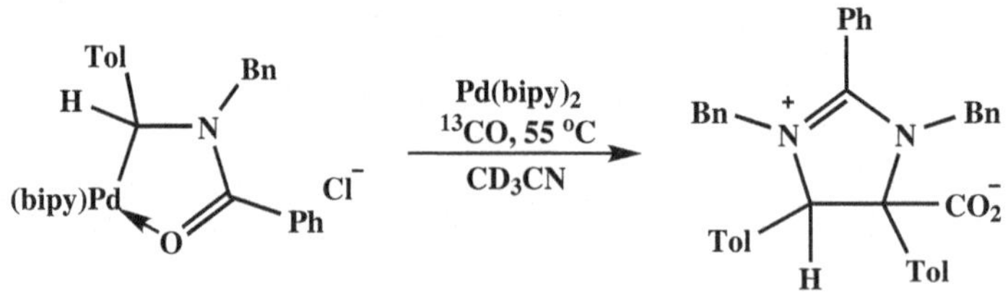

Scheme-16

The serotonin 5-HT3 receptor antagonist ondansetron (zofran) was produced by a totally different pathway. The tricyclic indole core was formed *via* a Pd-catalyzed intramolecular Heck reaction in a concise and short procedure **(Scheme 17)** [71-73].

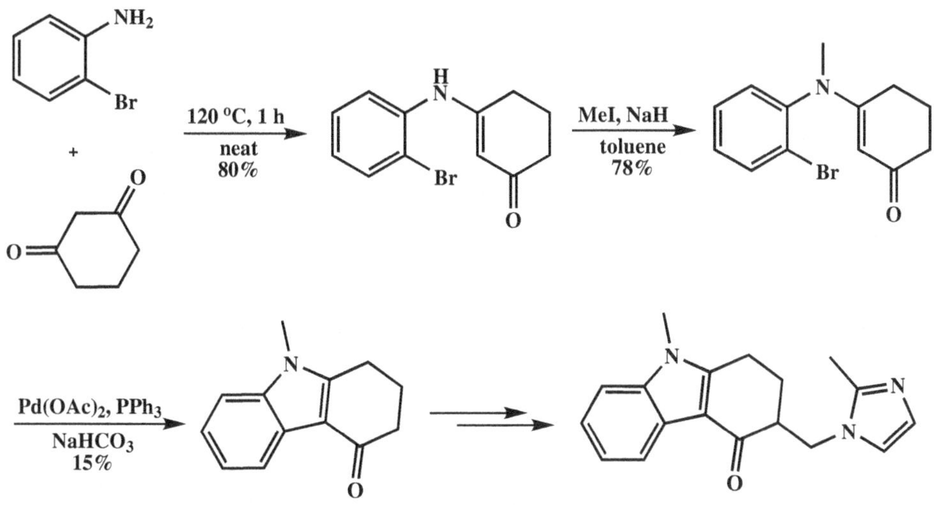

Scheme-17

The reactions involving bulky phosphine ligands occurred at comparable rates. The Pd benzoyl complex was formed as an intermediate immediately **(Scheme 18)**. However, the Pd benzoyl complex disappeared rapidly, and the phosphine was transformed into its protonated form quantitatively after one catalytic cycle [74]. Thus, to inhibit the immediate formation of inactive Pd black, phosphine played a critical role in initial stage of catalysis, but once the catalysis was underway it was a nonphosphine-bound Pd which mediated this reaction. The monitoring of stoichiometric reaction of imine and Pd benzoyl complex has shown that Pd benzoyl complex was cleanly converted into imidazoline and protonated phosphine. In this stoichiometric reaction Pd intermediates were not reported. The Pd benzoyl complex was coupled slowly with imine for the preparation of imidazoline, and then the Pd benzoyl complex was rapidly converted into product [75].

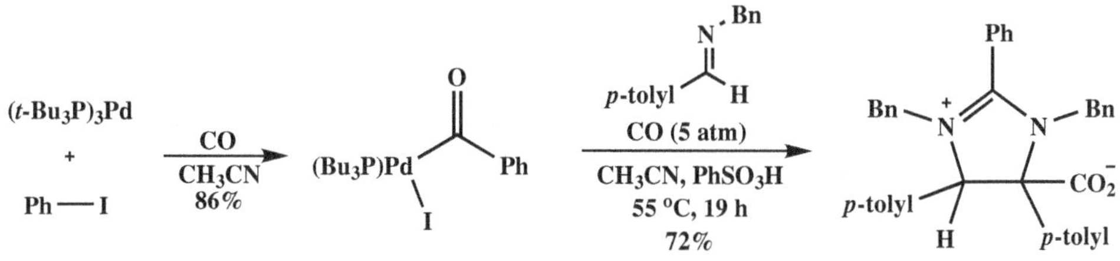

Scheme-18

Reactions catalyzed by different [SCS], [PCP], [NCN] and [S-CSe] pincer Pd complexes were reported [76]. All these complexes showed different diastereoselectivity (depending on the ligand) and excellent catalytic ability. Thus, optimal *cis* selectivity was displayed by electron-deficient phosphine complex, while a reversal of selectivity toward the *trans* isomer was exhibited by electron-rich selenide complexes **(Scheme 19)**. The [NCN] and [SCS] complexes also showed *trans* selectivity but in lower *de*. Their different behavior in catalytic cycle, rather than by electronic properties of ligand, was explained by differences in stereodirecting performance. The [NCN] and [SCS] pincer palladium complexes underwent insertion of an isocyanide into carbon-palladium bond. In contrast, [PCP] complexes were stable toward insertion [77-78]. Therefore, in these cases different species enter the catalytic cycle, which resulted in different diastereoselectivity [79].

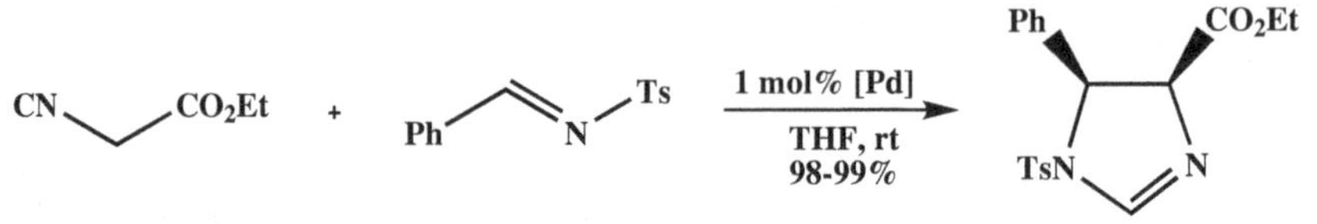

Scheme-19

Lloyd-Jones and Booker-Milburn [80] explained intermolecular diamination of 1,3-dienes and acyclic ureas to synthesize bicyclic or monocyclic urea in the presence of Pd catalyst combined with either oxygen or benzoquinone oxidant. For instance, urea was obtained in 82% yield from diene. These reactions involved the formation of *p*-allylpalladium complex intermediate. The first example reported for the diamination of conjugated dienes involved *N,N*-dialkylureas and dienes. A mixture of isomeric products was observed with isoprene in molecular O_2 or benzoquinone **(Scheme 20)** [81].

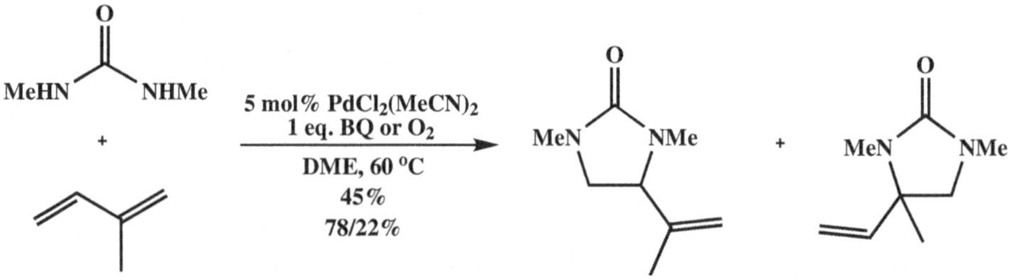

Scheme-20

Shi [82] in 2007 described the preparation of imidazolidin-2-ones by catalytic asymmetric diamination of conjugated dienes and trienes. Shi developed a much different pathway for the synthesis of cyclic ureas from 1,3-dienes or trienes. An intermediate was produced in 94% yield when conjugated diene was treated with di-*t*-butyldiaziridinone and Pd(PPh$_3$)$_4$ catalyst. This reaction occurred through oxidative addition of di-*t*-butyldiaziridinone to palladium(0), which underwent aminopalladation to produce allylpalladium complex. The urea product was formed upon reductive elimination from allylpalladium complex. An asymmetric variant of this conversion afforded products with 95% *ee*. A number of trienes and dienes were utilized. For the internal alkene of diene or triene, the diamination reaction was highly selective **(Scheme 21)**.

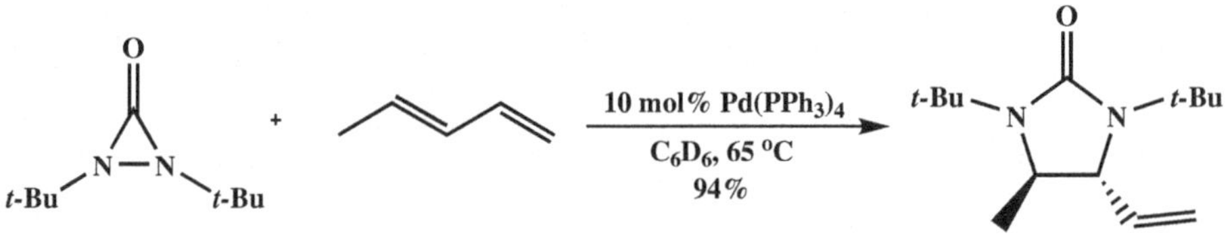

Scheme-21

Shi and co-workers [83] described the utility of conjugated diene for the preparation of imidazolidin-2-one with high regio-, diastereo and enantioselectivity in good yield through asymmetric diamination of terminal olefin in the presence of di-*tert*-butyldiaziridinone nitrogen source, Pd$_2$(dba)$_3$ catalyst and phosphorus amidite ligand **(Scheme 22)** [49].

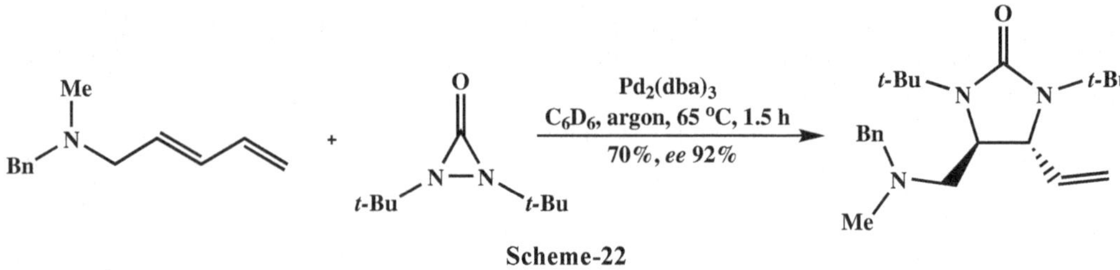

Scheme-22

Neither the use of chiral ligands nor chiral auxiliaries were particularly successful in achieving an asymmetric carboamination of *N*-allylureas. The best enantiomeric excess 53% was obtained through the use of (*R*)-(*S*)-Josiphos. The best diastereoselectivity 2:1 was observed with chiral auxiliaries. Other phosphoramidites besides (*R*)-monodentate phosphoramidite may be more successful for asymmetric cyclization. Shi [83] also demonstrated that large variations in enantioselectivity can be observed in palladium-catalyzed diamination reactions with different phosphoramidite ligands as shown in **Scheme 23**.

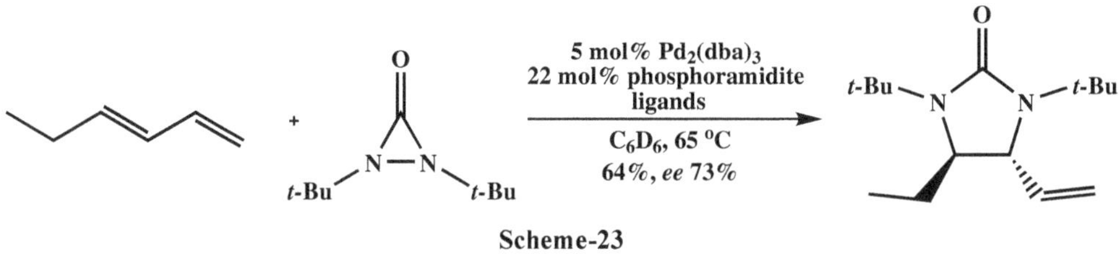

Scheme-23

A more direct route to 1,2-diamines was direct introduction of two nitrogen atoms onto an alkene. Diamination has until recently remained largely unexplored. This was in contrast to extensively studied catalytic dihydroxylation and aminohydroxylation reactions that have established themselves as valuable tools for synthetic chemists [84]. Early examples involved the use of stoichiometric metal reagents so remained far less practical than dihydroxylation and aminohydroxylation protocols, even though stereoselective examples were reported using either chiral auxiliaries or chiral Lewis acids [85-86]. Recent advances have enabled direct diamination of alkenes using transition metal (TM) derivatives in catalytic amounts. Shi and co-workers [82] reported enantioselective diamination of dienes and trienes using a palladium(0) catalyst, derived from phosphoramidite, and di-*tert*-butyldiaziridinone. The cyclic urea products were formed in excellent yield and enantioselectivity **(Scheme 24)**. The cleavage of *t*-Bu groups and urea could be achieved in high yield upon treatment with trifluoroacetic acid followed by hydrogen chloride.

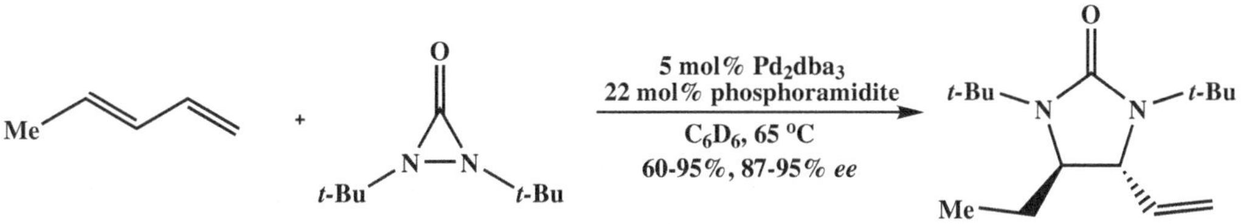

Scheme-24

In this conversion the heterolytic cleavage of B-B bond occurred rather than oxidative addition of diboron to metal as indicated by DFT calculations. Diaziridinone was utilized for the diamination of conjugated dienes (and trienes) in the presence of [(IPr)Pd(allyl)Cl] at 65 °C **(Scheme 25)** [87-88].

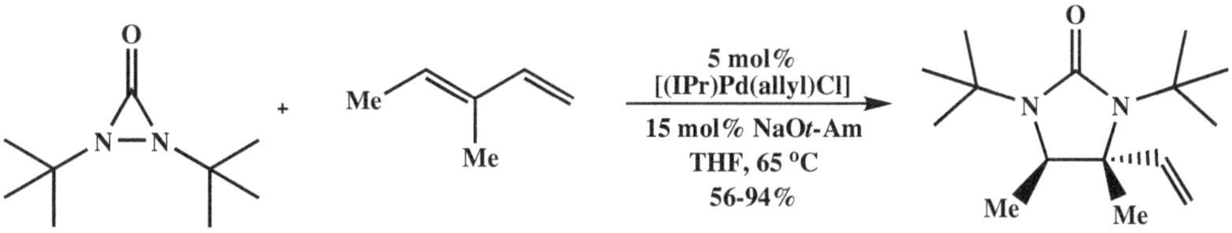

Scheme-25

Chiral NHC-palladium(0) complexes have been effective for asymmetric diamination reactions of conjugated dienes and trienes **(Scheme 26)** [89]. For example, treatment of di-*tert*-butylaziridinone and diene with *N*-heterocyclic carbene-palladium(0) complex afforded imidazolidin-2-one in 88% yield and 76% *ee*. As compared to palladium-phosphoramidite catalyst system described above, *N*-heterocyclic carbene-palladium(0) complexes can potentially serve as better catalysts, since these catalysts were potentially more stable and subtle changes to NHC structure seem to effect reactivity and enantioselectivites to a greater degree.

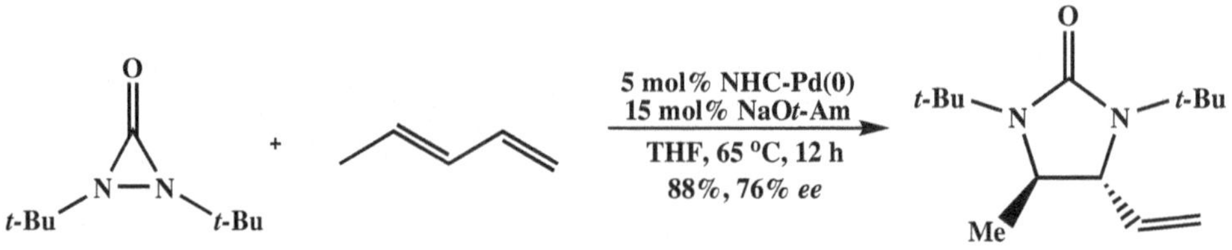

Scheme-26

Terminal alkene substrates were utilized in this reaction [90-91]. For instance, the target product was obtained from 1-hexene in 68% yield with Pd(PPh$_3$)$_4$ catalyst in the absence of solvent. In these reactions asymmetric induction has also been observed, and up to 94% *ee*'s were reported with a catalyst supported by chiral phosphoramidite ligand [92]. Mechanism of terminal alkene diamination reactions is not established yet, but still it seems that allylic carbon-hydrogen activation/amination was involved **(Scheme 27)**.

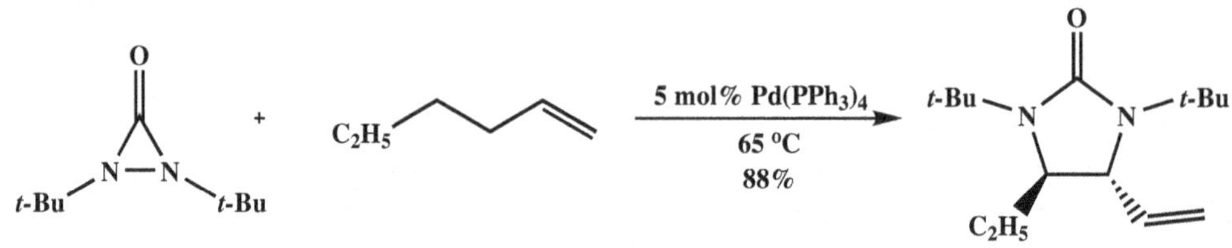

Scheme-27

The cyclic ureas and similar heterocycles were produced by reactions of vinylaziridines [93] or activated vinylcyclopropanes [94] with isocyanates and other heterocumulenes. For instance, Trost [95] reported the synthesis of urea with 99% *ee* in 82% yield through a dynamic kinetic asymmetric reaction of aziridine and phenylisocyanate. The isomerization resulted in interconversion of stereoisomers after oxidative addition of aziridine to palladium(0) **(Scheme 28)**.

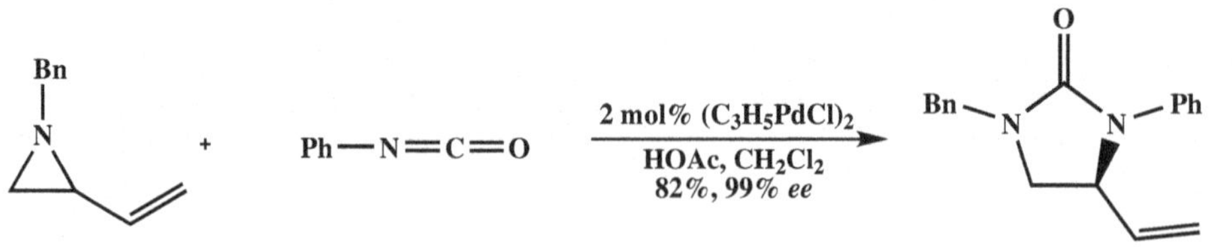

Scheme-28

Baeg and Alper [96] reported palladium-catalyzed [3+2]-cycloaddition reactions between activated heterocumulenes and aziridines like carbodiimides and isocyanates. Good yields of carbamates, ureas, and other heterocyclic compounds were obtained from these transformations. For instance, urea was formed in 72% yield when starting compound was reacted with phenylisocyanate. The reactions occurred through addition of aziridine to palladium(0), followed by insertion of isocyanate into palladium-nitrogen bond and carbon-carbon bond-forming reductive elimination **(Scheme 29)**.

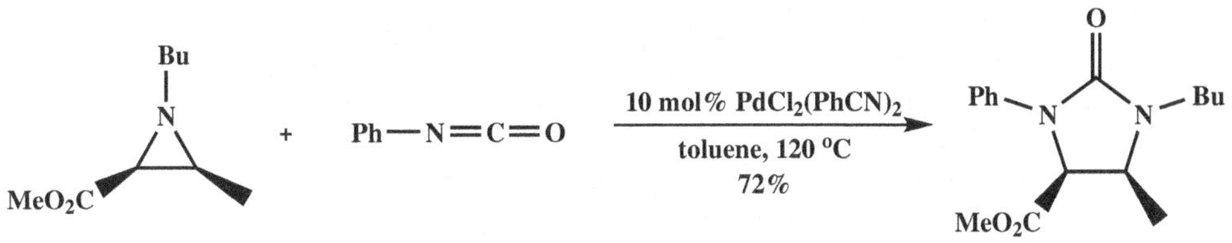

Scheme-29

The optically pure aziridines were synthesized from enantiomers of 2-phenyloxirane to determine the enantioselectivity of cycloaddition reaction. The (+)-1-*n*-butyl-3,4-diphenyli-midazolidin-2-one was formed in 82% yield from (*S*)-(+)-*n*-butyl-2-phenylaziridine and phenyl isocyanate *via* Pd(II)-catalyzed cycloaddition reaction **(Scheme 30)**. Similarly, when (*R*)-(-)-*n*-butyl-2-phenylaziridine was reacted with phenyl isocyanate, (-)-enantiomer was formed in 81% yield **(Scheme 31)**. These results have shown that Pd(II)-catalyzed cycloaddition reactions of aziridines and heterocumulenes proceeded enantiospecifically and with the retention of configuration of asymmetric center [97].

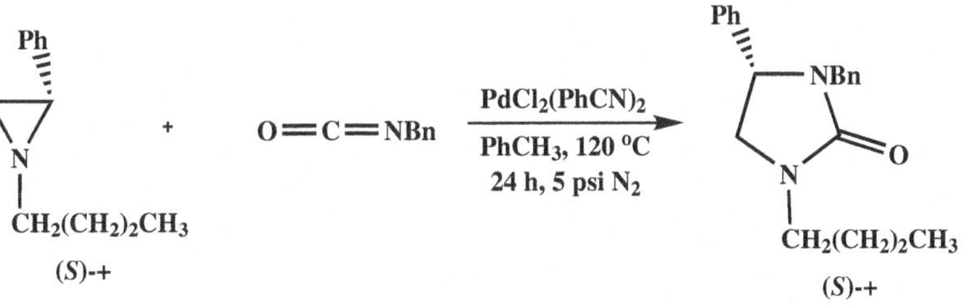

Scheme-30

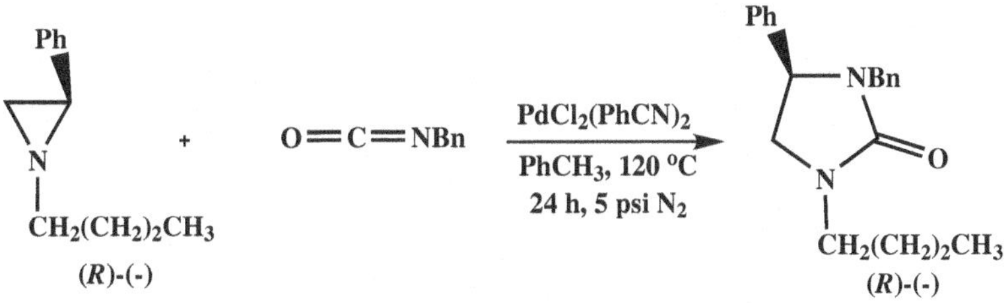

Scheme-31

An ester group containing *cis*-*n*-butyl-2-carboalkoxy-3-methylaziridines underwent cycloaddition reaction. The *cis*-*n*-butyl-3-(*p*-chlorophenyl)-4-carbomethoxy-5-methylimidazolidin-2-one was formed in 80% yield when cycloaddition of aziridine occurred with *p*-chlorophenyl isocyanate at 120 °C in PhMe for 20 h in catalytic amount of bis-(benzonitrile)palladium dichloride. The cycloaddition proceeded with retention of stereochemistry at heterocyclic carbon centers containing functional groups. The reaction was both stereo- and regiospecific. Good yields of thiazolidinimines were observed when aryl isocyanates and isothiocyanates were treated with aziridine in (PhCN)$_2$PdCl$_2$ **(Scheme 32)** [97-98].

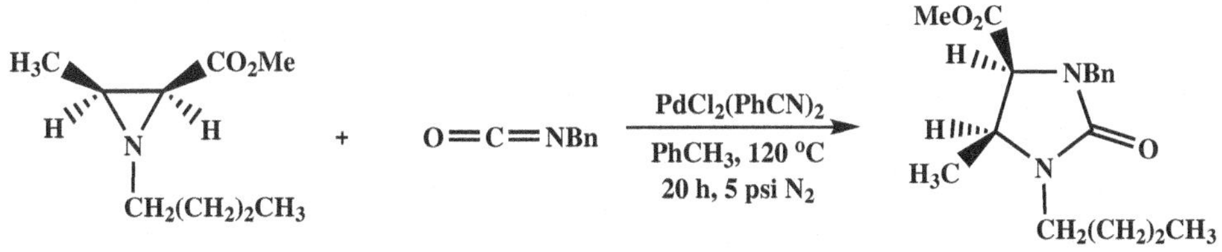

Scheme-32

A number of different methods have been used for the synthesis of 3-aminotetrahydroquinoline. Lombardo and co-workers [99-100] used hydrogenation of 3-aminoquinoline in the synthesis of farnesyltransferase inhibitors (**Scheme 33**). The drawbacks of this method were low yields obtained for hydrogenation and the products were formed racemically and, therefore, required a further chiral resolution step to obtain optically pure products.

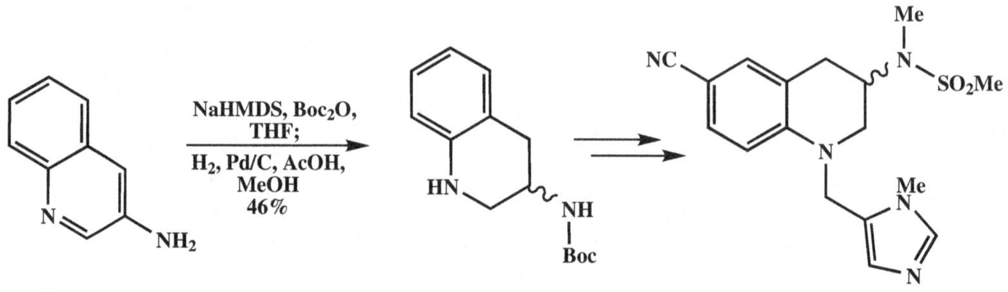

Scheme-33

Scarborough and Stahl [101] synthesized 2,4-disubstituted pyrrolidines *via* oxidative coupling of *N*-allyl tosylamides with butyl vinyl ether or many styrene derivatives in the presence of palladium(II) catalyst. The palladium catalyst was re-oxidized with molecular O_2 and copper(II)-co-catalyst. The beneficial effects of many non-traditional co-catalysts such as methyl acrylate, catechol, and 1,5-cyclooctadiene were also evaluated on reactions. Wolfe and co-workers [102-103] reacted allylamines, through $Pd_2(dba)_3$-Xanthphos induced carboamination of *N*-allylureas, for the synthesis of substituted imidazolidin-2-ones in two steps (**Scheme 34**). The use of *S*-Phos (2-dicyclohexylphosphino-2′,6′-dimethoxybiphenyl) prevented the formation of mixtures of regioisomeric product and minimized the *N*-arylation of substrate [49].

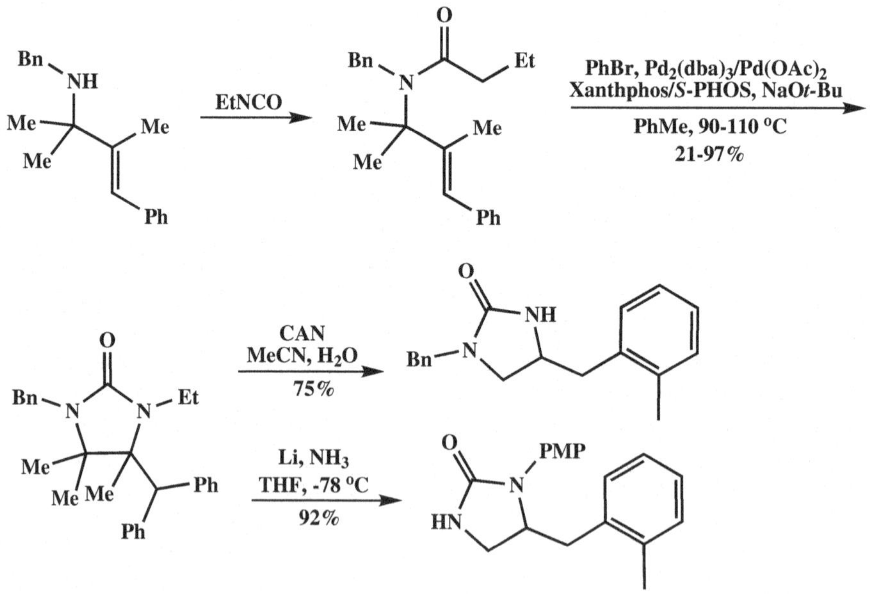

Scheme-34

Thomas and co-workers [104] reported the formation of imidazoles in high enantiomeric excess when substituted allylamine underwent palladium(0)-catalyzed amino-Heck reaction (**Scheme 35**) [49].

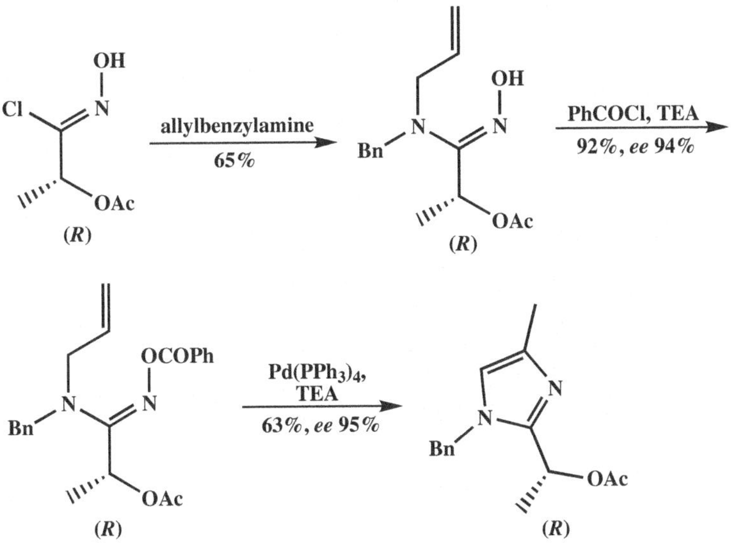

Scheme-35

High regioselectivity of products was observed with other 1,3-dienes in amination process **(Scheme 36)**. Benzoquinone acted as a superior re-oxidant in comparison to oxygen and avoided the not desired Wacker-type side process. For the progress of this reaction both a weakly coordinating solvent and a chloride containing palladium(II) catalyst were essential [81, 105-107].

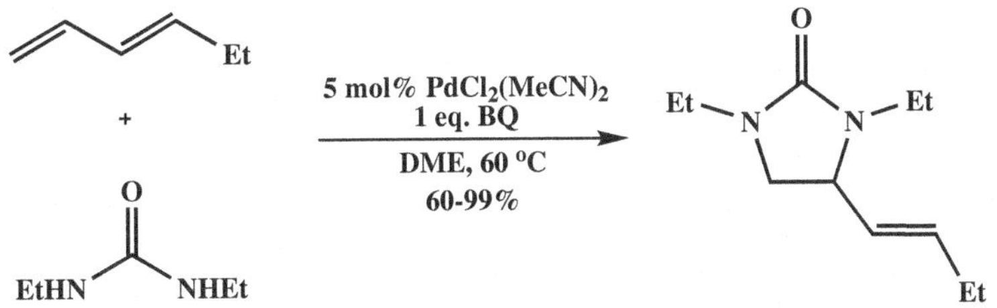

Scheme-36

The haloamination of allylic amines and allylic alcohol provided halomethyl-substituted imidazolinones and oxazolidinones, respectively, in the presence of *p*-toluenesulfonyl isocyanate and cupric chloride/palladium acetate/lithium chloride. High chemo-, regio-, and diastereo-selectivities were afforded in this reaction **(Scheme 37)** [81, 108].

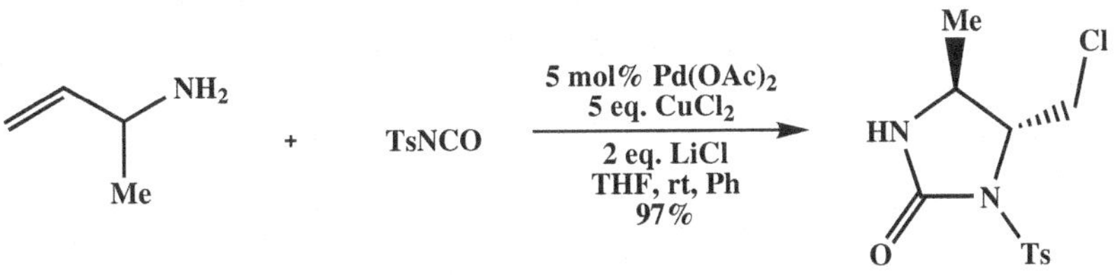

Scheme-37

The heterocycles were produced *via* intra- and intermolecular carbon-heteroatom bond forming reactions with alkenyl aziridines [109-110]. These substrates were utilized for the synthesis of heterocycles by two main protocols. Firstly, alkenyl aziridines underwent intramolecular allylation. In second pathway, an intermolecular cycloaddition of vinyl aziridines occurred with heterocumulenes, like carbodiimides, isocyanates, and isothiocyanates **(Scheme 38)** [111-115].

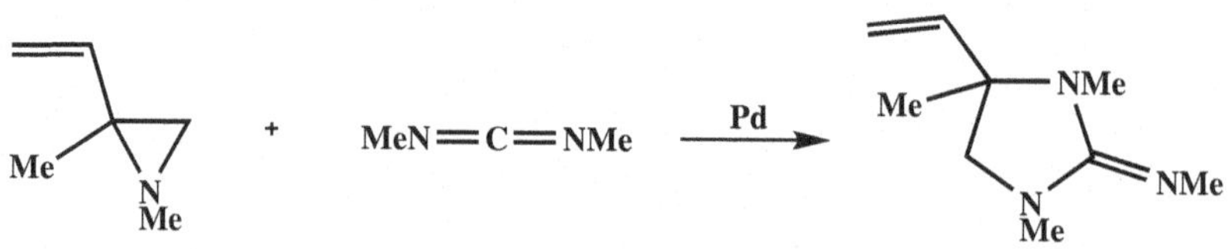

Scheme-38

Broggini [116a] reported intramolecular carboamination of allenamides in the presence of palladium catalyst for the preparation of 4-imidazolidinones **(Scheme 39)**. Optically enriched α-amino allenamides were used in this reaction, and the reaction progressed *via* a palladium-catalyzed carbopalladation-5-*exo-dig* amination reaction through Pd π-allyl intermediates (carbonylated). The tricyclic fused-ring imidazolidinones were afforded in this work *via* intramolecular carbopalladation of allenamides [116b].

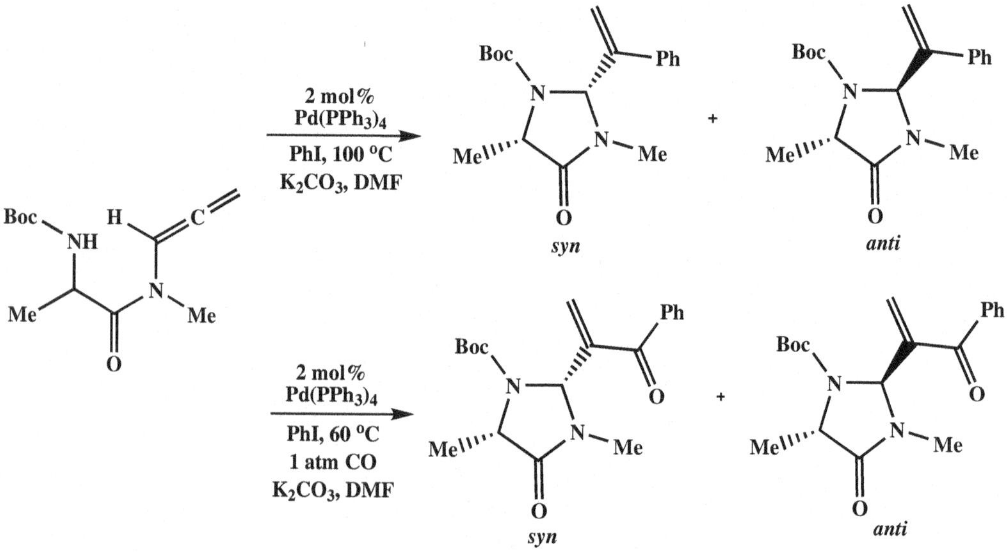

Scheme-39

A non-oxidative approach toward the asymmetric synthesis of *N*-heterocycles was palladium(II)-catalyzed alkene aminopalladation involving substrates bearing allylic acetates. These reactions no longer required oxidant, but substrates become more complex. Nonetheless, treatment of starting compound with catalytic amount of FOP catalyst afforded ureas, amides and oxazolidinones in high yield and enantioselectivities. Aminopalladation of starting compound proceeded through palladium-alkyl intermediate and subsequent β-acetoxy elimination provided *N*-heterocycles and regenerated the active catalyst **(Scheme 40)** [117].

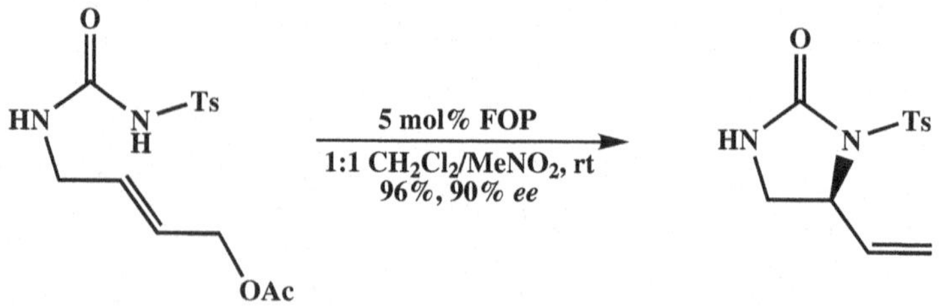

Scheme-40

Use of 1-allyl-3-ethyl-1-phenylurea greatly improved selectivity in these reactions. Previous experience in Wolfe group [118-119] suggested that outcome of carboaminations was largely dependent on the nature of phosphine ligand. Thus, a series of phosphine ligands was screened to determine which one would give highest selectivity and yield. Reaction of 1-allyl-3-ethyl-1-phenylurea with 4-Br-PhMe, Pd$_2$(dba)$_3$, phosphine ligand, and sodium *tert*-butoxide, in PhMe using phenanthrene as an internal NMR standard gave a mixture of three products including desired carboamination product, a formal oxidative amination product and a diaryl allylamine (**Scheme 41**) [120].

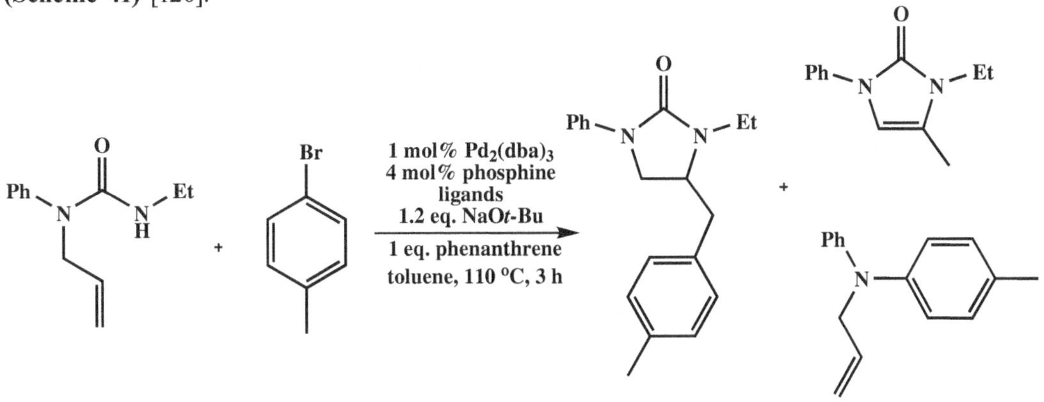

Scheme-41

Having optimized the reaction conditions with respect to phosphine ligand the scope of palladium-catalyzed carboamination of *N*-allylureas was explored (**Scheme 42**). Gratifyingly, it was found that 1-allyl-3-alkyl ureas successfully coupled with a variety of aryl halides to provide imidazolidin-2-ones. While good yields can be obtained for a variety of combinations of *N*-allylureas and aryl halides, reactions involving 2-bromoanisole and 4-bromoanisole were particularly challenging. The electron-donating ability of -OMe group may slow down oxidative addition, carbon-carbon bond forming reductive elimination, or olefin insertion, and allowed decomposition pathways to dominate [121]. Interestingly, the combination of 1-allyl-3-ethyl-1-phenyl urea and 4-bromobenzonitrile was expected to give a high yield for cyclized product but instead gave only a modest 43% yield. A product derived from competing *N*-arylation was also isolated (~35%). This was in marked contrast to the reaction of 1-allyl-3-benzyl-1-methyl urea with same aryl halide. The increased steric bulk of benzyl group relative to an ethyl group may serve to slow the rate of *N*-arylation.

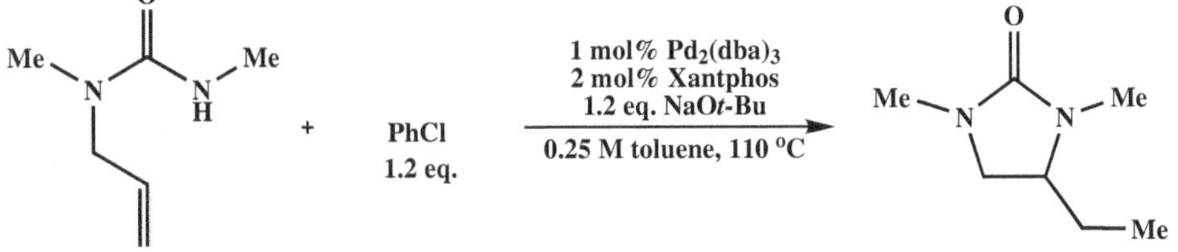

Scheme-42

In contrast to substrates having alkyl groups on cyclizing nitrogen, those with aryl groups on cyclizing nitrogen uniformly give excellent yields irrespective of the aryl halide used (**Scheme 43**). For example, replacement of Ph with Et on cyclizing nitrogen gave a 64% increase in yield for 4-bromoanisole. Likewise, with 2-bromonaphthalene, a 29% increase in yield was observed. This increase in yield could be explained by lack of a β-hydrogen for substrates having an aryl group on cyclizing nitrogen [122].

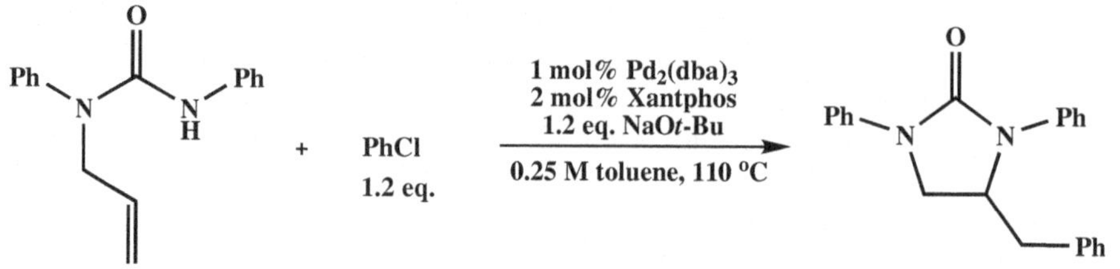

Scheme-43

There are several experiments that would provide a deeper understanding of this transformation and would expand its scope. For instance, a comparison of rate of carboamination of substrates which vary only in the configuration of alkene double bond (*Z* vs. *E*) may give useful information about transition state for the insertion of olefin into palladium-nitrogen bond. This implies that rate of carboamination of (*E*)-alkenes was greater than that of analogous (*Z*)-alkenes for *N*-allylureas (**Scheme 44**) [122].

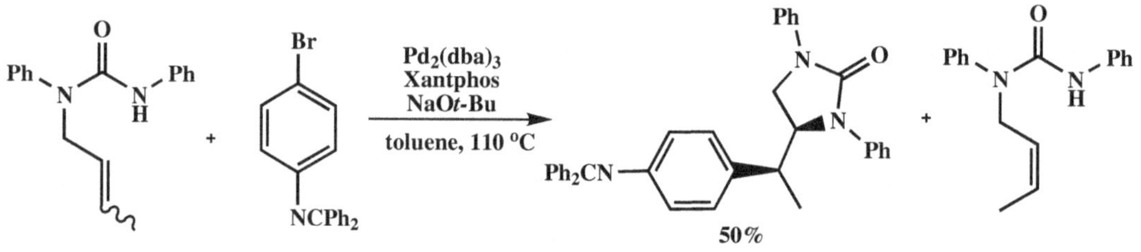

Scheme-44

Reactions of substrates that had substitution at terminal position of olefin proved to be more challenging. The reaction of (*E*)-1-benzyl-1-cinnamyl-3-(4-methoxyphenyl)urea with 4-bromobenzonitrile under standard reaction conditions only afforded 11% of desired cyclic urea due to competing hydroamination. However, previous work in the group led us believe that a weaker base, cesium carbonate, might also enable palladium-catalyzed carboamination [122]. Indeed, with the use of cesium carbonate, a competing base-mediated hydroamination pathway was completely shut down, and the desired carboamination product was formed in moderate yield. However, a 32% yield of (*E*)-1-benzyl-1-cinnamyl-3-(4-methoxyphenyl)urea, arising from a Heck reaction, was also generated. Further increases in yield of carboamination product were realized by employing palladium acetate and dioxane as palladium source and solvent respectively (**Scheme 45**).

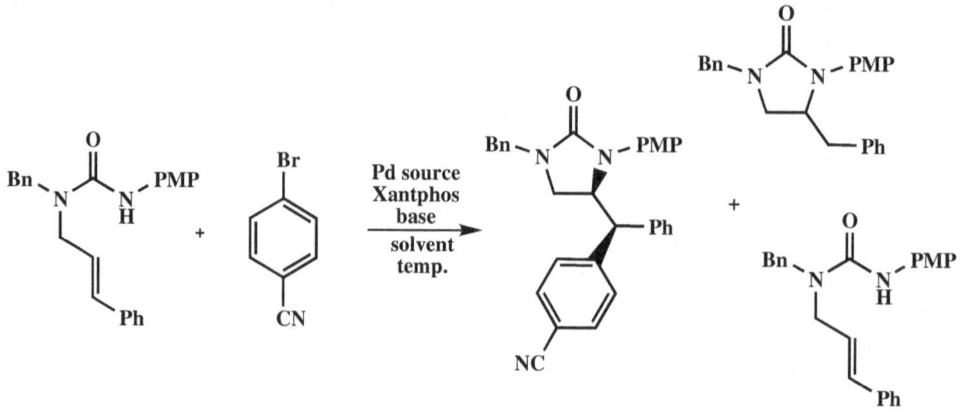

Scheme-45

In an attempt to gain more insight into the origin of higher yields obtained with *N*3-phenyl ureas, the sterically bulky 1-allyl-1-benzyl-3-*tert*-butylurea was produced. This substrate would have a *tert*-butyl group on cyclizing nitrogen. Thus, if the yield of cyclization was high for this substrate it would lend credence to the hypothesis that β-hydride elimination was responsible for lower yields seen for *N*3 alkyl ureas. Unfortunately, when this substrate was subjected to palladium catalysis the reaction proceeded to only 85% conversion after 20 h, and a by-product resulting from Heck arylation of olefin was observed in addition to desired carboamination product. This seems to indicate that steric hindrance of *tert*-butyl group on cyclizing nitrogen slowed the rate of carboamination considerably. As such, the increased yields observed with *N*3-phenyl substrates were presumably due to electronic effects **(Scheme 46)** [123].

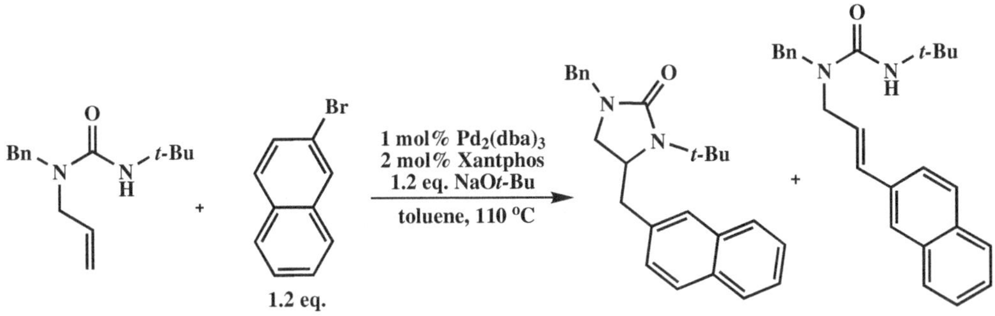

Scheme-46

Having demonstrated the carboamination of simple *N*-allylureas then the effect of substitution on allyl backbone was explored **(Scheme 47)**. It was found that 1,1-disubstituted olefins cleanly give 4,4-disubstituted imididazolidin-2-ones, which have a quaternary carbon, in high yield. The 4,5-disubstituted imidazolidin-2-ones were also generated in high yield from corresponding allylically substituted *N*-allylureas. Notably, formation of these 4,5-disubstituted imidazolidin-2-ones was complete in one hr. Modest to excellent diastereoselectivity was achieved. As the group at allylic position increased in size from methyl to isopropyl the diastereoselectivity correspondingly increased [124].

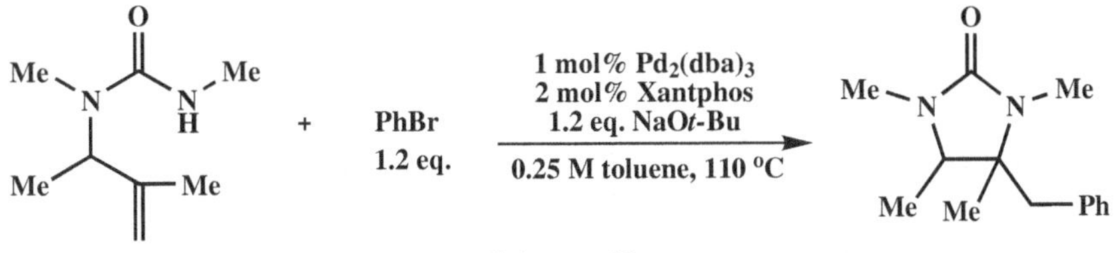

Scheme-47

As shown in **Scheme 48**, alkenyl halides can couple with a diverse set of *N*-allylureas to afford 4-monosubstituted, 4,4-disubstituted, and 4,5-disubstituted imidazolidin-2-ones in good to excellent yield similar to couplings with aryl bromides. Bicyclic imidazolildin-2-one was obtained as a 1.5:1 ratio of diastereomers compared to 11:1 ratio of diastereomers seen when coupling occurred with an aryl bromide [125].

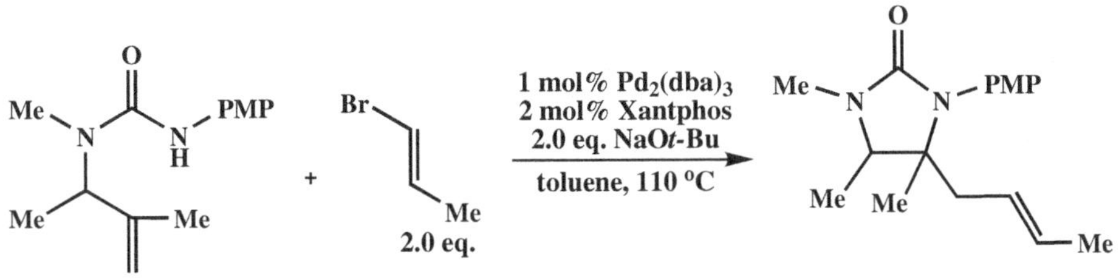

Scheme-48

It would be interesting to explore the carboamination of *N*-propargyl ureas for the synthesis of (*E*)- or (*Z*)-olefins by variation of phosphine ligand **(Scheme 49)** [126]. Other interesting products that could be formed from alkene-possessing urea substrates include spirocycles, tetrahydropyrimidinones, and hydantoins. Lastly, it would be interesting to pursue a tandem reaction which would incorporate two vinyl halide coupling partners.

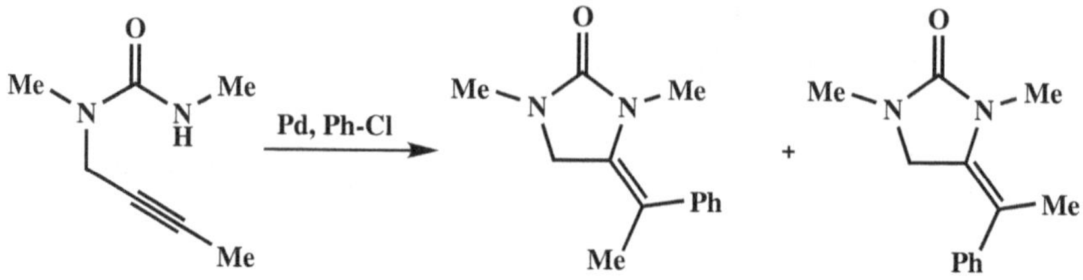

Scheme-49

In attempts to employ this strategy toward an asymmetric synthesis of imidazolidin-2-ones, the use of chiral phosphine ligands was explored. Reaction with 2-Br-PhMe was model system for determining the enantioselectivity associated with each phosphine ligand surveyed. With an achiral ligand, two products were expected to be formed in this reaction: (*S*)- and (*R*). It was hoped that with appropriate chiral ligand and reaction conditions either one of the products could be formed in preference to other **(Scheme 50)** [127].

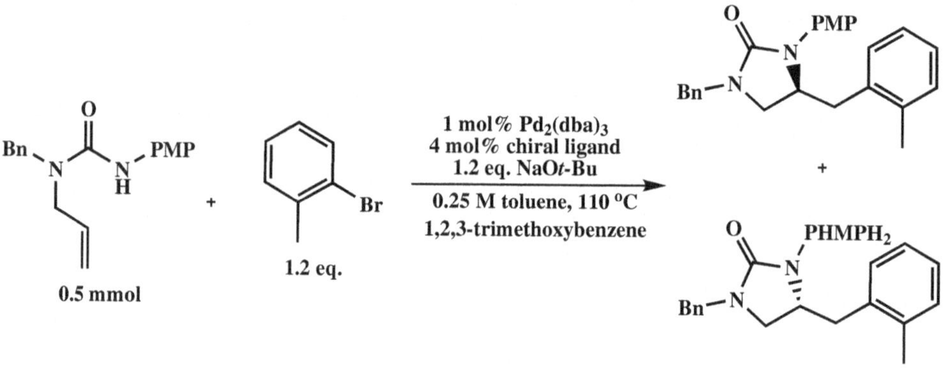

Scheme-50

The chiral auxiliaries were used to achieve high enantioselectivity in palladium-catalyzed carboamination of *N*-allylureas **(Scheme 51-52)**. Reaction of *N*-allylureas substrates resulted in a complex mixture of products. Replacement of Me group with Ph group on non-cyclizing nitrogen gave an approximately 30% yield of carboamination product, but as a 1:1 mixture of diastereomers. Use of α-methylbenzyl on *N*1 was also explored. Reaction using (*S*)-PHANEPHOS ((*S*)-(+)-4,12-bis(diphenylphosphino)-[2.2]-paracyclophane) resulted in a decrease in diastereoselectivity. This was likely due to a mismatch between (*S*)-(+)-4,12-bis(diphenylphosphino)-[2.2]-paracyclophane and chiral auxiliary [128].

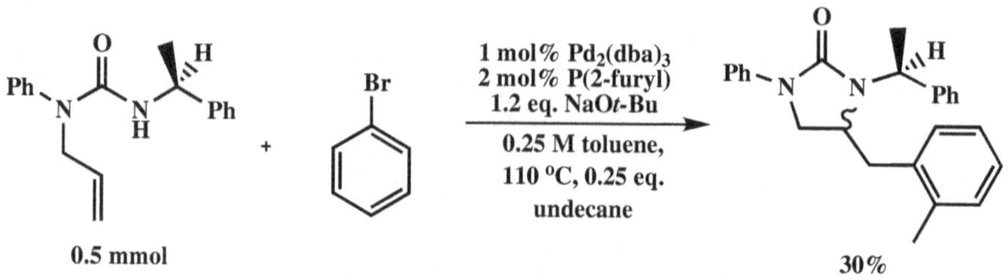

Scheme-51

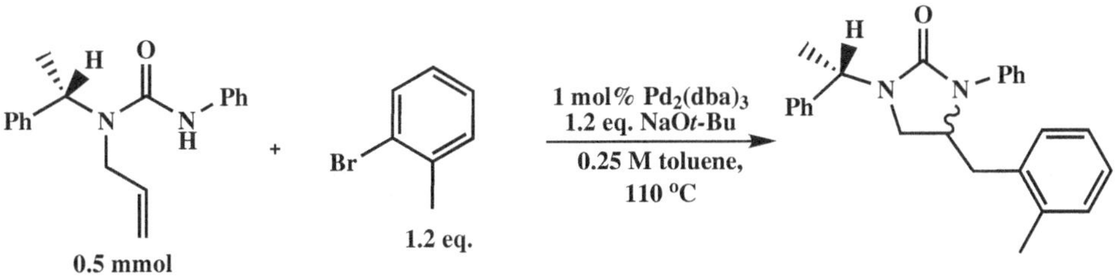

Scheme-52

A variety of electron-neutral and electron-poor aryl halides were coupled to *N*-allylguanidine to form imidazole under palladium-catalyzed carboamination conditions **(Scheme 53)**. Good yield (66%) of imidazole was obtained using 2-bromonapthalene as aryl halide. However, results for multiple trials were very inconsistent ranging from 19%-66%. This inconsistency may be due to variations in substrate purity for different batches. Reactions of 4-bromoacetophenone, 4-benzophenone, and 4-bromobenzonitrile with *N*-allylguanidine give imidazole in low yields ranging from 15-34% [129].

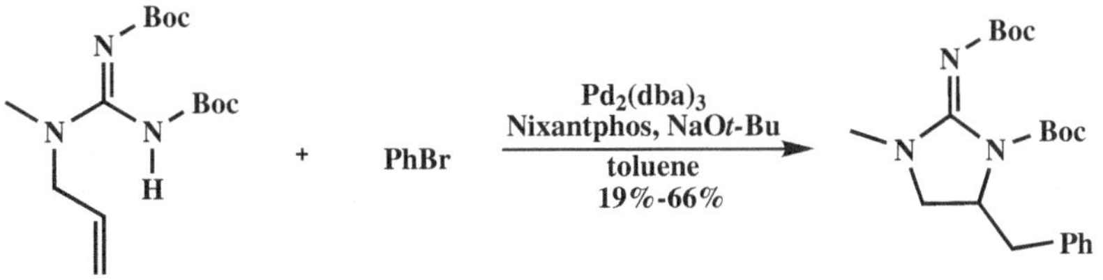

Scheme-53

The scope of reaction with respect to variation in *N*-allylguanidine component of the reaction was also briefly examined **(Scheme 54)**. In addition to substrate which has a *N*3 methyl group, substrates were prepared with benzyl and phenyl on non-cyclizing nitrogen (*N*3). These afforded lower yields than their methylated counterpart. For example, reaction of *N*-allylguanidine with 2-bromonaphthalene proceeded to give an approximately 4% yield of only carboamination product [130].

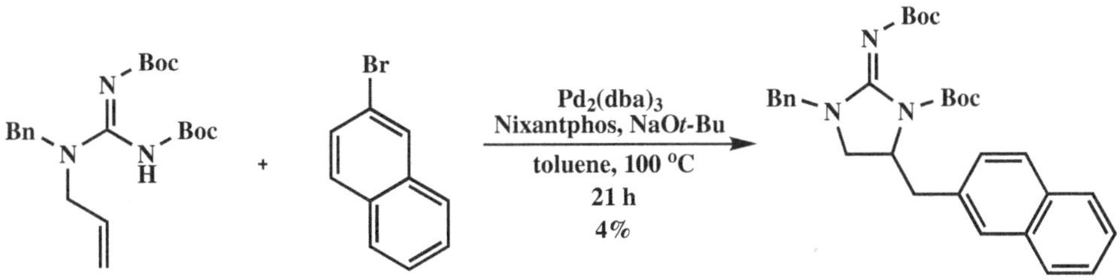

Scheme-54

The imidazolium salts as well as imidazolines were synthesized by this method. Imidazoline esters with different substituents were generated **(Scheme 55)** by coupling catalytic synthesis with de-protection [131]. For instance, the imidazoline was formed in 48% yield from imines and acid chloride when treated with BBr$_3$ (R1 = PMB). Alternatively, the 5-ester-substituted isomer was obtained from cycloaddition of *N*-allyl imines followed by Pd-catalyzed de-protection. This approach was modular and effective for the synthesis of polysubstituted imidazolines from acid chloride, simple imines, and carbon monoxide as compared to traditional protocols [132].

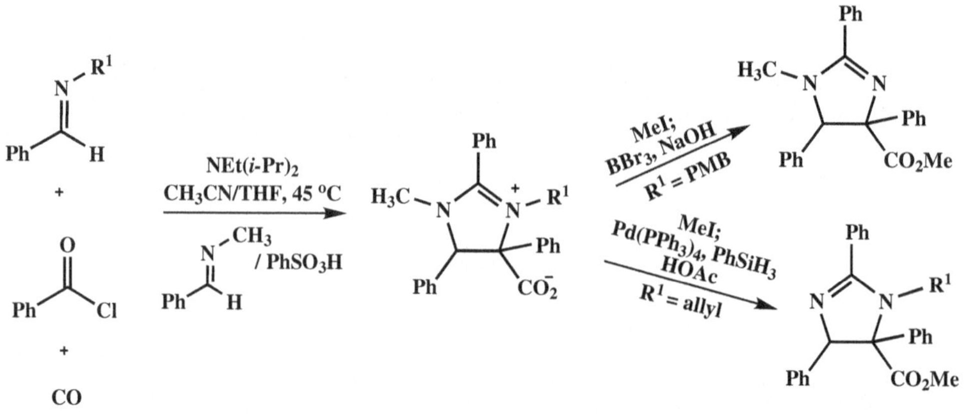

Scheme-55

Imidazoles constitue a useful class of heterocycles found in a diverse variety of pharmaceutically relevant products. While a number of approaches exist for the synthesis of imidazoles, these typically involve either the build-up of a polysubstituted precursor for cyclization, or the stepwise introduction of substituents on premade imidazoles. Each of these approaches are effective, however, they typically constitute multistep processes, where the product was built up one bond at a time. This can not only create significant waste, but also complicates structural diversification to tune properties. In principle, a more attractive approach to synthesize these complex structures would be to assemble them in a single step from multiple building blocks that are widely available. A Pd-catalyzed MCR, that considerd imidazole core as a coupling product of aryl halides, imines and carbon monoxide, was developed **(Scheme 56)** [132].

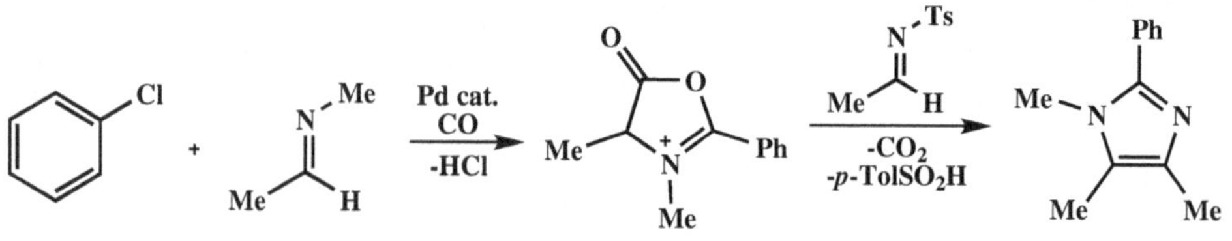

Scheme-56

A dipolar cycloaddition of münchnone intermediates with imines afforded imidazolinium salts. Arndtsen et al. [132] investigated a new highly active Pd catalyst for the improvement of already reported results. Moreover, polysubstituted imidazoliniums were obtained by this pathway through selective introduction of two different imines. The best results in terms of reaction yield and time were observed in the presence of palladacycle combined with di-*tert*-butyl-2-biphenylphosphine after evaluating a number of ligands and Pd pre-catalysts. Many imines and acid chlorides were utilized in this reaction. Only enolizable imines and those containing bulky nitrogen substituents were incompatible. A base (NEti-Pr$_2$) was added to reaction medium which favored the synthesis of münchnone intermediate in order to have four independent tunable substrates. After 16 h of heating at 45 °C, second imine was added along with PhSO$_3$H, which avoided the formation of β-lactam and catalyzed the dipolar cycloaddition **(Scheme 57-58)** [23].

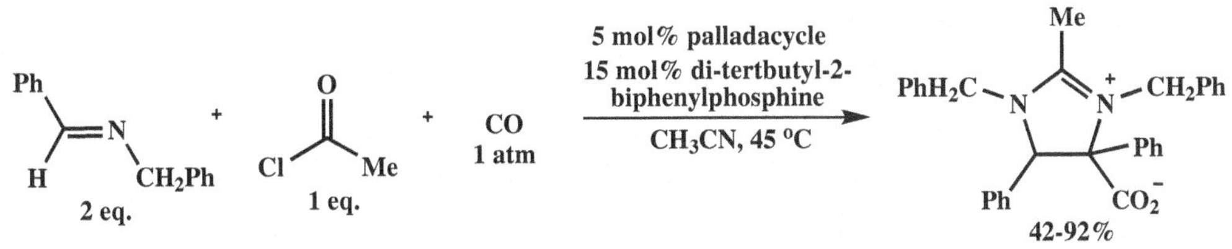

Scheme-57

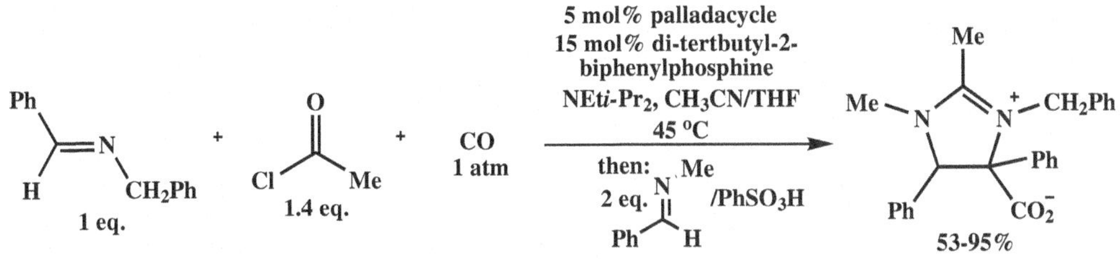

Scheme-58

The potential utility of this process was preparation of imidazoline (**Scheme 59-60**). Tepe and Sharma [133] have identified imidazoline as a potent sensitizer for the treatment of cancer. Good yield of imidazoline was obtained by this efficient Pd-catalyzed construction of imidazolinium salts followed by de-protection. An useful feature of this method was its tendency to afford variants of products in addition to synthesizing imidazoline. A new 5-carboxylic acid isomer of imidazoline was formed, through variation of position of protecting group on imines, from cycloaddition of same acid chloride and *N*-allyl imine [132].

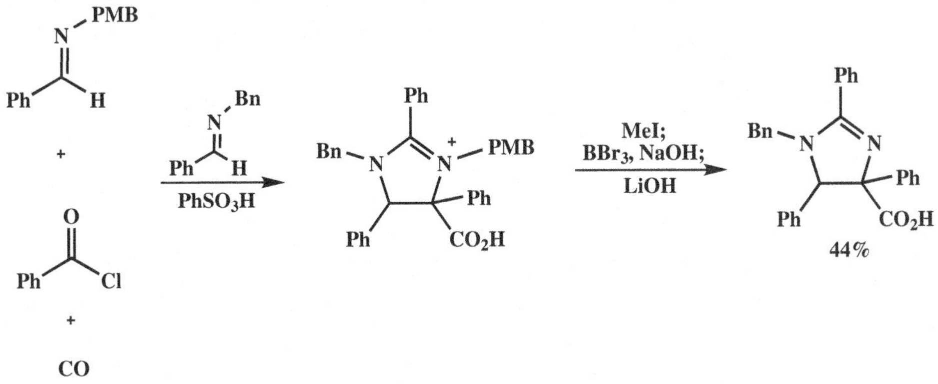

Scheme-59

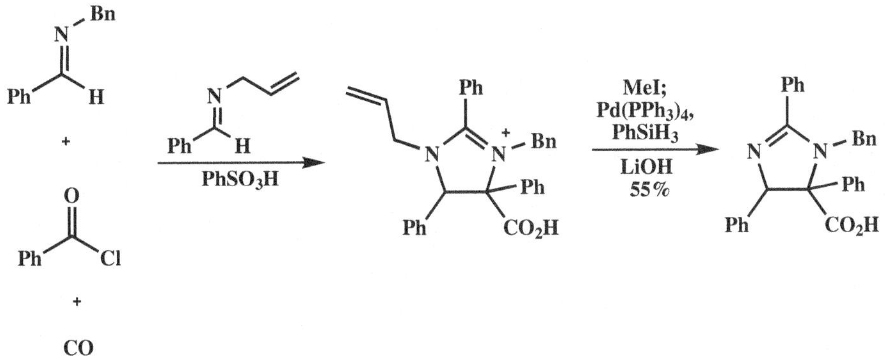

Scheme-60

A π-allylpalladium intermediate was produced by allene carbopalladation process with organic halides. The three-component adduct was formed from trapping of π-allylpalladium intermediate by intermolecular hetero- or carbonucleophiles. Ma and Jiao [134] used this pathway for the synthesis of five-membered *N*-heterocycles selectively from allene containing nucleophilic centers. Same authors carried out a three-component reaction of organic halides, 2,3-allenylamines, and isocyanates for the formation of substituted imidazolidinones in the presence of Pd catalyst [135]. The vinylic azacyclopropane or 2,5-dihydropyrrole derivatives were formed by carbopalladation of functionalized allene with ArI, followed by reaction of internal aza-nucleophile with highly electrophilic isocyanate derivative, before premature trapping of initially produced π-allylpalladium intermediate. Subsequently, a five-membered ring cyclization led to polysubstituted imidazolidinones in rather excellent selectivity and good yields **(Scheme 61)** [23].

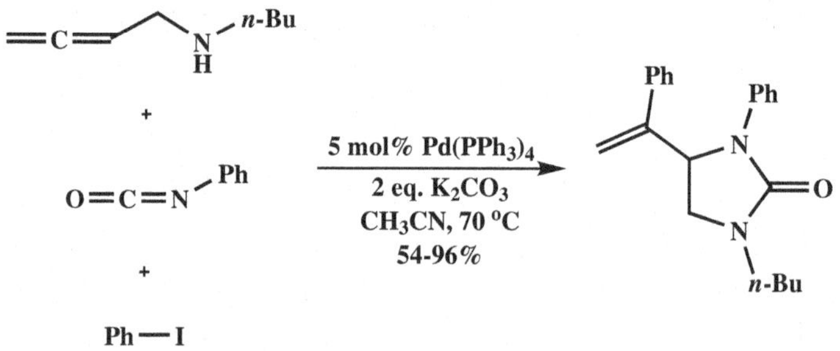

Scheme-61

After a careful screening using a starting substrate, it was found that a combination of 2 mol% Pd(PPh$_3$)$_4$, K$_2$CO$_3$ (4.0 eq.) and iodobenzene (1.5 eq.) in dimethylformamide, as reported by Kang [136], was ideal system to promote the desired transformation. These conditions were totally regioselective leading to imidazolidinones respectively in 55% and 16% yield **(Scheme 62)**.

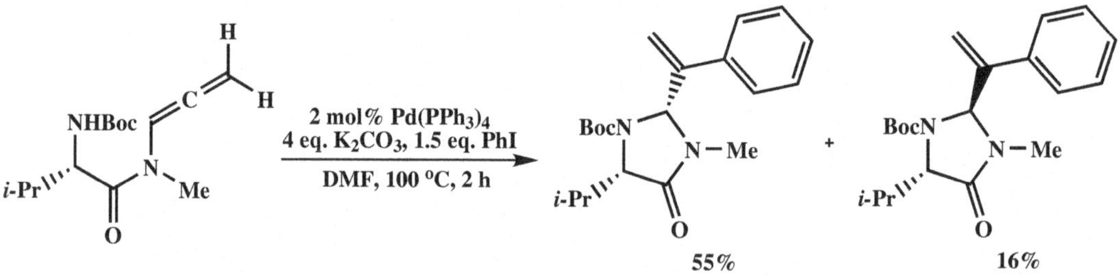

Scheme-62

Grubbs [137] during Ru-catalyzed ring-closing metathesis observed an asymmetric diamination based on chiral *N*-aryl-substituted NHC derived from (*R,R*)-diphenylethylenediamine. The imidazolium salts were synthesized from chiral diamine in two steps **(Scheme 63)** [138-140]. The imidazolium salts were treated with [Pd(allyl)Cl]$_2$ to deliver *N*-heterocyclic carbene-Pd(allyl)Cl complexes in the presence of potassium *tert*-butoxide in tetrahydrofuran [141-145]. The 1-(*p*-methoxyphenyl)butadiene and 1,3-hexadiene were used as substrates for asymmetric diamination with catalysts produced *in situ* from *N*-heterocyclic carbene-Pd(allyl) Cl complexes and NaO*t*-Am [146].

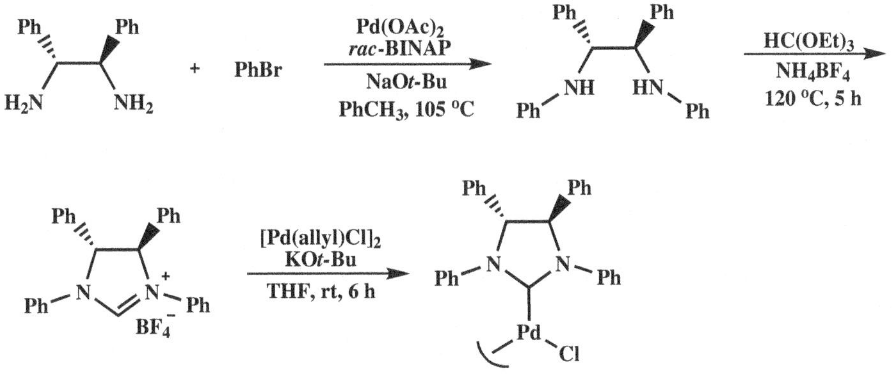

Scheme-63

Non-aromatic heterocycles can also be synthesized by this method. Intermediate can be trapped with a second equivalent of imine to form imidazoline carboxylates in good yield (**Scheme 64**) [147]. Imidazoline carboxylates can also be formed through initial catalytic formation of intermediate, followed by addition of a second, different imine. The latter provided a route to imidazoline carboxylates with independent control of five substituents (**Scheme 65**).

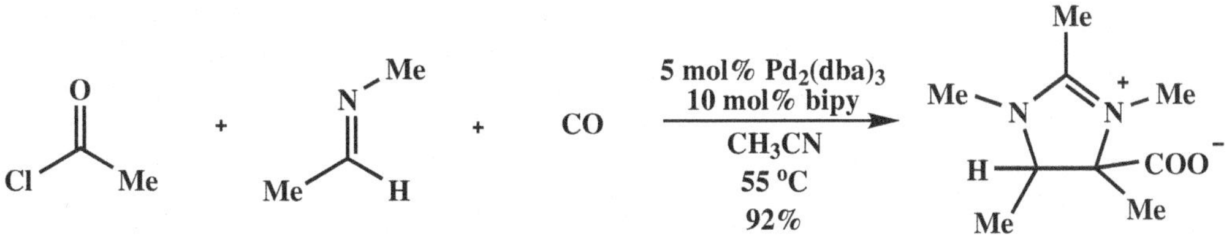

Scheme-64

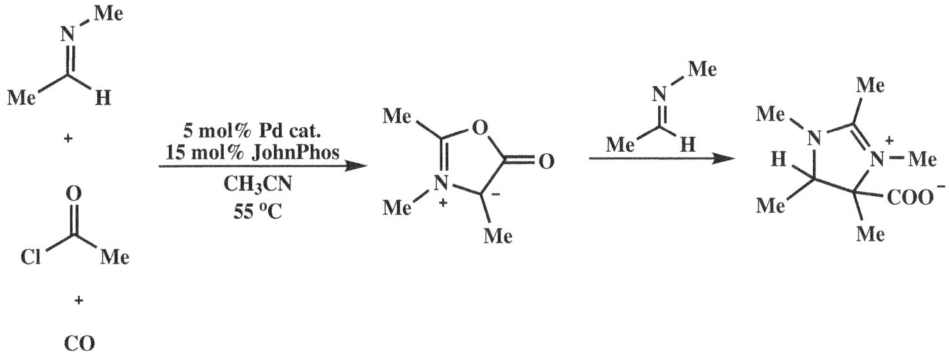

Scheme-65

The results presented in this method provided a number of opportunities for the efficient synthesis of new compounds. For example, as shown in **Scheme 66**, *in situ* trapping of münchnones (generated from carbonylation of α-alkoxyamides) with *N*-tosyl imines could provide a direct synthesis of substituted imidazoles [148].

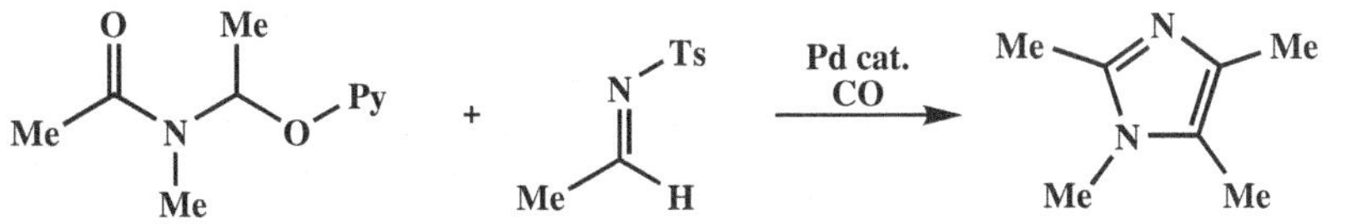

Scheme-66

The *O*-pentafluorobenzoylamidoximes were treated with Pd(PPh$_3$)$_4$ catalyst and TEA for the synthesis of 1-benzyl-4-methylimidazoles with different substituents at 2-position. C terminal imidazole possessing optically active amino acid mimetics were obtained in this reaction **(Scheme 67)** [149].

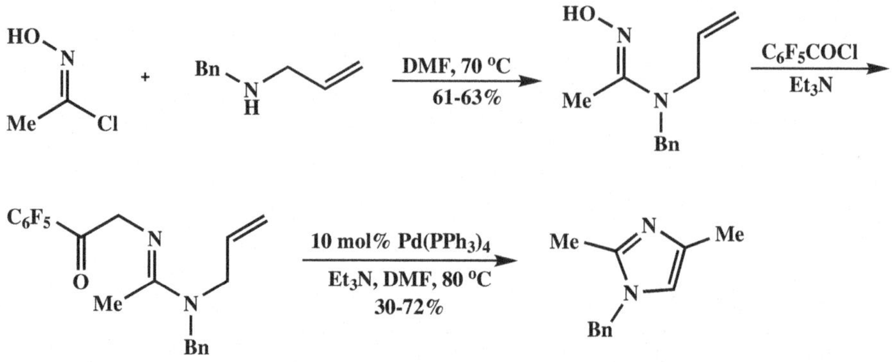

Scheme-67

The aldoximes (1:1, 75%) and *(E/Z)* (3:2, 72%) were formed from aliphatic aldehydes and hydroxylamine with pyridine. The hydroxamoyl chlorides were formed when aldoximes were separately reacted with *N*-chlorosuccinimide at 70 °C in dry dimethylformamide. The *in situ* formed hydroxamoyl chlorides were treated with *N*-allyl benzyl amine in dimethylformamide to afford (*E/Z*)-amidoximes predominantly (63%) and (61%) as single isomers, tentatively assigned as *E*-configuration **(Scheme 68)**. In a different procedure, aldoximes were reacted with *N*-chlorosuccinimide and the obtained crude product was analyzed by 1H NMR which indicated that hydroxamoyl chloride was obtained as a single isomer, characterized and tentatively assigned *E*-configuration. The sample of hydroxamoyl chlorides was then reacted with *N*-allyl benzyl amine as per *in situ* experiment to give the identical isomer of (*E/Z*)-amidoximes. Modeling studies of (*E/Z*)-amidoximes also suggested the population of amidoximes to be in lower energy (*E*)-conformation. This was attributed to intramolecular bonding between electron deficient oxime hydrogen and electron-rich phenyl rings [150].

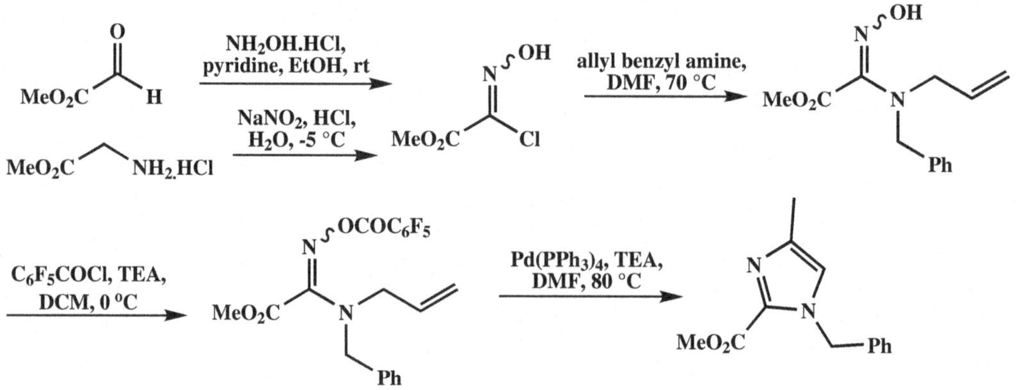

Scheme-68

A variety of heteroaryl and aryl bromides, as well as alkenyl bromides containing *N*-allylureas were effective for carboamination reactions **(Scheme 69)**. *Trans*-4,5-disubstituted imidazolidin-2-ones were obtained in good to excellent diastereoselectivities from an allylic substituent containing substrates. The palladium-catalyzed carboamination of *N*-allylureas was also performed with 1,1- or 1,2-disubstitued alkenes containing substrates **(Scheme 70-71)**. There was net *syn*-addition across the double bond in these reactions. When N1-atom contains an aromatic group, the imidazolidin-2-one products were formed in best yields. The protecting groups were selectively cleaved from product employing CAN or lithium/ammonia when two nitrogen atoms were protected with a *p*-methoxyphenyl group and a benzyl group, respectively [151-152a, b].

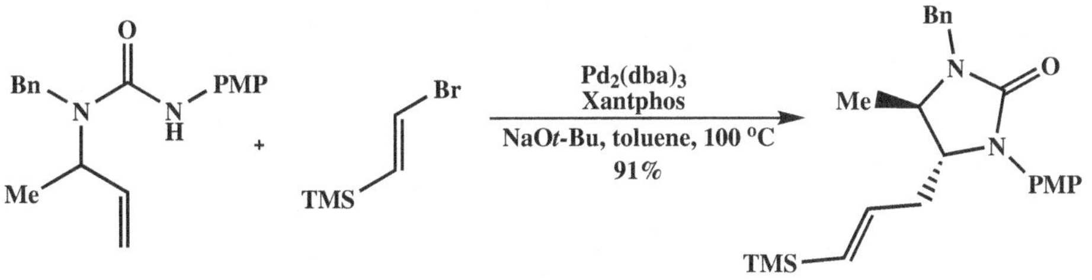

Scheme-69

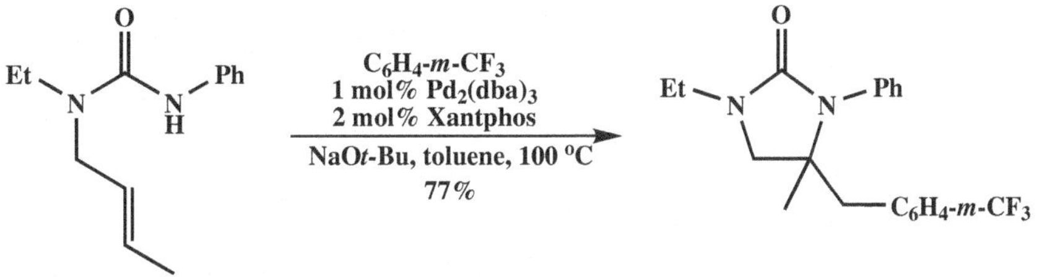

Scheme-70

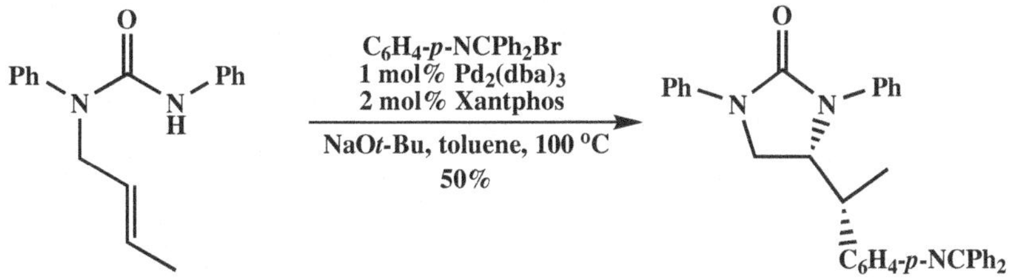

Scheme-71

Several cyclic guanidines exhibit potent biological activity and represent important medicinal targets. Cyclic guanidines can be produced using many of same techniques that are used for the synthesis of imidazolidin-2-ones. The rhodium-catalyzed C-H amination of an acyclic guanidine to form a cyclic guanidine was demonstrated. Intramolecular and intermolecular diaminations to generate cyclic guanidines have also been shown by Shi [153] **(Scheme 72)**.

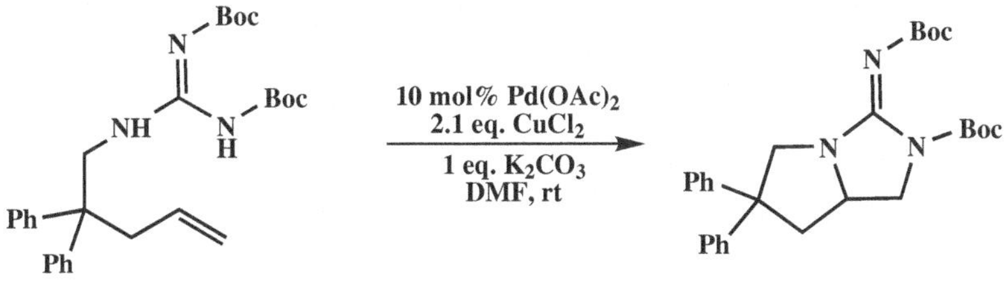

Scheme-72

4.5   Palladium assisted synthesis of five-membered 1,2-*N,N*-polyheterocycles

The *o*-alkynylhalothiophene or *o*-alkynylhalopyridine substrates were employed to afford heterocyclic derivatives like thienopyrroles and 7-azaindoles, respectively [154]. From same *o*-alkynylhaloarene other heterocyclic compounds were also synthesized. Halland and Lindenschmidt [155] utilized this aspect for the elegant preparation of 2*H*-indazoles **(Scheme 73)**. The *N,N*-disubstituted hydrazine was produced regioselectively *via* initial intermolecular amination of a monosubstituted hydrazine in the presence of Pd catalyst. The dihydroindazole intermediates were formed *via* intramolecular hydroamination. The dihydroindazole was isomerized to aromatic 2*H*-indazole spontaneously. A number of functional groups were tolerated. These precursors also afforded more complex polycyclic products. The *o*-alkynylhaloarene acted as substrates for the preparation of 5*H*-cyclopenta[*c*]quinolines [156-157].

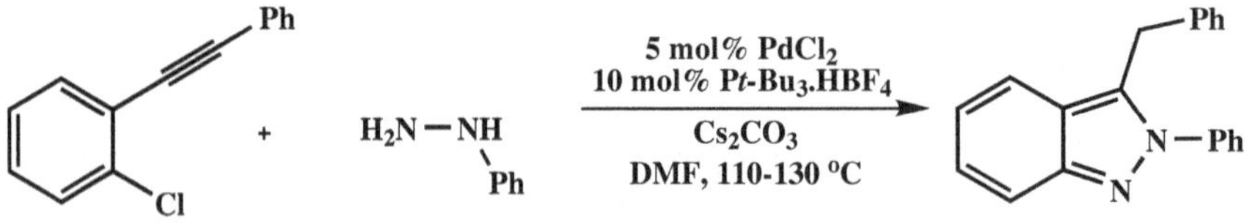

Scheme-73

For the synthesis of indazole many methods have been observed which employed transition metal catalysts particularly Pd [158-161]. For instance, indazole was produced *via* palladium-catalyzed amination [162-165]. Transition metal-catalyzed conventional cyclization afforded very effective and convenient one-step method for ring homologation and provided heterocyclic compounds which are either poorly available or un-accessible [50, 166]. The conditions optimized for 2-bromohydrazones were employed to other more reactive 2-iodophenyl hydrazones. The cyclization of 2-iodophenyl hydrazones with aryl isocyanates in the presence of Pd catalyst under MWI afforded 1*H*-indazole derivatives. The above developed optimal conditions were also applicable to the preparation of 1-arylamide substituted 1*H*-indazoles. The reaction was selectivity affected significantly by substituent on aryl isocyanates and aryl hydrazones. The less bulky hydrazones showed higher reactivity in the synthesis of five-membered ring as compared to the formation of seven-membered ring products. Good yields of 1-arylamide substituted 1*H*-indazoles were obtained when 2-iodophenyl hydrazones were utilized in this reaction. For example, moderate yields of 1-arylamide substituted 1*H*-indazoles were observed upon mixing of hydrazone with aryl isocyanates. The arylhydrazone was employed under above reaction conditions to afford good yields of indazoles with full transformation and high selectivity **(Scheme 74)** [167].

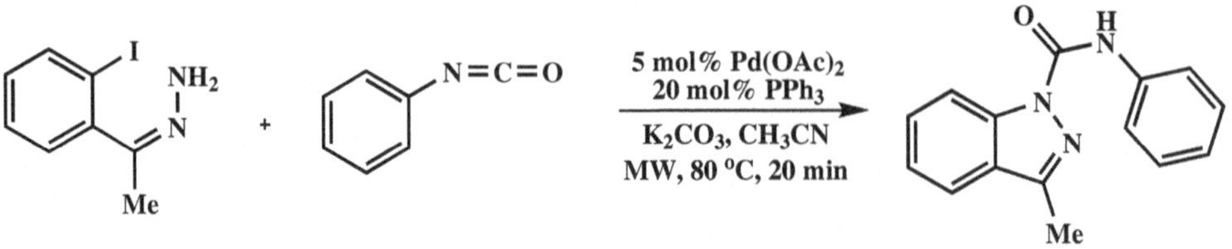

Scheme-74

Hoshina, Muraki, and co-workers [168] used hydrazones for the synthesis of indazole rings. Despite of studies, the preparation of tetrahydroisoquinolines and indolines from easily accessible phenylpropylamines and phenylethylamines by carbon-hydrogen activation remained an unsolved problem due to sluggish reactions proceeding through six- and seven-membered palladacycles **(Scheme 75)** [169-171].

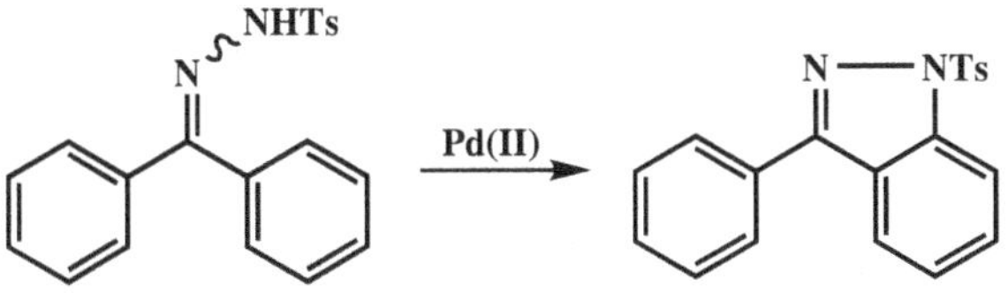

Scheme-75

Inamoto and co-workers [172] projected a synthetic method of indazole derivatives from benzophenione tosylhydrazones using catalytic amount of palladium acetate in the presence of copper acetate and AgOCOCF$_3$ in dimethylsulphoxide **(Scheme 76)**.

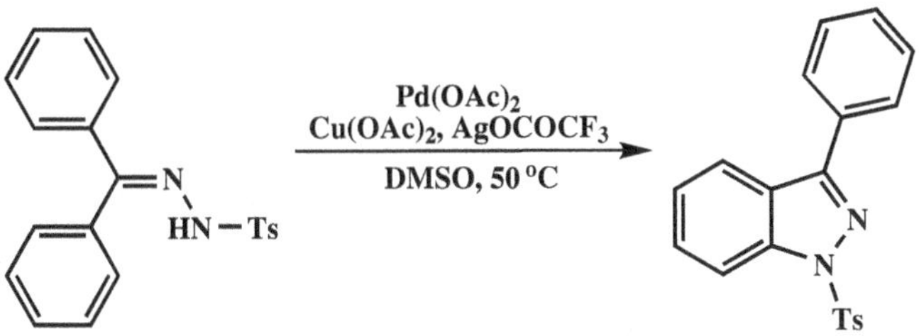

Scheme-76

Grigg [173] synthesized small and large *N*-heterocycles *via* palladium-catalyzed hydrostannylation-carbopalladation/cyclization, in which cyclization occurred at α-allenic carbon **(Scheme 77)**. The allylstannanes were obtained as a mixture of *E/Z* isomers from allenamides with highly regioselective Pd [palladium(0) or palladium(II) could be operative]-catalyzed hydrostannylations. Both *E/Z* isomeric allylstannanes underwent an oxidative addition, carbopalladation/cyclization, and elimination in the presence of palladium(0). Moderate to good yields of final products were observed as elimination of *n*-Bu$_3$SnPdX was faster than β-hydride (HPdX) elimination [116b].

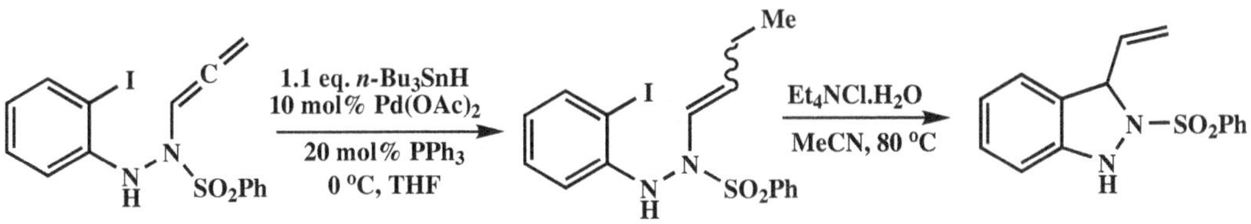

Scheme-77

The carbonylation and reductive *N*-hetero-cyclization of 2-nitrostyrenes with CO afforded indoles in moderate to good yields in the presence of elemental selenium (an efficient catalyst) [174]. The natural product arcyriaflavin-A was synthesized by a new synthetic protocol based on a nitrene insertion [175]. A variety of heterocycles were obtained from *o*-nitroaromatics by reductive *N*-heteroannulation with transition metal catalyst. For instance, *N*-(2-nitrobenzylidene) amine was used for the formation of 1-phenyl-2*H*-indazole **(Scheme 78)**.

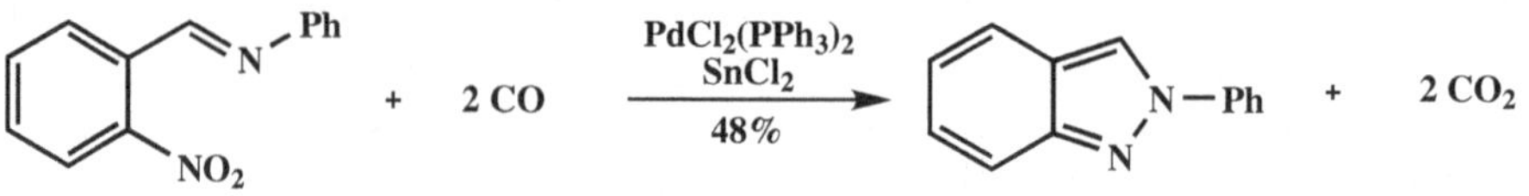

Scheme-78

The *N*-aryl-*N*-(*o*-bromobenzyl)hydrazines were cyclized in the presence of Pd acetate and 1,1'-bis(diphenylphosphino)ferrocene for the synthesis of indazole **(Scheme 79)** [176]. Same products were obtained by cyclization of [*N*-aryl-*N*-(*o*-bromobenzyl)-hydrazinato-*N*]-triphenylphosphonium bromides [177-181].

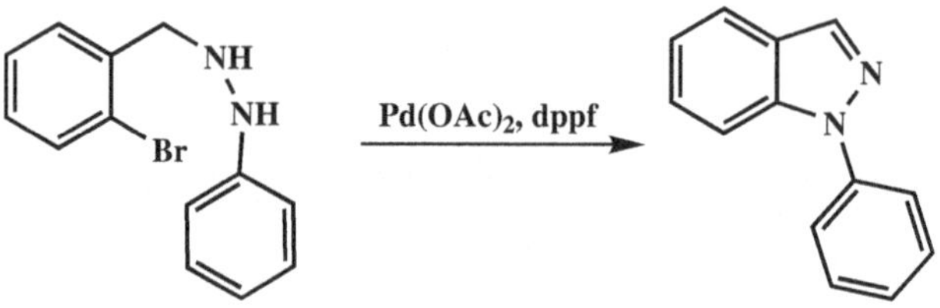

Scheme-79

The tandem hydrazine cross-coupling-condensation for the synthesis of NH-indazoles was also possible from 2-chlorobenzaldehydes under appropriate conditions with palladium mixtures **(Scheme 80)**. Now the scope of this conversion is not broad, therefore the utilization of 2-chloroacetophenones or tosylates as starting materials was unsuccessful [182-183].

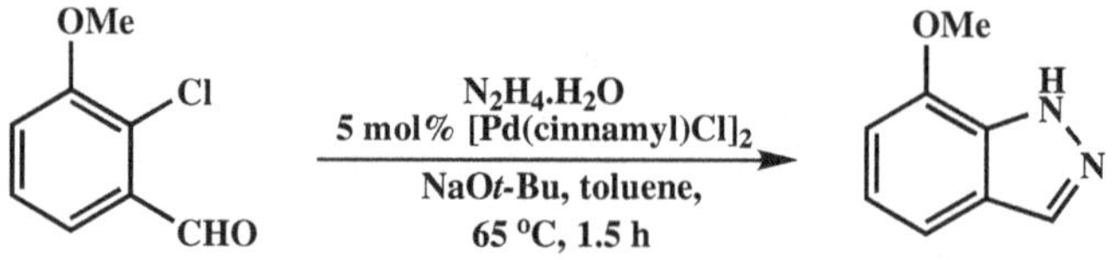

Scheme-80

4.6 Palladium assisted synthesis of five-membered 1,3-*N*,*N*-polyheterocycles

Aryl nonaflates were used as thermally stable arylating agents by Buchwald et al. [184] providing fast reactions ranging from 1-45 min. In favorable cases 99% yield was observed by coupling of aromatic amines in the presence of Pd, phosphine ligands under MW heating [185a-b]. The amination of azaheteroaryl chlorides and bromides was also observed which occurred efficiently within 10 min under standard reaction conditions and MWI [186]. Brain and Steer [187] used an amidine moiety as *N*-nucleophile for the preparation of benzimidazoles through an intramolecular cyclization process **(Scheme 81)**. Weigand and Pelka [188] reported MW enhanced aminations of aryl bromides and chlorides in the presence of amine resins as nitrogen nucleophile. The sluggish reaction (reflux 18 h), employing polystyrene Rink resin and electron-poor bromides and chlorides, was conducted within 15 min using a sealed vessel method at 130 °C with dimethoxyethane/*t*-BuOH 1:1 as solvent. This technique with high-speed provided equal yields as reported with much slower protocol under oil bath heating. Aryl chlorides were more reluctant to participate in amination than most other aryl pseudohalides/halides. Caddick and co-workers [189] studied the influence of Pd-NHC catalysts in fast MW-promoted reactions in order to tackle the problem. Anisyl and *P*-tolyl chloride were treated with aliphatic and aromatic amines to afford good yields at 160 °C heating within 6 min. Maes and co-workers [190] reacted anisyl, aliphatic amines and phenyl or tolyl chlorides with a phosphine ligand and a strong base to afford the desired products after heating at 110-200 °C for 10 min.

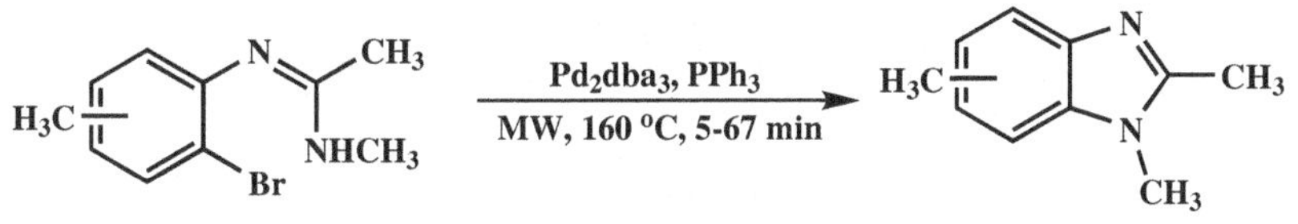

Scheme-81

Willis et al. [157] synthesized a number of 2-substituted benzimidazoles from *N*-(*o*-halophenyl)imidoyl chlorides in the presence of Pd-based catalysts **(Scheme 82)**. The optimal ligand for the method was bulky adamantyl-substituted monophosphane under MWI. Excellent yields of functionalized benzimidazole were obtained.

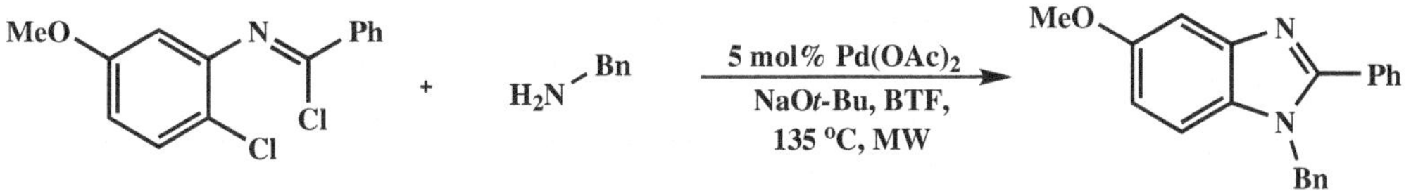

Scheme-82

Unlike other substrates, α-(*o*-haloaryl) ketone and *o*-haloacetanilide substrates were not utilized for the preparation of indoles. Hypothetically, such structures were synthesized from α-(*o*-haloaryl) ketones, but this was not observed. A number of benzimidazoles were prepared employing protocols combining *o*-haloacetanilides with carbon-nitrogen bond-forming reactions. Zheng and Buchwald [191] described a Pd-catalyzed pathway **(Scheme 83)**. Good yields of a range of *N*-arylbenzimidazole products were afforded by the reaction of *o*-bromoacetanilides with anilines in the presence of a catalyst based on biphenyl ligand XPhos. The formation of reaction intermediates suggested that an intermolecular *N*-arylation followed by cyclization/ condensation occurred. Only anilines acted as nucleophiles, while with aryl chloride substrates alteration of conditions were needed to obtain good yields. This method was also carried out with Cu catalyst. Ma et al. [135] explained the synthesis of a variety of substituted benzimidazoles when *o*-iodoacetanilide was reacted with *o*-bromoacetanilide in the presence of a Cu catalyst. With pyridine-based substrate, an aza variant was also prepared. However, intramolecular cyclization/condensation step was promoted with the addition of acid and/or subsequent heating [157].

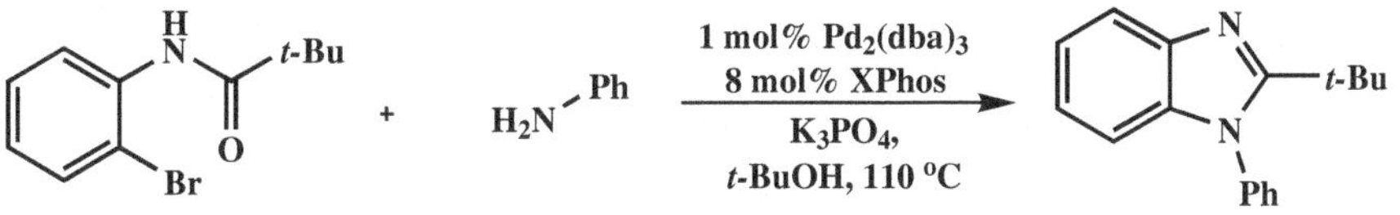

Scheme-83

Protection, nitration, de-protection and reduction of starting amine substrate were utilized for the incorporation of additional structural diversity in aniline. For example **Scheme 84** shows this phenomenon during the preparation of benzimidazole core of pantoprazole [73, 192].

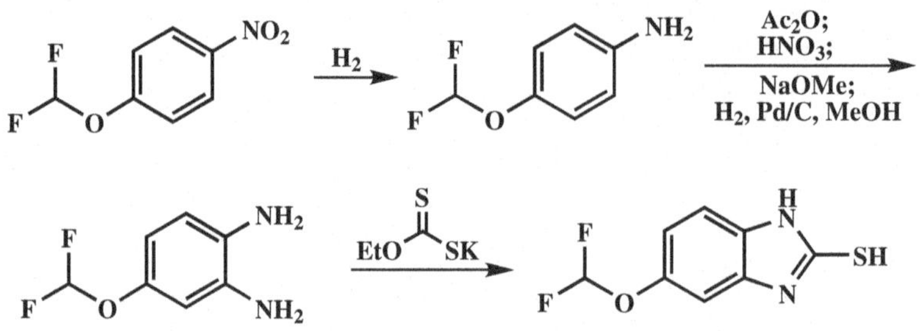

Scheme-84

The angiotensin II receptor antagonist, utilized for the treatment of bladder and heart diseases and hypertension, is telmisartan (micardis). A biphenyl unit and two linked benzimidazoles form the pharmacophore **(Scheme 85)**. The condensation reaction of a functionalized carbonyl compound and 1,2-diaminobenzene produced benzimidazoles. However, lower yields and many by-products were obtained in case of telmisartan due to the presence of other inherent functional groups like ester. Another disadvantage of initially reported pathway was that the reaction occurred in multistep manner (8 steps, 21% overall yield) [73, 193].

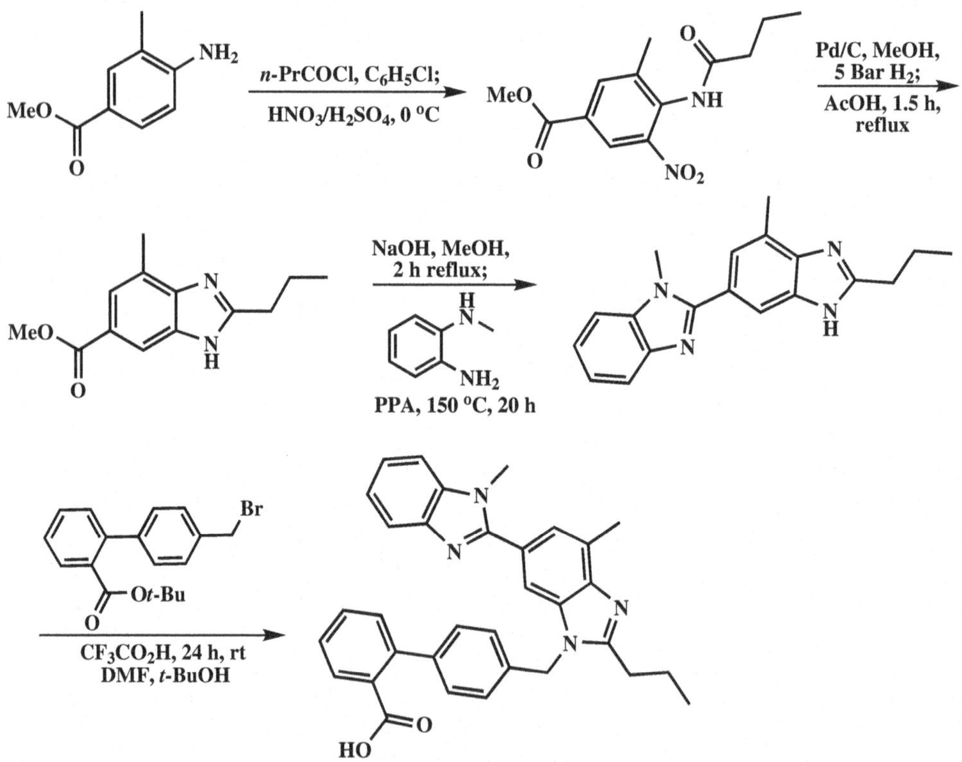

Scheme-85

The highly substituted nitrobenzene derivative was reduced to aniline with Pd under basic conditions. The formed aniline then underwent ring closure to benzimidazole [194]. The hydrolysis of methyl ester also proceeded under same reaction conditions which allowed the incorporation of second imidazole group in subsequent condensation step. The methyl ester was isolated as hydrochloride salt in 85% yield from sterically directed alkylation of free imidazole nitrogen in basic media with required biphenyl derivative. Finally, telmisartan was obtained in 50% yield (as compared to 21% in previous cases) from hydrolysis of methyl ester **(Scheme 86)** [73].

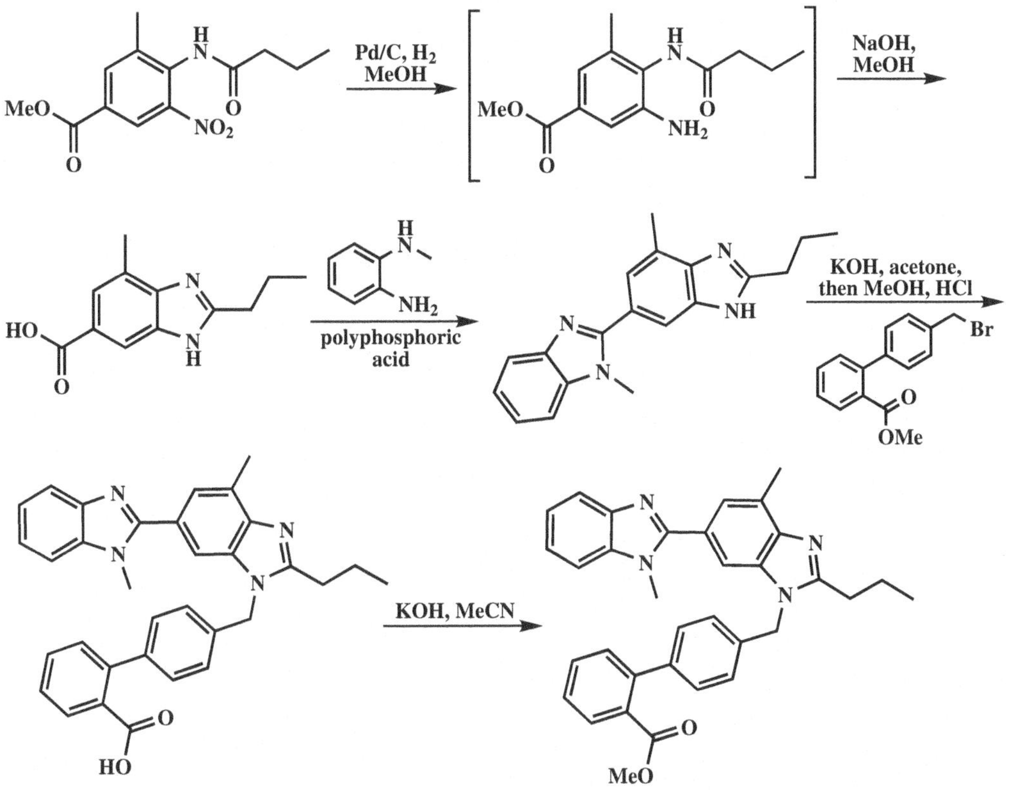

Scheme-86

The amide was formed in 56% yield when (S)-6,6′-dimethoxybiphenyl-2,2′-diamine was reacted with acetic anhydride at rt (25 °C) in CH_3COOH and dichloromethane. The NO_2 compound was synthesized in 98% yield when amide was coupled with 2-bromonitrobenzene in the presence of $Pd_2(dba)_3$ as catalyst and bis-[2-(diphenylphosphino)phenyl]ether as a ligand in cesium carbonate. The amino compound was provided in 98% yield upon reduction of NO_2 compound with palladium-carbon/hydrogen for 8 h. The benzimidazole was afforded in 83% yield by subsequent cyclization with triethyl *o*-formate in the presence of PTSA catalyst for 5 h at 100 °C. The benzimidazolium salt was synthesized in quantitative yields by quaternization of benzimidazole ring upon heating with methyl iodide in CH_3CN **(Scheme 87)** [195].

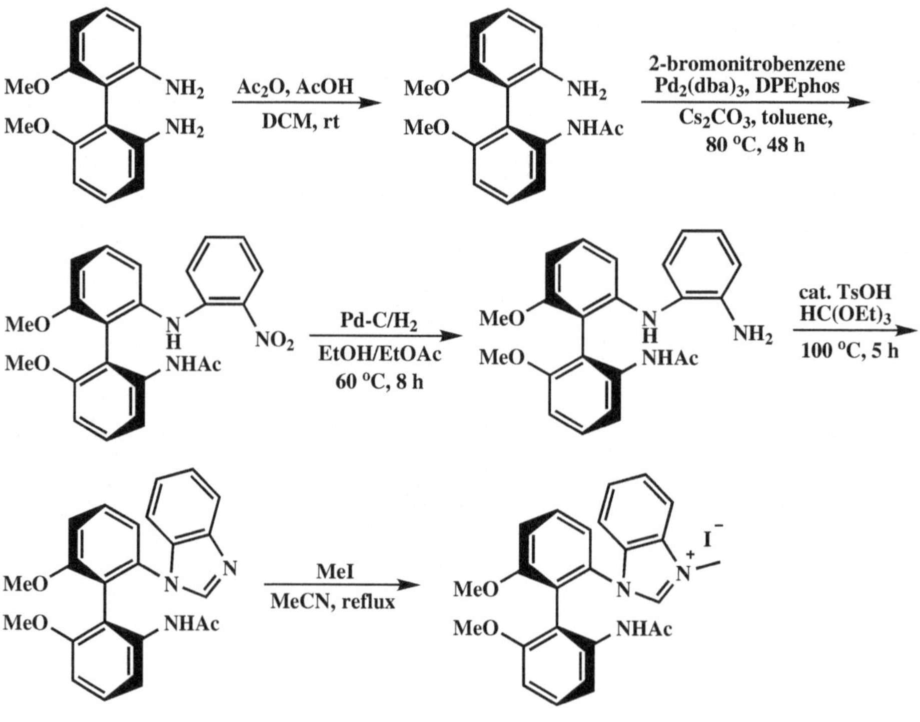

Scheme-87

The (S)-6,6'-dimethoxybiphenyl-2,2'-diamine was reacted with adamantane-2-carbonyl chloride for the synthesis of N-heterocyclic carbene-gold complex in dichloromethane and triethylamine at rt (25 °C) to provide 71% yield of amide. The N-heterocyclic carbene-gold complex was successfully prepared in 45% yield for the synthesis of products **(Scheme 88)** [195].

The protocols for the preparation of heterocyclic compounds employed Pd carbonylation which involved the formal carbon monoxide insertion into a palladium-heteroatom bond through either an outer-sphere or inner-sphere mechanism [196]. The carbonylation reactions of 1,2-diamines or 1,2-amino alcohols produced ureas and isoxazolidines in the presence of palladium catalyst [197-199]. For instance, Gabriele et al. [200] used a palladium iodide/ potassium iodide/air catalyst system for the production of oxazolidin-2-ones in high yields. Similarly, 1,3-dihydrobenzoimidazol-2-one was formed in 70% yield from diamine [201]. The carbon monoxide insertion into Pd amido complex formed carbon heteroatom bond, followed by intramolecular trapping of resulting acylpalladium intermediate with second heteroatom. The palladium(II) catalyst was reduced to palladium(0), and catalytically active palladium(II) species was regenerated in the presence of air (O_2) **(Scheme 89)**.

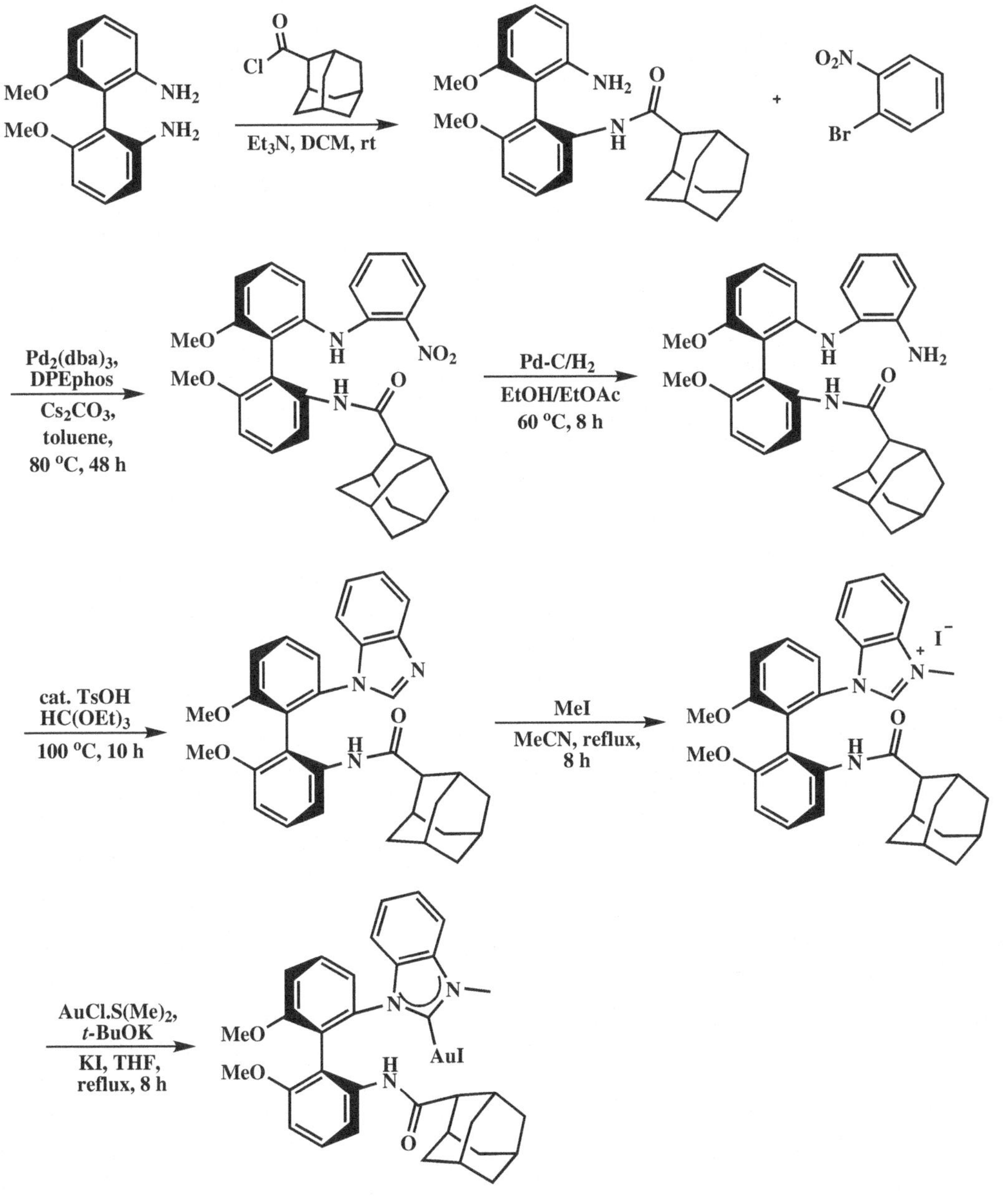

Scheme-88

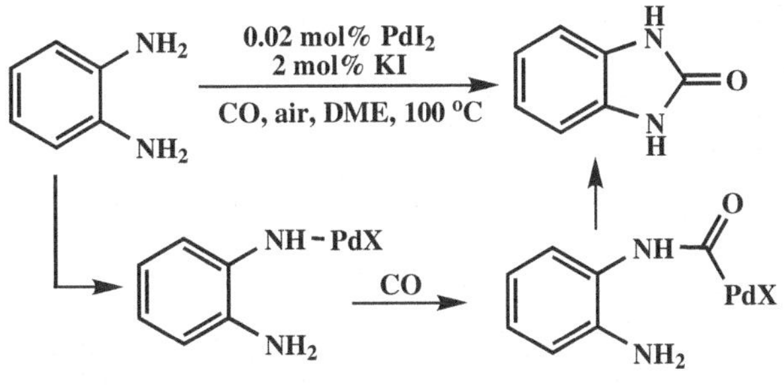

Scheme-89

Hubbard and co-workers [202] reported reductive *N*-heteroannulation of *N*-allyl-2-nitroanilines for the formation of 2-alkenyl substituted benzimidazoles in the presence of palladium catalyst with the help of reducing agent *i.e.* carbon monoxide (**Scheme 90**) [49].

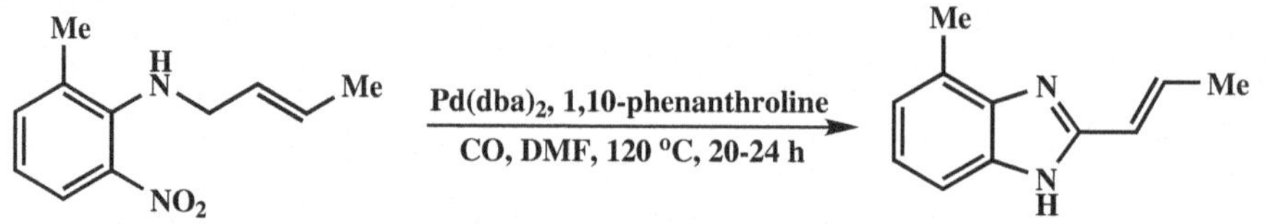

Scheme-90

By using Pd(PPh$_3$)$_4$ in the presence of triphenylphosphine in PhMe at 90 °C (microwave or conventional heating), better results were obtained with substituted aryl derivatives. Moreover the presence of additional triphenylphosphine was found to be crucial, probably acting as a stabilizing agent for intermediate thus avoiding the dealkylation process (**Scheme 91**) [203].

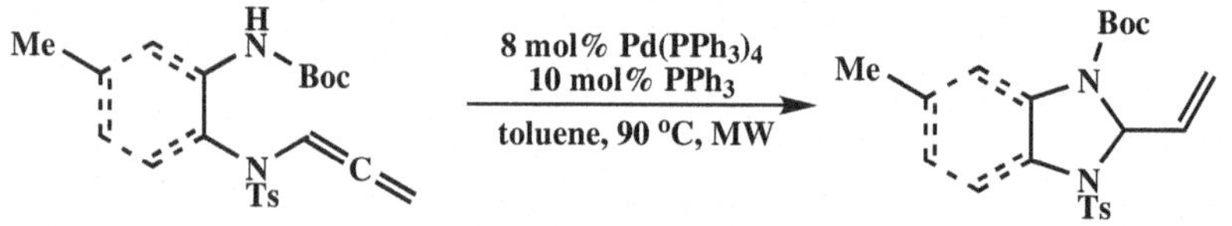

Scheme-91

The *N*-arylated five-, six- and seven-membered *N*-heterocycles were prepared with the use of sodium *tert*-butoxide as a base and SIPr as a ligand *via* sequential Pd-catalyzed intra- followed by intermolecular aryl amination (**Scheme 92**) [204].

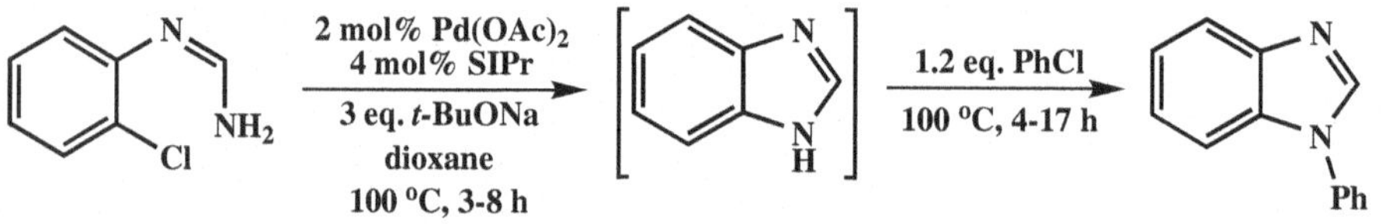

Scheme-92

The Pd-catalyzed intramolecular cyclization of arylbromide substituted guanidines and amidines produced aminobenzimidazoles and benzimidazoles, respectively (**Scheme 93**) [205]. Simple Pd$_2$dba$_3$/PPh$_3$ or Pd(PPh$_3$)$_4$ catalysts were sufficient to promote the cyclization of arylbromides. Polycyclic benzimidazoles and indazoles were also synthesized by this same synthetic protocol [206].

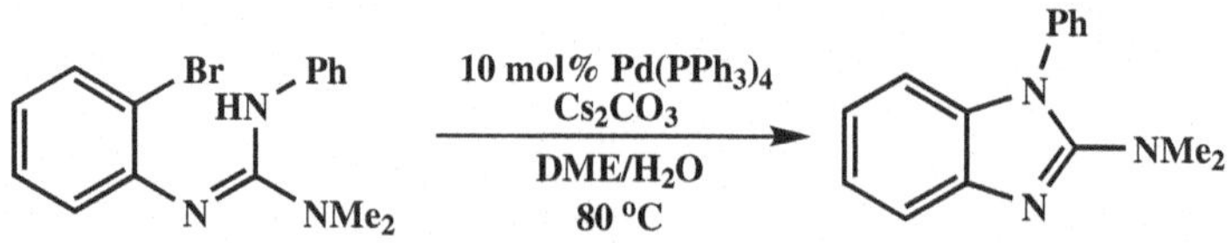

Scheme-93

REFERENCES

[1]   D. Castagnolo, F. Manetti, M. Radi, B. Bechi, M. Pagano, A. De Logu, R. Meleddu, M. Saddi and M. Botta. 2009. Synthesis, biological evaluation, and SAR study of novel pyrazole analogues as inhibitors of *Mycobacterium tuberculosis*: synthesis of rigid pyrazolones. Bioorg. Med. Chem. 17: 5716-5721.

[2] F.A. Pasha, M. Muddassar, M.M. Neaz and S.J. Cho. 2009. Pharmacophore and docking-based combined in-silico study of KDR inhibitors. J. Mol. Graph. Model. 28: 54-61.

[3] H.H. Zoorob, M.S. Elsherbini and W.S. Hamama. 2012. Utility of cyclododecanone as synthon to synthesize fused heterocycles. J. Org. Chem. 2: 63-68.

[4] K. Rehse, J. Kotthaus and L. Kadembashi. 2009. New 1*H*-pyrazole-4-carboxamides with anti-platelet activity. Arch. Pharm. Chem. Life Sci. 342: 27-33.

[5] G.P. Lahm, T.P. Selby, J.H. Freudenberger, T.M. Stevenson, B.J. Myres, G. Seburyamo, B.K. Smith, L. Flexner, C.E. Clark and D. Cordova. 2005. Insecticidal anthranilic diamides: a new class of potent ryanodine receptor activators. Bioorg. Med. Chem. Lett. 15: 4898-4906.

[6] K. Shalini, P.K. Sharma and N. Kumar. 2010. Imidazole and its biological activities: a review. Der Chemica Sinica 1: 36-47.

[7] K.G. Desai and K.R. Desai. 2006. Green route for the heterocyclization of 2-mercaptobenzimidazole into β-lactum segment derivatives containing -CONH- bridge with benzimidazole: screening *in vitro* anti-microbial activity with various microorganisms. Bioorg. Med. Chem. 14: 8271-8279.

[8] Z. Kazimierczuk, J.A. Upcroft, P. Upcroft, A. Gorska, B. Starosciak and A. Laudy. 2002. Synthesis, anti-protozoal and anti-bacterial activity of nitro- and halogeno-substituted benzimidazole derivatives. Acta Biochim. Pol. 49: 185-195.

[9] Z.M. Nofal, H.H. Fahmy and H.S. Mohamed. 2002. Synthesis, anti-microbial and molluscicidal activities of new benzimidazole derivatives. Arch. Pharm. Res. 25: 28-38.

[10] M. Pedini, B.G. Alunni, A. Ricci, L. Bastianini and E. Lepri. 1994. New heterocyclic derivatives of benzimidazole with germicidal activity-XII-Synthesis of *N*1-glycosyl-2-furyl benzimidazoles. Farmaco 49: 823-827.

[11] K.F. Ansari and C. Lal. 2009. Synthesis and biological activity of some heterocyclic compounds containing benzimidazole and β-lactam moiety. J. Chem. Sci. 121: 1017-1025.

[12] L. Garuti, M. Roberti and G. Gentilomi. 2000. Synthesis and anti-viral assays of some 2-substituted benzimidazoles *N*-carbamates. Farmaco 55: 35-39.

[13] D.P.A. Thakur, S.G. Wadodkar and C.T. Chopade. 2012. Synthesis and anti-inflammatory activity of some benzimidazole-2-carboxylic acids. Int. J. Drug Dev. Res. 4: 303-309.

[14] O.O. Guven, T. Erdogan, H. Goeker and S. Yildiz. 2007. Synthesis and anti-microbial activity of some novel phenyl and benzimidazole substituted benzyl ethers. Bioorg. Med. Chem. Lett. 17: 2233-2236.

[15] G.A. Kilcigil and N. Altanlar. 2006. Synthesis and anti-fungal properties of some benzimidazole derivatives. Turk J. Chem. 30: 223-228.

[16] M. Boiani and M. Gonzalez. 2005. Imidazole and benzimidazole derivatives as chemotherapeutic agents. Mini Rev. Med. Chem. 5: 409-424.

[17] L. Claisen. 1903. Zur kenntniss des propargylaldehyds und des phenylpropargylaldehyds. Ber. Dtsch. Chem. Ges. 36: 3664-3673.

[18] D.B. Grotjahn, S. Van, D. Combs, D.A. Lev, C. Schneider, M. Rideout, C. Meyer, G. Hernandez and L. Mejorado. 2002. New flexible synthesis of pyrazoles with different, functionalized substituents at C3 and C5. J. Org. Chem. 67: 9200-9209.

[19] B.C. Bishop, K.M.J. Brands, A.D. Gibb and D.J. Kennedy. 2004. Regioselective synthesis of 1,3,5-substituted pyrazoles from acetylenic ketones and hydrazines. Synthesis 1: 43-52.

[20] (a) B. Willy and T.J.J. Muller. 2008. Consecutive multi-component syntheses of heterocycles *via* palladium-copper catalyzed generation of alkynones. ARKIVOC (i): 195-208.
        (b) B. Willy and T.J.J. Muller. 2009. Multi-component heterocycle syntheses *via* catalytic generation of alkynones. Curr. Org. Chem. 13: 1777-1790.

[21] T.J.J. Muller and D.M. D'Souza. 2008. Diversity-oriented syntheses of functional π-systems by multicomponent and domino reactions. Pure Appl. Chem. 80: 609-620.

[22] B. Willy and T.J.J. Muller. 2008. Regioselective three-component synthesis of highly fluorescent 1,3,5-trisubstituted pyrazoles. Eur. J. Org. Chem. 24: 4157-4168.

[23] D. Bouyssi, N. Monteiro and G. Balme. 2011. Amines as key building blocks in Pd-assisted multicomponent processes. Beilstein J. Org. Chem. 7: 1387-1406.

[24]   M.S. Mohamed Ahmed, K. Kobayashi and A. Mori. 2005. One-pot construction of pyrazoles and isoxazoles with palladium-catalyzed four-component coupling. Org. Lett. 7: 4487-4489.

[25]   J.P. Stonehouse, D.S. Chekmarev, N.V. Ivanova, S. Lang, G. Pairaudeau, N. Smith, N.J. Stocks, S.I. Sviridov and L.U. Utkina. 2008. One-pot four-component reaction for the generation of pyrazoles and pyrimidines. Synlett 1: 100-104.

[26]   F. Xie, G. Cheng and Y. Hu. 2006. Three-component, one-pot reaction for the combinatorial synthesis of 1,3,4-substituted pyrazoles. J. Comb. Chem. 8: 286-288.

[27]   H.A. DeWald, S. Lobbestael and B.P.H. Poschel. 1981. Pyrazolodiazepines. 4-Aryl-1,6,7,8-tetrahydro-1,3-dialkylpyrazolo[3,4-e][1,4]diazepines as anti-depressant agents. J. Med. Chem. 24: 982-987.

[28]   N.K. Terret, A.S. Bell, D. Brown and P. Ellis. 1996. Sildenafil (Viagra^{TM}), a potent and selective inhibitor of type 5 cGMP phosphodiesterase with utility for the treatment of male erectile dysfunction. Bioorg. Med. Chem. Lett. 6: 1819-1824.

[29]   (a) S.M. Landge, A. Schmidt, V. Outerbridge and B. Torok. 2007. Synthesis of pyrazoles by a one-pot tandem cyclization-dehydrogenation approach on Pd/C/K-10 catalyst. Synlett 10: 1600-1604.
       (b) A. Das, A. Kulkarni and B. Torok. 2012. Environmentally benign synthesis of heterocyclic compounds by combined microwave-assisted heterogeneous catalytic approaches. Green Chem. 14: 17-34.

[30]   J.A. Fritz, J.S. Nakhla and J.P. Wolfe. 2006. A new synthesis of imidazolidin-2-ones via Pd-catalyzed carboamination of N-allylureas. Org. Lett. 8: 2531-2534.

[31]   G.S. Lemen, N.C. Giampietro, M.B. Hay and J.P. Wolfe. 2009. Influence of hydroxylamine conformation on stereocontrol in Pd-catalyzed isoxazolidine-forming reactions. J. Org. Chem. 74: 2533-2540.

[32]   J. Peng, W. Lin, S. Yuan and Y. Chen. 2007. Palladium-catalyzed highly stereoselective synthesis of N-aryl-3-arylmethylisoxazolidines via tandem arylation of O-homoallylhydroxylamines. J. Org. Chem. 72: 3145-3148.

[33]   J. Peng, D. Jiang, W. Lin and Y. Chen. 2007. Palladium-catalyzed sequential one-pot reaction of aryl bromides with O-homoallylhydroxylamines: synthesis of N-aryl-β-amino alcohols. Org. Biomol. Chem. 5: 1391-1396.

[34]   K.G. Dongol and B.Y. Tay. 2006. Palladium(0)-catalyzed cascade one-pot synthesis of isoxazolidines. Tetrahedron Lett. 47: 927-930.

[35]   N.C. Giampietro and J.P. Wolfe. 2008. Stereoselective synthesis of cis- or trans-3,5-disubstituted pyrazolidines via Pd-catalyzed carboamination reactions: use of allylic strain to control product stereochemistry through N-substituent manipulation. J. Am. Chem. Soc. 130: 12907-12911.

[36]   (a) W. Zhang. 2003. Fluorous technologies for solution-phase high-throughput organic synthesis. Tetrahedron 59: 4475-4489.
       (b) W. Zhang. 2006. Microwave-enhanced high-speed fluorous synthesis. Top. Curr. Chem. 266: 145-166.

[37]   W. Zhang, C.H.-T. Chen, Y. Lu and T. Nagashima. 2004. A highly efficient microwave-assisted Suzuki coupling reaction of aryl perfluorooctylsulfonates with boronic acids. Org. Lett. 6: 1473-1476.

[38]   P. Nun, J. Martinez and F. Lamaty. 2009. Solvent-free microwave-assisted Suzuki-Miyaura coupling catalyzed by PEPPSI-i-Pr. Synlett 11: 1761-1764.

[39]   M. Kitamura, S. Zaman and K. Narasaka. 2001. Synthesis of spiro imines from oximes by palladium-catalyzed cascade reaction. Synlett 974-976.

[40]   S. Zaman, M. Kitamura and K. Narasaka. 2003. Synthesis of polycyclic imines by palladium-catalyzed domino cyclization of di- and trienyl ketone O-pentafluorobenzoyloximes. Bull. Chem. Soc. Jpn. 76: 1055-1062.

[41]   M. Kitamura, S. Chiba, O. Saku and K. Narasaka. 2002. Palladium-catalyzed synthesis of 1-azaazulenes from cycloheptatrienylmethyl ketone O-pentafluorobenzoyl oximes. Chem. Lett. 31: 606-607.

[42]   S. Chiba, M. Kitamura, O. Saku and K. Narasaka. 2004. Synthesis of 1-azaazulenes from cycloheptatrienylmethyl ketone O-pentafluorobenzoyloximes by palladium-catalyzed cyclization. Bull. Chem. Soc. Jpn. 77: 785-796.

[43]   A.A. Aly, A.B. Brown, T.I. El-Emary, A.M.M. Ewas and M. Ramadane. 2009. Hydrazinecarbothioamide group in the synthesis of heterocycles. ARKIVOC (i): 150-197.

[44]   I.H. Gilbert, D.C. Rees, A.K. Crockett and R.C.F. Jones. 1995. Imidazolines as amide bond replacements. Tetrahedron 51: 6315-6335.

[45]   S. Pivsa-Art, T. Satoh, Y. Kawamura, M. Miura and M. Nomura. 1998. Palladium-catalyzed arylation of azole compounds with aryl halides in the presence of alkali metal carbonates and the use of copper iodide in the reaction. Bzlll. Clzern. Soc. Jprz. 71: 467-473.

[46]   B.A. Arndtsen. 2009. Metal-catalyzed one-step synthesis: towards direct alternatives to multistep heterocycle and amino acid derivative formation. Chem. Eur. J. 15: 302-313.

[47]   A.R. Siamaki and B.A. Arndtsen. 2006. A direct, one step synthesis of imidazoles from imines and acid chlorides: a palladium catalyzed multicomponent coupling approach. J. Am. Chem. Soc. 128: 6050-6051.

[48]   P.D. Croce, R. Rerraccioli and C. La Rosa. 1999. Reaction of mesoionic compounds deriving from cyclic *N*-acyl-α-aminoacids with *N*-(phenylmethylene)benzenesulfonamide. Tetrahedron 55: 201-210.

[49]   S. Nag and S. Batra. 2011. Applications of allylamines for the syntheses of aza-heterocycles. Tetrahedron 67: 8959-9061.

[50]   D.M. D'Souza and T.J.J. Muller. 2007. Multi-component syntheses of heterocycles by transition-metal catalysis. Chem. Soc. Rev. 36: 1095-1108.

[51]   J.L. Davis, R. Dhawan and B.A. Arndtsen. 2004. Imines in Stille-type cross-coupling reactions: a multicomponent synthesis of α-substituted amides. Angew. Chem. Int. Ed. 43: 590-594.

[52]   H.B. Lee and B. Balasubramanian. 2000. 2,6-Bis[4-(*p*-dihexylaminostyryl)styryl]anthracene derivatives with large two-photon cross sections. Org. Lett. 7: 323-326.

[53]   K.H. Bleicher, F. Gerber, Y. Wuthrich, A. Alanine and A. Capretta. 2002. Parallel synthesis of substituted imidazoles from 1,2-aminoalcohols. Tetrahedron Lett. 43: 7687-7690.

[54]   C.F. Claiborne, N.J. Liverton and K.T. Nguyen. 1998. An efficient synthesis of tetrasubstituted imidazoles from *N*-(2-oxo)-amides. Tetrahedron. Lett. 39: 8939-8942.

[55]   D.E. Frantz, L. Morency, A. Soheili, J.A. Murry, E.J.J. Grabowski and R.D. Tillyer. 2004. Synthesis of substituted imidazoles *via* organocatalysis. Org. Lett. 6: 843-846.

[56]   A.R. Siamaki, D.A. Black and B.A.J. Arndtsen. 2008. Palladium-catalyzed carbonylative cross-coupling with imines: a multicomponent synthesis of imidazolones. Org. Chem. 73: 1135-1138.

[57]   D.A. Black and B.A. Arndtsen. 2005. Copper-catalyzed cross-coupling of imines, acid chlorides, and organostannanes: a multicomponent synthesis of α-substituted amides. J. Org. Chem. 70: 5133-5138.

[58]   D.A. Black, R.E. Beveridge and B.A. Arndtsen. 2008. Copper-catalyzed coupling of pyridines and quinolines with alkynes: a one-step, asymmetric route to functionalized heterocycles. J. Org. Chem. 73: 1906-1910.

[59]   L. Ackermann and A. Althammer. 2007. Domino N-H/C-H bond activation: palladium-catalyzed synthesis of annulated heterocycles using dichloro(hetero)arenes. Angew. Chem. Int. Ed. 46: 1627-1629.

[60]   A.J. von Wangelin, H. Neumann, D. Gordes, S. Klaus, D. Strubing and M. Beller. 2003. Multicomponent coupling reactions for organic synthesis: chemoselective reactions with amide-aldehyde mixtures. Chem. Eur. J. 9: 4286-4294.

[61]   S.T. Staben and N. Blaquiere. 2010. Four-component synthesis of fully substituted 1,2,4-triazoles. Agnew. Chem. Int. Ed. 49: 325-328.

[62]   S. Maiti, S. Biswas and U. Jana. 2010. Iron(III)-catalyzed four-component coupling reaction of 1,3-dicarbonyl compounds, amines, aldehydes, and nitroalkanes: a simple and direct synthesis of functionalized pyrroles. J. Org. Chem. 75: 1674-1683.

[63]   M. Whiting and V.V. Fokin. 2006. Copper-catalyzed reaction cascade: direct conversion of alkynes into *N*-sulfonylazetidin-2-imines. Angew. Chem. Int. Ed. 45: 3157-3161.

[64]   D. Grassi, C. Dolka, O. Jackowski and A. Alexakis. 2013. Copper-free asymmetric allylic alkylation with a Grignard reagent: design of the ligand and mechanistic studies. Chem. Eur. J. 19: 1466-1475.

[65]   R.D. Dghaym, K.J. Yaccato and B.A. Arndtsen. 1998. The novel insertion of imines into a late-metal-carbon σ-bond: developing a palladium-mediated route to polypeptides. Organometallics 17: 4-6.

[66]   J.H. Groen, J.G.P. Delis, P.W.N.M. van Leeuwen and K. Vrieze. 1997. Kinetic study of the insertion of norbornadiene into palladium-carbon bonds of complexes containing the rigid bidentate nitrogen ligand bis(arylimino)acenaphthene. Organometallics 16: 68-77.

[67] R. van Asselt, E.E.C.G. Gielens, R.E. Rulke, K. Vrieze and C.J. Elsevier. 1994. Rigid bidentate nitrogen ligands in organometallic chemistry and homogeneous catalysis. Insertion of carbon monoxide and alkenes into palladium-carbon bonds of complexes containing rigid bidentate nitrogen ligands: the first example of isolated complexes in stepwise successive insertion reactions on the way to polyketones. J. Am. Chem. Soc. 116: 977-985.

[68] J.S. Brumbaugh, R.R. Whittle, M. Parvez and A. Sen. 1990. Insertion of olefins into palladium(II)-acyl bonds. Mechanistic and structural studies. Organometallics 9: 1735-1747.

[69] K. Severin, R. Bergs and W. Beck. 1998. Biometallorganische chemie - übergangsmetallkomplexe mit α-aminosäuren und peptiden. Angew. Chem. 110: 1722-1743.

[70] N. Kaur. 2018. Ultrasound-assisted green synthesis of five-membered *O*- and *S*-heterocycles. Synth. Commun. 48: 1715-1738.

[71] L.J. Hoyos, M. Primet and H. Praliaud. 1992. Sulfur poisoning and regeneration of palladium-based catalysts. Dehydrogenation of cyclohexane on Pd/Al_2O_3 and $Pd/SiO_2-Al_2O_3$ catalysts. J. Chem. Soc. Faraday Trans. 88: 113-119.

[72] H. Iida, Y. Yuasa and C. Kibayashi. 1980. Intramolecular cyclization of enaminones involving arylpalladium complexes. Synthesis of carbazoles. J. Org. Chem. 45: 2938-2942.

[73] M. Baumann, I.R. Baxendale, S.V. Ley and N. Nikbin. 2011. An overview of the key routes to the best selling 5-membered ring heterocyclic pharmaceuticals. Beilstein J. Org. Chem. 7: 442-495.

[74] M.R. Netherton and G.C. Fu. 2001. Air-stable trialkylphosphonium salts: simple, practical, and versatile replacements for air-sensitive trialkylphosphines. Applications in stoichiometric and catalytic processes. Org. Lett. 3: 4295-4298.

[75] S. Bontemps, J.S. Quesnel, K. Worrall and B.A. Arndtsen. 2011. Palladium-catalyzed aryl iodide carbonylation as a route to imidazoline synthesis: design of a five-component coupling reaction. Angew. Chem. Int. Ed. 50: 8948-8951.

[76] J. Aydin, K.S. Kumar, L. Eriksson and K.J. Szabo. 2007. Palladium pincer complex-catalyzed condensation of sulfonimines and isocyanoacetate to imidazoline derivatives. Dependence of the stereoselectivity on the ligand effects. Adv. Synth. Catal. 349: 2585-2594.

[77] M. Gagliardo, N. Selander, N.C. Mehendale, G. van Koten, R.J.M. Klein Gebbink and K.J. Szabo. 2008. Catalytic performance of symmetrical and unsymmetrical sulfur-containing pincer complexes: synthesis and tandem catalytic activity of the first PCS-pincer palladium complex. Chem. Eur. J. 14: 4800-4809.

[78] N.C. Mehendale, J.R.A. Sietsma, K.P. de Jong, C.A. van Walree, R.J.M. Klein Gebbink and G. van Koten. 2007. PCP- and SCP-pincer palladium complexes immobilized on mesoporous silica: application in C-C bond formation reactions. Adv. Synth. Catal. 349: 2619-2630.

[79] A.V. Gulevich, A.G. Zhdanko, R.V.A. Orru and V.G. Nenajdenko. 2010. Isocyanoacetate derivatives: synthesis, reactivity, and application. Chem. Rev. 110: 5235-5331.

[80] G.L.J. Bar, G.C. Lloyd-Jones and K.I. Booker-Milburn. 2005. Pd(II)-catalyzed intermolecular 1,2-diamination of conjugated dienes. J. Am. Chem. Soc. 127: 7308-7309.

[81] E.M. Beccalli, G. Broggini, M. Martinelli and S. Sottocornola. 2007. C-C, C-O, C-N Bond formation on sp^2 carbon by Pd(II)-catalyzed reactions involving oxidant agents. Chem. Rev. 107: 5318-5365.

[82] H. Du, B. Zhao and Y. Shi. 2007. A facile Pd(0)-catalyzed regio- and stereoselective diamination of conjugated dienes and trienes. J. Am. Chem. Soc. 129: 762-763.

[83] H. Du, W. Yuan, B. Zhao and Y. Shi. 2007. Catalytic asymmetric diamination of conjugated dienes and triene. J. Am. Chem. Soc. 129: 11688-11689.

[84] F. Cardona and A. Goti. 2009. Metal-catalyzed 1,2-diamination reactions. Nature Chem. 1: 269-275.

[85] D. Lucet, T. Le Gall and C. Mioskowski. 1998. The chemistry of vicinal diamines. Angew. Chem. Int. Ed. 37: 2580-2627.

[86] S.R.S.S. Kotti, C. Timmons and G. Li. 2006. Vicinal diamino functionalities as privileged structural elements in biologically active compounds and exploitation of their synthetic chemistry. Chem. Biol. Drug Des. 67: 101-114.

[87] L. Xu, H. Du and Y. Shi. 2007. Diamination of conjugated dienes and trienes catalyzed by *N*-heterocyclic carbine-Pd(0) complexes. J. Org. Chem. 72: 7038-7041.

[88] S. Diez-Gonzalez, N. Marion and S.P. Nolan. 2009. *N*-Heterocyclic carbenes in late transition metal catalysis. Chem. Rev. 109: 3612-3676.

[89] L. Xu and Y.J. Shi. 2008. Chiral *N*-heterocyclic carbene-Pd(0)-catalyzed asymmetric diamination of conjugated dienes and triene. Org. Chem. 73: 749-751.

[90] H. Du, W. Yuan, B. Zhao and Y. Shi. 2007. A Pd(0)-catalyzed diamination of terminal olefins at allylic and homoallylic carbons *via* formal C-H activation under solvent-free conditions. J. Am. Chem. Soc. 129: 7496-7497.

[91] B. Wang, H. Du and Y. Shi. 2008. A palladium-catalyzed dehydrogenative diamination of terminal olefins. Angew. Chem. Int. Ed. 47: 8224-8227.

[92] H. Du, B. Zhao and Y. Shi. 2008. Catalytic asymmetric allylic and homoallyic diamination of terminal olefins *via* formal C-H activation. J. Am. Chem. Soc. 130: 8590-8591.

[93] D.C.D. Butler, G.A. Inman and H. Alper. 2000. Room temperature ring-opening cyclization reactions of 2-vinylaziridines with isocyanates, carbodiimides, and isothiocyanates catalyzed by [Pd(OAc)$_2$]/PPh$_3$. J. Org. Chem. 65: 5887-5890.

[94] K. Yamamoto, T. Ishida and J. Tsuji. 1987. Palladium(0)-catalyzed cycloaddition of activated vinylcyclopropanes with aryl isocyanates. Chem. Lett. 16: 1157-1158.

[95] B.M. Trost and D.R. Fandrick. 2003. Dynamic kinetic asymmetric cycloadditions of isocyanates to vinylaziridines. J. Am. Chem. Soc. 125: 11836-11837.

[96] J.-O. Baeg and H. Alper. 1994. Novel palladium(II)-catalyzed cyclization of aziridines and sulfur diimides. J. Am. Chem. Soc. 116: 1220-1224.

[97] J.-O. Baeg, C. Bensimon and H. Alper. 1995. The first enantiospecific palladium-catalyzed cycloaddition of aziridines and heterocumulenes. Novel synthesis of chiral five-membered ring heterocycles. J. Am. Chem. Soc. 117: 4700-4701.

[98] L. Wang, S. Peng and J. Wang. 2011. Palladium-catalyzed cascade reactions of coumarins with alkynes: synthesis of highly substituted cyclopentadiene fused chromones. Chem. Commun. 47: 5422-5424.

[99] L. Nallan, K.D. Bauer, P. Bendale, K. Rivas, K. Yokoyama, C.P. Horney, P.R. Pendyala, D. Floyd, L.J. Lombardo, D.K. Williams, A. Hamilton, S. Sebti, W.T. Windsor, P.C. Weber, F.S. Buckner, D. Chakrabarti, M.H. Gelb and W.C. van Voorhis. 2005. Protein farnesyltransferase inhibitors exhibit potent anti-malarial activity. J. Med. Chem. 48: 3704-3713.

[100] L.J. Lombardo, A. Camuso, J. Clark, K. Fager, J. Gullo-Brown, J.T. Hunt, I. Inigo, D. Kan, B. Koplowitz, F. Lee, K. McGlinchey, L. Qian, D. Ricca, G. Rovnyak, S. Traeger, J. Tokarski, D.K. Williams, L.I. Wu, Y. Zhao, V. Manne and R.S. Bhide. 2005. Design, synthesis, and structure-activity relationships of tetrahydroquinoline-based farnesyltransferase inhibitors. Bioorg. Med. Chem. Lett. 15: 1895-1899.

[101] C.C. Scarborough and S.S. Stahl. 2006. Synthesis of pyrrolidines *via* palladium(II)-catalyzed aerobic oxidative carboamination of butyl vinyl ether and styrenes with allyl tosylamides. Org. Lett. 8: 3251-3254.

[102] J.A. Fritz and J.P. Wolfe. 2008. Stereoselective synthesis of imidazolidin-2-ones *via* Pd-catalyzed alkene carboamination. Scope and limitations. Tetrahedron 64: 6838-6852.

[103] B.R. Rosen, J.E. Ney and J.P. Wolfe. 2010. Use of aryl chlorides as electrophiles in Pd-catalyzed alkene difunctionalization reactions. J. Org. Chem. 75: 2756-2759.

[104] P.J. Thomas, A.T. Axtell, J. Klosin, W. Peng, C.L. Rand, T.P. Clark, C.R. Landis and K.A. Abboud. 2007. Asymmetric hydroformylation of vinyl acetate: application in the synthesis of optically active isoxazolines and imidazoles. Org. Lett. 9: 2665-2668.

[105] T. Antonsson, A. Heumann and C. Moberg. 1986. Selective formation of substituted cyclopentane derivatives from hexa-1,5-dienes *via* oxidative cyclization in the presence of Pd(OAc)$_2$-MnO$_2$-benzoquinone as catalyst. J. Chem. Soc. Chem. Commun. 7: 518-520.

[106] A. Heumann and C. Moberg. 1988. Palladium-catalyzed addition of chiral nucleophiles to non-conjugated dienes: enantioselective oxidative cyclization of *cis*-1,2-divinylcyclohexane. J. Chem. Soc. Chem. Commun. 23: 1516-1519.

[107] T. Antonsson, C. Moberg, L. Tottie and A. Heumann. 1989. Palladium-catalyzed oxidative cyclization of 1,5-dienes. Influence of different substitution patterns on the regio- and stereochemistry of the reaction. J. Org. Chem. 54: 4914-4929.

[108] A. Lei, X. Lu and G. Liu. 2004. A novel highly regio- and diastereoselective haloamination of alkenes catalyzed by divalent palladium. Tetrahedron Lett. 45: 1785-1788.

[109] B.M. Trost. 1989. Cyclizations *via* palladium-catalyzed allylic alkylation. Angew. Chem. Int. Ed. Engl. 28: 1173-1192.

[110] I. van Wijngaarden, C.G. Kruse, J.A.M. van der Heyden and M.T.M. Tulp. 1988. 2-Phenylpyrroles as conformationally restricted benzamide analogs. A new class of potential anti-psychotics. J. Med. Chem. 31: 1934-1940.

[111] R.C. Larock, E.K. Yum and M.D. Refvik. 1998. Synthesis of 2,3-disubstituted indoles *via* palladium catalyzed annulation of internal alkynes. J. Org. Chem. 63: 7652-7662.

[112] T. Beresneva, A. Mishnev, E. Jaschenko, I. Shestakova, A. Gulbe and E. Abele. 2012. Palladium-catalyzed synthesis of novel tetra- and penta-cyclic biologically active benzopyran- and pyridopyran-containing heterocyclic systems. ARKIVOC (ix): 185-194.

[113] C. Larksarp and H. Alper. 1997. Palladium(0)-catalyzed asymmetric cycloaddition of vinyloxiranes with heterocumulenes using chiral phosphine ligands: an effective route to highly enantioselective vinyloxazolidine derivatives. J. Am. Chem. Soc. 119: 3709-3715.

[114] C. Larksarp and H. Alper. 1999. Synthesis of 1,3-oxazine derivatives by palladium-catalyzed cycloaddition of vinyloxetanes with heterocumulenes. Completely stereoselective synthesis of bicyclic 1,3-oxazines. J. Org. Chem. 64: 4152-4158.

[115] Y. Noguchi, H. Uchiro, T. Yamada and S. Kobayashi. 2001. Synthetic study of polyoxypeptin: stereoselective synthesis of (2S,3R)-3-hydroxy-3-methylproline. Tetrahedron Lett. 42: 5253-5256.

[116] (a) E.M. Beccalli, G. Broggini, F. Clerici, S. Galli, C. Kammerer, M. Rigamonti and S. Sottocornola. 2009. Palladium-catalyzed domino carbopalladation/5-*exo*-allylic amination of α-amino allenamides: an efficient entry to enantiopure imidazolidinones. Org. Lett. 11: 1563-1566.
       (b) T. Lu, Z. Lu, Z.-X. Ma, Y. Zhang and R.P. Hsung. 2013. Allenamides: a powerful and versatile building block in organic synthesis. Chem. Rev. 113: 4862-4904.

[117] L.E. Overman and T.P. Remarchuk. 2002. Catalytic asymmetric intramolecular aminopalladation: enantioselective synthesis of vinyl-substituted 2-oxazolidinones, 2-imidazolidinones, and 2-pyrrolidinones. J. Am. Chem. Soc. 124: 12-13.

[118] M.B. Bertrand and J.P. Wolfe. 2005. Stereoselective synthesis of N-protected pyrrolidines *via* Pd-catalyzed reactions of γ-(N-acylamino) alkenes and γ-(N-Boc-amino) alkenes with aryl bromides. Tetrahedron 61: 6447-6459.

[119] J. Ney and J.P. Wolfe. 2005. Selective synthesis of 5- or 6-aryl octahydrocyclopenta[b]pyrroles from a common precursor through control of competing pathways in a Pd-catalyzed reaction. J. Am. Chem. Soc. 127: 8644-8651.

[120] V. Kotov, C.C. Scarborough and S.S. Stahl. 2007. Palladium-catalyzed aerobic oxidative amination of alkenes: development of intra- and intermolecular aza-Wacker reactions. Inorg. Chem. 46: 1910-1923.

[121] D. Culkin and J.F. Hartwig. 2004. Carbon-carbon bond-forming reductive elimination from arylpalladium complexes containing functionalized alkyl groups. Influence of ligand steric and electronic properties on structure, stability, and reactivity. Organometallics 23: 3398-3416.

[122] M.B. Bertrand, J.D. Neukom and J.P. Wolfe. 2008. Mild conditions for Pd-catalyzed carboamination of N-protected hex-4-enylamines and 1-, 3-, and 4-substituted pent-4-enylamines. Scope, limitations, and mechanism of pyrrolidine formation. J. Org. Chem. 73: 8851-8860.

[123] T.E. Muller, K.C. Hultzsch, M. Yus, F. Foubelo and M. Tada. 2008. Hydroamination: direct addition of amines to alkenes and alkynes. Chem. Rev. 108: 3795-3892.

[124] J. Seayad, A. Tillack, C.G. Hartung and M. Beller. 2002. Base-catalyzed hydroamination of olefins: an environmentally friendly route to amines. Adv. Synth. Catal. 344: 795-813.

[125] R.W. Hoffman. 1989. Allylic 1,3-strain as a controlling factor in stereoselective transformations. Chem. Rev. 89: 1841-1860.

[126] J.S. Nakhla, J.W. Kampf and J.P. Wolfe. 2006. Intramolecular Pd-catalyzed carboetherification and carboamination. Influence of catalyst structure on reaction mechanism and product stereochemistry. J. Am. Chem. Soc. 128: 2893-2901.

[127] Y. Gnas and F. Glorius. 2006. Chiral auxiliaries - principles and recent applications. Synthesis 12: 1899-1930.

[128] N.D. Buezo, O.G. Mancheno and J.C. Carretero. 2000. The 2-(*N,N*-dimethylamino)phenylsulfinyl group as an efficient chiral auxiliary in intramolecular Heck reactions. Org. Lett. 2: 1451-1454.

[129] K. Feichtinger, C. Zapf, H.L. Sings and M. Goodman. 1998. Diprotected triflylguanidines: a new class of guanidinylation reagents. J. Org. Chem. 63: 3804-3805.

[130] Y.F. Yong, J.A. Kowalski and M.A. Lipton. 1997. Facile and efficient guanylation of amines using thioureas and Mukaiyama's reagent. J. Org. Chem. 62: 1540-1542.

[131] L. Djakovitch, M. Wagner, C.G. Hartung, M. Beller and K. Koehler. 2004. Pd-catalyzed Heck arylation of cycloalkenes- studies on selectivity comparing homogeneous and heterogeneous catalysts. J. Mol. Catal. A: Chem. 219: 121-130.

[132] K. Worrall, B. Xu, S. Bontemps and B.A. Arndtsen. 2011. A palladium-catalyzed multicomponent synthesis of imidazolinium salts and imidazolines from imines, acid chlorides, and carbon monoxide. J. Org. Chem. 76: 170-180.

[133] V. Sharma, S. Peddibhotla and J.J. Tepe. 2006. Sensitization of cancer cells to DNA damaging agents by imidazolines. J. Am. Chem. Soc. 128: 9137-9143.

[134] S. Ma and N. Jiao. 2002. Pd0-catalyzed three-component tandem double-addition-cyclization reaction: stereoselective synthesis of *cis*-pyrrolidine derivatives. Angew. Chem. Int. Ed. 41: 4737-4740.

[135] W. Shu, Q. Yu, G. Jia and S. Ma. 2011. Palladium-catalyzed three-component reaction of 2,3-allenyl amines, isocyanates, and organic halides: a diversified assembly of imidazolidinones. Chem. Eur. J. 17: 4720-4723.

[136] S.K. Kang and K.J. Kim. 2001. Palladium(0)-catalyzed carbonylation-coupling-cyclization of allenic sulfonamides with aryl iodides and carbon monoxide. Org. Lett. 3: 511-514.

[137] T.J. Seiders, D.W. Ward and R.H. Grubbs. 2001. Enantioselective ruthenium-catalyzed ring-closing metathesis. Org. Lett. 3: 3225-3228.

[138] J.J. van Veldhuizen, S.B. Garber, J.S. Kingsbury and A.H. Hoveyda. 2002. A recyclable chiral Ru catalyst for enantioselective olefin metathesis. Efficient catalytic asymmetric ring-opening/cross metathesis in air. J. Am. Chem. Soc. 124: 4954-4955.

[139] T.W. Funk, J.M. Berlin and R.H. Grubbs. 2006. Highly active chiral ruthenium catalysts for asymmetric ring-closing olefin metathesis. J. Am. Chem. Soc. 128: 1840-1846.

[140] R.E. Giudici and A.H. Hoveyda. 2007. Directed catalytic asymmetric olefin metathesis. Selectivity control by enoate and ynoate groups in Ru-catalyzed asymmetric ring-opening/cross-metathesis. J. Am. Chem. Soc. 129: 3824-3825.

[141] D.R. Jensen and M.S. Sigman. 2003. Palladium catalysts for aerobic oxidative kinetic resolution of secondary alcohols based on mechanistic insight. Org. Lett. 5: 63-65.

[142] T. Chen, J-J. Jiang, Q. Xu and M. Shi. 2007. Axially chiral NHC-Pd(II) complexes in the oxidative kinetic resolution of secondary alcohols using molecular oxygen as a terminal oxidant. Org. Lett. 9: 865-868.

[143] M.S. Viciu, R.F. Germaneau and S.P. Nolan. 2002. Well-defined, air-stable (NHC)Pd(Allyl)Cl (NHC = *N*-heterocyclic carbene) catalysts for the arylation of ketones. Org. Lett. 4: 4053-4056.

[144] M.S. Viciu, R.F. Germaneau, O. Navarro-Fernandez, E.D. Stevens and S.P. Nolan. 2002. Activation and reactivity of (NHC)Pd(allyl)Cl (NHC = *N*-heterocyclic carbene) complexes in cross-coupling reactions. Organometallics 21: 5470-5472.

[145] M.R. Chaulagain, G.J. Sormunen and J. Montgomery. 2007. New *N*-heterocyclic carbene ligand and its application in asymmetric nickel-catalyzed aldehyde/alkyne reductive couplings. J. Am. Chem. Soc. 129: 9568-9569.

[146] N. Marion, O. Navarro, J. Mei, E.D. Stevens, N.M. Scott and S.P. Nolan. 2006. Modified (NHC) Pd(allyl)Cl (NHC = *N*-heterocyclic carbene) complexes for room-temperature Suzuki-Miyaura and Buchwald-Hartwig reactions. J. Am. Chem. Soc. 128: 4101-4111.

[147] R.D. Dghaym, R. Dhawan and B.A. Arndtsen. 2001. The use of carbon monoxide and imines as peptide derivative synthons: a facile palladium-catalyzed synthesis of α-amino acid derived imidazolines. Angew. Chem. Int. Ed. 40: 3228-3230.

[148] R. Dhawan and B.A. Arndtsen. 2004. Palladium-catalyzed multicomponent coupling of alkynes, imines, and acid chlorides: a direct and modular approach to pyrrole synthesis. J. Am. Chem. Soc. 126: 468-469.

[149] S. Zaman, K. Mitsuru and A.D. Abell. 2005. Synthesis of trisubstituted imidazoles by palladium-catalyzed cyclization of O-pentafluorobenzoylamidoximes: application to amino acid mimetics with a C-terminal imidazole. Org. Lett. 7: 609-611.

[150] M. Yanagisawa, H. Kurihara, S. Kimura, Y. Tomobe, M. Kobayashi, Y. Mitsui, Y. Yazaki, K. Goto and T. Masaki. 1988. A novel potent vasoconstrictor peptide produced by vascular endothelial cells. Nature 332: 411-415.

[151] N.J. Tom, W.M. Simon, H.N. Frost and M. Ewing. 2004. De-protection of a primary Boc group under basic conditions. Tetrahedron Lett. 45: 905-906.

[152] (a) J.P. Wolfe. 2006. Stereoselective synthesis of saturated heterocycles *via* Pd-catalyzed alkene carboetherification and carboamination reactions. Synlett 4: 571-582.
(b) J.P. Wolfe. 2008. Stereoselective synthesis of saturated heterocycles *via* Pd-catalyzed alkene carboetherification and carboamination reactions. Synlett 19: 2913-2937.

[153] B. Zhao, H. Du and Y. Shi. 2008. Cu(I)-catalyzed cycloguanidination of olefins. Org. Lett. 10: 1087-1090.

[154] C.B. Lavery, R. McDonald and M. Stradiotto. 2012. Efficient palladium-catalyzed synthesis of substituted indoles employing a new (silanyloxyphenyl)phosphine ligand. Chem. Commun. 48: 7277-7279.

[155] N. Halland, M. Nazare, O. R'Kyek, J. Alonso, M. Urmann and A. Lindenschmidt. 2009. A general and mild palladium-catalyzed domino reaction for the synthesis of 2H-indazoles. Angew. Chem. 121: 7011-7014.

[156] Y. Luo, X. Pan and J. Wu. 2011. Efficient synthesis of 5H-cyclopenta[c]quinoline derivatives *via* palladium-catalyzed domino reactions of o-alkynylhalobenzene with amine. Org. Lett. 13: 1150-1153.

[157] C.J. Ball and M.C. Willis. 2013. Cascade palladium- and copper-catalyzed aromatic heterocycle synthesis: the emergence of general precursors. Eur. J. Org. Chem. 3: 425-441.

[158] A. Schmidt, A. Beutler and B. Snovvdovych. 2008. Recent advances in the chemistry of indazoles. Eur. J. Org. Chem. 24: 4073-4095.

[159] N.F. Sandra, F. Joan-Carles, F. Pilar, E. Paul and A. Fernando. 2008. Solid phase preparation of 1,3-disubstituted indazole derivatives. QSAR Comb. Sci. 27: 1267-1273.

[160] N. Haddad and J. Baron. 2002. Novel application of the palladium-catalyzed N-arylation of hydrazones to a versatile new synthesis of pyrazoles. Tetrahedron Lett. 43: 2171-2173.

[161] M.Y.W. Toshihide and N. Masakazu. 2000. A new palladium-catalyzed intramolecular cyclization: synthesis of 1-aminoindole derivatives and functionalization of their carbocylic rings. Angew. Chem. Int. Ed. 39: 2501-2504.

[162] J.J. Song and N.K. Yee. 2000. A novel synthesis of 2-aryl-2H-indazoles *via* a palladium-catalyzed intramolecular amination reaction. Org. Lett. 2: 519-521.

[163] K. Inamoto, M. Katsuno, T. Yoshino, Y. Arai, K. Hiroya and T. Sakamoto. 2007. Synthesis of 3-substituted indazoles and benzoisoxazoles *via* Pd-catalyzed cyclization reactions: application to the synthesis of nigellicine. Tetrahedron 63: 2695-2711.

[164] S.P. McClintock, N. Forster, R. Herges and M.M. Haley. 2009. Synthesis of α-ketoester- and α-hydroxyester-substituted isoindazoles *via* the thermodynamic coarctate cyclization of ester-terminated azo-ene-yne systems. J. Org. Chem. 74: 6631-6636.

[165] G.L. Dou and D.Q. Shi. 2009. Efficient and convenient synthesis of indazol-3(2H)-ones and 2-amino-benzonitriles. J. Comb. Chem. 11: 1073-1077.

[166] F. Bellina and R. Rossi. 2010. Transition metal-catalyzed direct arylation of substrates with activated sp^3-hybridized C-H bonds and some of their synthetic equivalents with aryl halides and pseudohalides. Chem. Rev. 110: 1082-1146.

[167] C. Dong, L. Xie, X. Mou, Y. Zhong and W. Su. 2010. Facile synthesis of 1,3,4-benzotriazepines and 1-arylamide-1*H*-indazoles *via* palladium-catalyzed cyclization of aryl isocyanates and aryl hydrazones under microwave irradiation. Org. Biomol. Chem. 8: 4827-4830.

[168] H. Togo, Y. Hoshina, T. Muraki, H. Nakayama and M. Yokoyama. 1998. Study on radical amidation onto aromatic rings with (diacyloxyiodo)arenes. J. Org. Chem. 63: 5193-5200.

[169] A. Lazareva and O. Daugulis. 2006. Direct palladium-catalyzed *ortho*-arylation of benzylamines. Org. Lett. 8: 5211-5213.

[170] S.A. Reed and M.C. White. 2008. Catalytic intermolecular linear allylic C-H amination *via* heterobimetallic catalysis. J. Am. Chem. Soc. 130: 3316-3318.

[171] J.-J. Li, T.-S. Mei and J.-Q. Yu. 2008. Synthesis of indolines and tetrahydroisoquinolines from arylethylamines by PdII-catalyzed C-H activation reactions. Angew. Chem. 120: 6552-6555.

[172] K. Inamoto, T. Saito, M. Katsuno, T. Sakamoto and K. Hiroya. 2007. Palladium-catalyzed C-H activation/intramolecular amination reaction: a new route to 3-aryl/alkylindazoles. Org. Lett. 9: 2931-2934.

[173] R. Grigg and J.M. Sansano. 1996. Sequential hydrostannylation-cyclization of δ- and ω-allenyl aryl halides. Cyclization at the proximal carbon. Tetrahedron 52: 13441-13454.

[174] Y. Nishiyama, R. Maema, K. Ohno, M. Hirose and N. Sonoda. 1999. Synthesis of indoles: selenium-catalyzed reductive *N*-heterocyclization of 2-nitrostyrenes with carbon monoxide. Tetrahedron Lett. 40: 5717-5720.

[175] M. Adeva, F. Buono, E. Caballeno, M. Medarde and F. Tome. 2000. New synthetic approach to arcyriaflavin-A and unsymmetrical analogs. Synlett 6: 832-834.

[176] J.J. Song and N.K. Yee. 2001. Synthesis of 1-aryl-1*H*-indazoles *via* the palladium-catalyzed cyclization of *N*-aryl-*N'*-(*o*-bromobenzyl)hydrazines and [*N*-aryl-*N'*-(*o*-bromobenzyl)-hydrazinato-*N'*]-triphenylphosphonium bromides. Tetrahedron Lett. 42: 2937-2940.

[177] G. Kirsch, S. Hesse and A. Comel. 2004. Synthesis of five- and six-membered heterocycles through palladium-catalyzed reactions. Curr. Org. Synth. 1: 47-63.

[178] N. Halland, M. Nazare, O. Rkyek, J. Alonso, M. Urmann and A. Lindenschmidt. 2009. A general and mild palladium-catalyzed domino reaction for the synthesis of 2*H*-indazoles. Angew. Chem. Int. Ed. 48: 6879-6882.

[179] N. Halland, M. Nazare, J. Alonso, O. R'kyek and A. Lindenschmidt. 2011. A general and mild domino approach to substituted 1-aminoindoles. Chem. Commun. 47: 1042-1044.

[180] R. Martin, R.M. Rivero and S.L. Buchwald. 2006. Domino Cu-catalyzed C-N coupling/hydroamidation: a highly efficient synthesis of nitrogen heterocycles. Angew. Chem. Int. Ed. 45: 7079-7082.

[181] P.G. Alsabeh, R.J. Lundgren, L.E. Longobardi and M. Stradiotto. 2011. Palladium-catalyzed synthesis of indoles *via* ammonia cross-coupling-alkyne cyclization. Chem. Commun. 47: 6936-6938.

[182] R.J. Lundgren and M. Stradiotto. 2010. Palladium-catalyzed cross-coupling of aryl chlorides and tosylates with hydrazine. Angew. Chem. Int. Ed. 49: 8686-8690.

[183] R.J. Lundgren, K.D. Hesp and M. Stradiotto. 2011. Design of new 'DalPhos' P,N-ligands: applications in transition-metal catalysis. Synlett 17: 2443-2458.

[184] R.E. Tundel, K.W. Anderson and S.L. Buchwald. 2006. Expedited palladium-catalyzed amination of aryl nonaflates through the use of microwave-irradiation and soluble organic amine bases. J. Org. Chem. 71: 430-433.

[185] (a) B.U.W. Maes, K.T.J. Loones, G.L.F. Lemiere and R.A. Dommisse. 2003. The first rapid palladium-catalyzed aminations of (azahetero)aryl chlorides under temperature-controlled microwave heating. Synlett 12: 1822-1825.
      (b) P. Nilsson, K. Olofsson and M. Larhed. 2006. Microwave-assisted and metal-catalyzed coupling reactions. Top. Curr. Chem. 266: 103-144.

[186] J.-N. Heo, Y.S. Song and B.T. Kim. 2005. Microwave-promoted synthesis of amino-substituted 2-pyridone derivatives *via* palladium-catalyzed amination reaction. Tetrahedron Lett. 46: 4621-4625.

[187] C.T. Brain and J.T. Steer. 2003. An improved procedure for the synthesis of benzimidazoles, using palladium-catalyzed aryl-amination chemistry. J. Org. Chem. 68: 6814-6816.

[188] K. Weigand and S. Pelka. 2003. Microwave-assisted Pd(0)-catalyzed amination of aryl halides on solid support. Mol. Divers. 7: 181-184.

[189] A.J. McCarroll, D.A. Sandham, L.R. Titcomb, A.K. Lewis, F.G.N. Cloke, B.P. Davies, A. Perez de Santana, W. Hiller and S. Caddick. 2003. Studies on high-temperature amination reactions of aromatic chlorides using discrete palladium-*N*-heterocyclic carbene (NHC) complexes and *in situ* palladium/imidazolium salt protocols. Mol. Divers. 7: 115-123.

[190] B.U.W. Maes, K.T.J. Loones, S. Hostyn, G. Diels and G. Rombouts. 2004. Rapid palladium-catalyzed aminations of aryl chlorides with aliphatic amines under temperature-controlled microwave heating. Tetrahedron 60: 11559-11564.

[191] N. Zheng, K.W. Anderson, X. Huang, H.N. Nguyen and S.L. Buchwald. 2007. A palladium-catalyzed regiospecific synthesis of *N*-aryl benzimidazoles. Angew. Chem. 119: 7653-7656; Angew. Chem. Int. Ed. 46: 7509-7512.

[192] G. Rainer, R. Riedel, J. Senn-Biffinger, K. Klemm, H. Schaefer and V. Figaia. Fluoroalkoxysubstituted pyridylmethylthio-(or sulfinyl)-benzimidazoles. Eur. Patent 134400B1, March 24, 1993.

[193] U.J. Ries, G. Mihm, B. Narr, K.M. Hasselbach, H. Wittneben, M. Entzeroth, J.C.A. van Meel, W. Wienen and N.H. Hauel. 1993. 6-Substituted benzimidazoles as new nonpeptide angiotensin II receptor antagonists: synthesis, biological activity, and structure-activity relationships. J. Med. Chem. 36: 4040-4051.

[194] K.S. Reddy, N. Srinivasan, C.R. Reddy, N. Kolla, Y. Anjaneyulu, S. Venkatraman, A. Bhattacharya and V.T. Mathad. 2007. An efficient and impurity-free process for telmisartan: an anti-hypertensive drug. Org. Process Res. Dev. 11: 81-85.

[195] L. Liu, F. Wang, W. Wang, M. Zhao and M. Shi. 2011. Synthesis of chiral mono(*N*-heterocyclic carbene) palladium and gold complexes with a 1,1'-biphenyl scaffold and their applications in catalysis. Beilstein J. Org. Chem. 7: 555-564.

[196] B. Gabriele, G. Salerno, M. Costa and G.P. Chiusoli. 2003. Recent developments in the synthesis of heterocyclic derivatives by PdI_2-catalyzed oxidative carbonylation reactions. J. Organomet. Chem. 687: 219-228.

[197] I. Chiarotto and M. Feroci. 2001. Palladium-catalyzed electrochemical carbonylation of 2-amino-1-alkanols to oxazolidin-2-ones under very mild conditions. Tetrahedron Lett. 42: 3451-3453.

[198] F. Li and C. Xia. 2004. Synthesis of 2-oxazolidinone catalyzed by palladium on charcoal: a novel and highly effective heterogeneous catalytic system for oxidative cyclocarbonylation of β-aminoalcohols and 2-aminophenol. J. Catal. 227: 542-546.

[199] B. Gabriele, P. Plastina, G. Salerno, R. Mancuso and M. Costa. 2007. An unprecedented Pd-catalyzed, water-promoted sequential oxidative aminocarbonylation-cyclocarbonylation process leading to 2-oxazolidinones. Org. Lett. 9: 3319-3322.

[200] B. Gabriele, R. Mancuso, G. Salerno and M. Costa. 2003. An improved procedure for the palladium-catalyzed oxidative carbonylation of β-amino alcohols to oxazolidin-2-ones. J. Org. Chem. 68: 601-604.

[201] B. Gabriele, G. Salerno, R. Mancuso and M. Costa. 2004. Efficient synthesis of ureas by direct palladium-catalyzed oxidative carbonylation of amines. J. Org. Chem. 69: 4741-4750.

[202] J.W. Hubbard, A.M. Piegols and B.C.G. Soederberg. 2007. Palladium-catalyzed *N*-heteroannulation of *N*-allyl- or *N*-benzyl-2-nitrobenzenamines: synthesis of 2-substituted benzimidazoles. Tetrahedron 63: 7077-7085.

[203] C.F. Bender and R.A. Widenhoefer. 2005. Platinum-catalyzed intramolecular hydroamination of unactivated olefins with secondary alkylamines. J. Am. Chem. Soc. 127: 1070-1071.

[204] T. Jeffery. 1984. Palladium-catalyzed vinylation of organic halides under solid liquid-phase transfer conditions. J. Chem. Soc. Chem. Commun. 19: 1287-1289.

[205] G. Evindar and R.A. Batey. 2003. Copper- and palladium-catalyzed intramolecular aryl guanidinylation: an efficient method for the synthesis of 2-aminobenzimidazoles. Org. Lett. 5: 133-136.

[206] C. Venkatesh, S.G.M. Sundaram, H. Ila and H. Junjappa. 2006. Palladium-catalyzed intramolecular *N*-arylation of heteroarenes: a novel and efficient route to benzimidazo[1,2-*a*]quinolines. J. Org. Chem. 71: 1280-1283.

Five-Membered Poly and Fused O-Heterocycles

5.1 Introduction

Heterocycles are important bioactive molecules found in nature. These heterocycles possess significant physiological applications [1-2]. Among these heterocycles oxygen-containing heterocycles are found to have good biological activity. In past few decades, the preparation of these heterocycles has attracted the attention of chemists because of their broad applicability [3a-f]. Oxygen-containing heterocycles are very abundant in nature due to their presence in various natural products like hormones, vitamins, and alkaloids. These *O*-heterocycles are also important from an industrial point of view especially for the preparation of dyes, pharmaceuticals, herbicides, and pesticides [4-7].

The benzofuran moiety is present in various natural bioactive compounds like analogues of furochromonone (inhibit platelet aggregation by inhibiting cyclic AMP phosphodiesterase), furocoumarin heraclenol isolated from *Cymopterus watsonii*, DOPA D-2 antagonist (selective agonist with potency 25 times greater than morphine), Khellin (acts as a potent coronary vasodilator), and benzo[*b*]-furo[3,4-*d*]furan-1-one scaffold found in various naturally occurring products, which have a wide range of biological effects [8-11].

In recent yrs, the field of heterocyclic chemistry has been revolutionized with the use of transition metal catalyst. To achieve greater levels of molecular complexity and better functional group compatibilities various research groups have focused on the development of general protocols which use easily available starting substrates under mild reaction conditions. This goal involved the introduction of molecular rearrangement steps into transition metal-catalyzed cycloisomerization reactions [12-16]. This method affords an important advantage in comparison to alternative pathways in the synthesis of heterocyclic compounds with new substituents. This chapter covers the most important advances in palladium assisted syntheses of five-membered *O*-heterocycles.

5.2 Palladium assisted synthesis of five-membered poly and fused *O*-heterocycles

5.3 Synthesis of five-membered *O*-polyheterocycles

The preparation of alkyl aryl ethers from aryl halides in one-pot protocol and synthesis of substituted benzofurans through a palladium-catalyzed phenol formation/cyclization method from 2-chloroaryl alkynes were explained. Heterocyclic compounds were generated from *o*-alkynylhaloarenes in carbon-oxygen bond-forming reactions. The phenols were produced from aryl halides under mild conditions by Pd- and Cu-catalyzed hydroxylation protocol. Buchwald et al. [17] employed Pd-catalyzed phenol synthesis for the preparation of benzofurans (**Scheme 1**). The *o*-hydroxyalkynylarene intermediates were produced from the reaction of *o*-alkynylchloroarene with KOH and Pd catalyst derived from Buchwald's bulky *t*-Bu-XPhos ligand. *In situ* cyclization provided excellent yields of heterocyclic products. The same reaction was also carried out under MWI [18-20].

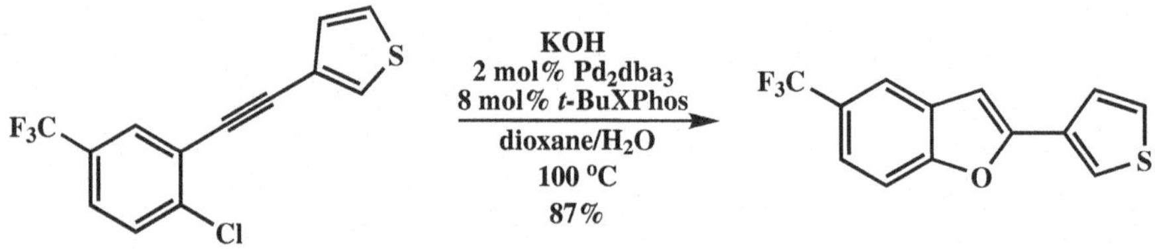

KOH
2 mol% Pd$_2$dba$_3$
8 mol% *t*-BuXPhos

dioxane/H$_2$O
100 °C
87%

Scheme-1

The drawback of cyclization-anion capture protocol was that most cascades were two-component processes. If poly-component processes were achieved by extension of relay phase with incorporation of both intra- and intermolecular segments, the shortcoming was circumvented. The synthesis of ester was an example of a three-component reaction (**Scheme 2**). A number of three-component reactions were performed with carbon monoxide (1 atm) in combination with anionic and MR groups of capture agents [21-24].

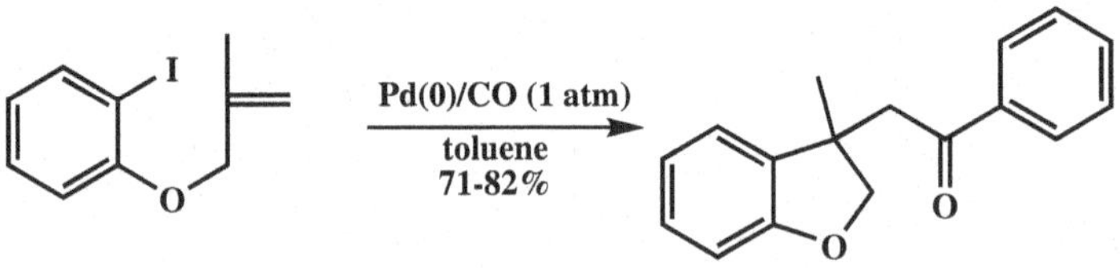

Pd(0)/CO (1 atm)

toluene
71-82%

Scheme-2

Larock [25] demonstrated the utility of this increasingly popular catalytic reaction in the synthesis of a number of lactones by intramolecular allylic oxidation of alkenoic acids (**Scheme 3**).

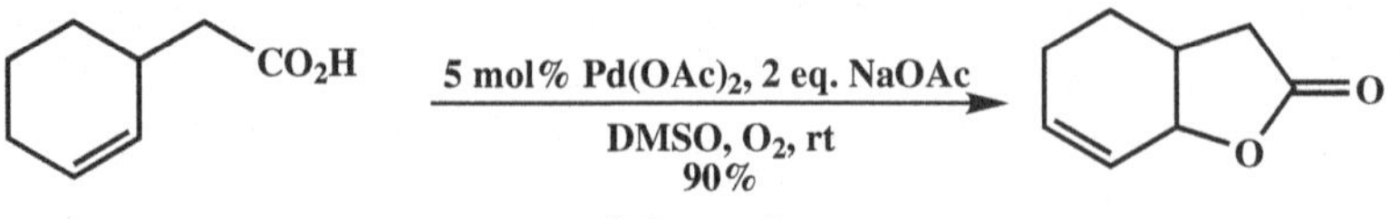

5 mol% Pd(OAc)$_2$, 2 eq. NaOAc

DMSO, O$_2$, rt
90%

Scheme-3

The heterocyclic compounds were generated *via* Pd-catalyzed cyclization of alkynes with nucleophilic centers in proximity to the triple bond. Balme et al. [26] and Yung et al. [27]

produced benzofurans by an intramolecular 5-*endo-dig* cyclization. Cacchi et al. [28] has extended this protocol by a prefix oxidative addition of a vinyl triflate followed by CO insertion. The 3-alkylidenebenzofuranones mixtures of *E*- and *Z*-isomers were obtained by embedding CO in heterocyclic compound, unlike earlier observations under carbonylative conditions [29]. The reductive elimination terminated the sequence after subsequent intramolecular alkyne insertion **(Scheme 4)** [30].

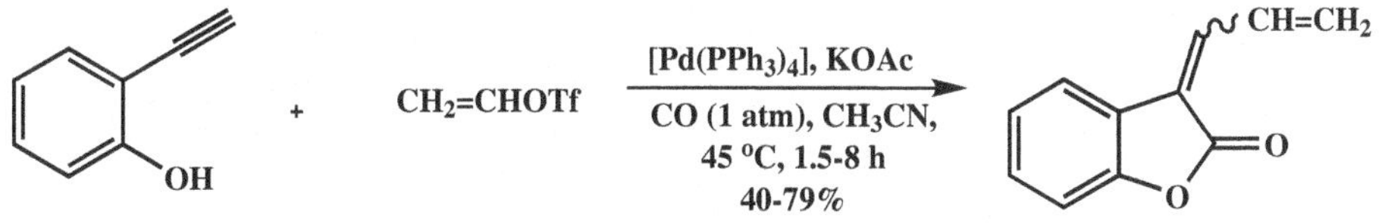

Scheme-4

The oxygenated stereocenters were delivered by Wacker-type oxidative cyclization. A number of dihydrobenzofurans were prepared in the presence of *in situ* produced carbene/palladium catalyst. High yields of pure cyclized products were reported with [Pd(TFA)$_2$] and IMes. The mixtures bearing the desired product and its six-membered ring isomer were obtained with Pd salts possessing acetate or chloride ligands. The palladium-*N*-heterocyclic carbene catalysts were also applied in Wacker-type oxidations [31], for example the aerobic Wacker cyclization of allyl-phenol derivatives in the presence of palladium catalyst [32]. Many *N*-heterocyclic carbene ligands with IMes and Pd(TFA)$_2$ were evaluated and afforded superior results. The reaction used 5 mol% of *in situ* generated Pd(IMes)(TFA)$_2$ in PhMe at 80 °C under an O$_2$ atmosphere **(Scheme 5)** [33].

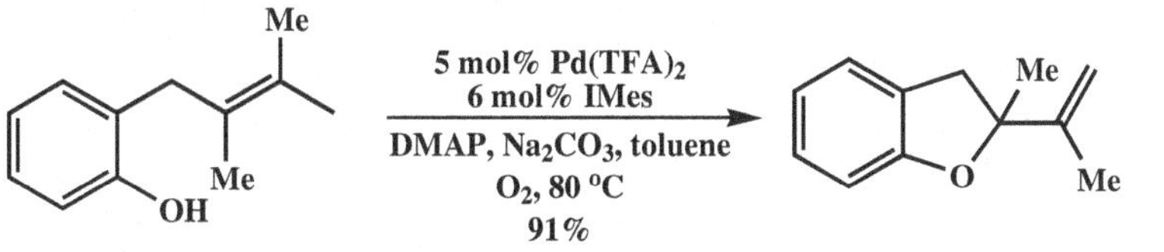

Scheme-5

Muniz [34] reported an intramolecular cyclization of 2-allylphenols **(Scheme 6)**. The palladium(II)-carbene catalysts were prepared *in situ* by complexation of *N*-heterocyclic carbene to Pd(OCOCF$_3$)$_2$. High yields of 2,3-dihydrobenzofurans were obtained in the presence of palladium(II)-carbene catalysts. The reaction needed an oxygen atmosphere for catalyst reoxidation and a basic reaction medium to maintain the catalyst activity [35].

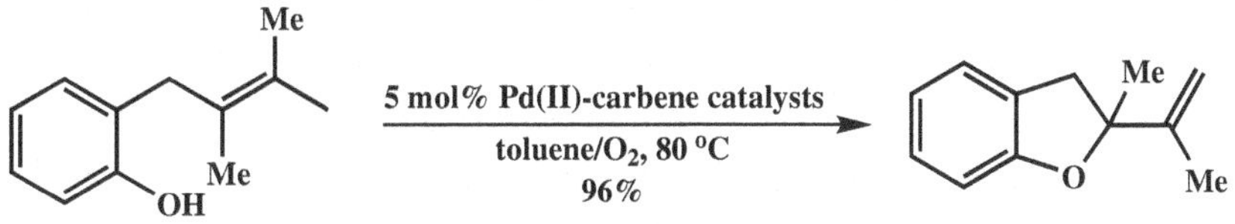

Scheme-6

The ring closure of aryl 2-bromobenzyl ketones was carried out for the preparation of 2-arylbenzofurans with IPr/[Pd$_2$(dba)$_3$] [36]. Nevertheless, nature of aryl influenced the outcome of reaction strongly, although a clear trend was established **(Scheme 7)** [33].

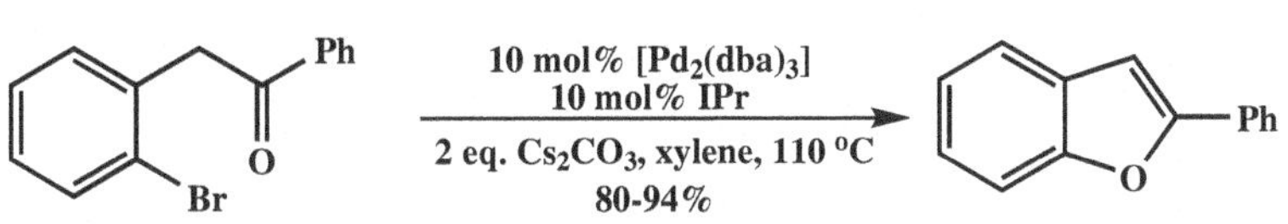

Scheme-7

Du and co-workers [37] produced a range of 3-chalcogenbenzo[*b*]furans in moderate to excellent yields with palladium chloride and iodine **(Scheme 8)**. An intermediate was formed *in situ* by the reaction of disulfides with iodine and then the intermediate underwent electrophilic addition in 5-*endo-dig* manner. The 3-sulfenylbenzofurans were formed from annulation of produced compound followed by loss of methyl group as methyl iodide [38].

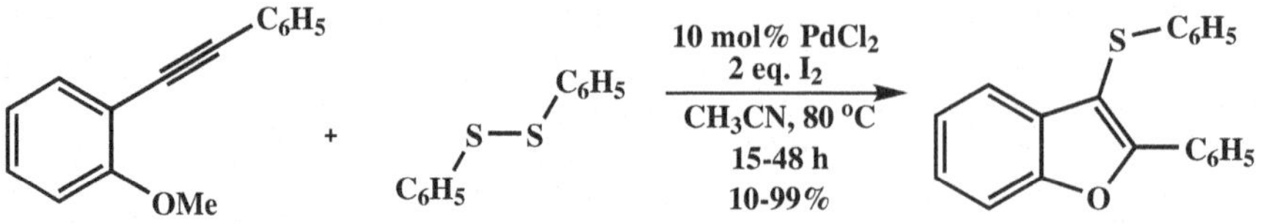

Scheme-8

The allylaryl ethers were used for the synthesis of electron-rich heterocycles such as highly substituted dihydrobenzofurans and benzofurans under acidic conditions (*t*-AmOH-acetic acid 4:1) with palladium acetate, a pyridine ligand, and benzoquinone oxidant in the presence or absence of base (0.00-1.0 eq. sodium acetate) **(Scheme 9-10)** [39]. Mechanism has suggested that *o*-aryl-palladation occurred through olefin insertion and α-hydride elimination. The reaction sequence was classified as Fujiwara-Moritani/oxidative Heck cyclization [35].

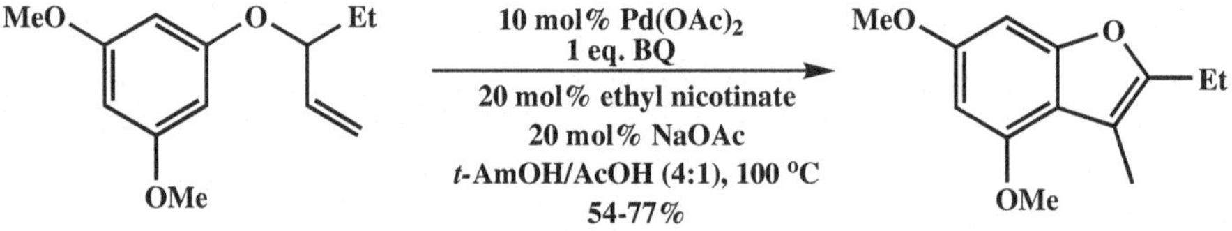

Scheme-9

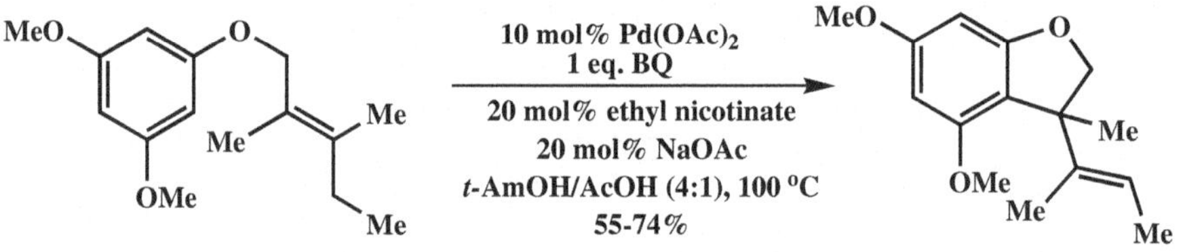

Scheme-10

The Pd-catalyzed asymmetric heterocyclization was explained. Uozumi et al. [40-43] used Pd(OCOCF$_3$)$_2$ catalyst, coordinated with chiral BOXAX (3,3′-disubstituted 2,2′-bis(oxazolyl)-1,1′-binaphthyls) based on 1,1-binaphthyl backbone for improving the enantioselectivity of cyclization of 2-allylphenols up to 90-97% *ee* **(Scheme 11)**. To clarify the stereochemistry of oxypalladation step authors published deuterium-labeling studies in 2004. The cyclization occurred with a predominantly *syn*-stereochemistry with regard to Pd and O$_2$ without chloride ion, while with chloride the outcome was mainly *anti* [35].

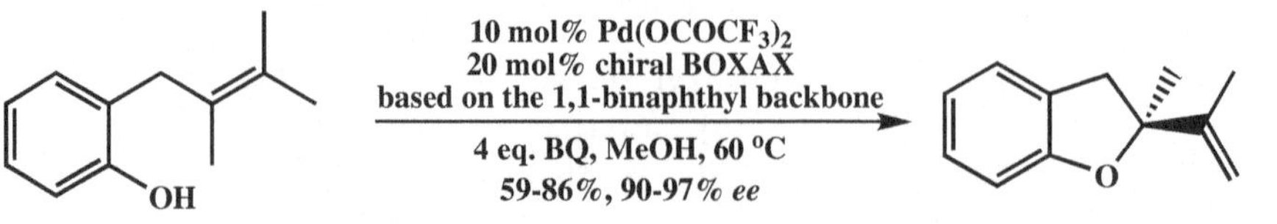

Scheme-11

Excellent yields of benzofurans were produced with 10 mol% Pd(OCOCF$_3$)$_2$, MS3 Å in PhMe and calcium hydroxide under oxygen atmosphere at 80 °C **(Scheme 12)** [44-45]. Specially, the presence of (-)-sparteine provided a high degree of enantioselectivity (90% *ee*) [35].

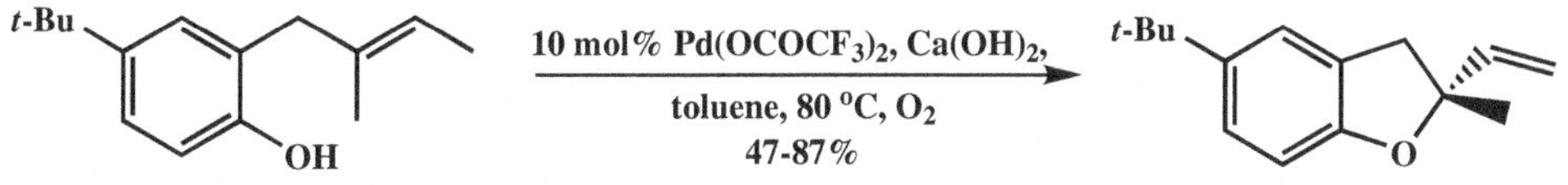

Scheme-12

The benzofuran derivatives were produced from aryl allyl ethers by cyclization in the presence of PdCl$_2$(MeCN)$_2$ and benzoquinone in dioxane **(Scheme 13)** [46]. An *o*-allylphenol was formed by a Claisen rearrangement of palladium-complexed olefin, and phenoxide anion nucleophile attacked palladium-coordinated olefin; finally, the catalytic cycle was completed by α-hydride elimination from *o*-alkylpalladium complex. The substituted chromenes were obtained from aryl homoallyl ethers under same conditions [35].

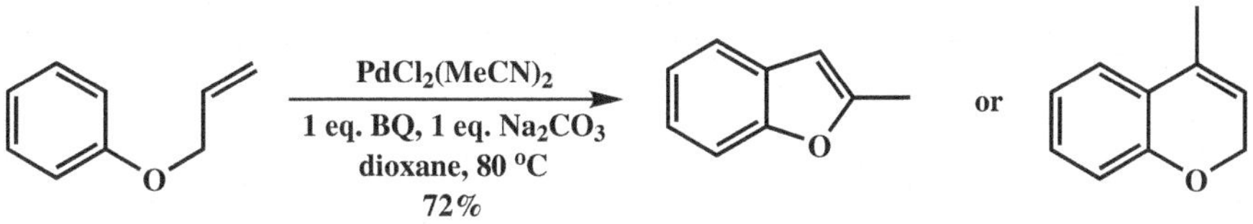

Scheme-13

The 5,7 and 5,6 fused ring systems were obtained in an intramolecular 1,4-addition of 1,3-cycloheptadienes and 1,3-cyclohexadienes, respectively in the presence of nucleophiles such as carbamates, tosylamides, and alcohols [47-48]. The nucleophiles were added across the diene in a stereo- and regiospecific manner in the presence of an external nucleophile such as halide or acetate **(Scheme 14)** [35].

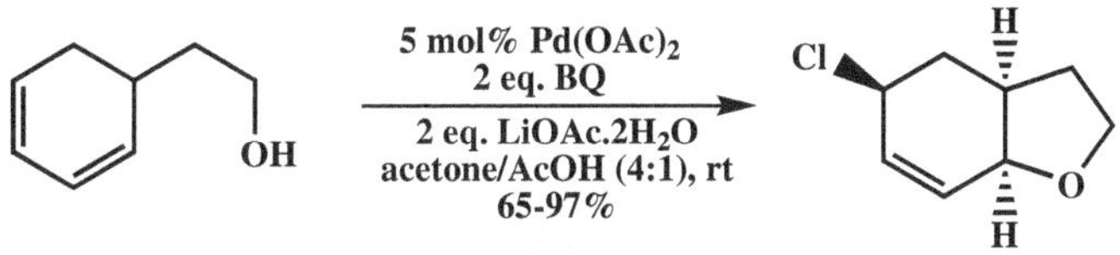

Scheme-14

The 1,3-cyclodienes containing a 2-hydroxyalkyl chain by stereocontrolled palladium(II)-catalyzed 1,4-additions synthesized a variety of fused THFs with 5 mol% of palladium acetate, acetone, benzoquinone, and acetic acid solvent **(Scheme 15)** [48]. The absence or presence of lithium chloride determined the stereoselective outcome. In the presence of lithium chloride, a 20% ratio promoted the formation of a *cis*-acetoxylation product, while in the absence of LiCl a *trans* acetoxylation product was produced. With 2 eq. of lithium chloride, chloride was incorporated as a nucleophile instead of acetoxy group. Similarly, fused tetrahydropyrans were formed stereoselectively when 3-hydroxyalkyl-1,3-cycloalkadienes were used [35, 49].

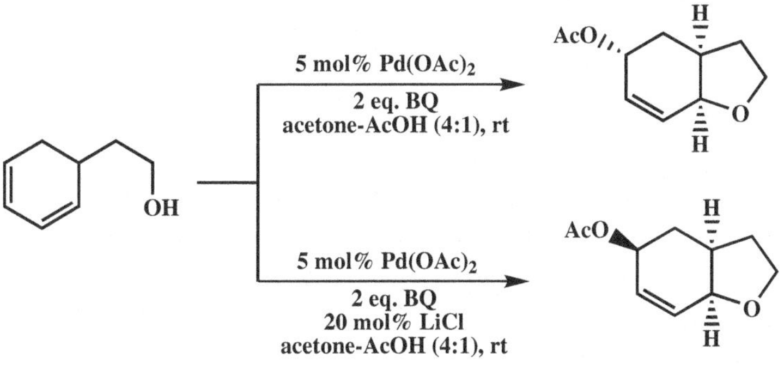

Scheme-15

The intramolecular 1,4-oxidative functionalization of conjugated dienes containing a carboxylic group was reported. Backvall et al. [50-52] synthesized acetoxylated *cis*-fused lactone *via* an intramolecular cyclization of cyclohexadienylacetic acid **(Scheme 16)**. This highly stereo- and regioselective reaction occurred by successive intramolecular and intermolecular nucleophilic attacks. First, there was an *anti* intramolecular attack of carboxylate on Pd-complexed diene. An allylpalladium complex was formed on cyclization. The allylpalladium complex was attacked intermolecularly by CH_3COOH, which led to reported stereochemistry. The intermolecular attack of CH_3COOH was controlled by manipulating the reaction conditions, to end up with either a *syn-* or *anti* lactone. Natural products such as paeonilactone A and B were also synthesized by this reaction [35, 53-54].

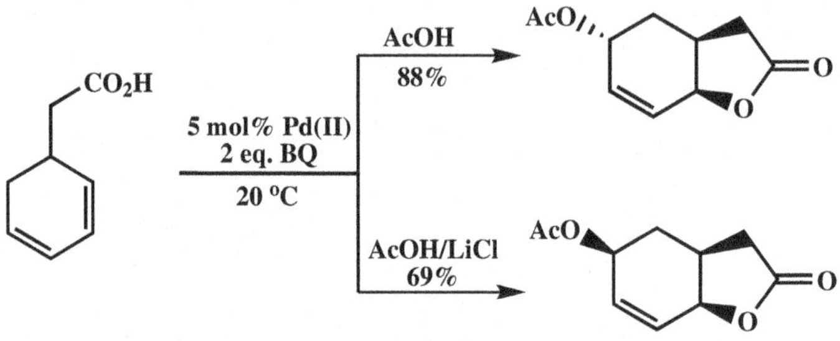

Scheme-16

Backvall [55] reported oxypalladation/cyclization of 5-(2-hydroxyethyl)-1,3-cyclohexadiene in the presence of a $MeCO_2X$ to synthesize bicyclic products **(Scheme 17)**. The $MeCO_2X$ species influenced the *cis/trans* ratio of products. *Cis* product was favored with carboxylic acids and *trans* isomers were favored with salts of carboxylic acids [35].

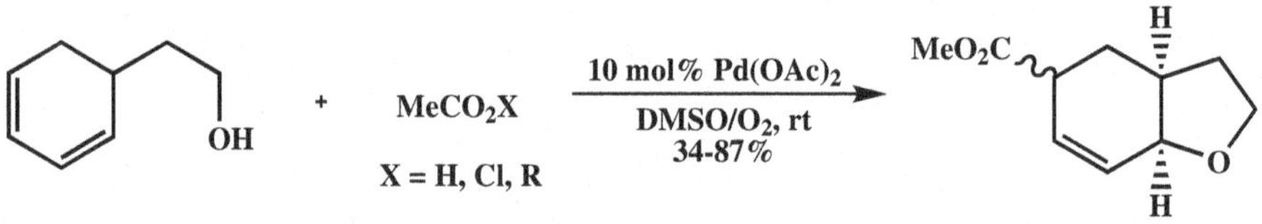

Scheme-17

The Pd-catalyzed intramolecular benzannulation pathway afforded phthalide and 3,4-dihydroisocoumarin **(Scheme 18)** [56]. The reaction occurred *via* the formation of palladacycle followed by reductive elimination of Pd(0).

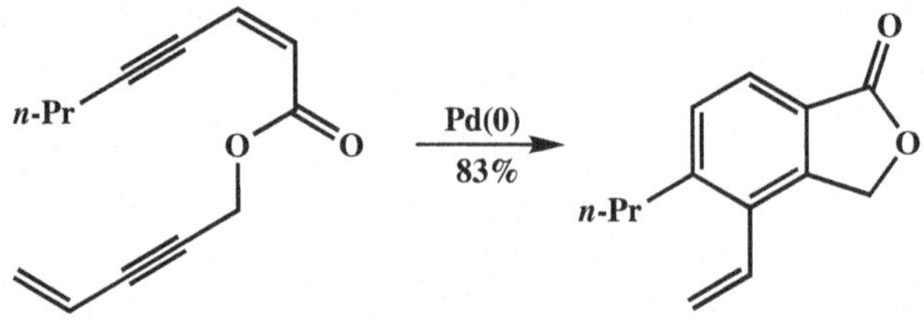

Scheme-18

Bouyssi and Balme [57] described the synthesis of indanylide phthalide *via* Pd-catalyzed bicyclization of *o*-alkynylbenzoic acid. The indanylide phthalide acted as a substrate for the core of fredericamycin A, in 64% yield **(Scheme 19)**. However this aspect was difficult to apply to compound, as four products were produced in this reaction. The optimization of nature of bases and catalysts have shown that compound was formed in 64% yield when the reaction was carried out in dimethylsulphoxide in the presence of palladium acetate, cesium carbonate, sodium borohydride, and triphenylphosphine [58].

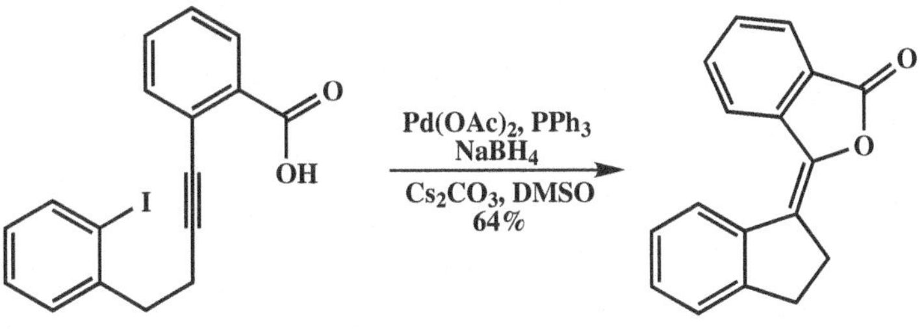

Scheme-19

Buchwald and co-workers [59-60] reported the synthesis of *O*-heterocycles *via* an intramolecular carbon-oxygen bond formation in the presence of Pd catalyst **(Scheme 20)**.

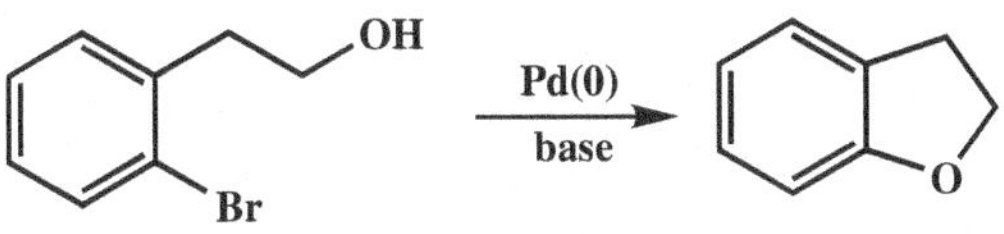

Scheme-20

The conversion of *O*-allyl 2-nitrophenyl ether was conducted with carbon monoxide in the presence of palladium catalyst under basic conditions. Surprisingly, 2,3,3-trimethyl-7-nitro-2,3-dihydrobenzofuran was obtained as a major product in the presence of palladium catalyst from *O*-allyl 2-nitrophenyl ether with TEA as a base **(Scheme 21)** [61].

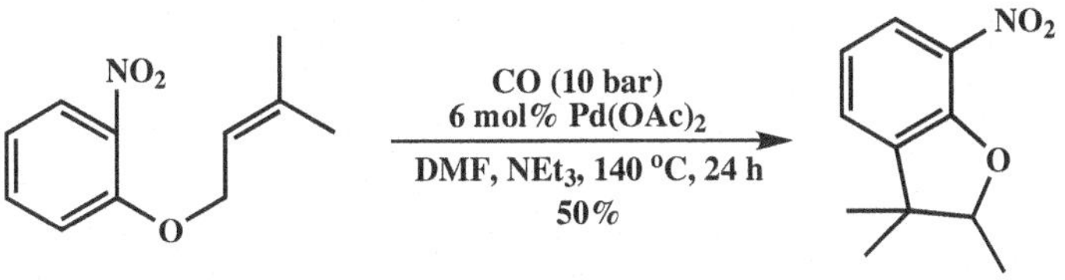

Scheme-21

The incorporation of acetylenes in heterocycles by these new protocols was expected to find widespread applications in the synthesis of organic materials and bioactive compounds. An intramolecular oxyalkynylation of olefins [62-63] in the presence of benziodoxolone-based hypervalent iodine reagents as well as gold-catalyzed alkynylation of pyrrole and indole heterocycles were performed **(Scheme 22)** [64].

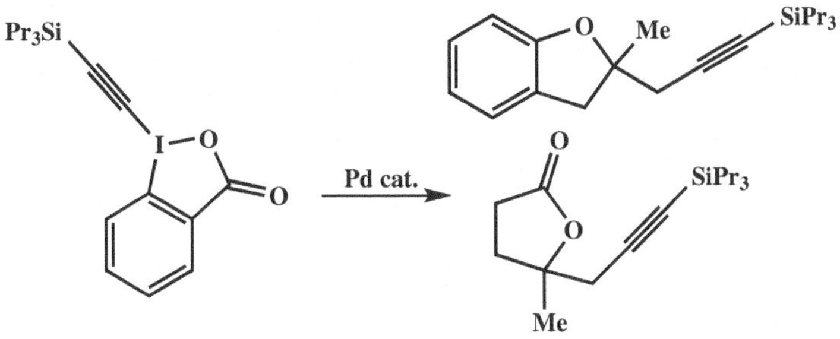

Scheme-22

A variety of substituted derivatives were cyclized to afford the 2-trimethylsilylbenzofuran in high yields with TMG **(Scheme 23)** [65]. The 2-trimethylsilylbenzofuran was synthesized directly in coupling reaction with combined utilization of SiO_2 and 1,1,3,3-tetramethylguanidine. The 3-iodobenzofurans were synthesized when cyclization agent was iodine [66]. With trimethylsilyl or H, the benzofuran was not produced. Here, iodination occurred on aromatic ring. The possibility of further coupling reactions was opened due to the presence of iodine on benzofuran ring. The 2-substituted benzofurans were obtained upon cyclization with Pd in K_2CO_3 [54, 58].

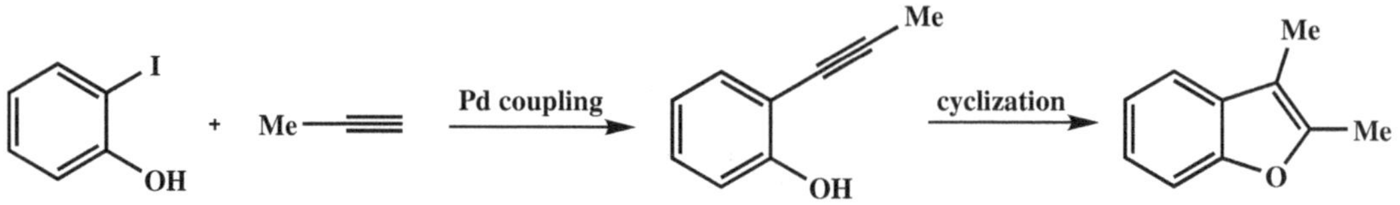

Scheme-23

Balme [67] reported that *O*-allylated precursor (alternative to external allylic substrates) underwent cyclization to form the 3-allyl indoles **(Scheme 24)**. A Pd-allyl complex was formed on activation of carbon-oxygen bond with $Pd(PPh_3)_4$, which then mediated the cyclization and subsequent reductive elimination of functionalized compound. In this intramolecular rearrangement other substrates (like propargylic units) also participated, which formed either propargyl or allenyl substituted benzofurans [68].

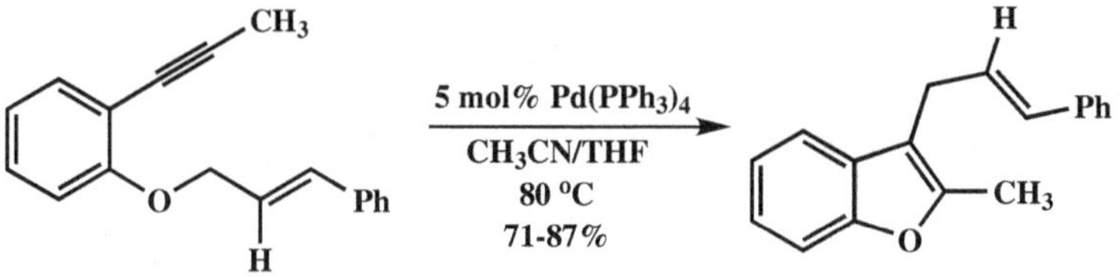

Scheme-24

Two different protocols were involved in Pd chemistry for the preparation of 2,3-dihydrobenzofurans. The protocols were based on cyclization forming cyclic ethers. This method involved an internal ether formation between a bromide and an alcohol **(Scheme 25)** [58, 69-71].

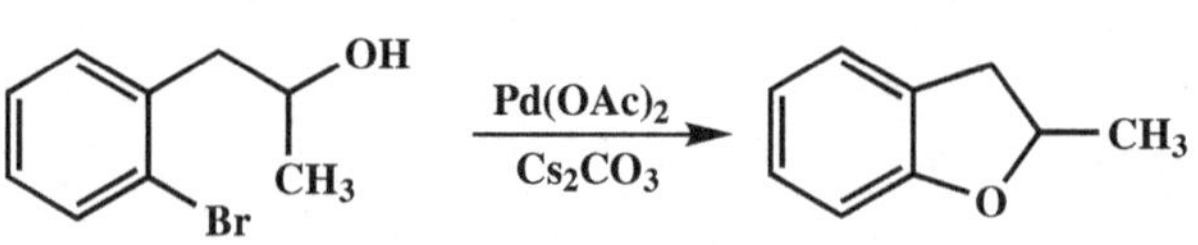

Scheme-25

The isocoumarins or 3-alkylidenephtalides were obtained from *o*-alkynylbenzoic acids depending on conditions. Sonogashira coupling of alkynes with halogenobenzoic acids, nonaflates or triflates afforded *o*-alkynylbenzoic acids [72]. Sashida and co-workers [73] synthesized isocoumarins from *o*-ethynylbenzoic acids by cyclization in catalytic amounts of Pd species. The predominant strategy was 6-*endo*-cyclization but 5-*exo* process occurred when a bulky group was present at the end of triple bond **(Scheme 26)**. The 3-substituted isoquinolin-1-ones were produced from *o*-ethynylbenzamides unless substituent was a bulky group (no cyclization occurred) [58].

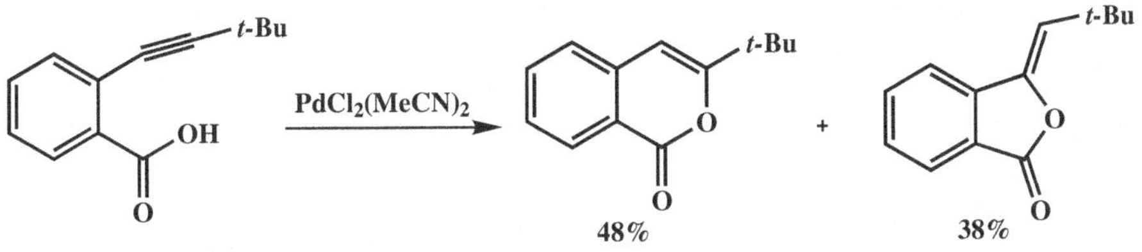

Scheme-26

Yu et al. [74] used Pd coordinating auxiliaries for carboxylic acids in dehydrogenation of alkyl groups. Fagnou et al. [75-77] used a little different strategy where a moiety was utilized ideal for oxidative addition built into the reagent in close proximity to carbon-hydrogen bond. The palladium(II) complexes were formed by oxidative addition in which Pd was in close proximity to a sp^3 carbon-hydrogen bond when halide substituents were present on aromatic systems. The carbon-hydrogen bond was activated by proton abstraction carried out by a pivalate or carbonate ligand on Pd, giving it character of an electrophilic substitution mechanism, and finally ring-closing was conducted **(Scheme 27)**. A similar reaction was reported by Baudoin et al. [78] for the preparation of benzocyclobutenes.

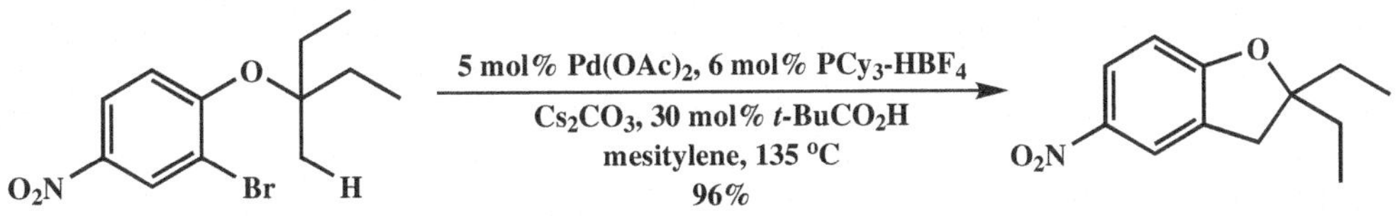

Scheme-27

The original Larock protocol was performed with easily reusable, recyclable, and separable heterogeneous Pd catalysts [79]. In 2009, Batail and co-workers [80] described this approach first time with the aim of developing an additive-free (*i.e.*, salt- and ligand-free) Larock indole synthesis. The heterogeneous Pd catalysts were easily homemade [Pd(NH$_3$)$_4$]/NaY catalyst (prepared by ion exchange of a NaY zeolite using a 0.1 M aqueous solution of [Pd(NH$_3$)$_4$]Cl$_2$ according to [81-82], 3.8% wt) or commercially available palladium/carbon. The 2,3-diphenylindole was formed in 70% yield when 2-iodoaniline was coupled with diphenylacetylene in sodium carbonate and dimethylformamide in the presence of 2 mol% of palladium/carbon for 14 h at 120 °C. Excellent yields of indoles were afforded upon extending the methodology to many alkynes and 2-iodoanilines **(Scheme 28)**. Higher chemical yields were reported with homemade [Pd(NH$_3$)$_4$]/NaY catalyst with the exception of 2-iodoaniline for which palladium/carbon exhibited a higher activity. The benzofurans were also prepared by this method starting from 2-iodophenol. The [Pd(NH$_3$)$_4$]/NaY or palladium/carbon catalyst was reusable up to 5 and 3 times, respectively [83].

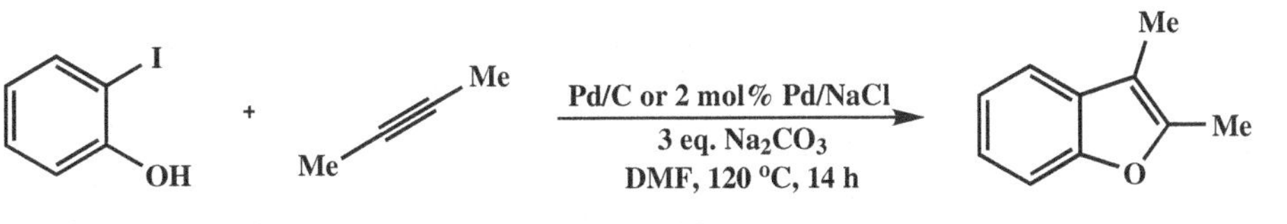

Scheme-28

The 4-methylthiazole and bromoarene were used for the reaction development and optimization. The nature of ligand and base influenced the regioselectivity and yield of arylation. For instance, significant amounts of desired product were not obtained, with DavePhos, in the presence of potassium phosphate or cesium carbonate base. The product was formed in 21%

yield and low regioselectivity with potassium carbonate. The use of JohnPhos did not provide any change in reaction yield. The regioisomer was afforded with a 3:1 regioisomeric ratio in 31% yield and an inversion in direct arylation regioselectivity at thiazole was observed when tri-*tert*-butylphosphine was utilized. On the other hand, with X-Phos a little improved yield of 33% was reported but favored the formation of regioisomer in 8:1 ratio **(Scheme 29)** [84-88].

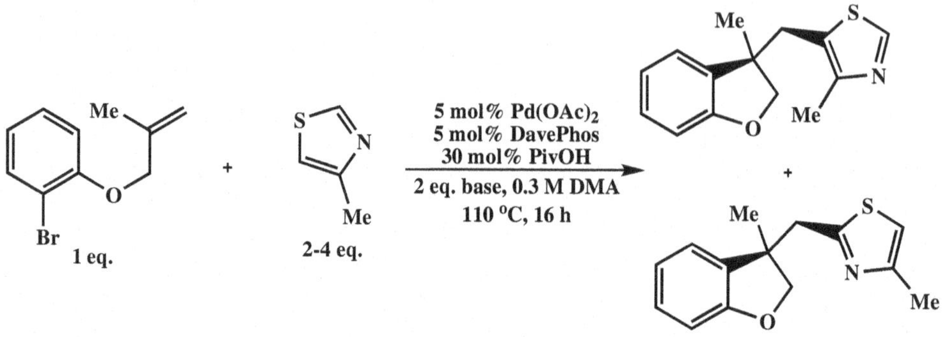

Scheme-29

Dyker [89] explained the preparation of a palladacyclic intermediate through a carbon-hydrogen activation of *o*-methoxy group of intermediate. The Pd(IV) intermediate was obtained when palladacyclic intermediate was reacted with vinylbromide. Then after reductive elimination, Pd(IV) intermediate formed the Pd intermediate. The following intramolecular carbopalladation and subsequent β-hydride elimination produced the product, which underwent isomerization **(Scheme 30)**.

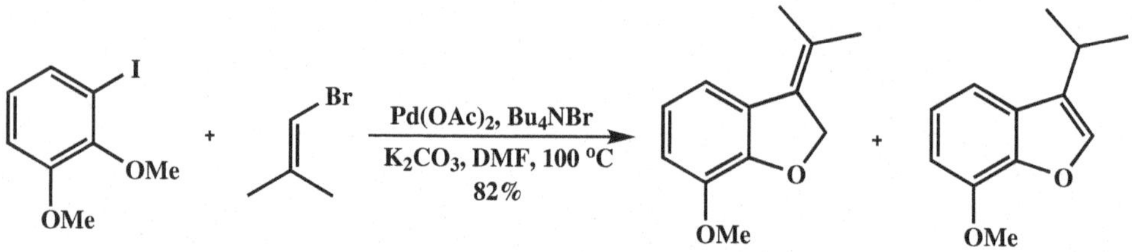

Scheme-30

The phenols and bromoalkynes underwent addition/Pd-catalyzed carbon-hydrogen bond functionalization for the synthesis of benzo[*b*]furans in one-pot synthetic protocol. The (*Z*)-2-bromovinyl phenyl ethers were produced exclusively by addition of phenols to bromoalkynes. Subsequently, 2-substituted benzo[*b*]furans were afforded in good yields by intramolecular cyclization through Pd-catalyzed direct carbon-hydrogen bond functionalizations **(Scheme 31)** [90].

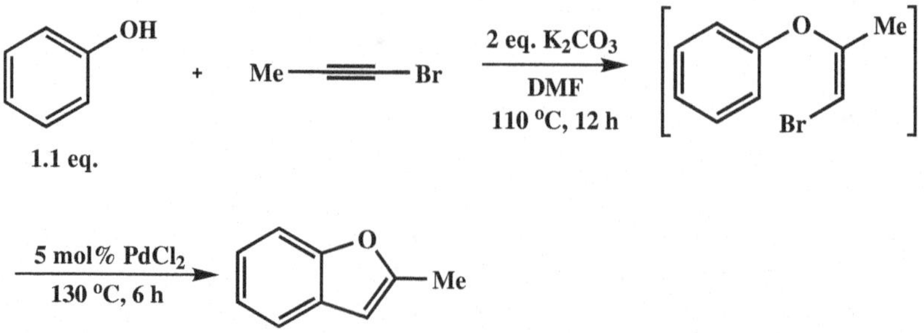

Scheme-31

Hydroxyterphenylphosphine was an effective ligand for a palladium-catalyzed one-pot benzo[*b*]furan synthesis from 2-chlorophenols and alkynes **(Scheme 32)** [91].

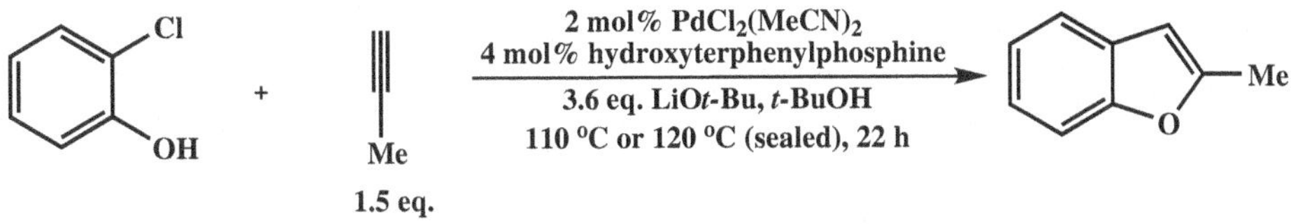

Scheme-32

The synthesis of benzofurans by this one-pot synthetic method in the presence of Pd-catalyzed enolate arylation provided a wide range of substrate scope and afforded moderate yields of differentially substituted benzofurans. The formation of natural product eupomatenoid in three steps was also carried out with this protocol **(Scheme 33)** [92].

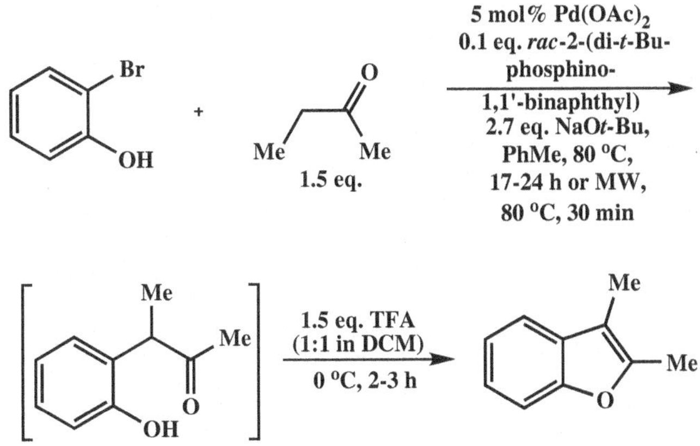

Scheme-33

Yu [93] reported that hydroxyl directed carbon-hydrogen activation/carbon-oxygen bond formation was developed for the synthesis of dihydrobenzofuran. The dihydrobenzofurans were obtained in good yield by cyclization of tertiary alcohols with palladium acetate in the presence of iodobenzene diacetate oxidant. This reaction afforded a new protocol for the preparation of dihydrobenzofurans, including spirocyclic analogues, a method that was potentially applicable to the synthesis of natural product **(Scheme 34)**.

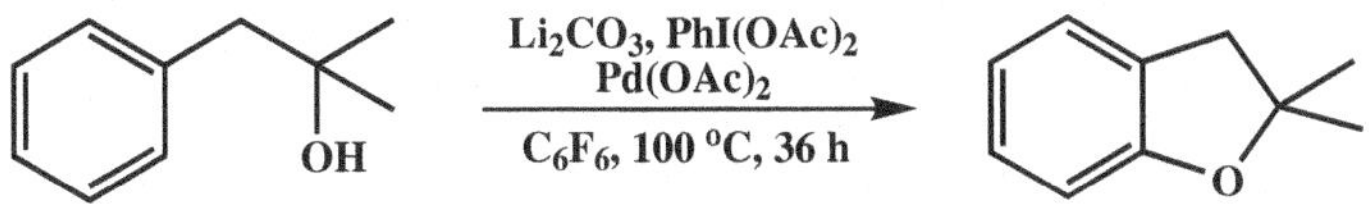

Scheme-34

Aromatic C-O synthesis was developed by mirroring the development of Pd-catalyzed protocols to generate aromatic C-N bonds and oxygen possessing aromatic heterocycle was synthesized with this strategy. The 2-aryl substituted ketones were cyclized to benzofurans **(Scheme 35)** [94]. The reaction proceeded similar to indole syntheses, where *in situ* formed enolate underwent cyclization *via* Pd-catalyzed oxidative addition of aryl-chloride or aryl-bromide bond. This conversion was equally employed to synthesize benzothiophenes from thioketones.

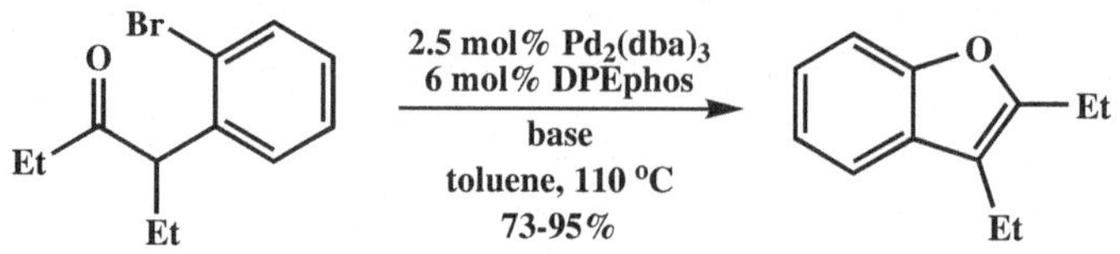

Scheme-35

The *o*-iodophenols afforded an effective precursor for the synthesis of benzofurans **(Scheme 36-37)** [95-97]. These reactions need higher reaction temperatures because of lower nucleophilicity of phenolic oxygen. Nevertheless, similar regioselectivity was found here as with indole synthesis, and in particular, 2-silyl-subsituted benzofuran were often obtained with high selectivity [98-99].

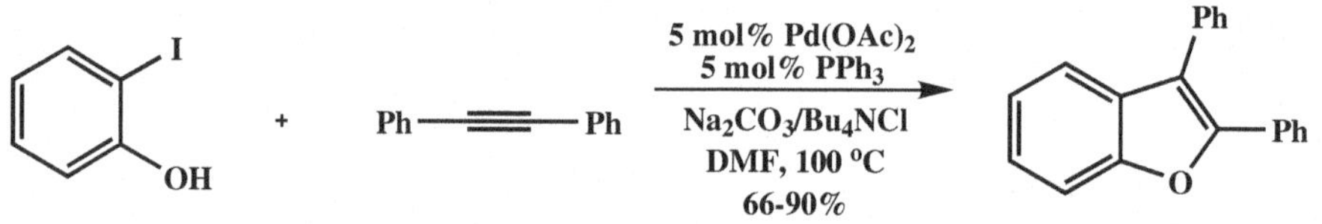

Scheme-36

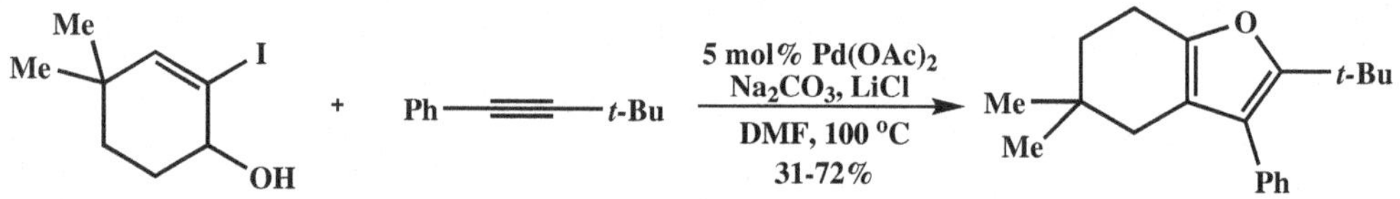

Scheme-37

The nucleophilic addition across the *in situ* formed dichloroacetylene formed (*E*)-1,2-dichlorovinyl ethers starting from easily available trichloroethylene. The organoboronic acids and dichlorovinyl ethers through a one-pot, sequential Suzuki-Miyaura coupling/intramolecular direct arylation afforded a number of benzofurans from cheap easily accessible compounds in only two steps. This protocol was also applied for the synthesis of indoles from dichlorovinyl amides **(Scheme 38)** [100].

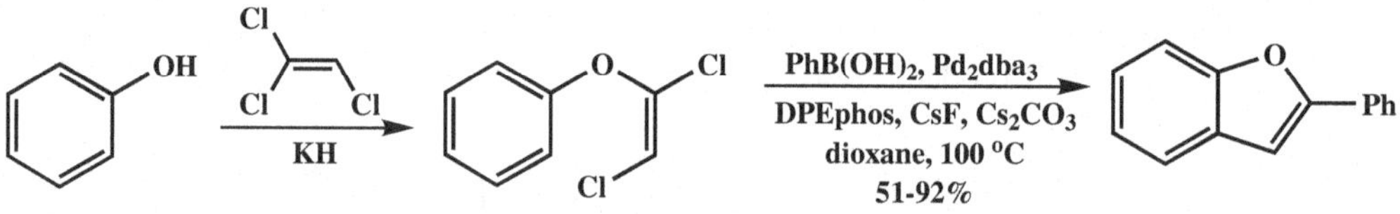

Scheme-38

5.4   Synthesis of five-membered fused *O*-heterocycles

There was a net inversion of geometry with respect to starting olefin in palladium-catalyzed oxidation reaction for the stereospecific transformation of enynes into cyclopropyl ketones. On the basis of these results a mechanism was proposed which indicated the involvement of cyclopropane-forming step by nucleophilic attack of a tethered olefin onto palladium(IV)-carbon bond **(Scheme 39)** [101].

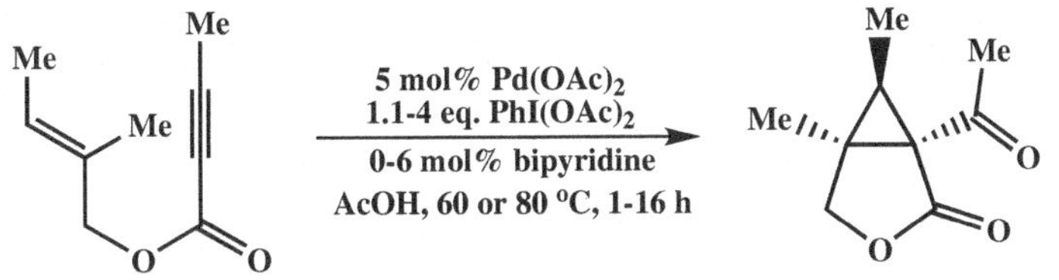

Scheme-39

Beller and Tse [102], and Sanford [103] independently described the cyclopropanation at a palladium(IV) center to transform 1,6-enynes into bicyclo-[3.1.0]hexanes **(Scheme 40)**. Carbon-carbon bond-forming reactions occurred with power of higher-oxidation-state Pd catalysis which was not possible *via* conventional palladium(II) catalysis. A related conversion was developed by Yin and Liu [104] for the synthesis of chloro-substituted lactones when reaction occurred in the presence of CH_3COOH under aerobic conditions in large amounts of LiCl. Here the opposite relative configuration of products was observed to a direct reductive elimination from within the coordination sphere of palladium(IV) catalyst [105-107].

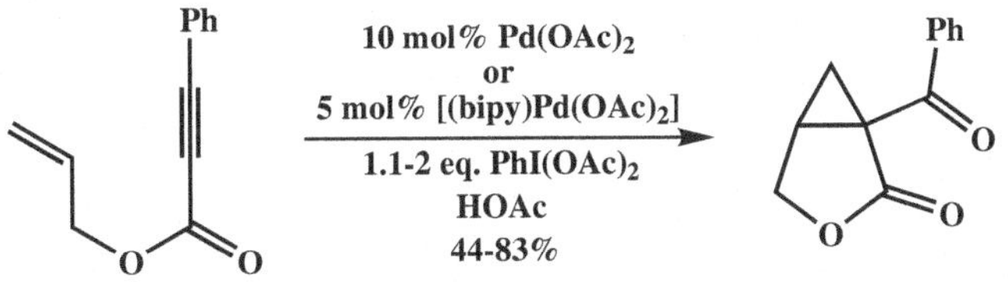

Scheme-40

The bicyclic unsaturated ethers were produced *via* palladium(II)-catalyzed intramolecular cyclization of cyclic alkenols in the presence of molecular O_2 (oxidant) **(Scheme 41)** [108]. The reaction of substrate with palladium acetate catalyst in O_2/dimethylsulphoxide at rt afforded most promising results. The reaction was inhibited with potassium carbonate or lithium chloride [35].

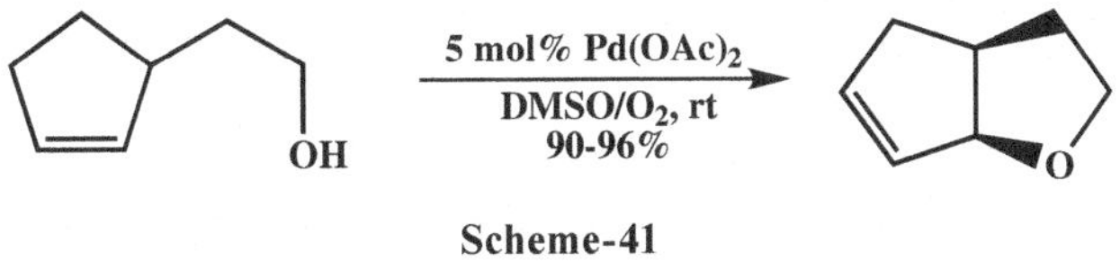

Scheme-41

The 2-cycloalkenylacrylic acids were reacted with palladium acetate and sodium acetate in the presence of tetrahydrofuran in molecular O_2 to afford good yields of *exo*-methylene butyro-lactones **(Scheme 42)** [35, 109].

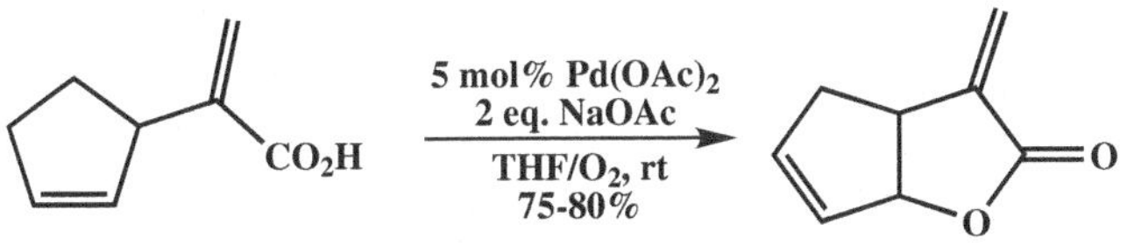

Scheme-42

The tertiary alcohols containing pendant internal alkenes formed THF when reaction conditions were slightly modified. Good results were observed with these more sterically encumbered substrates in the presence of 4-10 mol% of P(*o*-tol)$_3$, 1-2.5 mol% of Pd$_2$(dba)$_3$, at 110 °C [110-112]. The reaction occurred when aryl group and oxygen atom were added across the carbon-carbon double in *syn*-manner. The products with >20:1 dr, and both fused bicyclic were provided from cyclic alkenes **(Scheme 43)** [113].

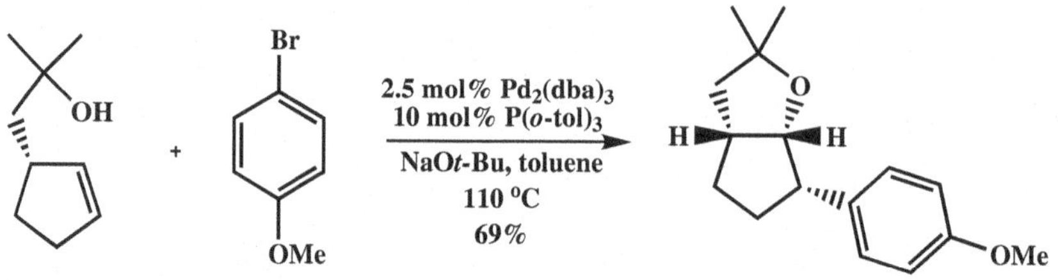

Scheme-43

Oh [114] catalyzed cascade cyclization of starting substrate for the synthesis of furan derivatives in the presence of Pd complexes. The reaction involved initial formation of a palladium-hydride bond, which mediated the sequential insertion of alkyne units to construct the product **(Scheme 44)**. A formal hydride addition formed an enolate anion in the presence of formate. The formed enolate anion underwent cyclization to form the furan [115].

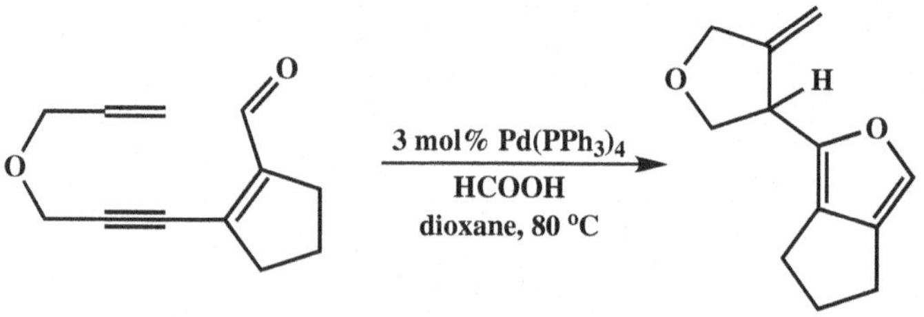

Scheme-44

The intermediacy of α-allyl species in transformation was ruled out based on two observations; firstly, when an equimolar mixture of olefins were subjected to palladium(II)-mediated oxidation conditions, suggesting a difference in reaction mechanisms. Secondly, no scrambling or loss of deuterium content was observed upon oxidation of bis-deuterated olefins, giving lactones **(Scheme 45)** [116].

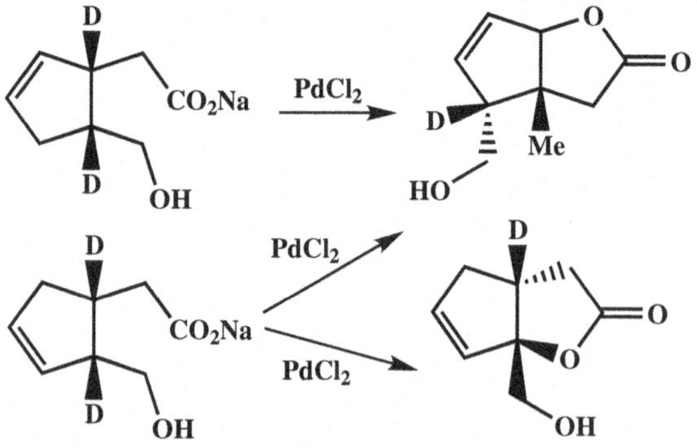

Scheme-45

The benzoannulated enol lactone acted as a key intermediate for the preparation of anti-ulcer agent [117]. High yield of benzoannulated enol lactone was obtained by cyclocarbonylation of *o*-allylbenzyl chloride in the presence of Pd catalyst and TEA **(Scheme 46)** [118a-b].

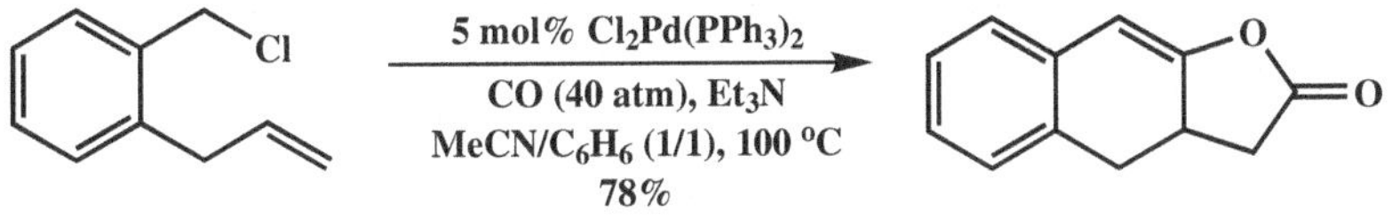

Scheme-46

Intramolecular enolate *O*-arylation was a popular tactic in a number of syntheses. α-(*o*-Haloaryl)ketone substrates were useful in conjunction with carbon-oxygen bond-forming reactions. Willis et al. [119] reported the use of such protocol. The intramolecular carbon-oxygen bond formation was influenced with the use of a Pd catalyst derived from bidentate ligand bis-[2-(diphenylphosphino)phenyl]ether **(Scheme 47)**. Excellent yields of a variety of 2,3-substituted benzofurans (tricyclic product) were obtained [20].

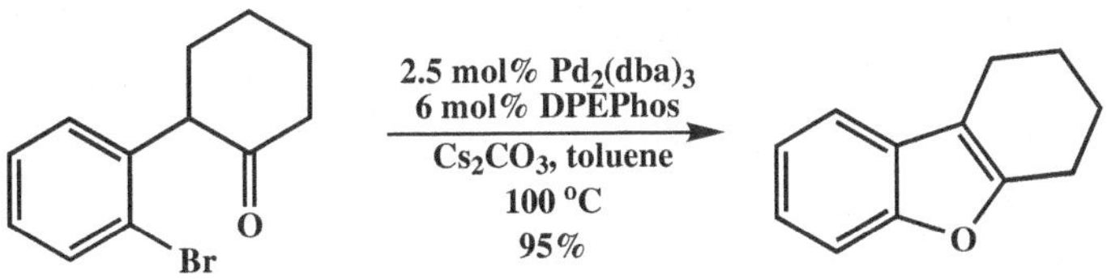

Scheme-47

Liu et al. [120] through a Pd-catalyzed phenol-directed carbon-hydrogen activation/carbon-oxygen cyclization reaction developed an intramolecular Csp^2-O bond formation. The reaction occurred *via* a palladium(0)/palladium(II) catalytic cycle in the presence of air as a oxidant. The turnover-limiting step was carbon-oxygen reductive elimination in place of carbon-hydrogen activation. An anionic ligand acted as a proton shuttle and the phenol group coordinated with palladium(II) as a neutral donor to promote the carbon-hydrogen activation. This reaction tolerated a number of substituents and for the preparation of substituted dibenzofurans it was complementary to previous protocols **(Scheme 48)** [121].

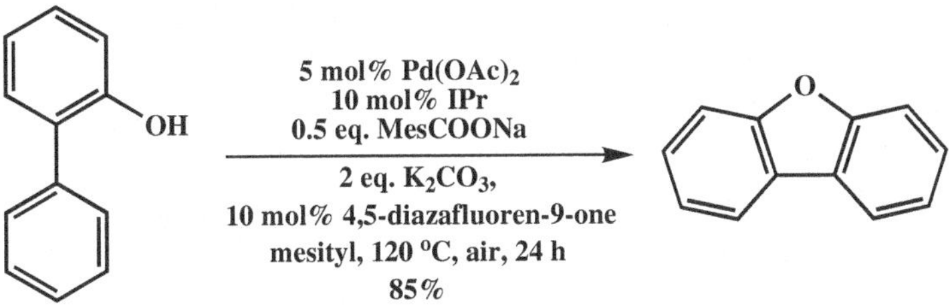

Scheme-48

Ames [122] described one of the earliest instances of intramolecular direct arylation in early 1980s. The 2-bromophenyl phenyl ethers were reacted at 170 °C in dimethylaniline in the presence of palladium acetate and sodium carbonate to synthesize various functionalized dibenzofurans **(Scheme 49)**. Good yields of desired products were obtained with both electron-withdrawing and electron-donating substituents under reaction conditions. The carbazole and fluorenone products were observed in high yields with iodobenzophenone and (iodophenyl) phenylamine [123]. Regioselective carbon-hydrogen bond functionalizations have been achieved in intramolecular systems. Here, regioselectivity originated from steric factors, such that the sterically allowed ring was formed. A seminal report by Ames showed the intramolecular direct arylation of 2-bromophenyl phenyl ethers to form dibenzofurans. Both electron rich and deficient substituents were well tolerated. Furthermore, the conditions were extended to incorporate substrates with varying linkages (NH, CO, OCO, NRCO, SO$_2$NR), forming both five- and six-membered rings.

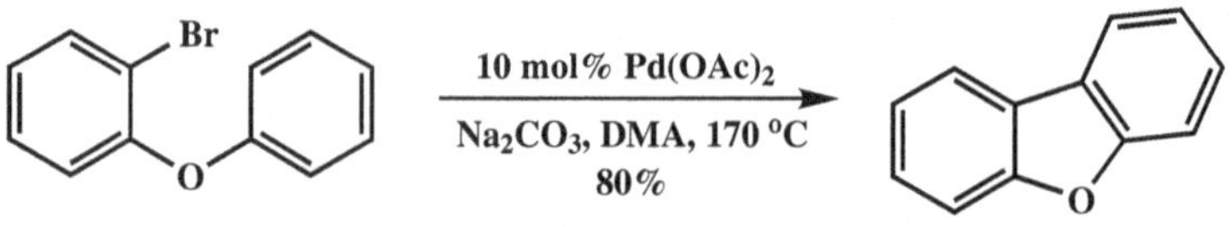

Scheme-49

Ames [123] described the pyridine involving first intramolecular direct arylation reaction in 1980. The tricyclic compounds were obtained in low yield (10%) when 2-(2-bromophenoxy) pyridine was treated with palladium acetate and sodium carbonate **(Scheme 50)**.

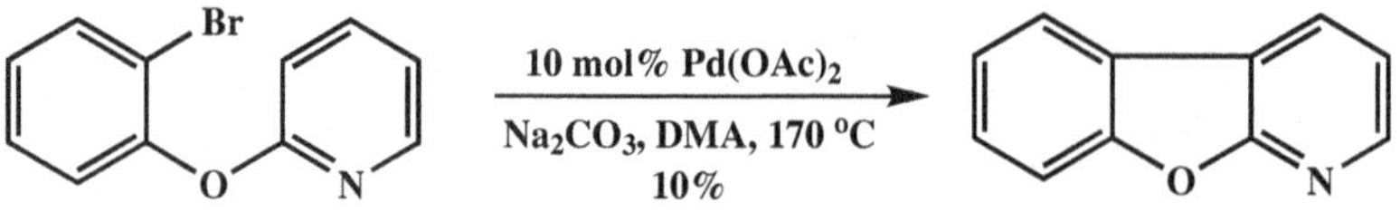

Scheme-50

Larock [124] synthesized carbazoles by one-pot two-step method conveniently. The addition of *o*-iodoaniline to a benzyne intermediate occurred in the first step. The benzyne intermediate was produced *in situ* from silylaryl triflates in the presence of cesium fluoride. The carbazole was formed when *N*-arylated *o*-iodoaniline underwent a Pd-catalyzed intramolecular direct arylation. Good yields of a number of NH and *N*-substituted carbazoles were afforded using this strategy **(Scheme 51)**. In addition, dibenzofurans and *N*-possessing six-membered rings were formed from phenol and benzylamines derivatives, respectively.

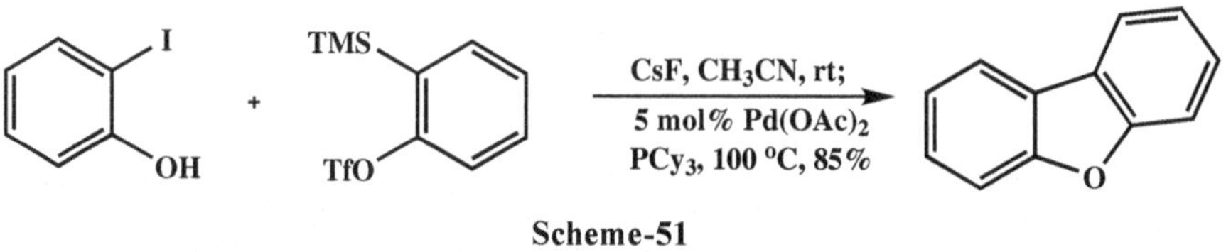

Scheme-51

Larock [125-126] produced fused polycycles *via* Pd migration/arylation protocol. An arylpalladium intermediate was generated through a Pd-catalyzed carbon-hydrogen activation/1,4-palladium migration. The formed arylpalladium intermediate then underwent carbon-carbon bond formation by intramolecular direct arylation **(Scheme 52)**.

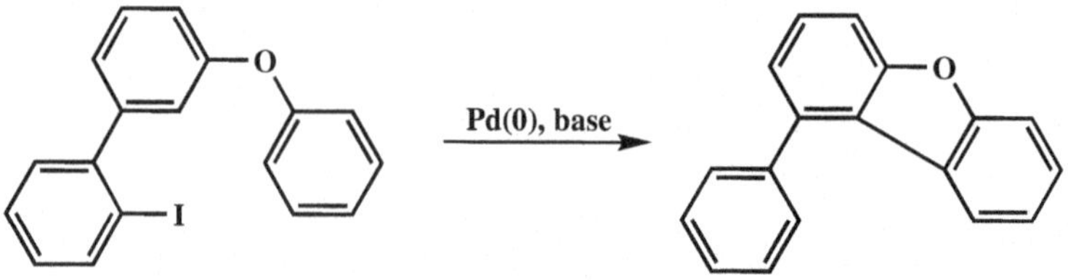

Scheme-52

This protocol involved double Pd migration/direction arylation process. The 2-iodo-5-phenoxybiphenyl under reaction conditions provided phenyldibenzofuran in 88% yield **(Scheme 53)** [126].

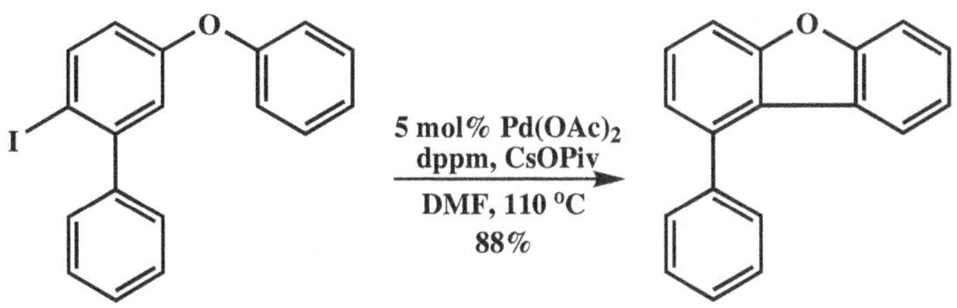

Scheme-53

The mechanism of this reaction has proposed the oxidative insertion of Pd into PhI, followed by 1,4-migration of Pd to phenyl functionality by carbon-hydrogen activation. The *o*-phenoxy Pd species was produced with bond rotation followed by 1,4-migration. The desired phenyldibenzofuran was formed when *o*-phenoxy Pd species underwent direct arylation **(Scheme 54)** [126].

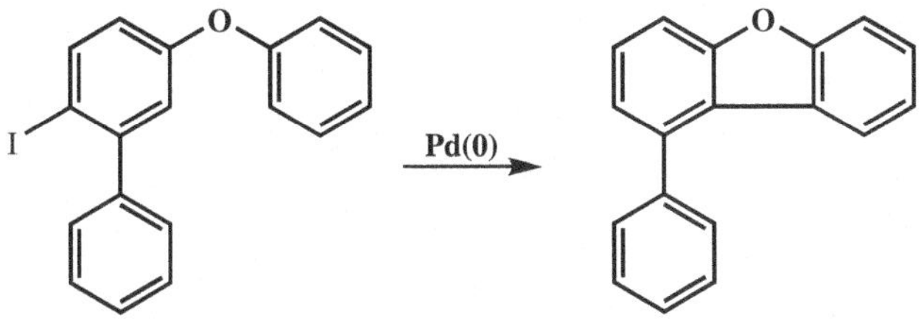

Scheme-54

The reaction conditions were optimized with 5 mol% of 1,2-bis(diphenylphosphino)methane, 5 mol% of palladium acetate, and CsOPiv at 100 °C in dimethylformamide. The reaction was successful in the presence of a highly soluble cesium pivalate base. Poor yields of desired phenyldibenzofurans were obtained with benzylbiphenyls, while excellent yields were reported when phenoxybiphenyls were used **(Scheme 55)**. The poor reactivity of benzyl moiety as compared to electron-rich oxygen-substituted phenyl ring of a phenoxybiphenyl system resulted in low yields of substrates. The formation of six-membered ring was not as favorable as the five-membered ring. From the benzyl phenyl ether, six-membered ring was formed with 60:40 mixture (the desired compound to reduced product). The difficulty in synthesizing a seven-membered ring palladacycle prior to reductive elimination was the reason of poor result [127].

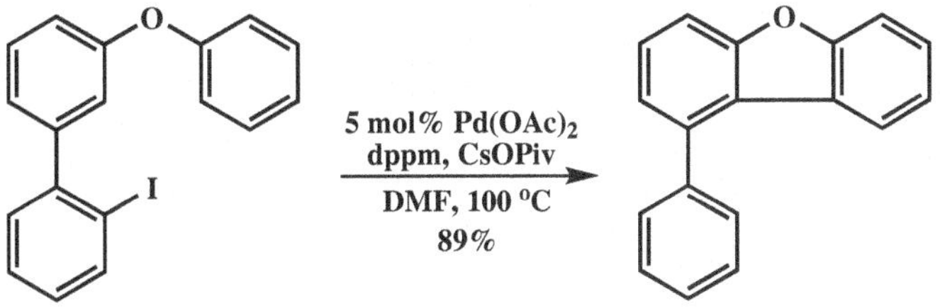

Scheme-55

Dibenzofurans were produced in this reaction **(Scheme 56)** [128]. Low yield (30%) of isomeric dibenzofurans was reported when 3-iodophenyl phenyl ether was reacted with 1-phenyl-1-butyne. There was a significant increase in yield (80%) with a more electron rich substrate possessing a –OMe substituent on iodoarene functionality, presumably due to arene's increased ability to facilitate the vinyl to aryl Pd migration.

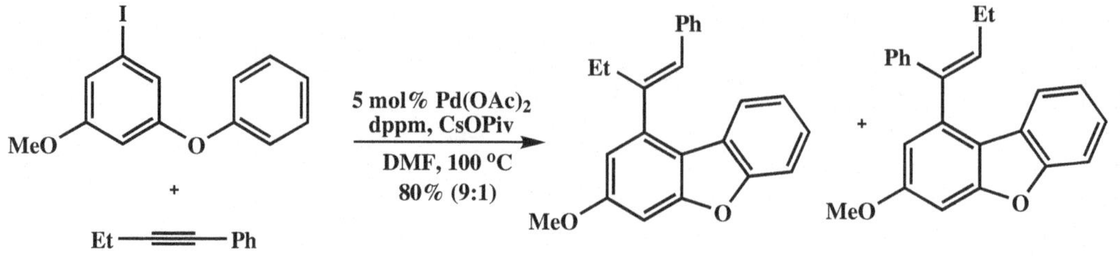

Scheme-56

The development of domino reactions have become a prominent field of research in organic synthesis as a strategy to construct complex and functionally diverse molecules from simple starting materials with less time, cost and undesirable waste. A progress was reported towards the development of a one-pot, domino procedure involving asymmetric rhodium-catalyzed ring-opening of oxabicyclic alkenes followed by a Pd-catalyzed carbon-oxygen coupling reaction to form novel dihydrobenzofuran derivatives with high enantio- and diastereoselectivities **(Scheme 57)**.

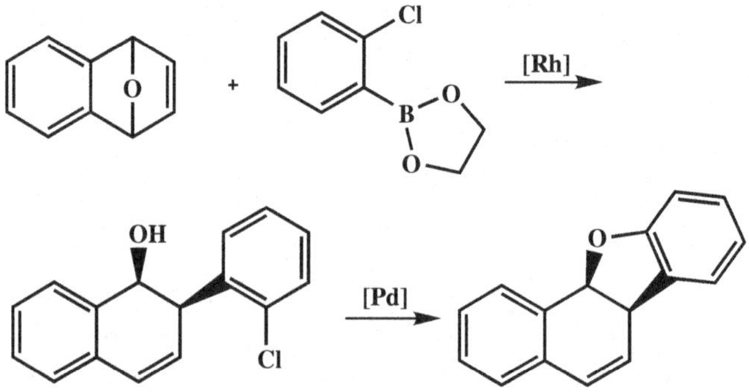

Scheme-57

Yue and Li [129] described the synthesis of benzo[4,5]furopyridines in high yields when diiodides were reacted with hexamethylditin in $PdCl_2(PPh_3)_2$ **(Scheme 58)**.

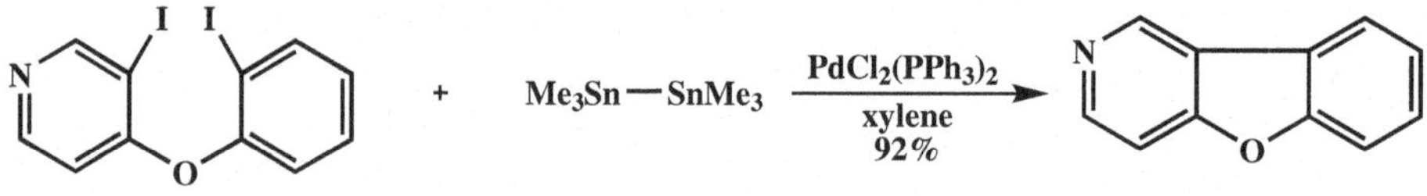

Scheme-58

The pyridine-possessing heterocycles, natural products, and synthetic intermediates were formed *via* an intramolecular Heck reaction **(Scheme 59)** [130-134].

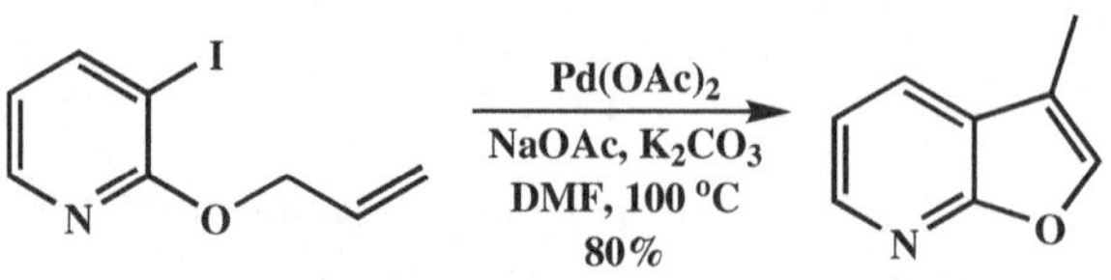

Scheme-59

Grigg et al. [24, 135] on the basis of multi-component "cascade molecular queuing processes" of allenes and/or CO as reactive substrates have synthesized heterocyclic compound. Heterocyclic chemistry has employed both intra- and intermolecular variations. An allene, unsaturated halide, and heterocyclic enols were reacted with the help of palladium(0) catalyst and base and subsequently, TFA was added to conclude the sequence by cyclization of allylation product, for the successful synthesis of annelated dihydrofurans (**Scheme 60**). The nucleophilic displacement at allyl-palladium occurred either by C- or O-allylation with a subsequent [3,3]-sigmatropic rearrangement [136a-b]. The electronic nature of aryl substituent affected the acid catalyzed cyclization. The cyclization was hampered with electron-withdrawing groups by destabilizing the carbocation intermediate [30].

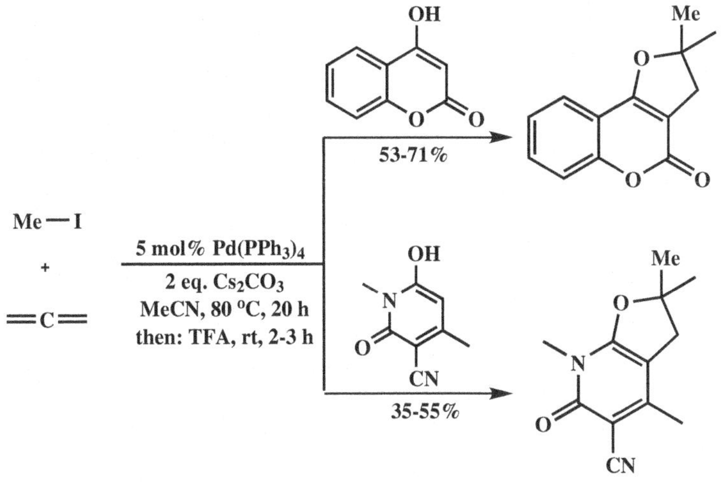

Scheme-60

The 4-(aryloxy)-5-iodopyrimidines were synthesized in one-step and in good yields from phenol and 4-chloro-5-iodopyrimidine *via* Pd-catalyzed intramolecular arylation of pyrimidine [137]. Moderate to good yields of benzo[4,5]furo[2,3-*d*]pyrimidine were obtained when iodopyrimidine was coupled to tethered aryl group (**Scheme 61**). This protocol has many disadvantages such as six-membered ring synthesized from 4-(benzyloxy)-5-iodopyrimidine did not provide the cyclized product and no cyclized adduct was obtained when strong electron-withdrawing groups (*i.e.*, nitro) were present on phenoxy ring.

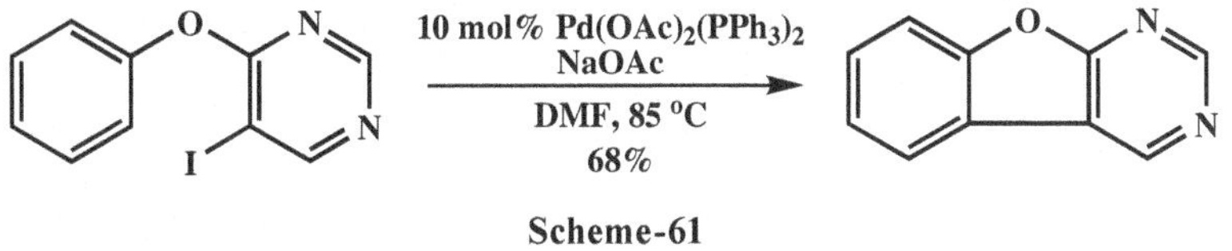

Scheme-61

The pyridazinone underwent intramolecular direct arylation reaction (**Scheme 62**) [138]. The substrates possessing halogen on either the pyridazinone or arene moiety afforded good yields of cyclized product. This protocol was also suitable for substrates which bear oxygen or nitrogen tether.

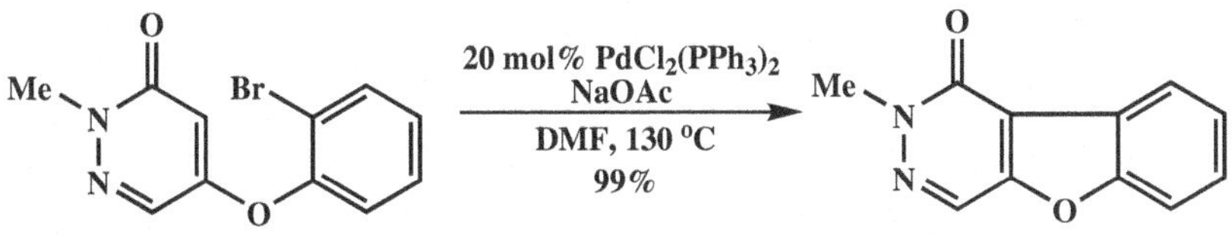

Scheme-62

Ames et al. [139] described the preparation of benzofuro[3,2-*c*]cinnoline *via* Pd-catalyzed intramolecular direct arylation reaction **(Scheme 63)**. The intramolecular direct arylations of arene carbon-hydrogen bonds with aryl halides were reported in many examples. Some examples are there for direct arylation with heteroaryl halides.

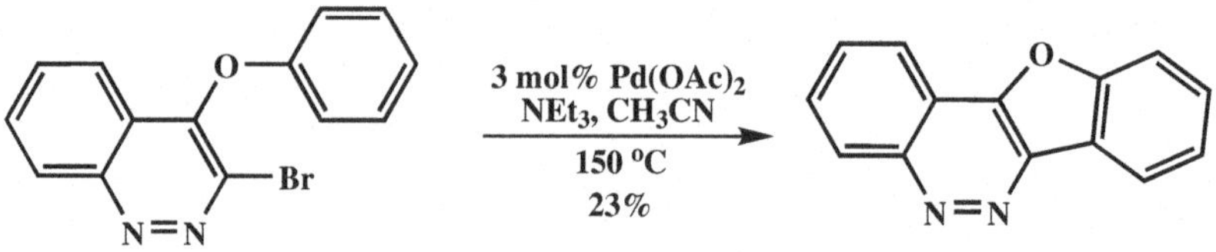

Scheme-63

The dibenzofuran was prepared from diaryl ether by this tandem migratory coupling **(Scheme 64)** [140]. As suggested by mechanism, the reaction occurred through carbopalladation followed by a 1,4-palladium migration. Then the direct arylation of diaryl ether afforded target product.

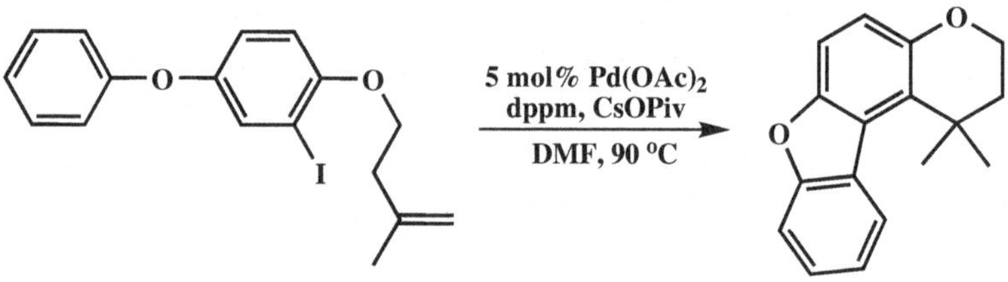

Scheme-64

A one-pot double-alkylation-alkenylation process was reported in the presence of palladium catalyst. Good yields of a series of symmetrical and unsymmetrical *N*-, *O*-, *S*- and silicon-containing tricyclic heterocycles were obtained under MWI. The tricyclic mescaline analogue was also synthesized by this tandem process which involved two intramolecular norbornene mediated *o*-alkylations, followed by an intermolecular Mizoroki-Heck reaction. Two complex steroidal fragments were linked through an olefinic double bond by Heck-type coupling of a vinyl triflate with a monosubstituted olefin in 77% yield under optimized reaction conditions (*i.e.* with base under single-mode MW conditions) **(Scheme 65)** [141].

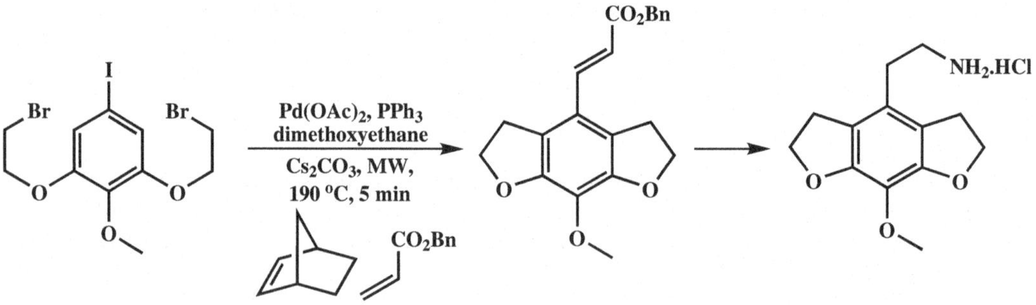

Scheme-65

The taiwanins C and E were synthesized from key intermediate aryl naphthalene derivative. The [2+2+2] co-cyclization of diyne and benzyne species produced from starting substrate formed the aryl naphthalene intermediate in the presence of Pd(0) catalyst **(Scheme 66)** [142-144].

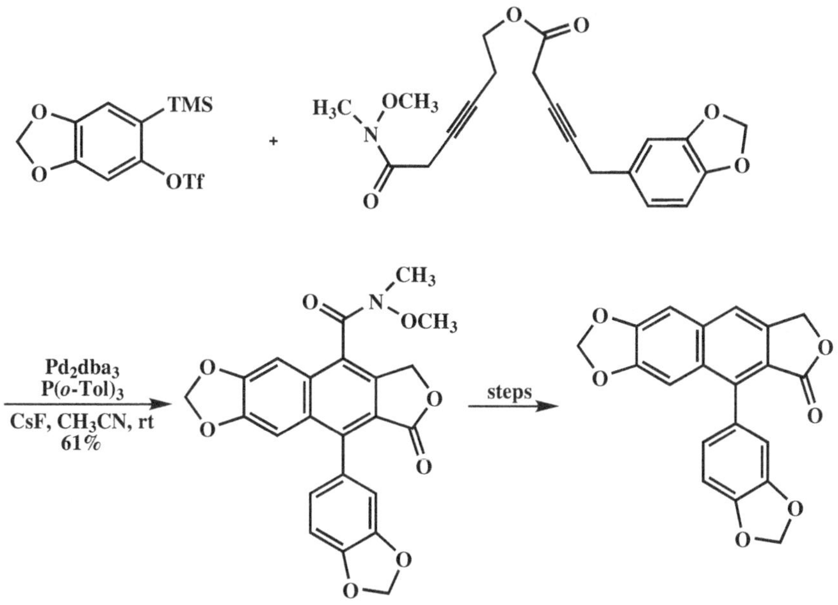

Scheme-66

Cyclic olefin containing substrates were examined in the intramolecular carboetherification reaction. Cyclic olefin containing substrates were prepared in 5 steps *via* condensation of *N,N*-dimethylhydrazine with cyclopentanone, followed by deprotonation with BuLi and alkylation with 2-bromobenzyl bromide. Hydrolysis afforded ketone, which was treated with lithium diisopropylamide followed by PhSeBr [145]. Oxidation and α-elimination of alkyl selenide provided enone. Reduction of enone with 9-BBN (9-borabicyclo[3.3.1]nonane) provided allylic alcohol and the stereochemistry of major diastereomer was confirmed by a NOESY-2D experiment of major diastereomer as shown in **Scheme 67**. The major diastereomer was converted to ester *via* a Johnson *o*-ester Claisen reaction. Reduction with lithium aluminum hydride afforded substrate. The carboetherification reaction was conducted under standard conditions to yield THF in good yield and excellent diastereoselectivity in six steps from cyclopentanone.

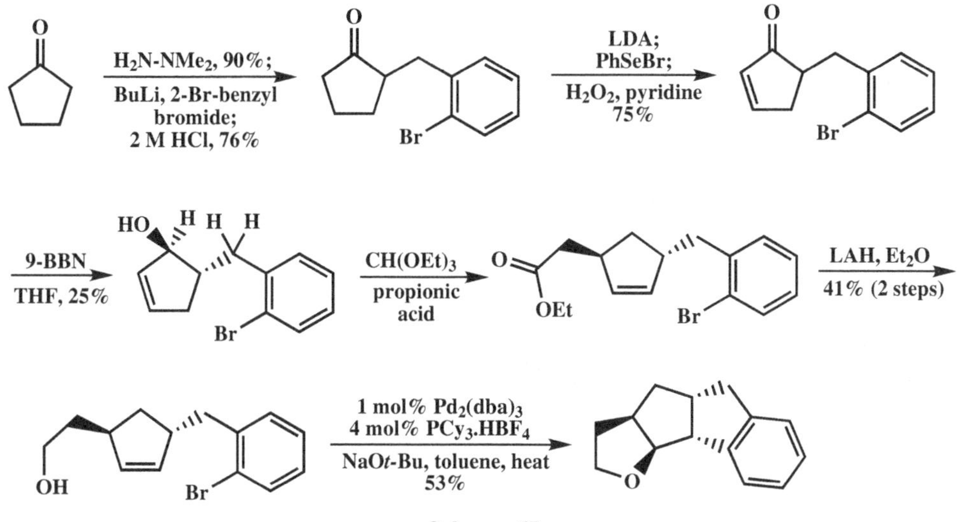

Scheme-67

The 3-carbomethoxy derivatives were synthesized by carbonylative cyclization reaction in the presence of CO and Pd catalyst in MeOH [146]. This protocol was extended to the synthesis of benzo[*b*]furo[3,4-*d*]furanones **(Scheme 68)** [58].

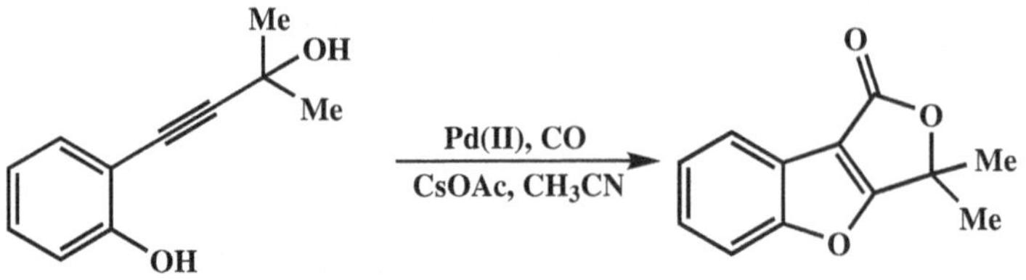

Scheme-68

Tetra- and pentacyclic *N*-fused heterocycles were afforded by this efficient Pd-catalyzed intramolecular carbopalladation/cyclization reaction. Moderate to excellent yields of polycyclic pyrroloheterocycles were obtained in this conversion occurring through Pd-catalyzed coupling of aryl halides with internal propargylic ethers or esters followed by *5-endo-dig* cyclization **(Scheme 69)** [147].

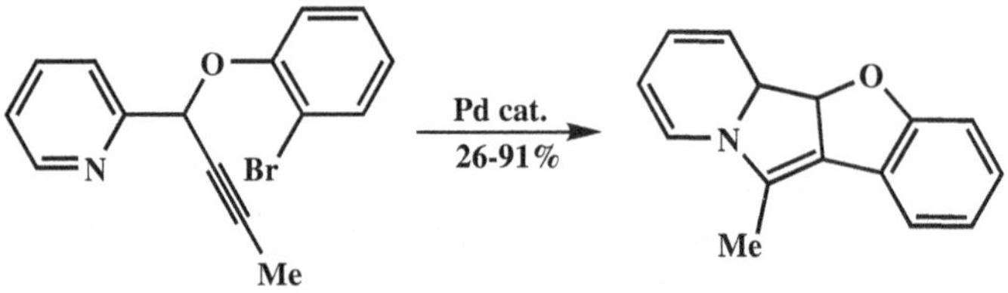

Scheme-69

Usually not a good control of "pair" selectivity nor regioselectivity was observed in intermolecular [2+2+2] cyclotrimerization of alkynes to synthesize benzene derivatives. Polysubstituted benzenes were produced in highly regiocontrolled manner *via* cyclic cascade carbometalation **(Scheme 70)** [118a-b, 148-151].

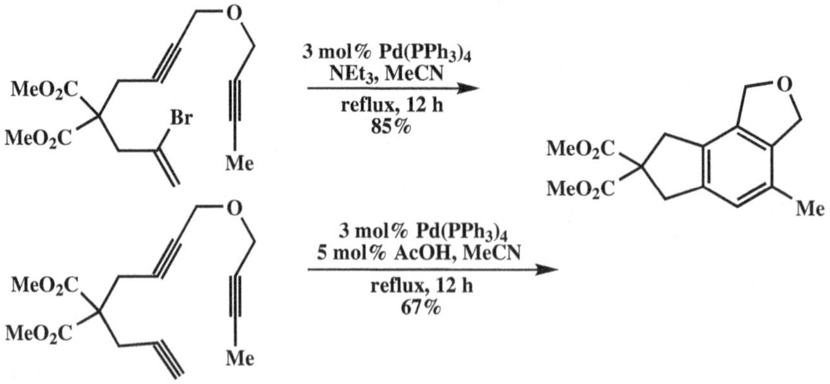

Scheme-70

REFERENCES

[1]   D.A. Horton, G.T. Bourne and M.L. Smythe. 2003. The combinatorial synthesis of bicyclic privileged structures or privileged substructures. Chem. Rev. 103: 893-930.

[2]   A.T. Balaban, D.C. Oniciu and A.R. Katritzky. 2004. Aromaticity as a cornerstone in heterocyclic chemistry. Chem. Rev. 104: 2777-2812.

[3]   (a) N. Kaur. 2014. Palladium-catalyzed approach to the synthesis of five-membered *O*-heterocycles. Inorg. Chem. Commun. 49: 86-119.

(b) N. Kaur and D. Kishore. 2014. Nitrogen-containing six-membered heterocycles: solid-phase synthesis. Synth. Commun. 44: 1173-1211.

(c) N. Kaur and D. Kishore. 2014. Solid-phase synthetic approach toward the synthesis of oxygen-containing heterocycles. Synth. Commun. 44: 1019-1042.

(d) N. Kaur. 2014. Microwave-assisted synthesis of five-membered *O*-heterocycles. Synth. Commun. 44: 3483-3508.

(e) N. Kaur. 2014. Microwave-assisted synthesis of five-membered *O,N*-heterocycles. Synth. Commun. 44: 3509-3537.

(f) N. Kaur. 2014. Microwave-assisted synthesis of five-membered *O,N,N*-heterocycles. Synth Commun. 44: 3229-3247.

[4]   J. Morris, D.G. Wishka, W.R. Humphrey, A.H. Lin, A.L. Wiltse, C.W. Benjamin, R.R. Gorman and R.J. Shebuski. 1994. Synthesis and biological activity of a potent anti-platelet 7- amino furochromone. Bioorg. Med. Chem. Lett. 4: 2621-2626.

[5]   A.S.K. Hashmi and G.J. Hutchings. 2006. Gold catalysis. Angew. Chem. Int. Ed. 45: 7896-7936.

[6]   A.S.K. Hashmi. 2007. Gold-catalyzed organic reactions. Chem. Rev. 107: 3180-3211.

[7]   H.C. Shen. 2008. Recent advances in syntheses of heterocycles and carbocycles *via* homogeneous gold catalysis. Heteroatom addition and hydroarylation reactions of alkynes, allenes, and alkenes. Tetrahedron. 64: 3885-3903.

[8]   L. Gil, D. Compère, B. Guilloteau-Bertin, A. Chiaroni and C. Marazano. 2000. An enantioselective entry to substituted 6-membered nitrogen heterocycles from chiral pyridinium salts *via* selective epoxidation of tetrahydropyridine intermediates. Synthesis 14: 2117-2126.

[9]   A. Padwa and S. Bur. 2004. The Pummerer reaction: methodology and strategy for the synthesis of heterocyclic compounds. Chem. Rev. 104: 2401-2432.

[10]   F. Arico, U. Toniolo and P. Tundo. 2012. 5-Membered *N*-heterocyclic compounds by dimethyl carbonate chemistry. Green Chem. 14: 58-61.

[11]   A.S. Dudnik, N. Chernyak and V. Gevorgyan. 2010. Copper-, silver-, and gold-catalyzed migratory cycloisomerizations leading to heterocyclic five-membered rings. Aldrichimica Acta 43: 37-46.

[12]   Z. Li, C. Brouwer and C. He. 2008. Gold-catalyzed organic transformations. Chem. Rev. 108: 3239-3265.

[13]   A. Fürstner and P.W. Davies. 2007. Catalytic carbophilic activation: catalysis by platinum and gold pi acids. Angew. Chem. Int. Ed. 46: 3410-3449.

[14]   S.R. Chemler and P.H. Fuller. 2007. Heterocycle synthesis by copper facilitated addition of heteroatoms to alkenes, alkynes and arenes. Chem. Soc. Rev. 36: 1153-1160.

[15]   F. Monnier and M. Taillefer. 2008. Catalytic C-C, C-N, and C-O Ullmann-type coupling reactions: copper makes a difference. Angew. Chem. Int. Ed. 47: 3096-3099.

[16]   A. Arcadi. 2008. Alternative synthetic methods through new developments in catalysis by gold. Chem. Rev. 108: 3266-3325.

[17]   K.W. Anderson, T. Ikawa, R.E. Tundel and S.L. Buchwald. 2006. The selective reaction of aryl halides with KOH: synthesis of phenols, aromatic ethers, and benzofurans. J. Am. Chem. Soc. 128: 10694-10695.

[18]   M.C. Willis. 2007. Palladium-katalysierte kupplung von ammoniak und hydroxid mit arylhalogeniden: die direkte synthese von primären anilinen und phenolen. Angew. Chem. 119: 3470-3472.

[19]   V. Guilarte, M. Pilar-Castroviejo, E. Alvarez and R. Sanz. 2011. Combined directed *o*-zincation and palladium-catalyzed strategies: synthesis of 4,n-dimethoxy-substituted benzo[*b*]furans. Beilstein J. Org. Chem. 7: 1255-1260.

[20]   C.J. Ball and M.C. Willis. 2013. Cascade palladium- and copper-catalyzed aromatic heterocycle synthesis: the emergence of general precursors. Eur. J. Org. Chem. 425-441.

[21]   R. Grigg and V. Sridharan. 1994. Spirocycles *via* palladium-catalyzed cascade cyclization-carbonylation-anion capture processes. Tetrahedron Lett. 34: 7471-7474.

[22] B. Gabriele, R. Mancuso, E. Lupinacci, L. Veltri, G. Salerno and C. Carfagna. 2011. Synthesis of benzothiophene derivatives by Pd-catalyzed or radical-promoted heterocyclodehydration of 1-(2-mercaptophenyl)-2-yn-1-ols. J. Org. Chem. 76: 8277-8286.

[23] R. Grigg, B. Putnikovic and C. Urch. 1996. Palladium catalyzed ter- and tetra-molecular queuing processes. One-pot routes to 3-spiro-2-oxindoles and 3-spiro-2(3*H*)-benzofuranones. Tetrahedron Lett. 37: 695-698.

[24] R. Grigg and V. Sridharan. 1998. Heterocycles *via* Pd catalyzed molecular queuing processes. Relay switches and the maximization of molecular complexity. Pure Appl. Chem. 70: 1047-1057.

[25] R.C. Larock and T.R. Hightower. 1993. Synthesis of unsaturated lactones *via* palladium-catalyzed cyclization of alkenoic acids. J. Org. Chem. 58: 5298-5300.

[26] E. Bossharth, P. Desbordes, N. Monteiro and G. Balme. 2003. Palladium-mediated three-component synthesis of furo[2,3-*b*]pyridones by one-pot coupling of 3-iodopyridones, alkynes, and organic halides. Org. Lett. 5: 2441-2444.

[27] B.L. Flynn, E. Hamel and M.K. Jung. 2002. One-pot synthesis of benzo[*b*]furan and indole inhibitors of tubulin polymerization. J. Med. Chem. 45: 2670-2673.

[28] A. Arcadi, S. Cacchi, M. Del Rosario, G. Fabrizi and F. Marinelli. 1996. Palladium-catalyzed reaction of *o*-ethynylphenols, *o*-((trimethylsilyl)ethynyl)phenyl acetates, and *o*-alkynylphenols with unsaturated triflates or halides: a route to 2-substituted-, 2,3-disubstituted-, and 2-substituted-3-acylbenzo[*b*]furans. J. Org. Chem. 61: 9280-9288.

[29] N. Henaff and A. Whiting. 1999. A convergent stereoselective total synthesis of racemic phthoxazolin A. Org. Lett. 1: 1137-1139.

[30] D.M. D'Souza and T.J.J. Muller. 2007. Multi-component syntheses of heterocycles by transition-metal catalysis. Chem. Soc. Rev. 36: 1095-1108.

[31] J.M. Takacs and X.-T. Jiang. 2003. The Wacker reaction and related alkene oxidation reactions. Curr. Org. Chem. 7: 369-396.

[32] V.I. Timokhin, N.R. Anastasi and S.S. Stahl. 2003. Dioxygen-coupled oxidative amination of styrene. J. Am. Chem. Soc. 125: 12996-12997.

[33] S. Diez-Gonzalez, N. Marion and S.P. Nolan. 2009. *N*-Heterocyclic carbenes in late transition metal catalysis. Chem. Rev. 109: 3612-3676.

[34] K. Muniz. 2004. Palladium-carbene catalysts for aerobic, intramolecular Wacker-type cyclization reactions. Adv. Synth. Catal. 346: 1425-1428.

[35] E.M. Beccalli, G. Broggini, M. Martinelli and S. Sottocornola. 2007. C-C, C-O, C-N Bond formation on sp^2 carbon by Pd(II)-catalyzed reactions involving oxidant agents. Chem. Rev. 107: 5318-5365.

[36] J. Farago and A. Kotschy. 2009. Synthesis of benzo[*b*]furans by palladium-NHC catalyzed ring closure of *o*-bromobenzyl ketones. Synthesis 1: 85-90.

[37] H.-A. Du, X.-G. Zhang, R.-Y. Tang and J.-H. Li. 2009. PdCl$_2$-promoted electrophilic annulation of 2-alkynylphenol derivatives with disulfides or diselenides in the presence of iodine. J. Org. Chem. 74: 7844-7848.

[38] P.T. Parvatkar, P.S. Parameswaran and S.G. Tilve. 2012. Recent developments in the synthesis of five- and six-membered heterocycles using molecular iodine. Chem. Eur. J. 18: 5460-5489.

[39] H. Zhang, E.M. Ferreira and B.M. Stoltz. 2004. Direct oxidative Heck cyclizations: intramolecular Fujiwara-Moritani arylations for the synthesis of functionalized benzofurans and dihydrobenzofurans. Angew. Chem. Int. Ed. 43: 6144-6148.

[40] Y. Uozumi, K. Kato and T. Hayashi. 1997. Catalytic asymmetric Wacker-type cyclization. J. Am. Chem. Soc. 119: 5063-5064.

[41] Y. Uozumi, K. Kato and T. Hayashi. 1998. Cationic palladium/boxax complexes for catalytic asymmetric Wacker-type cyclization. J. Org. Chem. 63: 5071-5075.

[42] T. Hayashi, K. Yamasaki, M. Mimura and Y. Uozumi. 2004. Deuterium-labeling studies establishing stereochemistry at the oxypalladation step in Wacker-type oxidative cyclization of an *o*-allylphenol. J. Am. Chem. Soc. 126: 3036-3037.

[43] Y. Uozumi, H. Kyota, K. Kato, M. Ogasawara and T. Hayashi. 1999. Design and preparation of 3,3'-disubstituted 2,2'-bis(oxazolyl)-1,1'-binaphthyls (boxax): new chiral bis(oxazoline) ligands for catalytic asymmetric Wacker-type cyclization. J. Org. Chem. 64: 1620-1625.

[44] R.M. Trend, Y.K. Ramtohul, E.M. Ferreira and B.M. Stoltz. 2003. Palladium-catalyzed oxidative Wacker cyclizations in nonpolar organic solvents with molecular oxygen: a stepping stone to asymmetric aerobic cyclizations. Angew. Chem. Int. Ed. 42: 2892-2895.

[45] R.M. Trend, Y.K. Ramtohul and B.M. Stoltz. 2005. Oxidative cyclizations in a nonpolar solvent using molecular oxygen and studies on the stereochemistry of oxypalladation. J. Am. Chem. Soc. 127: 17778-17788.

[46] S.W. Youn and J.I. Eom. 2005. Facile construction of the benzofuran and chromene ring systems *via* PdII-catalyzed oxidative cyclization. Org. Lett. 7: 3355-3358.

[47] J.-E. Backvall and P.G. Andersson. 1990. Palladium-catalyzed stereocontrolled intramolecular 1,4-additions to cyclic 1,3-dienes involving amides as nucleophiles. J. Am. Chem. Soc. 112: 3683-3685.

[48] J.-E. Backvall and P.G. Andersson. 1992. Intramolecular palladium-catalyzed 1,4-addition to conjugated dienes. Stereoselective synthesis of fused tetrahydrofurans and tetrahydropyrans. J. Am. Chem. Soc. 114: 6374-6381.

[49] E.B. Koroleva, J.-E. Backvall and P.G. Andersson. 1995. Palladium-catalyzed stereo-controlled *endo*-cyclization of 3-hydroxypropyl-1,3-cyclohexadiene leading to versatile fused tetrahydropyrans. Tetrahedron Lett. 36: 5397-5400.

[50] J.-E. Backvall, P.G. Andersson and J.O. Vagberg. 1989. Stereocontrolled lactonization reactions *via* palladium-catalysis. Tetrahedron Lett. 30: 137-140.

[51] J.-E. Backvall, K.L. Granberg, P. Andersson, R. Gatti and A. Gogoll. 1993. Stereocontrolled lactonization reactions *via* palladium-catalyzed 1,4-addition to conjugated dienes. J. Org. Chem. 58: 5445-5451.

[52] J.-E. Backvall, R. Gatti and H.E. Shink. 1993. Enzyme and palladium catalysis as a powerful combination in asymmetric transformations of meso-2-alkene-1,4-diol derivatives. Application to enantiodivergent synthesis of (R)- and (S)-(2,4-cycloalkadienyl)acetic acids. Synthesis 3: 343-348.

[53] M. Ronn, P.G. Andersson and J.-E. Backvall. 1998. Enantiocontrolled formal total synthesis of paeonilactone A and B from (S)-(+)-carvone. Acta Chem. Scand. 52: 524-527.

[54] C. Jonasson, M. Ronn and J.-E. Backvall. 2000. An enantioselective route to paeonilactone A *via* palladium- and copper-catalyzed reactions. J. Org. Chem. 65: 2122-2126.

[55] M. Ronn, P.G. Andersson and J.-E. Backvall. 1997. Application of O_2/DMSO as reoxidant in the Pd(II)-catalyzed 1,4-oxidation of 5-substituted 1,3-cyclohexadienes. Acta Chem. Scand. 51: 773-777.

[56] T. Kawasaki, S. Saito and Y. Yamamoto. 2002. Synthesis of phthalides and 3,4-dihydroisocoumarins using the palladium-catalyzed intramolecular benzannulation strategy. J. Org. Chem. 67: 2653-2658.

[57] D. Bouyssi and G. Balme. 2001. New palladium-catalyzed access to 3-(1'-indanylidene) phthalide, precursor of the core of fredericamycin A. Synlett 7: 1191-1193.

[58] G. Kirsch, S. Hesse and A. Comel. 2004. Synthesis of five- and six-membered heterocycles through palladium-catalyzed reactions. Curr. Org. Synth. 1: 47-63.

[59] M. Palucki, J.P. Wolfe and S.L. Buchwald. 1996. Synthesis of oxygen heterocycles *via* a palladium-catalyzed C-O bond-forming reaction. J. Am. Chem. Soc. 118: 10333-10334.

[60] S. Kuwabe, K.E. Torraca and S.L. Buchwald. 2001. Palladium-catalyzed intramolecular C-O bond formation. J. Am. Chem. Soc. 123: 12202-12206.

[61] E. Merisor, J. Conrad, S. Mika and U. Beifuss. 2007. Microwave-assisted reductive cyclization of *N*-allyl 2-nitroanilines: a new approach to substituted 1,2,3,4-tetrahydroquinoxalines. Synlett 13: 2033-2036.

[62] J.P. Brand, J. Charpentier and J. Waser. 2009. Direct alkynylation of indole and pyrrole heterocycles. Angew. Chem. Int. Ed. 48: 9346-9349.

[63] J.P. Brand and J. Waser. 2010. Direct alkynylation of thiophenes: cooperative activation of TIPS-EBX with gold and Brønsted acids. Angew. Chem. Int. Ed. 49: 7304-7307.

[64] S. Nicolai, S. Erard, D.F. Gonzalez and J. Waser. 2010. Pd-catalyzed intramolecular oxyalkynylation of alkenes with hypervalent iodine. Org. Lett. 12: 384-387.

[65] I. Candiani, S. DeBernardinis, W. Cabri, M. Marchi, A. Bedeschi and S. Penco. 1993. A facile one-pot synthesis of polyfunctionalized 2-unsubstituted benzo[*b*]furans. Synlett. 4: 269-270.

[66] A. Arcadi, S. Cacchi, G. Fabrizi, F. Marinelli and L. Moro. 1999. A new approach to 2,3-disubstituted benzo[*b*]furans from *o*-alkynylphenols *via* 5-*endo-dig*-iodocyclization/palladium-catalyzed reactions. Synlett 9: 1432-1434.

[67] N. Monteiro and G. Balme. 1998. Palladium-catalyzed allylating heteroannulation of *o*-alkynyl-allyloxybenzenes. A route to 2-substituted-3-allylbenzo[*b*]furans. Synlett 7: 746-747.

[68] N. Yongpruksa, N.L. Calkins and M. Harmata. 2011. Efficient palladium-catalyzed *N*-arylation of sulfoximine with aryl chlorides. Chem. Commun. 47: 7665-7667.

[69] P. Liou and C-Y. Cheng. 2000. Total synthesis of (±)-desoxycodeine-D: a novel route to the morphine skeleton. Tetrahedron Lett. 41: 915-918.

[70] C. Morice, M. Domostoj, K. Briner, A. Mann, J. Suffert and C-W. Wermuth. 2001. Synthesis of constrained arylpiperidines using intramolecular Heck or radical reactions. Tetrahedron Lett. 42: 6499-6502.

[71] S-I. Kuwabe, K.E. Toracca and S.L. Buchwald. 2001. Pd(II)-catalyzed hydroxyl-directed C-H activation/C-O cyclization: expedient construction of dihydrobenzofurans. J. Am. Chem. Soc. 49: 12203-12205.

[72] S. Hesse and G. Kirsch. 2003. Synthesis of new furocoumarin analogues *via* cross-coupling reaction of triflate. Tetrahedron Lett. 44: 97-99.

[73] H. Sashida and A. Kawamukai. 1999. Palladium-catalyzed intramolecular cyclization of *o*-ethynyl-benzoic acids and *o*-ethynylbenzamides: preparation of isocoumarins and isoquinolin-1-ones. Synthesis 7: 1145-1148.

[74] R. Giri, N. Maugel, B.M. Foxman and J.-Q. Yu. 2008. Dehydrogenation of inert alkyl groups *via* remote C-H activation: converting a propyl group into a π-allylic complex. Organometallics 27: 1667-1670.

[75] M. Lafrance, S.I. Gorelsky and K. Fagnou. 2007. High-yielding palladium-catalyzed intramolecular alkane arylation: reaction development and mechanistic studies. J. Am. Chem. Soc. 129: 14570-14571.

[76] B. Liegault and K. Fagnou. 2008. Palladium-catalyzed intramolecular coupling of arenes and unactivated alkanes in air. Organometallics 27: 4841-4843.

[77] S. Rousseaux, M. Davi, J. Sofack-Kreutzer, C. Pierre, C.E. Kefalidis, E. Clot, K. Fagnou and O. Baudoin. 2010. Intramolecular palladium-catalyzed alkane C-H arylation from aryl chlorides. J. Am. Chem. Soc. 132: 10706-10716.

[78] M. Chaumontet, R. Piccardi, N. Audic, J. Hitce, J.-L. Peglion, E. Clot and O. Baudoin. 2008. Synthesis of cyclobutenes by palladium-catalyzed C-H activation of methyl groups: method and mechanistic study. J. Am. Chem. Soc. 130: 15157-15166.

[79] C.J. Engelin and P. Fristrup. 2011. Palladium catalyzed allylic C-H alkylation: a mechanistic perspective. Molecules 16: 951-969.

[80] N. Batail, A. Bendjeriou, T. Lomberget, R. Barret, V. Dufaud and L. Djakovitch. 2009. First heterogeneous ligand- and salt-free Larock indole synthesis. Adv. Synth. Catal. 351: 2055-2062.

[81] L. Djakovitch and K. Koehler. 1999. Heterogeneously catalyzed Heck reaction using palladium modified zeolites. J. Mol Catal. A: Chem. 142: 275-284.

[82] L. Djakovitch and K. Koehler. 2001. Heck reaction catalyzed by Pd-modified zeolites. J. Am. Chem. Soc. 123: 5990-5999.

[83] L. Djakovitch, N. Batail and M. Genelot. 2011. Recent advances in the synthesis of *N*-containing heteroaromatics *via* heterogeneously transition metal catalyzed cross-coupling reactions. Molecules 16: 5241-5267.

[84] R.T. Ruck, M.A. Huffman, M.M. Kim, M. Shevlin, W.V. Kandur and I.W. Davies. 2008. Palladium-catalyzed tandem Heck reaction/C-H functionalization- preparation of spiro-indane-oxindoles. Angew. Chem. Int. Ed. 47: 4711-4714.

[85] G. Satyanarayana, C. Maichle-Mossmer and M.E. Maier. 2009. Formation of pentacyclic structures by a domino sequence on cyclic enamides. Chem. Commun. 12: 1571-1573.

[86] Y. Hu, C. Yu, D. Ren, Q. Hu, L. Zhang and D. Cheng. 2009. One-step synthesis of the benzocyclo [penta- to octa-]isoindole core. Angew. Chem. Int. Ed. 48: 5448-5451.

[87] M. Beaudoin and J.P. Wolfe. 2007. Palladium-catalyzed synthesis of cyclopentane-fused benzo-cyclobutenes *via* tandem directed carbopalladation/C-H bond functionalization. Org. Lett. 9: 3073-3075.

[88] O. Rene, D. Lapointe and K. Fagnou. 2009. Domino palladium-catalyzed Heck-intermolecular direct arylation reactions. Org. Lett. 11: 4560-4563.

[89] G. Dyker. 1993. Pd-catalyzed C-H activation of methoxy groups by aryl-tomethoxy 1,4-migration. J. Org. Chem. 58: 6426-6428.

[90] S. Wang, P. Li, L. Yu and L. Wang. 2011. Sequential and one-pot reactions of phenols with bromoalkynes for the synthesis of (Z)-2-bromovinyl phenyl ethers and benzo[*b*]furans. Org. Lett. 13: 5968-5971.

[91] J.-R. Wang and K. Manabe. 2010. Hydroxyterphenylphoshine- palladium catalyst for benzo[*b*]furan synthesis from 2-chlorophenols. Bifunctional ligand strategy for cross-coupling of chloroarenes. J. Org. Chem. 75: 5340-5342.

[92] C. Eidamshaus and J.D. Burch. 2008. One-pot synthesis of benzofurans *via* palladium-catalyzed enolate arylation with *o*-bromophenols. Org. Lett. 10: 4211-4214.

[93] X. Wang, Y. Lu, H.-X. Dai and J.-Q. Yu. 2010. Pd(II)-catalyzed hydroxyl-directed C-H activation/C-O cyclization: expedient construction of dihydrobenzofurans. J. Am. Chem. Soc. 132: 12203-12205.

[94] N. Kaur. 2018. Synthesis of six- and seven-membered heterocycles under ultrasound irradiation. Synth. Commun. 48: 1235-1258.

[95] R.C. Larock, E.K. Yum, M.J. Doty and K.K.C. Sham. 1996. Synthesis of aromatic heterocycles *via* palladium-catalyzed annulation of internal alkynes. J. Org. Chem. 60: 3270-3271.

[96] B.C. Bishop, I.F. Cottrell and D. Hands. 1997. Synthesis of 3-hydroxyalkylbenzo[*b*]furans *via* the palladium-catalyzed heteroannulation of silyl-protected alkynols with 2-iodophenol. Synthesis 11: 1315-1320.

[97] T. Konno, J. Chae, T. Ishihara and H. Yamanaka. 2004. A first regioselective synthesis of 3-fluoroalkylated benzofurans *via* palladium-catalyzed annulation of fluorine-containing internal alkynes with variously substituted 2-iodophenol. Tetrahedron 60: 11695-11700.

[98] M.L. Crawley, I. Goljer, D.J. Jenkins, J.F. Mehlmann, L. Nogle, R. Dooley and P.E. Mahaney. 2006. Regioselective synthesis of substituted pyrroles: efficient palladium-catalyzed cyclization of internal alkynes and 2-amino-3-iodoacrylate derivatives. Org. Lett. 8: 5837-5840.

[99] R.C. Larock, M.J. Doty and X. Han. 1998. Palladium-catalyzed heteroannulation of internal alkynes by vinylic halides. Tetrahedron Lett. 39: 5143-5146.

[100] P.G. Hultin. 2009. Modular construction of 2-substituted benzo[*b*]furans from 1,2-dichlorovinyl ethers. Org. Lett. 11: 5478-5481.

[101] L.L. Welbes, T.W. Lyons, K.A. Cychosz and M.S. Sanford. 2007. Synthesis of cyclopropanes *via* Pd(II/IV)-catalyzed reactions of enynes. J. Am. Chem. Soc. 129: 5836-5837.

[102] X. Tong, M. Beller and M.K. Tse. 2007. A palladium-catalyzed cyclization-oxidation sequence: synthesis of bicyclo[3.1.0]hexanes and evidence for S_N2 C-O bond formation. J. Am. Chem. Soc. 129: 4906-4907.

[103] T.W. Lyons and M.S. Sanford. 2009. Palladium (II/IV) catalyzed cyclopropanation reactions: scope and mechanism. Tetrahedron 65: 3211-3221.

[104] G. Yin and G. Liu. 2008. Palladium-catalyzed oxidative cyclization of enynes with hydrogen peroxide as the oxidant. Angew. Chem. Int. Ed. 47: 5442-5445.

[105] H. Liu, J. Yu, L. Wang and X. Tong. 2008. Cyclization-oxidation of 1,6-enyne derivatived from Baylis-Hillman adducts *via* Pd(II)/Pd(IV)-catalyzed reactions: stereoselective synthesis of multi-substituted bicyclo[3.1.0]hexanes and insight into reaction pathways. Tetrahedron Lett. 49: 6924-6928.

[106] T. Tsujihara, K. Takenaka, K. Onitsuka, M. Hatanaka and H. Sasai. 2009. Pd(II)/Pd(IV) catalytic enantioselective synthesis of bicyclo[3.1.0]hexanes *via* oxidative cyclization of enynes. J. Am. Chem. Soc. 131: 3452-3453.

[107] K. Muniz. 2009. High-oxidation-state palladium catalysis: new reactivity for organic synthesis. Angew. Chem. Int. Ed. 48: 2-14.

[108] M. Ronn, J.-E. Backvall and P.G. Andersson. 1995. Palladium(II)-catalyzed cyclization using molecular oxygen as reoxidant. Tetrahedron Lett. 36: 7749-7752.

[109] S. Jabre-Truffert and B. Waegell. 1997. Intramolecular acryloxypalladation - stereospecific synthesis of ring-fused unsaturated α-methylene-γ-butyrolactones. Tetrahedron Lett. 38: 835-836.

[110] M.B. Hay and J.P. Wolfe. 2005. Palladium-catalyzed synthesis of 2,1'-disubstituted tetrahydrofurans from γ-hydroxy internal alkenes. Evidence for alkene insertion into a Pd-O bond and stereochemical scrambling *via* β-hydride elimination. J. Am. Chem. Soc. 127: 16468-16476.

[111] M.B. Hay and J.P. Wolfe. 2006. Synthesis of polysubstituted tetrahydrofurans *via* Pd-catalyzed carboetherification reactions. Tetrahedron Lett. 47: 2793-2796.

[112] M.-C.P. Yeh, W.C. Tsao and L.-H. Tu. 2005. Palladium-catalyzed reaction of aryl bromides with 7-hydroxy-1,3-dienes. Organometallics 24: 5909-5915.

[113] J.P. Wolfe. 2006. Stereoselective synthesis of saturated heterocycles *via* Pd-catalyzed alkene carboetherification and carboamination reactions. Synlett 4: 571-582.

[114] C.H. Oh, H.M. Park and D.I. Park. 2007. Highly functionalized and stereocontrolled syntheses of 2-(2-methylenecycloalkyl)-furan derivatives by Pd-catalyzed cycloreduction. Org. Lett. 9: 1191-1193.

[115] T. Jeffery. 1985. Highly stereospecific palladium-catalyzed vinylation of vinylic halides under solid-liquid phase-transfer conditions. Tetrahedron Lett. 26: 2667-2670.

[116] B. Akermark, S. Hansson, T. Rein, J. Vagberg, A. Heumann and J.E. Bäckvall. 1989. Palladium-catalyzed allylic acetoxylation: an exploratory study of the influence of added acids. J. Organomet. Chem. 369: 433-444.

[117] G.Z. Wu, I. Shimoyama and E. Negishi. 1991. Palladium catalyzed carbonylative cyclization of *o*-allylbenzyl halides to produce benzo-annulated enol lactones and or bicyclo[3.3.0]hept-3-en-6-ones - an efficient route to U-68,215. J. Org. Chem. 56: 6506-6507.

[118] (a) I. Ojima, M. Tzamarioudaki, Z. Li and R.J. Donovan. 1996. Transition metal-catalyzed carbocyclizations in organic synthesis. Chem. Rev. 96: 635-662.
     (b) G. Vasapollo and G. Mele. 2006. Synthesis of heterocycles by transition metals-catalyzed cyclocarbonylation reactions. Curr. Org. Chem. 10: 1397-1421.

[119] M.C. Willis, D. Taylor and A.T. Gillmore. 2004. Palladium-catalyzed intramolecular *O*-arylation of enolates: application to benzo[*b*]furan synthesis. Org. Lett. 6: 4755-4757.

[120] B. Xiao, T.-J. Gong, Z.-J. Liu, J.-H. Liu, D.-F. Luo, J. Xu and L. Liu. 2011. Synthesis of dibenzofurans *via* palladium-catalyzed phenol-directed C-H activation/C-O cyclization. J. Am. Chem. Soc. 133: 9250-9253.

[121] Z. Shi, C. Zhang, C. Tanga and N. Jiao. 2012. Recent advances in transition-metal catalyzed reactions using molecular oxygen as the oxidant. Chem. Soc. Rev. 41: 3381-3430.

[122] D.E. Ames and A. Opalko. 1983. Synthesis of dibenzofurans by palladium-catalyzed intramolecular dehydrobromination of 2-bromophenyl phenyl ethers. Synthesis 3: 234-235.

[123] D.E. Ames and A. Opalko. 1984. Palladium-catalyzed cyclization of 2-substituted halogenoarenes by dehydrohalogenation. Tetrahedron 40: 1919-1925.

[124] Z. Liu and R.C. Larock. 2004. Synthesis of carbazoles and dibenzofurans *via* cross-coupling of *o*-iodoanilines and *o*-iodophenols with silylaryl triflates. Org. Lett. 6: 3739-3741.

[125] M.A. Campo, Q. Huang, T. Yao, Q. Tian and R.C. Larock. 2003. 1,4-Palladium migration *via* C-H activation, followed by arylation: synthesis of fused polycycles. J. Am. Chem. Soc. 125: 11506-11507.

[126] Q. Huang, M.A. Campo, T. Yaq, Q. Tian and R.C. Larock. 2004. Synthesis of fused polycycles by 1,4-palladium migration chemistry. J. Org. Chem. 69: 8251-8257.

[127] G. Bringmann, A. Wuzik, J. Kraus, K. Peters and E.-M. Peters. 1998. Synthesis and structure of a novel two fold lactone-bridged ternaphthyl. Tetrahedron Lett. 39: 1545-1548.

[128] C.-H. Cho, D.-I. Jung, B. Neuenswander and R.C. Larock. 2011. Parallel synthesis of a desketoraloxifene analogue library *via* iodocyclization/palladium-catalyzed coupling. ACS Comb. Sci. 13: 501-510.

[129] W.S. Yue and J.J. Li. 2002. A concise synthesis of all four possible benzo[4,5]furopyridines *via* palladium-mediated reactions. Org. Lett. 4: 2201-2203.

[130] P.J. Guiry and D. Kiely. 2004. The development of the intramolecular asymmetric Heck reaction. Curr. Org. Chem. 8: 781-794.

[131] A.B. Dounay and L.E. Overman. 2003. The asymmetric intramolecular Heck reaction in natural product total synthesis. Chem. Rev. 103: 2945-2964.

[132] M. Ikeda, S.A.A. El Bialy and T. Yakura. 1999. Synthesis of heterocycles using the intramolecular Heck reaction involving a 'formal' *anti*-elimination process. Heterocycles 51: 1957-1970.

[133] B. Chattopadhyay and V. Gevorgyan. 2012. Transition-metal-catalyzed denitrogenative trans-annulation: converting triazoles into other heterocyclic systems. Angew. Chem. Int. Ed. 51: 862-872.

[134] D. Yang, S. Burugupalli, D. Daniel and Y. Chen. 2012. Microwave-assisted one-pot synthesis of isoquinolines, furopyridines, and thienopyridines by palladium-catalyzed sequential coupling-imination-annulation of 2-bromoarylaldehydes with terminal acetylenes and ammonium acetate. J. Org. Chem. 77: 4466-4472.

[135] R. Grigg, M. Nurnabi and M.R.A. Sarkar. 2004. Dihydrofurocoumarin and dihydrofurodihydropyrid-2-one derivatives *via* palladium catalyzed cascades involving aryl/heteroaryl/vinyl iodides and allene followed by acid catalyzed cyclization. Tetrahedron 60: 3359-3373.

[136] (a) B. Nay, J.-F. Peyra and J. Vercauteren. 1999. Phenols as C- and O-nucleophiles in palladium-catalyzed allylic substitutions. Eur. J. Org. Chem. 9: 2231-2234.
   (b) L.E. Overman. 1984. Mercury(II) and palladium(II)-catalyzed [3,3]-sigmatropic rearrangements. Angew. Chem. Int. Ed. Engl. 23: 579-586.

[137] Y.-M. Zhang, T. Razler and P.F. Jackson. 2002. Synthesis of pyrimido[4,5-*b*]indoles and benzo[4,5]furo[2,3-*d*]pyrimidines *via* palladium-catalyzed intramolecular arylation. Tetrahedron Lett. 43: 8235-8239.

[138] B. Dajka-Halasz, K. Monsieurs, O. Elias, L. Karolykazy, P. Tapolcsanyi, B.U.W. Maes, Z. Riedl, G. Hajos, R.A. Dommisse, G.L.F. Lemiere, J. Kosmrlj and P. Matyus. 2004. Synthesis of 5*H*-pyridazino[4,5-*b*]indoles and their benzofurane analogues utilizing an intramolecular Heck-Type reaction. Tetrahedron 60: 2283-2291.

[139] D.E. Ames and D. Bull. 1982. Some reactions of 3-halogenocinnolines catalyzed by palladium compounds. Tetrahedron 38: 383-387.

[140] Q.H. Huang, A. Fazio, G.X. Dai, M.A. Campo and R.C. Larock. 2004. Pd-catalyzed alkyl to aryl migration and cyclization: an efficient synthesis of fused polycycles *via* multiple C-H activation. J. Am. Chem. Soc. 126: 7460-7461.

[141] W. Bonrath, M. Eggersdorfer and T. Netscher. 2007. Catalysis in the industrial preparation of vitamins and nutraceuticals. Catal. Today 121: 45-57.

[142] Y. Sato, T. Tamura and M. Mori. 2004. Arylnaphthalene lignans through Pd-catalyzed [2+2+2] cocyclization of arynes and diynes: total synthesis of taiwanins C and E. Angew. Chem. Int. Ed. 43: 2436-2440.

[143] S. Kotha, E. Brahmachary and K. Lahiri. 2005. Transition metal catalyzed [2+2+2] cycloaddition and application in organic synthesis. Eur. J. Org. Chem. 22: 4741-4767.

[144] J.-E. Backvall, P.G. Andersson, G.B. Stone and A. Gogoll. 1991. Synthesis of (+)-.α- and (+)-γ-lycorane *via* a stereocontrolled organopalladium route. J. Org. Chem. 56: 2988-2993.

[145] H.J. Reich, J.M. Renga and I.L. Reich. 1975. Organoselenium chemistry. Conversion of ketones to enones by selenoxide *syn* elimination. J. Am. Chem. Soc. 97: 5434-5447.

[146] Y. Hu and Z. Yang. 2001. Palladium-mediated intramolecular carbonylative annulation of *o*-alkynylphenols to synthesize benzo[*b*]furo[3,4-*d*]furan-1-ones. Org. Lett. 3: 1387-1390.

[147] D. Chernyak and V. Gevorgyan. 2010. Palladium-catalyzed intramolecular carbopalladation/cyclization cascade: access to polycyclic *N*-fused heterocycles. Org. Lett. 12: 5558-5560.

[148] Y. Zhang and E. Negishi. 1989. Palladium-catalyzed cascade carbometalation of alkynes and alkenes as an efficient route to cyclic and polycyclic structures. J. Am. Chem. Soc. 111: 3454-3456.

[149] J.M. Takacs and S. Chandramouli. 1990. Catalytic transition-metal-mediated tetraene carbo-cyclizations. A new carbocyclization *via* hydrosilylation? Organometallics 9: 2877-2880.

[150] J.M. Takacs and J. Zhu. 1990. Catalytic palladium-mediated tetraene carbocyclizations: enamine trapping reagents. Tetrahedron Lett. 31: 1117-1120.

[151] E. Negishi, L.S. Harring, Z. Owczarczyk, M.M. Mohamud and M. Ay. 1992. Cyclic cascade carbopalladation reactions as a route to benzene and fulvene derivatives. Tetrahedron Lett. 33: 3253-3256.

CHAPTER 6

Five-Membered O,N-Heterocycles

6.1 Introduction

Five-membered *N*-heterocyclic compounds are very important in a number of applications and occur in a diversity of drugs and natural products [1a-d]. Aromatic five-membered *N*-heterocycles containing one to four nitrogen atoms include pyrroles, pyrazoles, imidazoles, 1,2,3-triazoles, 1,2,4-triazoles, and tetrazoles. Additionally, aromatic *N*-heterocyclic compounds may possess another heteroatom, like oxygen in oxazoles, isoxazoles, 1,2,4-oxadiazoles, and 1,3,4-oxadiazoles [2-8].

Heterocycles, especially *N*- and *O*-containing heterocycles, are most important class of compounds in agrochemical and pharmaceutical industries. Isoxazolines are one of the key oxygen and nitrogen-containing five-membered heterocycles which exhibit biological and synthetic applications. Besides being starting materials for the synthesis of various multi-functional synthetic intermediates like oximes and α,β-unsaturated ketones, nitriles and β-hydroxyketones, γ-amino alcohols etc., isoxazolines are excellent precursors for *C*-disaccharides, β-amino acids, amino sugars, steroids, imino/amino polyols, and novel azaheterocycles. A spiroisoxazoline motif is an important constituent of various pharmacologically active natural products like aerothionin, calafianin, aerophobin and homoaerothionin. These *N,O*-heterocycles are employed as key building blocks in the construction of many unnatural and natural compounds including indolizine and quinolizidine tricycles, β-lactam anti-biotics, sarkomycin, testosterone, and biotin etc. Isoxazolines represent a unique class of pharmacophores present in various therapeutic agents and have diverse and interesting biological activities. Isoxazoline possessing cyclolignan derivatives exhibit potent immunosuppressive, anti-viral, and cytotoxic properties. The biological importance of isoxazolines is further proved from their anti-inflammatory, anti-microbial, anti-cancer, fibrinogen receptor antagonistic, anti-depressant and anti-HIV activities [9-14].

Oxazolidinones are anti-bacterial agents which display potent activity against a wide range of Gram-positive organisms. Linezolid drug is the only and first member of oxazolidinone series. AZD2563 and eperezolid are still potential drug candidates and they are used as structural precursors for modification [15-16].

6.2   Palladium assisted synthesis of five-membered *O,N*-heterocycles

6.3   Synthesis of five-membered 1,2-*O,N*-heterocycles

The aromatic nitrile oxides (a class of propargyl-type 1,3-dipoles) underwent 1,3-dipolar cycloaddition to provide isoxazoles [17]. Due to instablity of aromatic nitrile oxides, it was necessary to produce them *in situ* by dehydrochlorination of hydroximinoyl chlorides in the presence of a suitable base. This step was fully compatible with a preceding alkynone synthesis if TEA was used as a base. The acid chlorides were reacted with terminal alkynes under modified Sonogashira conditions at rt for 1 hr to afford alkynones, subsequently, TEA and hydroximinoyl chlorides were added. Moderate to excellent yields of isoxazoles were obtained after dielectric heating for 30 min. Among two possible regioisomers only one was produced **(Scheme 1)** [18]. This one-pot coupling-cycloaddition was conducted under mild conditions to afford isoxazole with excellent regio- and chemoselectivity. As a consequence of acid chlorides as halide coupling partner, hydroxy and amine groups were needed to be protected before the reaction. The use of acid chlorides was predominantly limited to (hetero)aromatic compounds and derivatives without α-hydrogens. Cyclopropyl substituent was tolerated in both steps with one exception. Electron poor as well as electron rich aromatic and aliphatic alkynes were utilized. Even heterocyclic alkynes were also utilized as starting substrates. The coupling procedure also occurred efficiently with silylated alkynes *i.e.* TMS acetylene. With respect to 1,3-dipolar nitrile oxide, polycyclic, electron-rich, heterocyclic and electron-deficient substituents were tolerated and reacted easily with alkynones. Alternatively, multi-component heterocyclic compound synthesis was conducted in the presence of Pd catalyst to synthesize keto-alkynes for cycloaddition reactions. Muller [19-21] has shown the importance of this method for the generation of a variety of aromatic heterocyclic compounds. Aromatic heterocycles were synthesized by trapping of substrate.

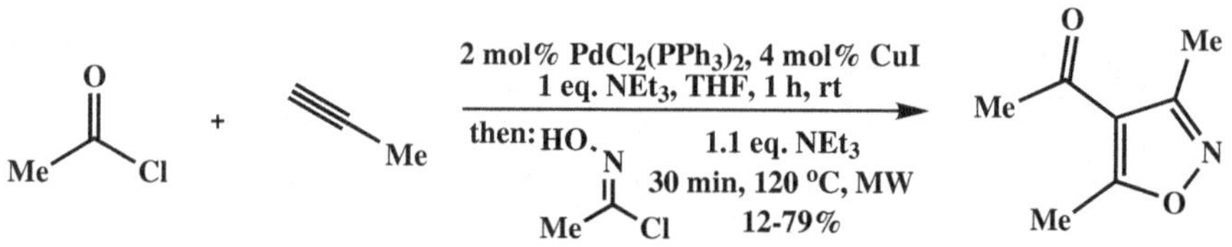

Scheme-1

Broggini and co-workers [22] described the synthesis of 4-spiroannulated tetrahydro-isoquinolines conveniently **(Scheme 2)** although yields were unsatisfactory. The prolonged heating of reaction without isocyanate resulted in isoquinolin-1-ones, which was the reason for low yields of spiroannulated products [23].

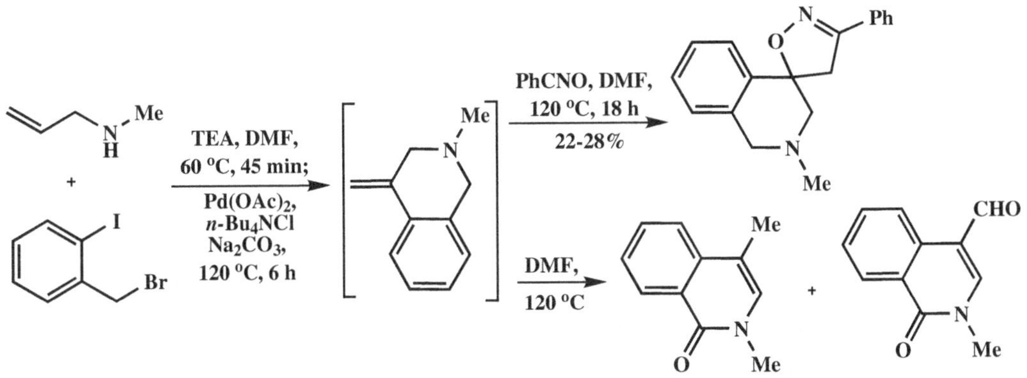

Scheme-2

In 2009, Zhang and Yu [24] explained palladium(II)-catalyzed hydroxylation of arenes with air or 1 atm of oxygen **(Scheme 3)**. Loh et al. [25] reported an oxime assisted intramolecular dioxygenation of alkenes in the presence of 1 atm of air (sole oxidant) and Pd catalyst under very mild conditions in 2010. The dioxygenation of olefin occurred readily at rt under 1 atm of molecular oxygen to afford dioxygenated products when oxime was treated with 24 mol% of 1,10-phenanthroline, 20 mol% of palladium acetate, and 10 eq. of acetic acid. The target products were provided in comparable yields with both aliphatic and aromatic groups. But lower yields were afforded when a bulky phenyl group or two methyl groups were present on CH_2 tether. The oxygen of hydroxyl group of products was originated from molecular oxygen as shown by isotopic labeling studies. This protocol used atmospheric oxygen for the efficient preparation of synthetically important compounds under extremely mild conditions [26]. Alexanian et al. [27-28] reported a similar inter- and intramolecular aerobic dioxygenation of alkenes under metal-free conditions employing hydroxamic acids.

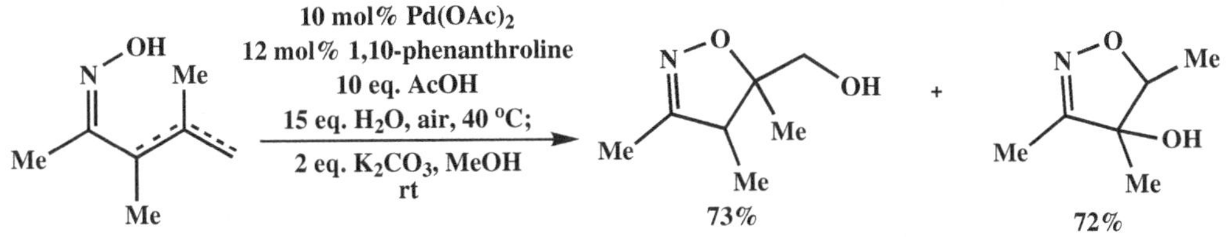

Scheme-3

Isoxazolylsilanols were synthesized from [3+2]-cycloaddition reaction of alkyl and aryl nitrile oxides and alkynyldimethylsilyl ethers. The 3,4,5-trisubstituted isoxazoles were obtained by cross-coupling reaction of heterocyclic silanols with a number of PhI. Rapid variation of substituents at 3, 4, and 5 positions of isoxazole was observed in this method **(Scheme 4)** [29].

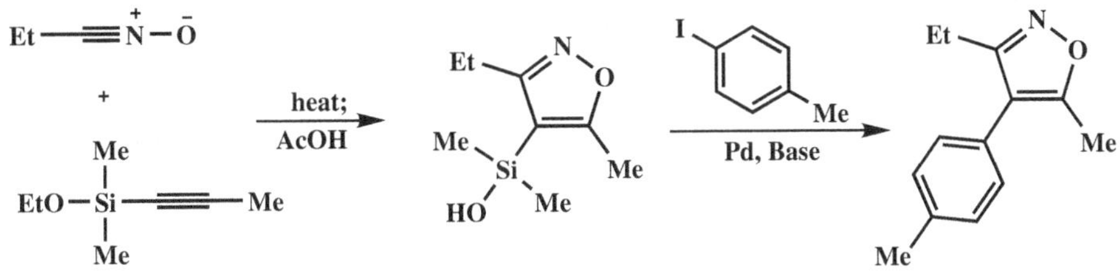

Scheme-4

The hydroamination process was applied to hydroxylamine derivative to confirm the effectiveness of procedure and vinyl isoxazolidine was obtained in good yield **(Scheme 5)** [30].

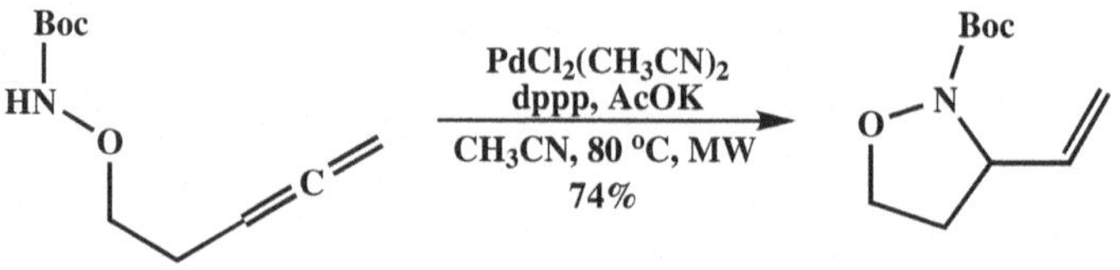

Scheme-5

The transformation of aryl chlorides as electrophiles in palladium-catalyzed alkene carboamination and carboetherification, prevented the formation of regiosisomieric mixtures and minimized the *N*-arylation with catalyst composed of palladium acetate and *S*-Phos (2-dicyclohexylphosphino-2′,6′-dimethoxybiphenyl). Many heterocyclic compounds, such as isoxazolidines, pyrrolidines, pyrazolidines, and tetrahydrofurans were efficiently produced with this protocol **(Scheme 6)** [31].

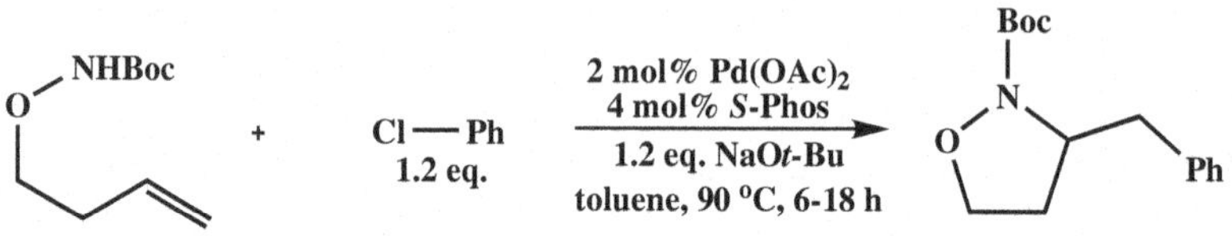

Scheme-6

Parsons et al. [32a] produced functionalized and fused isoxazolines by a MCR involving sequential [1+3]- and [2+3]-cycloadditions **(Scheme 7)**. In 1989, the original intramolecular reaction explained by same group was elaborated to include intermolecular versions and *in situ* formation of isocyanides. The *N*-(isoxazolylidene)alkylamines were synthesized by a sequential formation of isocyanide through ring-opening of epoxide with TMS cyanide followed by [1+3]-cycloaddition of isocyanide with nitroalkene. Nitrile oxide was produced by fragmentation of ring and then intermolecular 13DC of nitrile oxide with electron deficient dienophiles formed isoxazolines [32b].

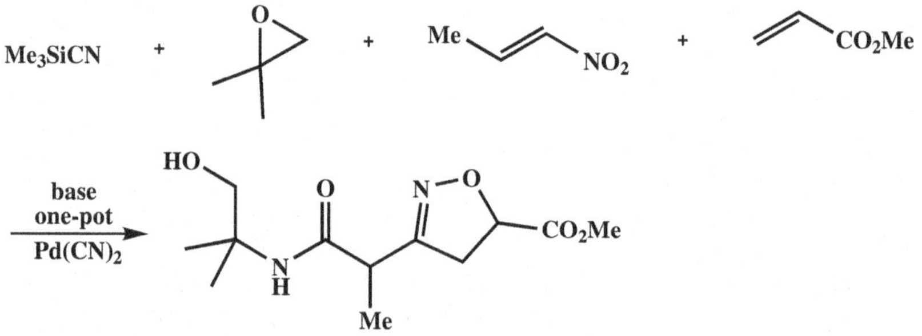

Scheme-7

Oximes and their derivatives are widely used in organic synthesis as key intermediates in the preparation of a variety of heterocycles [33]. Murahashi and co-workers [34] reported the transformation of unsaturated ketoxime into isoxazole on treatment with an equimolar amount of PdCh(PPh$_3$)$_2$ in the presence of 5 eq. of sodium phenoxide in benzene **(Scheme 8)**.

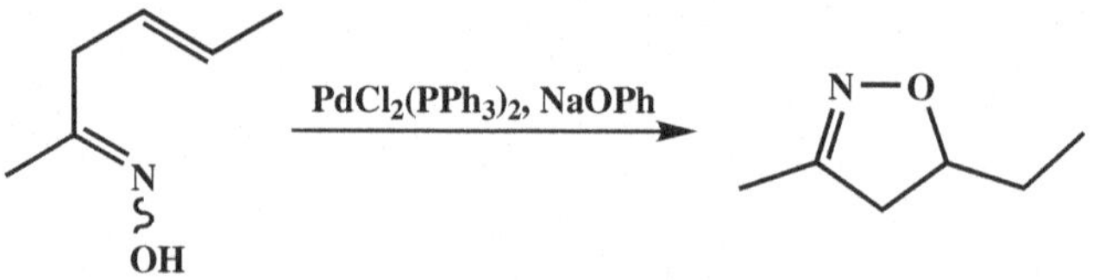

Scheme-8

An important ester group was obtained when Pd(II)-induced ring-closing occurred onto an alkene with subsequent carbon monoxide insertion **(Scheme 9)**. This method was based on previous work which utilized alcohols as intramolecular nucleophile [35]. The starting substrates were easy to synthesize. Due to high acidity of *N*-hydroxyphthalimide the homoallylic alcohols were transformed into *N*-phthaloyl hydroxylamines using Mitsunobu chemistry [36-38]. De-protection in Ing-Manske style with hydrazine provided a facile method completing in min at rt. Under Pd-catalyzed carbonylation conditions, the *N*-unsubstituted hydroxylamines did not react but the corresponding carbamates cyclized with complete stereoselectivity and efficiently. In this way only five-membered rings were generated [39].

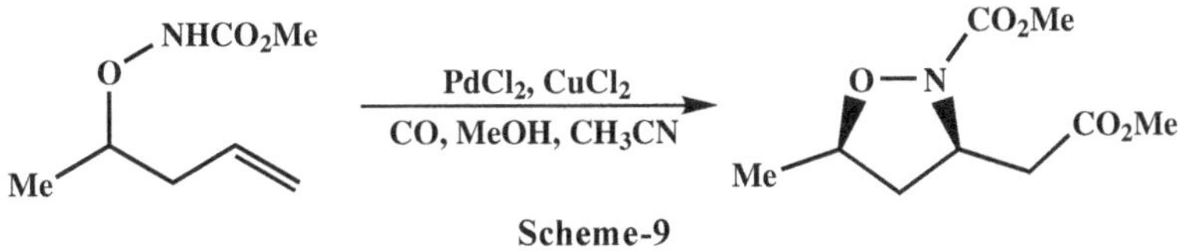

Scheme-9

Bates and Sa-Ei [40] synthesized isoooxazolidine in good yields when *O*-homoallylhydro-xyamines were reacted with CO and Pd catalyst in MeOH. The reaction of sulfonamide provided a 5:1 mixture of *cis-trans* diastereomers while the reaction of carbamate afforded only *cis* isomer diastereoselectively **(Scheme 10)**. The isoxazolidines were produced by cyclization of *O*-alkenylsubstituted hydroxylamines in the presence of palladium catalyst. For the success of this reaction an electron-withdrawing group on nitrogen was required [41].

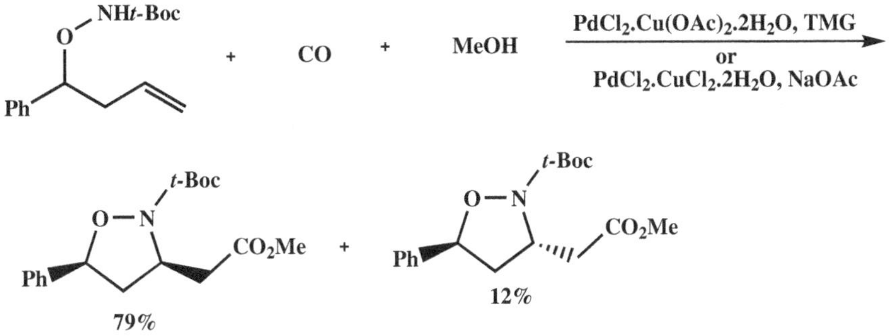

Scheme-10

Three steps such as sequential dipolar cycloaddition, Suzuki coupling and MW-induced amination were performed for the synthesis of highly functionalized isoxazoles **(Scheme 11)** [42].

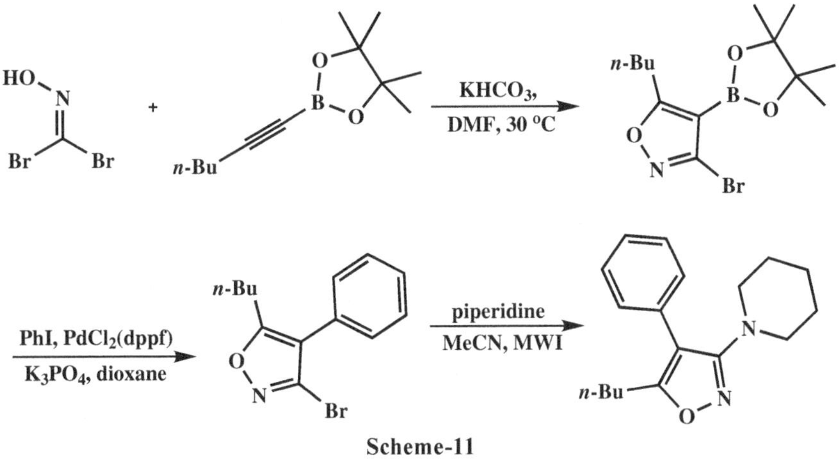

Scheme-11

The 1α,25-dihydoroxyvitamin D3-26,23-lactam was produced as depicted in **Scheme 12**. The protocols developed by Uskokovic and co-workers [43] were employed for the synthesis of nitrone in five steps from Inhoffen-Lythgoe diol (derived from vitamin D2). The isoxazoline with separable 4 isomers was obtained in 70% yield by 1,3-dipolar cycloaddition of nitrone with methyl metacrylate. The silyl ether of isoxazoline was de-protected with PTS to give isoxazoline-alcohol. The lactam was obtained in 90% yield upon reduction of isoxazoline-alcohol with hydrogen over palladium-carbon. The tertiary alcohol of lactam was protected as trimethylsilyl ether, after that the successive oxidation of secondary alcohol followed by Wittig reaction provided vinyl bromide. Trost [44] developed the coupling of vinyl bromide with compound (derived from (S)-malic acid) in the presence of Pd catalyst. Subsequently, 1α,25-dihydoroxyvitamin D3-26,23-lactam was formed in 50-60% yield upon de-protection of silyl ether with tetrabutylammonium fluoride and Dowex-50W.

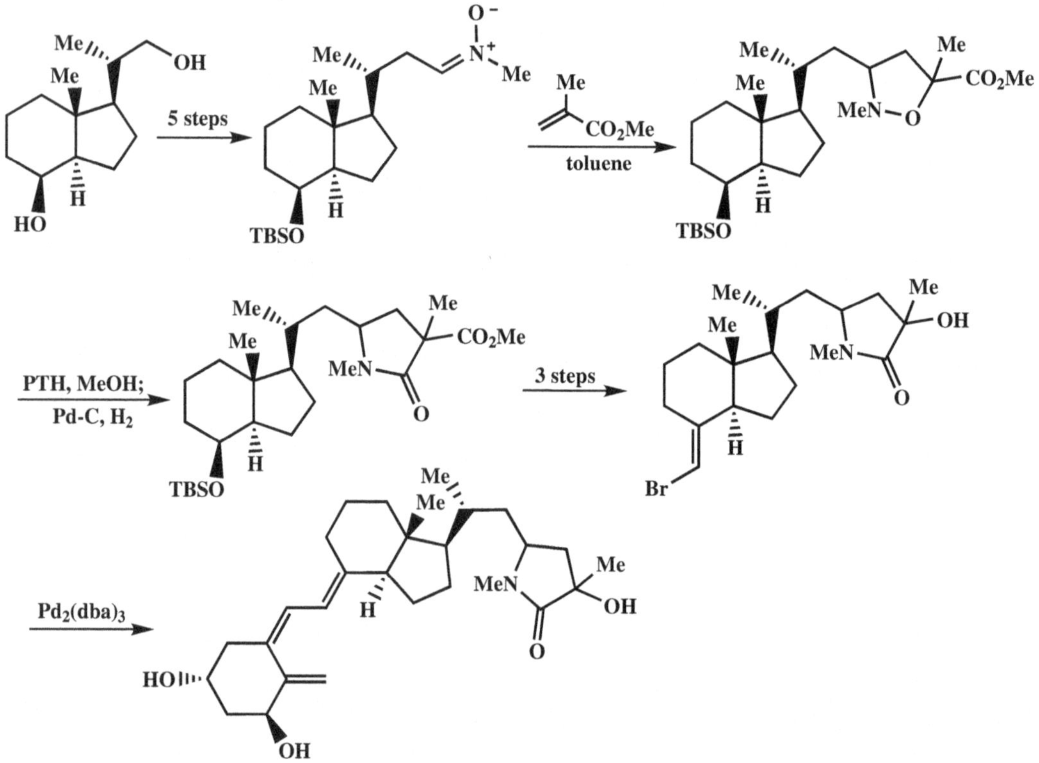

Scheme-12

6.4   Synthesis of five-membered 1,3-*O,N*-heterocycles

The amide protected propargyl amines were afforded upon amidation of propargyl amine with acid chlorides under mild reaction conditions. These propargylamides without isolation were reacted with acid chlorides to form the alkynone intermediates. Then, a proton catalyzed cycloisomerization afforded good yields of functionalized oxazoles *via* an amidation-coupling-cycloisomerization sequence **(Scheme 13)** [21, 45].

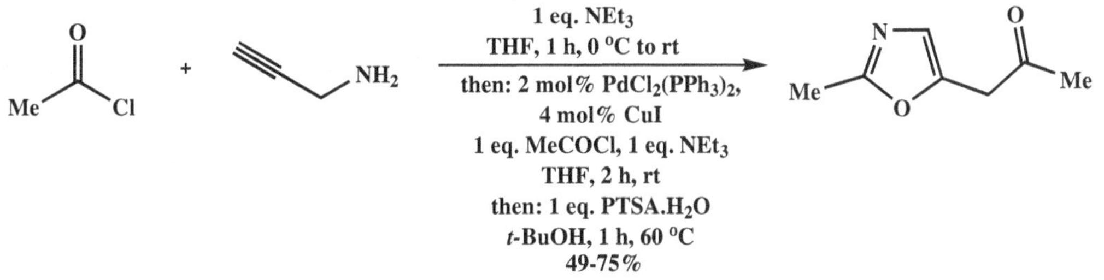

Scheme-13

Deprez and Sanford [46] reported synthetically useful organic conversions with the aid of Pd-catalyzed reactions of DIB ((diacetoxyiodo)benzene) and other hypervalent iodine reagents. Such palladium-catalyzed oxidation reactions, included the 1,2-aminooxygenation of olefinic substrates and the oxidative functionalization of carbon-hydrogen bonds [47-57]. Examples of these catalytic oxidations were intramolecular aminoacetoxylation in the reaction of γ-aminoolefins with (diacetoxyiodo)benzene in the presence of palladium acetate catalyst and the selective acetoxylation of carbon-hydrogen bonds adjacent to coordinating functional groups **(Scheme 14)** [58]. The main step in these catalytic reactions was the (diacetoxyiodo) benzene-promoted oxidation of palladium(II) to palladium(IV) species, as proved by isolation and X-ray structural identification of stable palladium(IV) complexes prepared by the reaction of PhI(O$_2$CPh)$_2$ with palladium(II) complexes possessing chelating 2-phenylpyridine ligands [59]. Many examples of chlorinations of organic substrates utilizing (dichloroiodo)benzene in the presence of palladium catalyst were reported [60-62a, b].

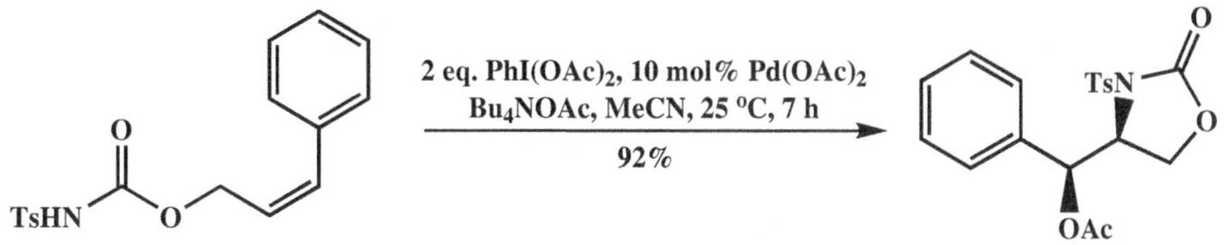

Scheme-14

Sorensen and Lee [63] reported a palladium(II)-catalyzed aminoacetoxylation of alkenes. Oxazolidinone was generated in 65% yield when starting substrate was treated with palladium acetate and iodobenzene diacetate. This conversion occurred through a palladium(II)/ palladium(IV) catalytic cycle that was initiated by *anti*-aminopalladation of alkene to provide an intermediate. The palladium(II) complex intermediate was oxidized to alkyl palladium(IV) intermediate with iodobenzene diacetate. The oxazolidinone was formed upon carbon-oxygen bond-forming reductive elimination of alkyl palladium(IV) intermediate **(Scheme 15)**.

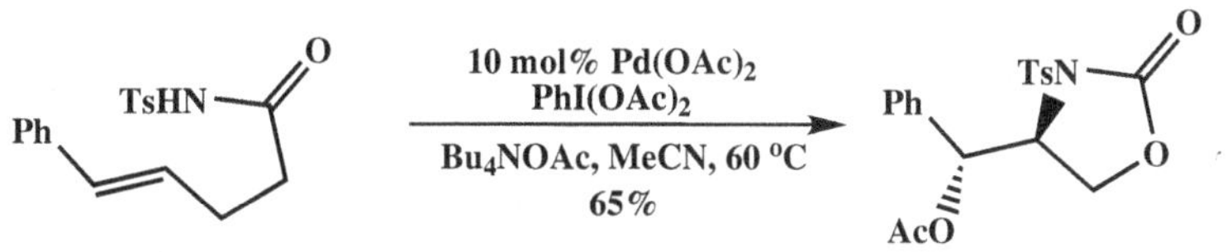

Scheme-15

There are several other classes of heterocycles that could potentially be generated from palladium-catalyzed carboamination reactions. There are several medicinal and synthetic uses for oxazolidin-2-ones. They represent an extremely important new class of anti-biotics and Evan's auxiliary (an oxizolidin-2-one) was one of the most important chiral auxiliaries for controlling stereochemistry. There are several known methods for their synthesis. As shown in **Scheme 16** they have been recently made from chiral precursors such as aziridines [64]. However, given the ever present threat of anti-biotic resistance it is crucial to develop new methods of developing oxiziolidin-2-ones, especially ones which allowed for rapid formation of multiple analogs. Palladium-catalyzed carboaminations would be particularly well suited for meeting this need as simple variation of aryl or vinyl halide coupling partner allowed for a library of compounds to be quickly generated.

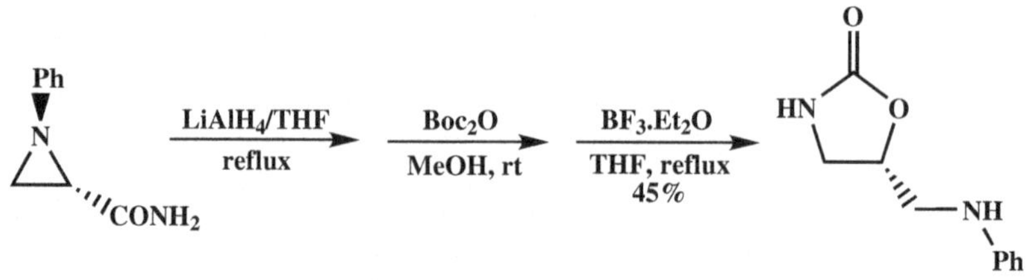

Scheme-16

Fraunhoffer and White [65] explained a palladium-catalyzed variant of oxidative carbamate carbon-hydrogen bond amination with palladium acetate, a quinone oxidant and a bissulfoxide ligand **(Scheme 17)**. Fraunhoffer and White [65] reported the formation of isoxazolidine through an allylpalladium complex by allylic carbon-hydrogen activation. Isoxazolidine was afforded in 72% yield when homoallylic carbamate was reacted with palladium acetate in phenylbenzoquinone and sulfoxide ligand. Larock [66] described the related conversion for the synthesis of indoline products. Studies suggested that amination occurred *via* a nucleophilic addition of carbamate into a (allyl)palladium(II) intermediate rather than *via* a palladium-nitrene. With substitution at the position of carbamate, amination occurred in good diastereoselectivities with *anti* product formed preferentially over *syn* product.

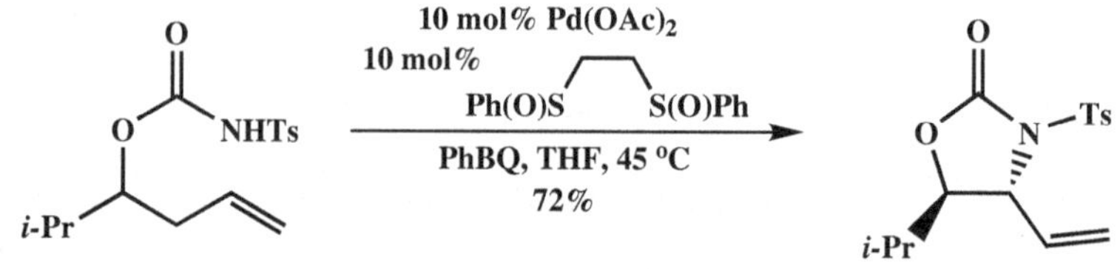

Scheme-17

The didmolamides A contain thiazole and oxazoline rings. The two cyclic hexapeptides were isolated from marine ascidian *Didemnum molle* collected in Madagascar [67]. Kelly and co-workers [68] described the biomimetic synthesis of thiazolines and was utilized in the total preparation of bistratamides E-J and dendroamide A which seems to be suitable for the generation of thiazole rings of didmolamides A and B. The thiazole was formed when *N*-acylated cysteine substrate was reacted, followed by oxidation of resulting thiazoline. With the application of this protocol You and Kelly [69] produced didmolamides A **(Scheme 18)**. The treatment of *N*-Fmoc-*S*-trityl-L-cysteine allyl ester dipeptide, followed by oxidation of formed thiazoline with activated manganese oxide and then the elimination of allyl ester protecting group in the presence of Pd catalyst provided thiazole-based amino acid building block in 92% yield. The Fmoc protecting group of supported thiazole was removed with 20% piperidine in dimethylformamide after the attachment of thiazole to Wang resin using 1-hydroxybenzotriazole and 2-(1*H*-benzotriazole-1-yl)-1,1,3,3-tetramethyluroniumhexafluorophosphate in diisopropylethylamine. The thiazole containing dipeptide was provided upon coupling of thiazole-based amino acid residue and resin-supported amine in the presence of 2-(1*H*-benzotriazole-1-yl)-1,1,3,3-tetramethyluroniumh exafluorophosphate/1-hydroxybenzotriazole. Finally, all the stereogenic centers of didmolamide A and the complete skeleton was synthesized by coupling of *N*-Fmoc-L-phenylalanine and *N*-Fmoc-allo-threonine under same coupling conditions. The thiazole-possessing triamide was formed upon de-protection of Fmoc group of *N*-Fmoc-L-phenylalanine and *N*-Fmoc-allo-threonine and cleavage of resin with 95% trifluoroacetic acid. The formed triamide underwent macrolactamization into macrolactam by employing a combination of 4-dimethylaminopyridine and PyBOP (*N,N*-bis(2-oxo-3-oxazolidinyl)phosphine). The didmolamide A was generated in 56% yield when macrolactam was treated with Burgess reagent [70].

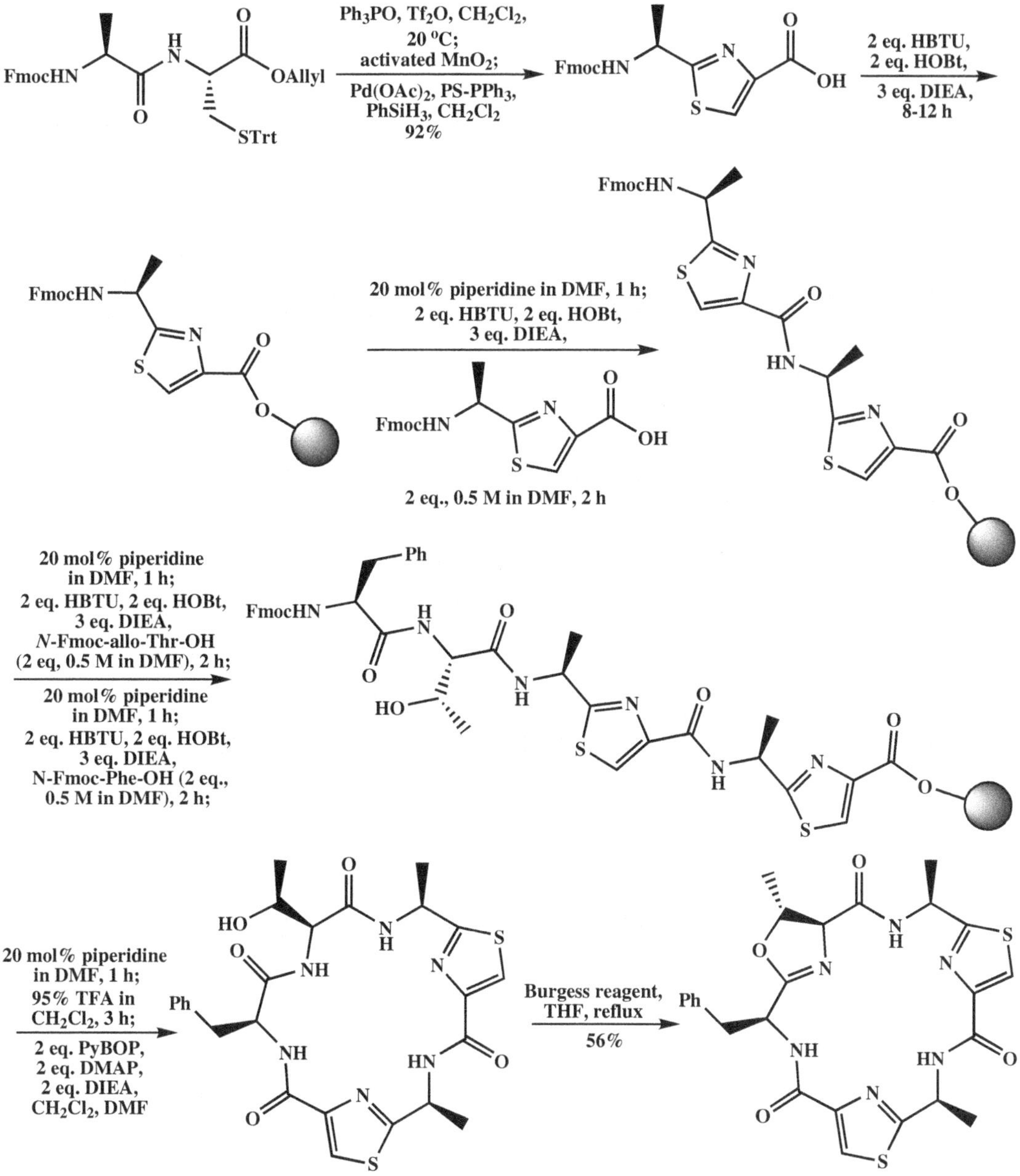

Tf$_2$O=(trifluoromethanesulfonic anhydride)

Scheme-18

Münchnone substrates were utilized for the preparation of biologically active molecules in turn münchnones were synthesized by a versatile catalytic pathway [71]. The acid chlorides and imines underwent oxidative addition to afford a highly active Pd intermediate which incorporated CO and after hydrogen chloride elimination produced the münchnone skeleton (**Scheme 19**) [72]. The most favorable conditions used Bu₄NBr as a halide source, a palladacyclic dimer for the stabilization of intermediates, relatively high pressures of carbon monoxide and non-nucleophilic base *N,N*-diisopropylethylamine [73]. However, α-amino acid derivatives were formed in quantitative yields by the addition of MeOH to reaction mixture. Dhawan and co-workers [74-75] explained the construction of münchnone when imine was reacted with benzoyl chloride and CO with the help of Pd catalyst. The reaction occurred through the formation of aciliminium salt, the insertion of carbon monoxide into carbon-palladium bond of intermediate, dehydrochlorination from resulting acylpalladium complex, and cyclization by attack of oxygen to electron-deficient carbonyl coordinated to Pd [76-77]. This reaction involved the coupling of imines and acid chlorides for the synthesis of *N*-acyl iminium salts. Then the *N*-acyl iminium salts upon oxidative addition to Pd can underwent carbonylation and cyclization. For instance, a variety of polysubstituted pyrroles were produced when the reaction was performed with alkynes [78-79].

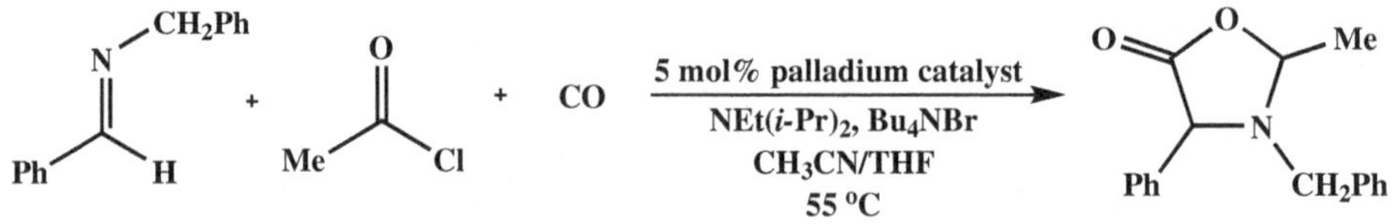

Scheme-19

The α-oxo lactams, through indium-mediated carbonyl-allenylation reactions under Barbier-type conditions, afforded starting substrates *i.e.* 2-azetidinone-tethered allenols [80]. The 1,2-bromoamidation of allenes occurred smoothly in the presence of Pd(II) catalyst, synthesizing spiranic oxazolidinone-β-lactams as single isomer (**Scheme 20**) [81-82].

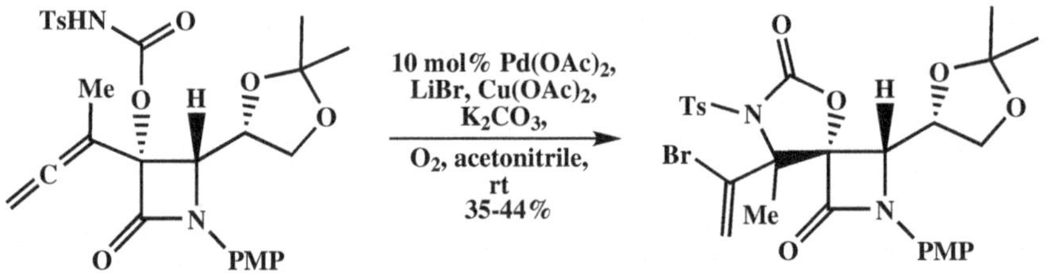

Scheme-20

Many carboamination reactions of aryl halides and alkyne-tethered amines were described in the presence of palladium(0) catalyst [83-86]. The reactions of alkynes occurred through *anti*-aminopalladation, although in some cases products were formed from *syn*-aminopalladation [87]. The carboamination reactions used aryl halides as coupling partners while other conversions employ other electrophiles, like acrylate derivatives (**Scheme 21**) [88-92].

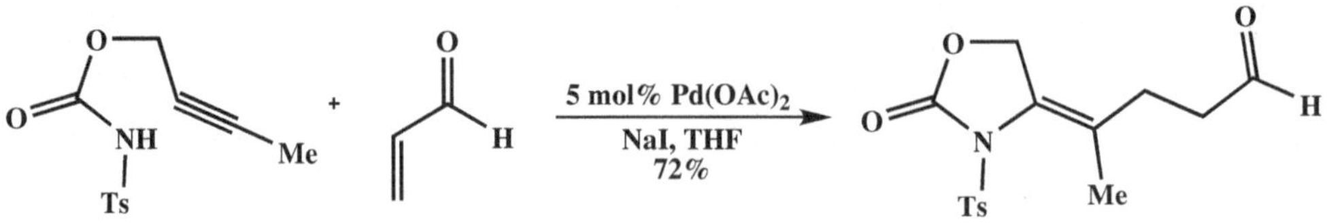

Scheme-21

Carboamination reactions of aryl or alkenyl halides and allenes were described in the presence of palladium(0) catalyst [93-98]. The mechanism involved alkene aminopalladation to explain these reactions. However, in various examples these reactions may involve π-allylpalladium intermediate. For comparison with the related reactions of alkenes and alkynes these transformations have been included in this section, due to this mechanistic ambiguity. Similar reactions which involve allylic halides have also been reported **(Scheme 22)** [99-100].

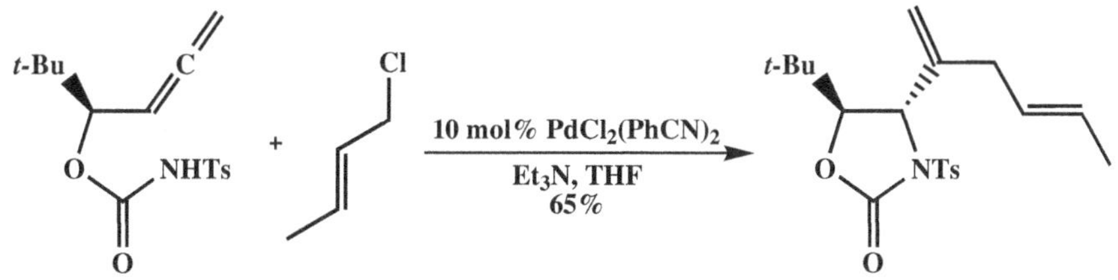

Scheme-22

Alkenyl aziridines and epoxides were utilized as electrophiles in reactions which occurred through intermediate π-allylpalladium complexes [101-102], including reactions that synthesized five-membered *N*-heterocycles [103-104]. The alkenyl epoxide was coupled with isocyanate to afford oxazolidin-2-one in quantitative yield with the aid of *in situ* produced catalyst from $P(Oi\text{-}Pr)_3$ and $Pd_2(dba)_3$. An intermediate was formed by oxidative addition of alkenyl epoxide to palladium(0) and the intermediate was reacted with isocyanate. The allylpalladium complex was trapped with pendant carbamate anion to form the product. When imines were utilized in place of isocyanates, the 1,3-oxazolidines were obtained [105]. The substituted pyrrolidines were synthesized from 2-vinyloxiranes containing tethered nitrogen nucleophiles **(Scheme 23)** [106-107].

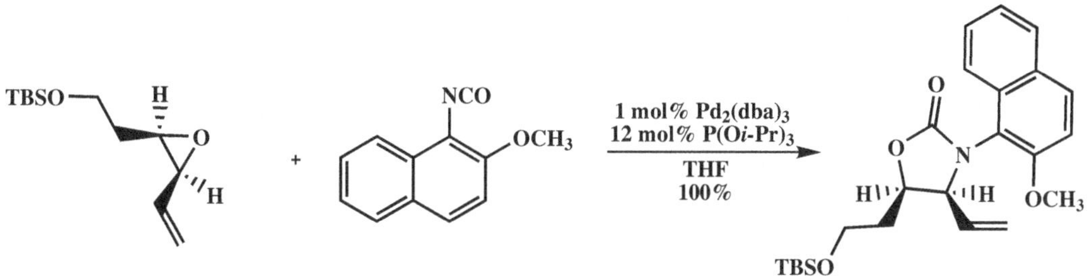

Scheme-23

Many protocols were developed for the construction of heterocyclic compounds using Pd carbonylation which involved carbon monoxide insertion into a palladium-heteroatom bond through either an outer-sphere or inner-sphere mechanism [108]. Many groups used this protocol for the synthesis of ureas and isoxazolidines *via* carbonylation reactions of 1,2-diamines or 1,2-amino alcohols in the presence of palladium catalyst [109-110]. Gabriele et al. [111-112] used a palladium iodide/potassium iodide/air catalyst system for the production of oxazolidin-2-ones in high yields. The oxazolidin-2-one was formed in 96% yield from amino alcohol substrate employing only 0.05 mol% of palladium iodide. The palladium(II) catalyst was reduced to palladium(0), and for the regeneration of catalytically active palladium(II) species, air (oxygen) was required **(Scheme 24)**.

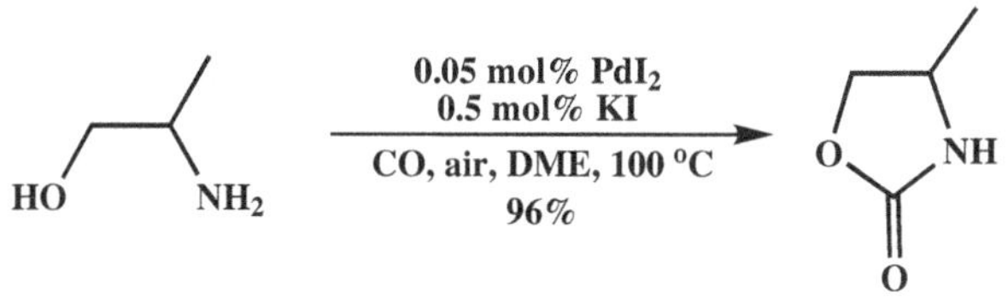

Scheme-24

Yoshida et al. [113] utilized (*E*)-4-(benzylamino)-2-butenyl methyl carbonates for the preparation of 5-vinyloxazolidinones in the presence of a palladium catalyst through a carbon dioxide fixation-elimination sequence. The DBU (1,8-diazabicyclo[5.4.0]undec-7-ene) was required for the efficient fixation of carbon dioxide. The yield decreased significantly in the presence of argon atmosphere because of the formation of aziridines **(Scheme 25)** [23].

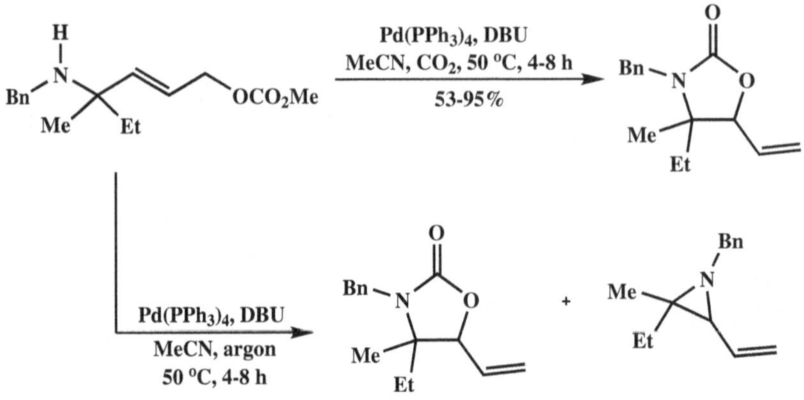

Scheme-25

Oshima et al. [114] reported a carboetherification reaction of *N*-allylacetamides with aryl halides for the synthesis of benzyl-substituted oxazolines in the presence of palladium catalyst, SPHOS ligand (C-45) and sodium *tert*-butoxide **(Scheme 26)** [23].

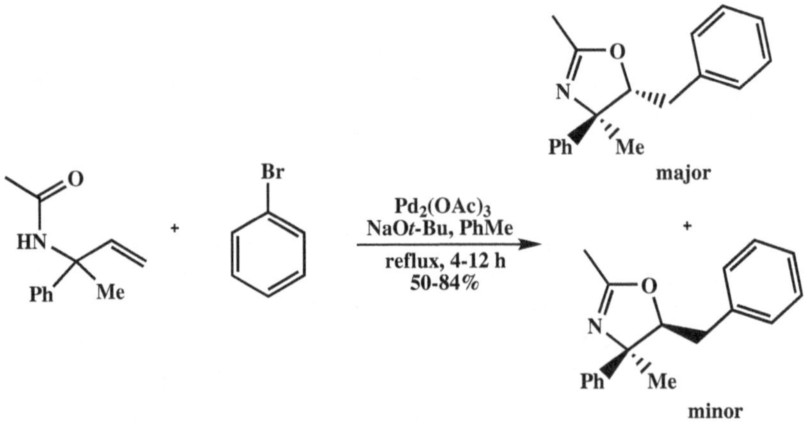

Scheme-26

Bacchi and co-workers [115] explained oxidative carbonylation of pro-2-ynylamides for the general and efficient preparation of 5-(alkoxylcarbonyl)methylene-3-oxazolines in the presence of Pd catalyst **(Scheme 27)**. The vinylpalladium intermediate was formed by nucleophilic attack of an oxygen atom of an amide group on an alkyne coordinated by Pd(II). The acylpalladium complex was formed upon insertion of carbon monoxide into carbon-palladium bond of vinylpalladium intermediate. Then, the methanolysis of acylpalladium complex afforded esters and palladium(0) catalyst. The palladium(II) was formed from oxidation of palladium(0) with molecular O_2, and thus the catalytic cycle operated well.

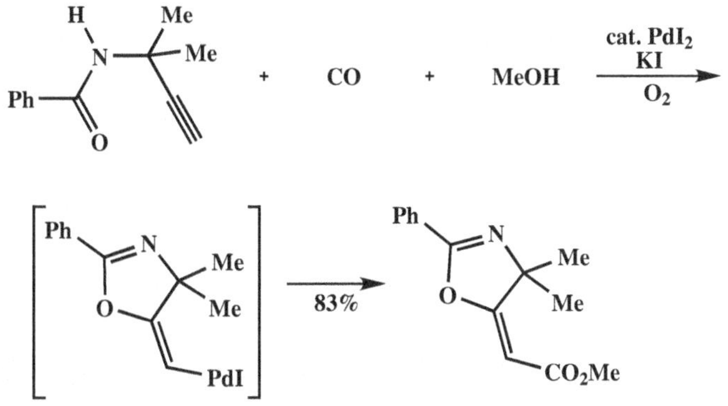

Scheme-27

Gabriele and co-workers [116-117] explained the Pd-catalyzed oxidative carbonylation of 2-amino-1-alkanols for the construction of 2-oxazolidinones **(Scheme 28)**. An intermediate *i.e.* aminocarbonyl Pd complex was produced, and subsequently 2-oxazolidinones were delivered upon ring closure.

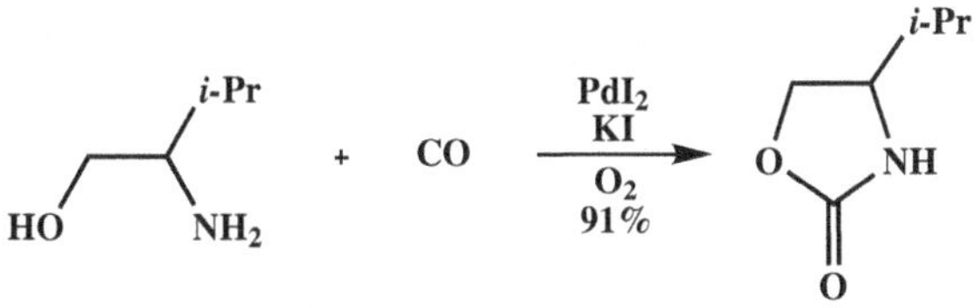

Scheme-28

Heterocycles were synthesized using alkenyl aziridines and epoxides *via* inter- and intramolecular carbon-heteroatom bond forming reactions [118-119]. Two main methods for the construction of heterocyclic compounds using these substrates, as shown in **Scheme 29**, are: (a) intramolecular allylation of alkenyl aziridines and epoxides and (b) intermolecular cycloaddition of vinyl aziridines and epoxides with heterocumulenes, like carbodiimides, isocyanates, and isothiocyanates [120-124].

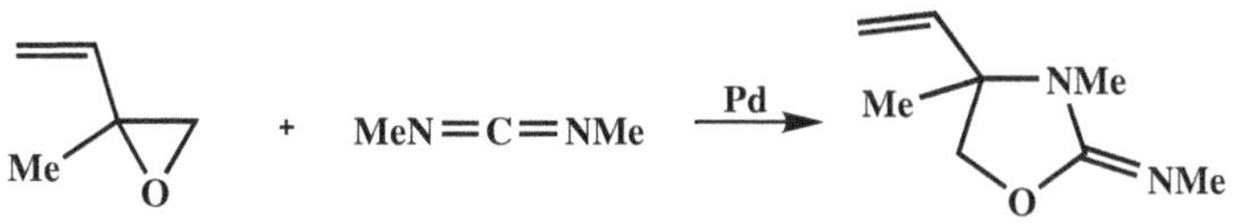

Scheme-29

The regioselective [3+2]-cycloaddition products *i.e.* 1,3-oxazolidine derivatives were synthesized in good to excellent yields *via* Pd-catalyzed intermolecular reaction of imines with vinyl oxirane **(Scheme 30)** [125].

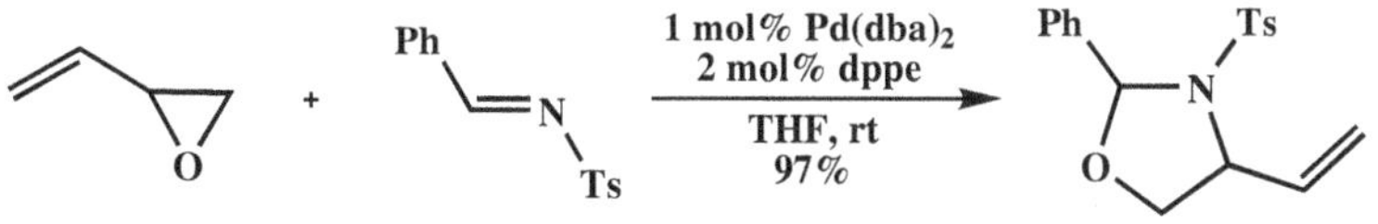

Scheme-30

A mixture of different allenamides was obtained with unsymmetrical biscarbamates from adducts. The oxidative addition of palladium(0) preferred less hindered propargyl carbon as suggested by ratios of allenamides with different substituents **(Scheme 31)** [126a-b].

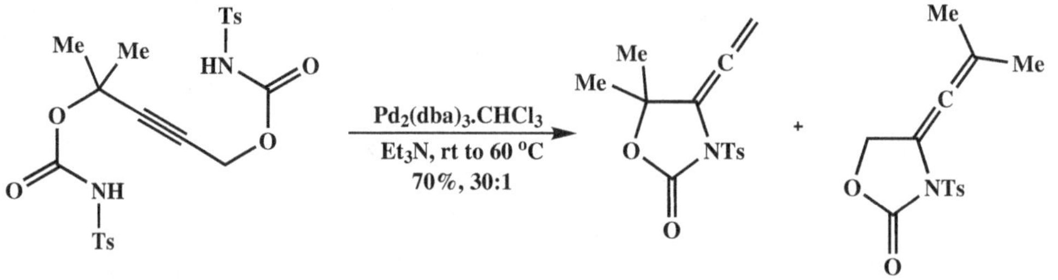

Scheme-31

A non-oxidative approach toward the asymmetric synthesis of *N*-heterocycles was palladium(II)-catalyzed alkene aminopalladation involving substrates bearing allylic acetates. In contrast to oxidative amination reactions described in **Scheme 32**, these transformations were terminated by *β*-elimination of allylic acetate. These reactions no longer require oxidant, but substrates become more complex. Nonetheless, treatment of starting compound with catalytic amount of catalyst afforded ureas, amides and oxazolidinones in high yield and enantioselectivities. Aminopalladation of starting compound proceeded through palladium-alkyl intermediate and subsequent *β*-acetoxy elimination provided *N*-heterocycles and regenerated the active catalyst [127].

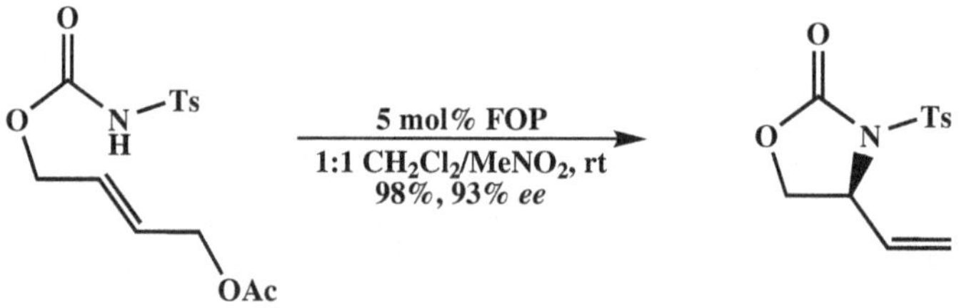

Scheme-32

In order to determine the optimal ligand to effect palladium-catalyzed carboamination of *O*-allylcarbamates, allyl phenylcarbamate was reacted with iodobenzene in the presence of ligands. The best yields of carboamination product were obtained with DPE Phos and P(2-furyl) phosphine. As it was evident from the results, about 50% of mass balance remained unaccounted. Control reactions demonstrated that substrate was susceptible to palladium and base catalyzed decomposition **(Scheme 33)** [128].

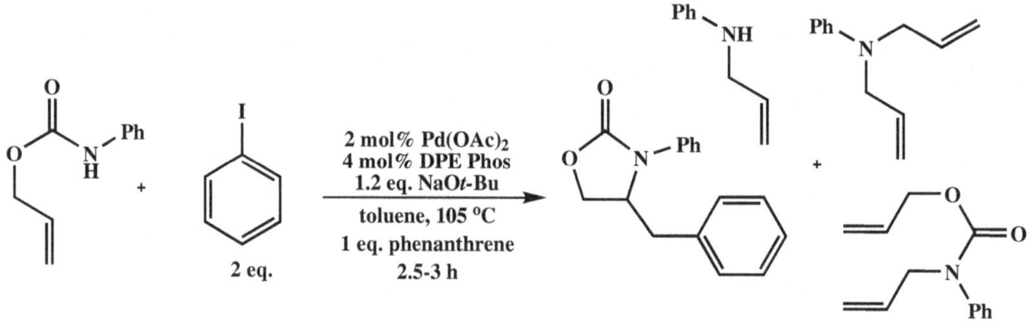

Scheme-33

Although in transition metal-catalyzed cross-coupling reactions the tolerance of activated epoxides has little precedent [129-130], Pericas [131] showed that the SPhos was optimal supporting ligand (high yield) in SMC of enantiomerically-pure epoxides. The straightforward synthesis of these compounds allowed rapid access to chiral *C*2 symmetrical bis(oxazolines) **(Scheme 34)**. The chiral *C*2 symmetrical bis(oxazolines) were useful ligands for asymmetric catalysis [132].

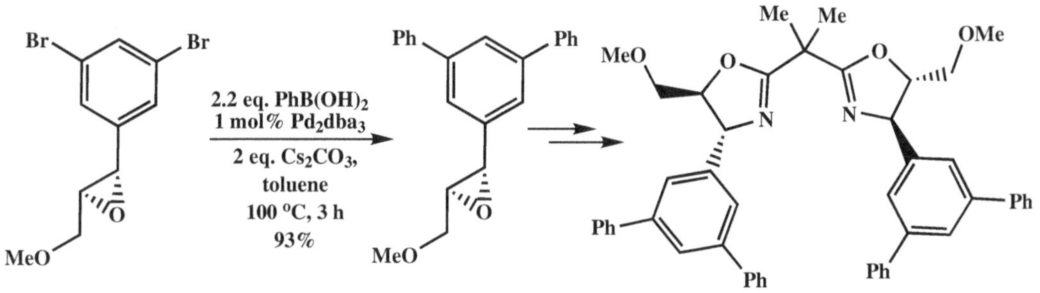

Scheme-34

The five- [133-138] and six-membered [139-140] *N*-heterocycles [141-144] were prepared *via* palladium-catalyzed carboamination reactions of amines containing pendant alkenes and alkenyl or aryl halides. However, the synthesis of seven-membered heterocyclic compounds through this pathway was quite challenging, as with increasing the ring size both reaction rates and yields diminished. This was due to two main problems associated with mechanism of these reactions: (a) competing synthesis of enamine side products, through β-hydride elimination from intermediate (b) due to stereoelectronic and entropic effects the *syn*-aminopalladation of alkene **(Scheme 35)** becomes more difficult. This protocol was not applied for the preparation of seven-membered rings previously, and the synthesis of seven-membered *N*-heterocycles through other alkene difunctionalization reactions in the presence of metal catalyst was very rare [145-147]. For instance, Michael reported a palladium(II)-catalyzed carbon-hydrogen activation/carboamination of a *N*-allyl-2-(aminomethyl)aniline derivative which provided a 3-substituted 1,4-benzodiazepine in modest yield (53%) [148-149].

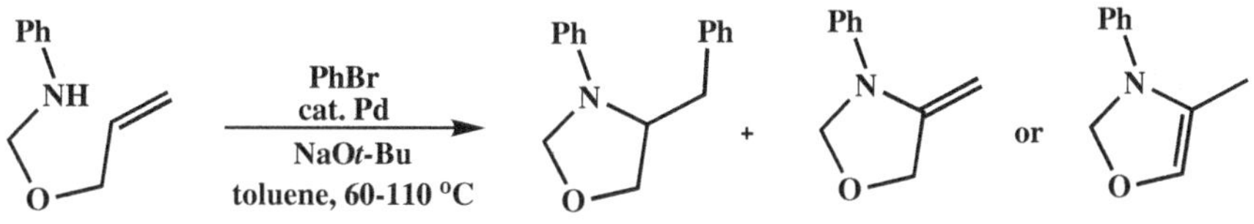

Scheme-35

The Pd-catalyzed carbonylation of organic halides provided an efficient route to construct carboxylic acids and their derivatives (*e.g.* esters and amides). These catalytic transformations were considered to proceed *via* Pd-acyl intermediates, which underwent reaction with nucleophiles in a fashion similar to acid chlorides. The carbonylation was exploited with acid chlorides to build up complex and useful structures, as acid chlorides were known to undergo transformations beyond ester and amide bond formation. This will describe the development in using PhI carbonylation to construct aryl-substituted heterocycles. This involved the reaction of catalytically generated Pd-acyl intermediates with imines to form *N*-acyl iminium salts, which underwent subsequent carbonylation, providing a route to synthesize 1,3-oxazolium-5-olates (münchnones). These 1,3-dipoles can undergo cycloaddition with a range of substrates to afford *N*-heterocycles (*e.g.* imidazolines and pyrroles) **(Scheme 36)** [149].

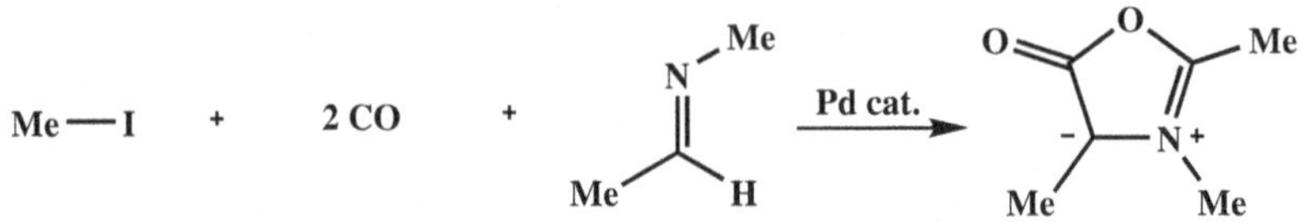

Me—I   +   2 CO   +   [structure: N-methyl ethylidenimine]   →[Pd cat.]   [structure: oxazoline product]

Scheme-36

This protocol outlined in **Scheme 37** was an improvement of Kende's method [150]. The propargyl alcohol under a modified method involving methyliodination [151] and Sonogashira coupling of starting compound with (trimethylsilyl)acetylene followed by manganese(IV) oxide oxidation synthesized aldehyde stereoselectively. The Kende's procedure [150] was followed for the transformation of aldehyde into iodoalkene through Reformatsky-type aldol reaction although the final diimide reduction was carried out using *o*-nitrobenzenesulfonyl hydrazide in place of hydrazine, which afforded high reproducibility. The preparation of stannane required for Stille coupling with iodoalkene started from 2,2-diethoxyethanol. The oxazole-2-thiol was formed by

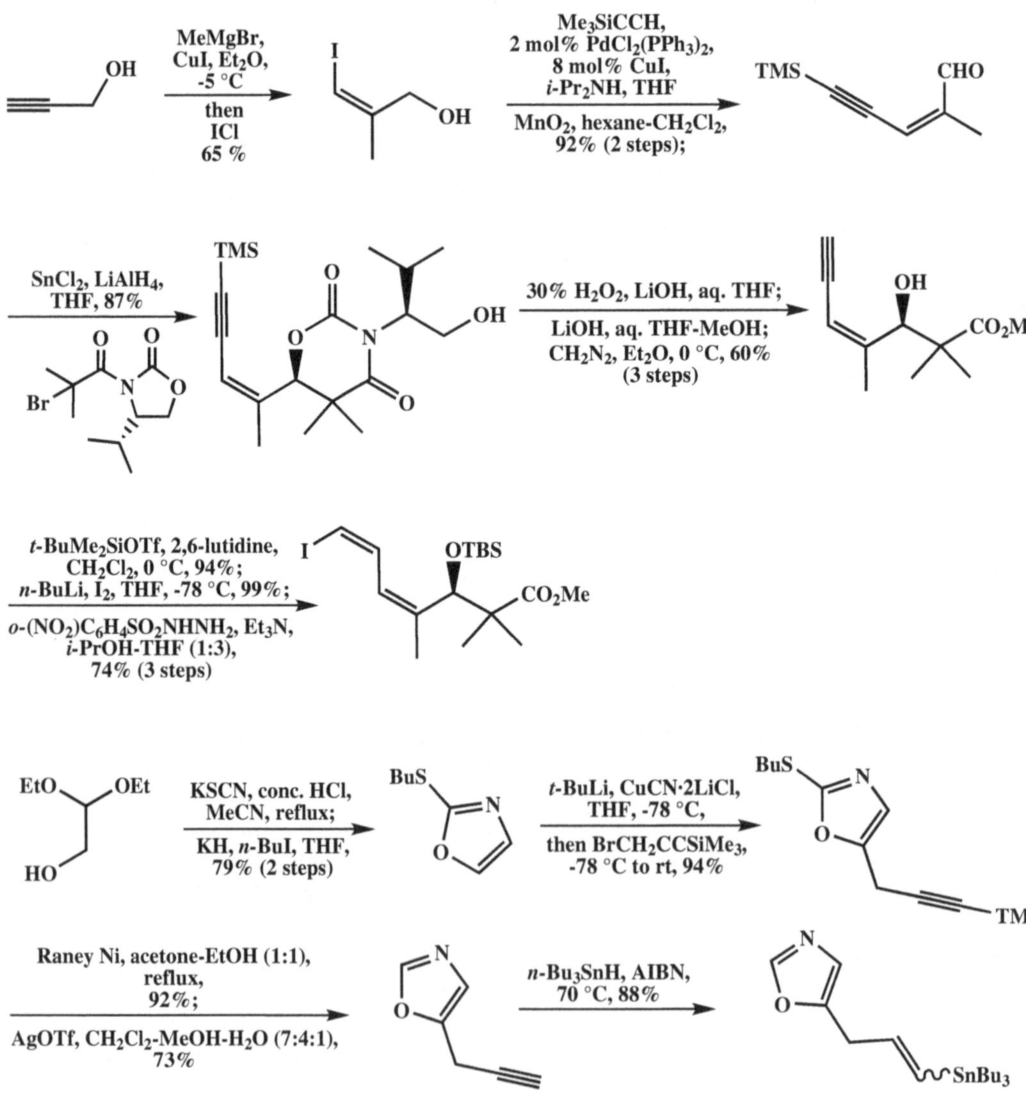

Scheme-37

the reaction of 2,2-diethoxyethanol with potassium thiocyanate under acidic conditions [152] and the formed oxazole-2-thiol underwent butylation to provide good yield of oxazole. A clean product was synthesized by propargylation [153-154] of oxazole in the presence of copper catalyst. The formed product upon desulfurization, desilylation, and hydrostannylation afforded stannane as a 6:1 *E/Z*-mixture [155].

Every soft metal-based Lewis acid which was capable of forming a complex with isocyano moiety can be utilized as a catalyst. This reaction was catalyzed by a number of metals **(Scheme 38)**. So far most commonly applied species are silver, copper, gold, and palladium. Many reactions using nickel, zinc, ruthenium, platinum, and rhodium catalysts were also reported. Asymmetric Au and Ag catalysts were utilized for the highly efficient enantioselective synthesis of oxazoline. Enantioselective platinum- and palladium-catalyzed reaction has been evaluated; however highly efficient catalyst systems were not found [156].

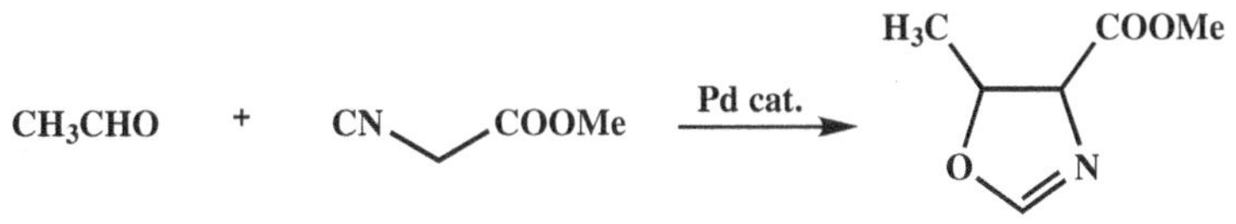

$$CH_3CHO \quad + \quad CN\diagdown\diagup COOMe \xrightarrow{\text{Pd cat.}}$$

Scheme-38

The 1,3-oxazin-2-ones and 1,3-oxazolidin-2-ones (containing an acrylate side-chain) were afforded under buffered conditions upon aminocarbonylation of allenic *N*-tosylcarbamates. The reaction afforded only *trans*-4,5-disubstituted heterocyclic compounds with high stereoselectivity **(Scheme 39)** [41, 157-158].

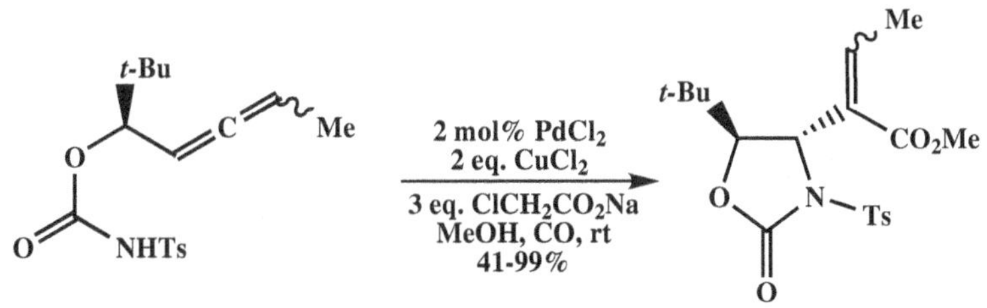

Scheme-39

The *N*-heterocycles were generated through palladium-catalyzed carbonylative sequence which involved Wacker-type *anti*-aminopalladation of alkynes, alkenes, or allenes. Danishefsky [159] used stoichiometric amounts of Pd for intramolecular alkene aminopalladation followed by carbonylation. Tamaru [160-163] developed the catalytic versions of these reactions, and extended the scope of this reaction for the construction of diverse *N*-heterocycles, such as imidazolidin-2-ones, oxazolidin-2-ones, isoxazolidines and pyrrolidines. For instance, the oxazolidin-2-one was synthesized in 70% yield when carbamate was treated with 5 mol% of palladium chloride and cupric chloride using trimethyl orthoacetate as solvent under carbon monoxide [164]. The heterocyclic compound was formed upon capture of acylpalladium intermediate with MeOH (produced *in situ* from trimethyl *o*-acetate). The functionalized *N*-heterocycles were synthesized when carbon monoxide was inserted into intermediate aminopalladium adducts. Specially, both the nitrogen atoms acted as nucleophiles when urea derivatives were used as substrates. *Endo*-carbamates showed a distinctive reactivity among other nitrogen nucleophiles and needed NaOAc as a buffer for the reaction **(Scheme 40)** [41].

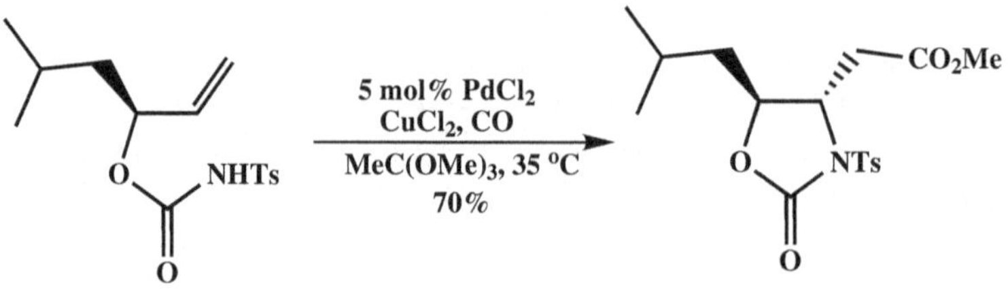

Scheme-40

The 2-aza-4-alkenols produced oxazolidines through oxypalladation and subsequent α-hydride elimination **(Scheme 41)** [165]. Only 5-*exo*-cyclization occurred in good yield with an excess of copper acetate as oxidant and palladium acetate as catalyst in dimethylsulphoxide. The use of molecular O_2 was investigated as a clean alternative to copper acetate in order to improve the oxidation step [166]. Dimethylsulphoxide played the role of stabilizing ligand of giant Pd clusters [41, 167].

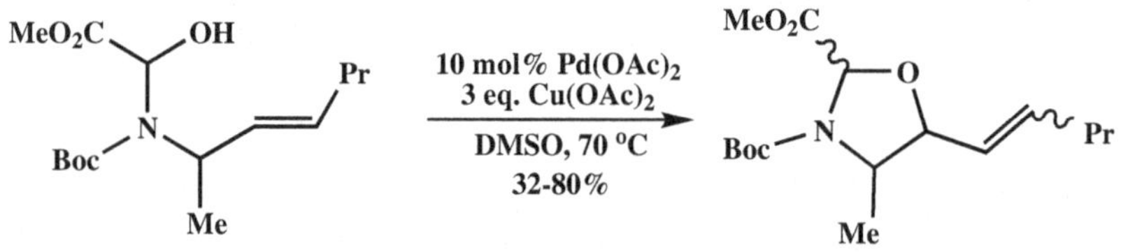

Scheme-41

The haloamination of allylic alcohol with *p*-toluenesulfonyl isocyanate synthesized halomethyl-substituted oxazolidinones in palladium acetate/cupric chloride/lithium chloride. The reaction occurred with high regio-, chemo-, and diastereoselectivity **(Scheme 42)** [41, 168].

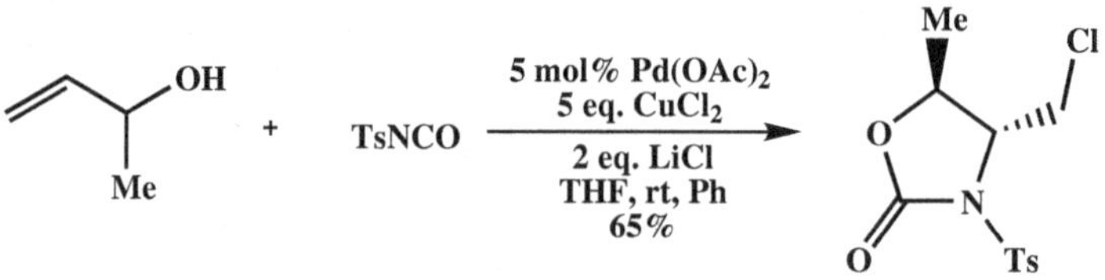

Scheme-42

Various examples of asymmetric palladium-catalyzed insertion reactions in the presence of chiral ligands are constituted by Heck reactions [169]. There are less common examples of enantioselective aminopalladation reactions. Again the Overman group [170] has demonstrated an enantioselective cyclization of an *O*-allylcarbamate to an oxazolidinone using an exotic bimetallic catalyst [171]. Zhu and Yang [172] provided examples of asymmetric aza-Wacker-type cyclizations using (-)-sparteine **(Scheme 43)**.

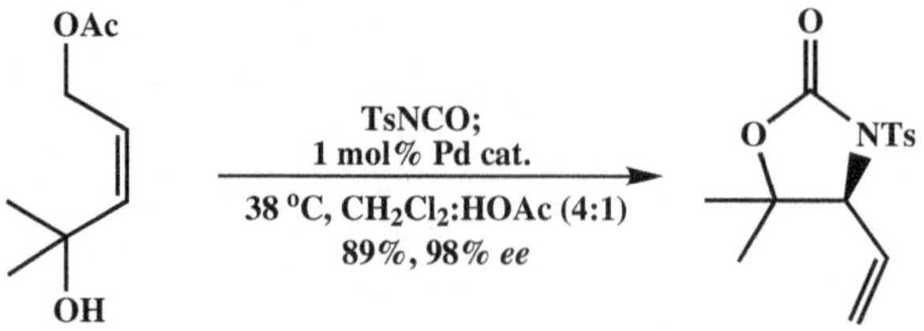

Scheme-43

The amidation of propargylamine with an acid chloride followed by cross-coupling with another acid chloride provided substituted oxazol-5-ylethanones by a three-component sequence.

Therefore, an amidation-coupling-cycloisomerization (ACCI) sequence was a diversity-oriented one-pot protocol for the synthesis of substituted oxazoles **(Scheme 44)** [173].

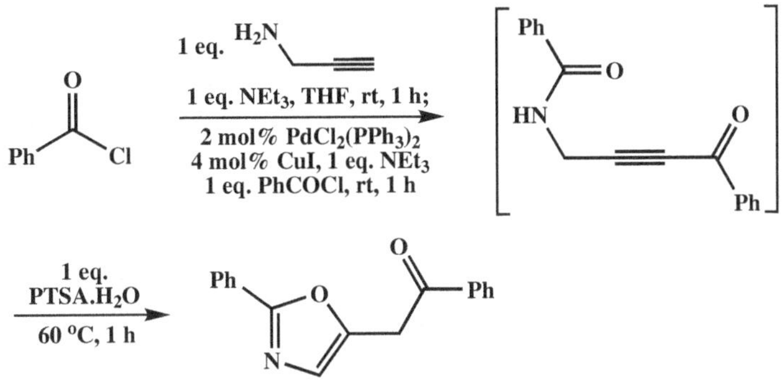

Scheme-44

This method was described in the presence of Cu catalyst, though palladium was required for the cyclization as a separate step [174]. The *t*-Bu sulfinamide was used as NH_3 surrogate with Pd catalyst for the synthesis of free NH indoles [175]. Ackermann's original procedure was modified in which an additional Cu- or Pd-catalyzed reaction was introduced. The 2-aminoindole derivatives were synthesized using *o*-haloaryl acetylenic bromides in two steps consisting of a Cu-catalyzed *N*-alkynylation followed by a separate Pd-catalyzed *N*-arylation and subsequent cyclization **(Scheme 45)** [176]. Good yields of functionalized products were obtained [177].

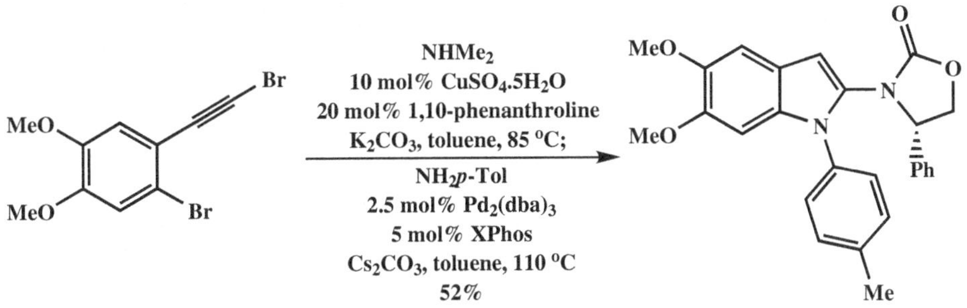

Scheme-45

The isocyanates used in this reaction were 2-methoxy-1-naphthyl isocyanates. As shown in **Scheme 46**, the same product was obtained from either isomer of initial vinyl epoxide in which the exclusive product (in 80-100% yield) was thermodynamically less stable isomer [178].

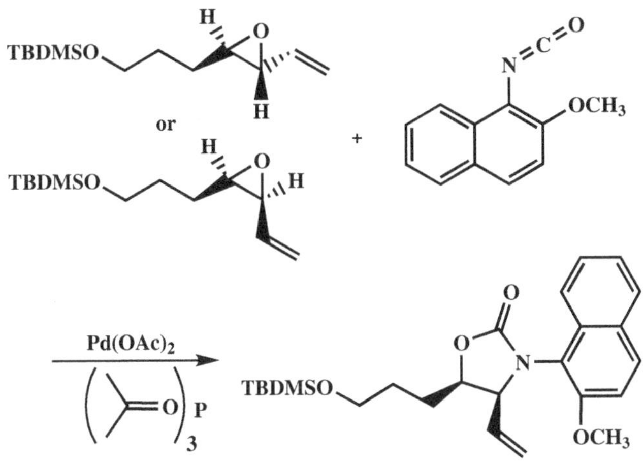

Scheme-46

The *N*-heterocycles were prepared through palladium(II)-catalyzed alkene aminopalladation, but involved substrates containing allylic hydroxy or allylic acetate groups [179-182]. The *β*-elimination of hydroxy or acetate group (rather than *β*-hydride elimination) terminated these conversions. This method alleviated the requirement of oxidants, but it needed slightly more complex substrates. This protocol was quite important for the generation of many natural products [183]. An interesting method for the asymmetric formation of oxazolidinones (in 91% *ee* and 81% yield) involved the treatment of tosylcarbamate with chiral palladium(II) catalyst (catalytic amounts) **(Scheme 47)** [184].

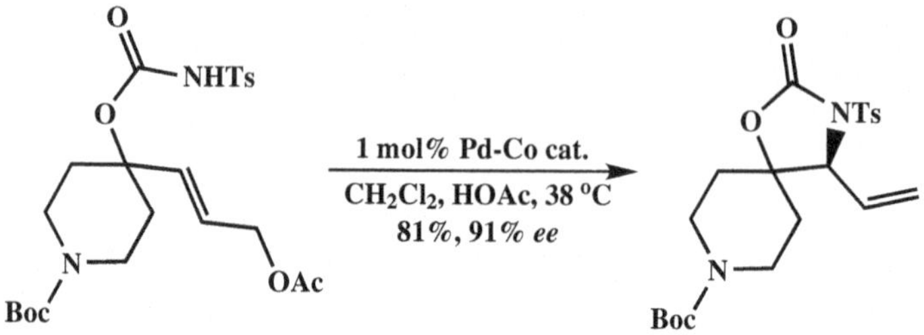

Scheme-47

6.5   Synthesis of five-membered *O,N*-polyheterocycles

For this purpose, *O*-allenylether of 2-aminophenol was chosen as suitable substrate and several reaction conditions were screened starting with the best found on indole derivatives. By changing different parameters such as solvent, catalyst and heating source, the reaction was optimized with PdCl$_2$(CH$_3$CN)$_2$ as catalyst in acetonitrile solvent under MW activation, to afford the desired vinyl derivative in high yield, providing a 5-*exo*-allylic hydroamination **(Scheme 48)** [185].

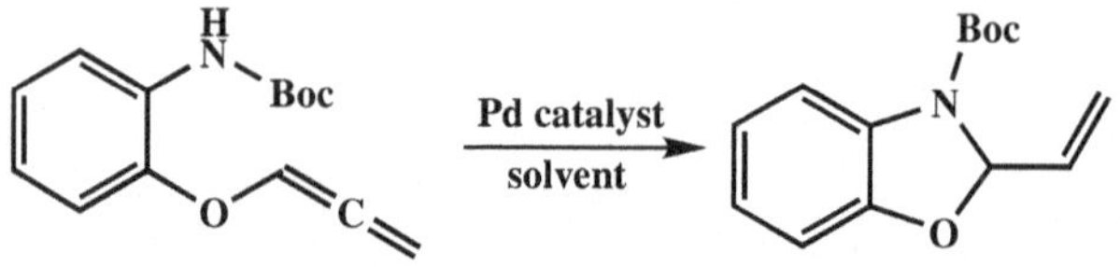

Scheme-48

By using Pd(PPh$_3$)$_4$ in the presence of 10 mol% triphenylphosphine in PhMe at 90 °C under conventional or microwave heating, the better results were obtained on substituted aryl derivatives. Moreover the presence of additional triphenylphosphine was found to be crucial, probably acting as a stabilizing agent for intermediate thus avoiding the dealkylation process **(Scheme 49)** [186].

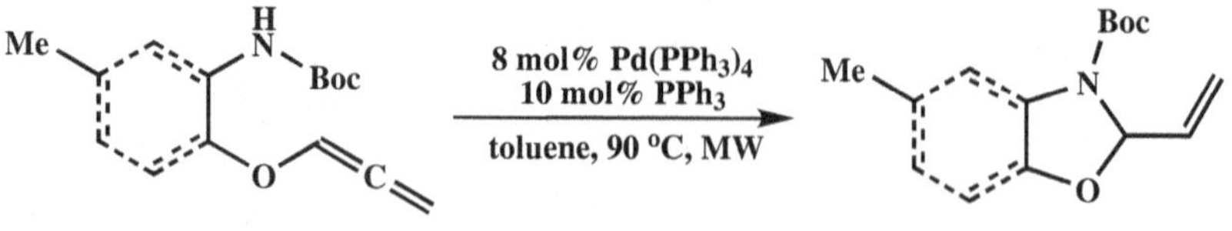

Scheme-49

A series of oxazolines was obtained in excellent yield by this convenient and efficient three-component coupling of amino alcohols, aryl halides, and *t*-Bu isocyanide in the presence of Pd catalyst. When 1,2-amino phenols were employed in place of amino alcohols the benzoxazoles were obtained **(Scheme 50)** [187].

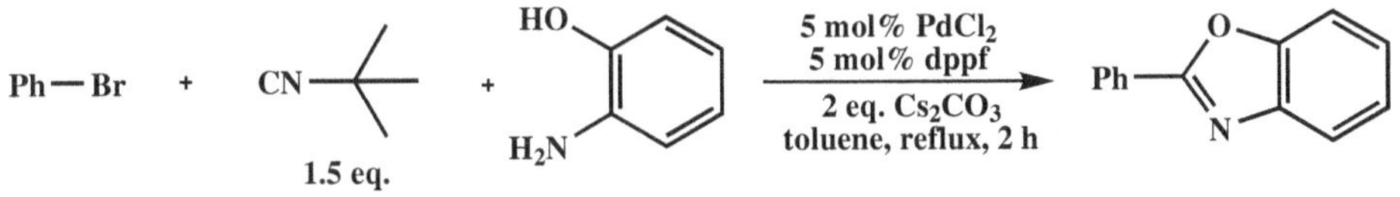

Scheme-50

The *N*-arylated five-, six- and seven-membered *N*-heterocycles were generated using sodium *tert*-butoxide as a base and *N,N′*-bis(2,6-diisopropylphenyl)dihydroimidazol-2-ylidene as a ligand for sequential Pd-catalyzed intra- followed by intermolecular aryl amination **(Scheme 51)** [188].

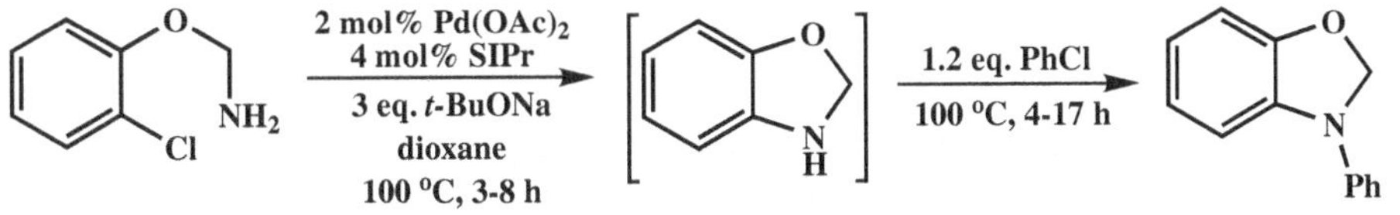

Scheme-51

The *gem*-dihaloalkenylaniline precursors were utilized. The highly functionalized indoles were prepared rapidly by intramolecular amination in the presence of Pd and/or Cu catalyst **(Scheme 52)**. The 2-heteroarylindoles were synthesized efficiently by direct carbon-hydrogen arylation processes [177, 189-195].

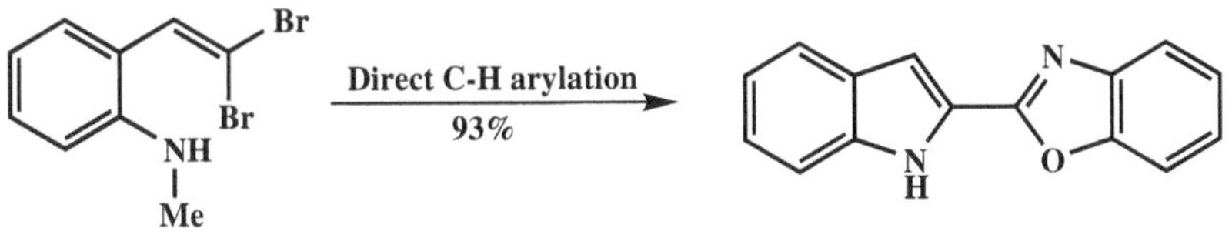

Scheme-52

Various transition metal catalysts including $Pd(PPh_3)_4$, $PdCl_2(PPh_3)_2$, $NiCl_2(PPh_3)_2$, $PtCl_2(PPh_3)_2$, $RuCl_2(PPh_3)_3$, and $RhCl(PPh_3)_3$ were utilized for the construction of indazoles from *N*-(2-nitro-benzylidene)amines under CO pressure [196-197]. It was found that 2*H*-indazoles were not produced in appreciable amounts in the presence of $Ru_3(CO)_{12}$ [198]. The reductive *N*-hetero-annulation of different nitroaromatics was carried out with transition metal catalyst in CO for the synthesis of other nitrogen heterocycles. Cenini [199] reported the catalytic reductive carbonylation of *o*-nitrobenzyl alcohols to prepare 1,4-dihydro-2*H*-3,1-benzoxyzin-2-one derivatives. In this type of reaction the selectivity of reaction was far superior with palladium(II) as compared to Ru catalyst [200-205]. The benzoxazol-2-one was synthesized by carbonylation of *o*-nitrophenol with mixed metal cluster-derived heterogeneous bimetallic catalysts like iron-palladium **(Scheme 53)** [206].

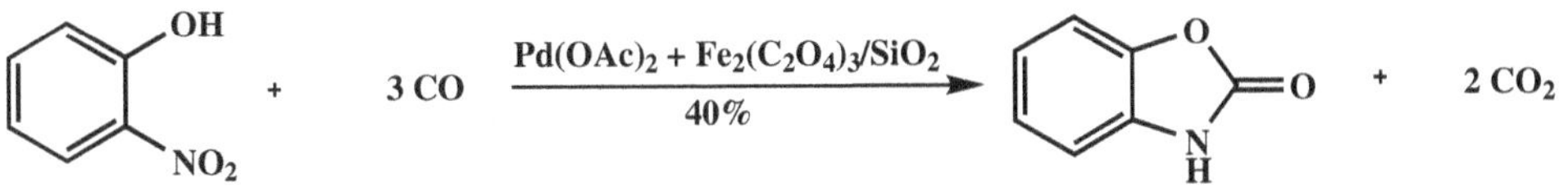

Scheme-53

The 2-(7-bromo-9,9-diethyl-2-fluorenyl)benzoxazole was synthesized by condensation of 2-bromo-7-formyl-9,9-diethylfluorene with 2-aminophenol. The 2-(7-(3-benzyloxydiphenylamino)-9,9-diethyl-2-fluorenyl)benzoxazole was formed when 2-(7-bromo-9,9-diethyl-2- fluorenyl) benzoxazole was reacted with 3-hydroxydiphenylamine in the presence of diphenylphos-phinoferrocene and Pd(dba)0. The 2-(7-(3-hydroxydiphenylamino)-9,9-diethyl-2-fluorenyl) benzoxazole was produced by debenzylation of 2-(7-(3-benzyloxydiphenylamino)-9,9-diethyl-2-fluorenyl)benzoxazole **(Scheme 54)** [207].

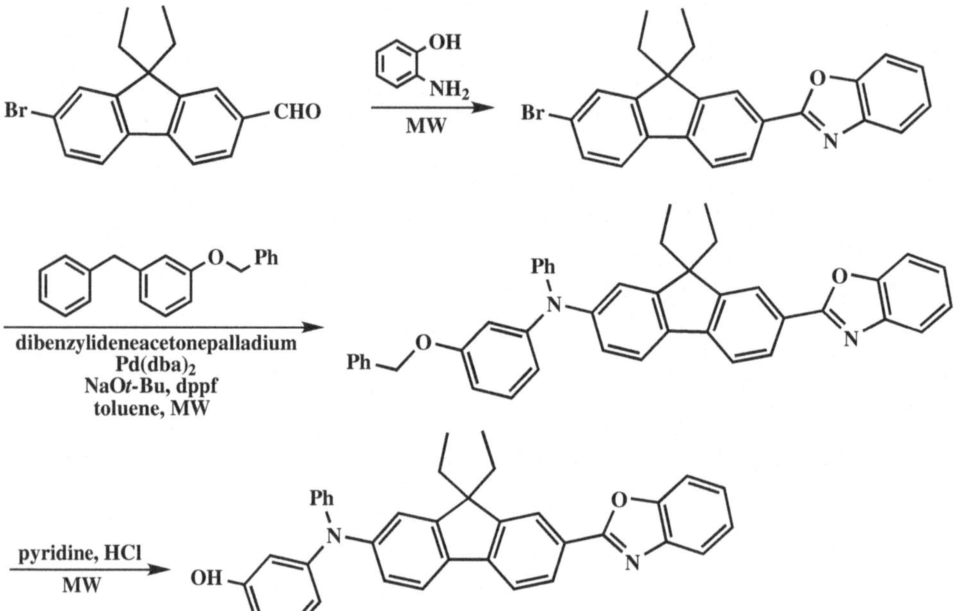

Scheme-54

6.6   Synthesis of five-membered *O,N*-heterocycles fused with aromatics

The benzodiazepine synthesis was not induced due to competitive nucleophilic attack on α-allyl complex by hydroxamate carbonyl oxygen **(Scheme 55)**. The nitrone underwent further reaction in the presence of many olefins in reaction mixture to afford the complex mixture of products. To avoid the competitive nucleophile problem the pKa of anthranilate NH was altered to facilitate a proton transfer from amine to hydroxamate at α-allyl complex stage. With this nucleophilicity of anthranilate nitrogen was increased and led to the synthesis of benzodiazepine. To lower the NH pKa, the amine was replaced with a sulfonamide [208].

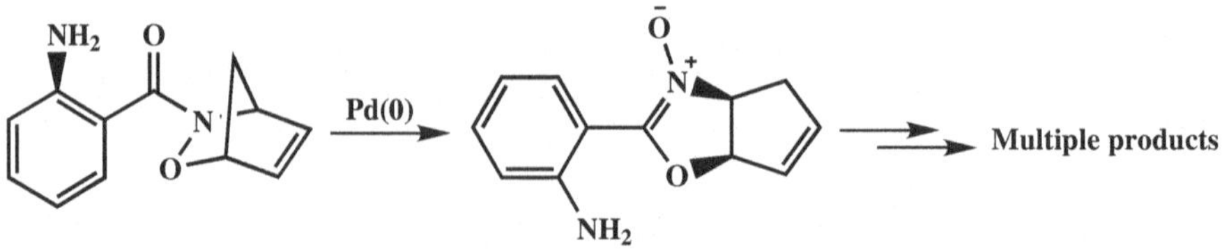

Scheme-55

The cyclopentene derivative was transformed to isoxazolidine to complement the traditional protocols for isoxazolidine synthesis. As shown in **Scheme 56**, using dipolar cycloaddition chemistry the major stereoisomer was produced with difficulty in this reaction [209-211], as nitrone would need to attack (with high regioselectivity in an electronically unbiased system) the more sterically hindered face of a 2-substituted cyclopentene dipolarophile [141, 212].

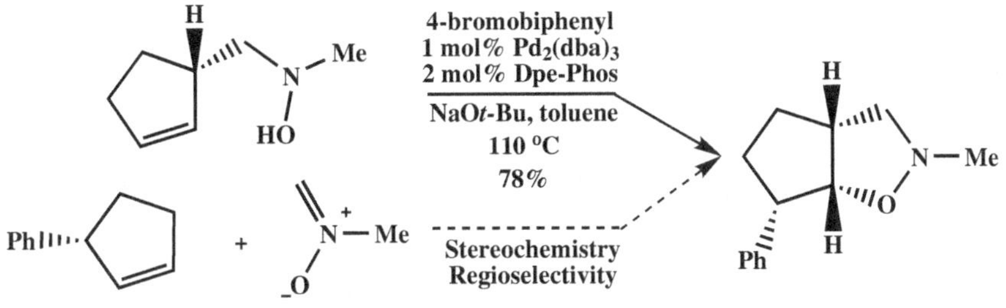

Scheme-56

6.7 Synthesis of five-membered *O,N*-heterocycles fused with other heterocycles

1,3-Oxazolidines are often employed as chiral auxiliaries in organic reactions and display unique biological activity in their own right. Therefore, myriad methods have been employed to synthesize diastereomerically pure 1,3-oxazolidines by condensation reactions of 1,2 amino alcohols and ketones **(Scheme 57)** [213-214]. However, stereoselectivity was often difficult to achieve, especially when the formation of 2,5-*cis*-1,3-oxazolidines was desired. To this end, various palladium-catalyzed methods and tandem reactions based on Michael additions have been developed [215-216]. Although the diastereoselectivity of these methods was high, carbon-carbon bond formation cannot be effected. Thus, a method that can achieve both high diastereoselectivity and concomitant carbon-heteroatom and carbon-carbon bond formation was required to produce libraries of 1,3-oxazolidine chiral auxiliaries for stereoselective syntheses.

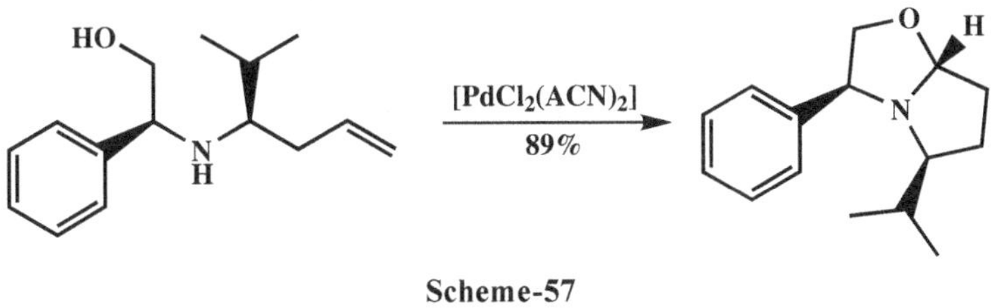

Scheme-57

Cochran [217] used substituted allylamine for the production of 7-tosyl-tetrahydro-1*H*-oxazolo[3,4-*a*]pyrazin-3(5*H*)-one in the presence of a halogenating agent, like *N*-bromosuccinimide or *N*-chlorosuccinimide and palladium catalyst **(Scheme 58)**. The method involved intramolecular haloamination followed by halide displacement by neighboring carbamate group [23].

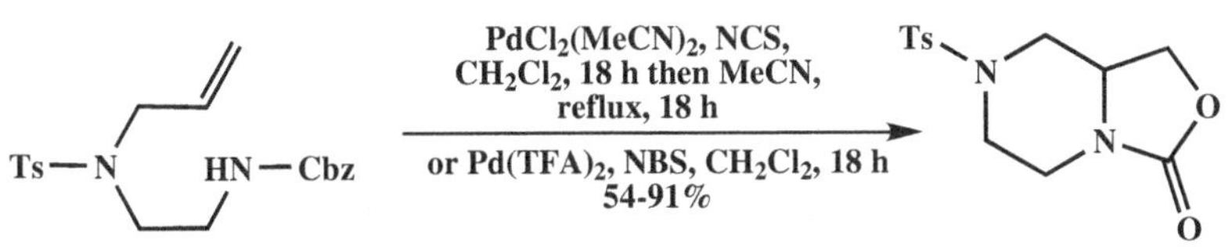

Scheme-58

REFERENCES

[1] (a) S. Cicchi, M. Cordero and D. Giomi. 2003. Five-membered ring systems: with O & N atoms. Prog. Heterocycl. Chem. 15: 261-283.
(b) N. Kaur. 2018. Copper catalysts in the synthesis of five-membered *N*-polyheterocycles. Curr. Org. Synth. 15: 940-971.
(c) N. Kaur. 2018. Recent developments in the synthesis of nitrogen-containing five-membered polyheterocycles using rhodium catalysts. Synth. Commun. 48: 2457-2474.
(d) N. Kaur. 2018. Ruthenium-catalyzed synthesis of five-membered *O*-heterocycles. Inorg. Chem. Commun. 99: 82-107.

[2] N. Sewald. 2003. Synthetic routes towards enantiomerically pure β-amino acids. Angew. Chem. Int. Ed. 42: 5794-5795.

[3] H.M.I. Osborn, N. Gemmell and L.M. Harwood. 2002. 1,3-Dipolar cycloaddition reactions of carbohydrate derived nitrones and oximes. J. Chem. Soc. Perkin Trans. 1 2419-2438.

[4] C. Thoms, R. Ebel and P. Proksch. 2006. Activated chemical defense in *Aplysina* sponges revisited. J. Chem. Ecol. 32: 97-123.

[5] T. Ogamino and S. Nishiyama. 2005. Synthesis and structural revision of calafianin, a member of the spiroisoxazole family isolated from the marine sponge *Aplysina gerardogreeni*. Tetrahedron Lett. 46: 1083-1086.

[6] C. Thoms, R. Ebel and P. Proksch. 2006. Sequestration and possible role of dietary alkaloids in the sponge-feeding mollusk *Tylodina perversa*. Prog. Mol. Subcell. Biol. 43: 261-275.

[7] N. Venkatesan, Y.J. Seo, E.K. Bang, S.M. Park, Y.S. Lee and B.H. Kim. 2006. Chemical modification of nucleic acids toward functional nucleic acid systems. Bull. Kor. Chem. Soc. 27: 613-630.

[8] C.A. Kontogiorgis and D. Hadjipavlou-Litina. 2004. Current trends in quantitative structure activity relationships on FXa inhibitors: evaluation and comparative analysis. Med. Res. Rev. 24: 687-747.

[9] M.L. Quan and R.R. Wexler. 2001. The design and synthesis of noncovalent factor Xa inhibitors. Curr. Top. Med. Chem. 1: 137-149.

[10] D. Simoni, G. Grisolia, G. Giannini, M. Roberti, R. Rondanin, L. Piccagli, R. Baruchello, M. Rossi, R. Romagnoli, F.P. Invidiata, S. Grimaudo, M.K. Jung, E. Hamel, N. Gebbia, L. Crosta, V. Abbadessa, A. Di Cristina, L. Dusonchet, M. Meli and M. Tolomeo. 2005. Heterocyclic and phenyl double-bond-locked combretastatin analogues possessing potent apoptosis-inducing activity in HL60 and in MDR cell lines. J. Med. Chem. 48: 723-736.

[11] Z. Mincheva, M. Courtois, J. Creche, M. Rideau and M.C. Viaud-Massuard. 2004. One-pot synthesis of functionalized 4,5-dihydroisoxazole derivatives *via* nitrile oxides and biological evaluation with plant cells. Bioorg. Med. Chem. 12: 191-197.

[12] M. Imran, S.A. Khan and N. Siddiqui. 2004. Therapeutic potential of 2-isoxazolines. Indian J. Pharm. Sci. 66: 377-381.

[13] A.G. Habeeb, P.N. Praveen Rao and E.E. Knaus. 2001. Design and synthesis of 4,5-diphenyl-4-isoxazolines: novel inhibitors of cyclooxygenase-2 with analgesic and anti-inflammatory activity. J. Med. Chem. 44: 2921-2927.

[14] C. Antczak, B. Bauvois, C. Monneret and J.C. Florent. 2001. A new acivicin prodrug designed for tumor-targeted delivery. Bioorg. Med. Chem. 9: 2843-2848.

[15] S.K. Bharti, G. Nath, R. Tilak and S.K. Singh. 2010. Synthesis, anti-bacterial and anti-fungal activities of some novel Schiff bases containing 2,4-disubstituted thiazole ring. Eur. J. Med. Chem. 45: 651-660.

[16] N. Selvakumar, G.G. Rajulu, K.C.S. Reddy, B.C. Chary, P.K. Kumar, T. Madhavi, K. Praveena, K.H.P. Reddy, M. Takhi, A. Mallick, P.V.S. Amarnath and S. Kandepu. 2008. Synthesis, SAR, and anti-bacterial activity of novel oxazolidinone analogues possessing urea functionality. Bioorg. Med. Chem. Lett. 18: 856-860.

[17] L. Djakovitch and P. Rouge. 2007. New homogeneously and heterogeneously [Pd/Cu]-catalyzed C3-alkenylation of free NH-indoles. J. Mol. Catal. A: Chem. 273: 230-239.

[18] B. Willy, F. Rominger and T.J.J. Muller. 2008. Novel microwave-assisted one-pot synthesis of isoxazoles by a three-component coupling-cycloaddition sequence. Synthesis 2: 293-303.

[19]   A.S. Karpov and T.J.J. Muller. 2003. New entry to a three-component pyrimidine synthesis by TMS-ynones *via* Sonogashira coupling. Org. Lett. 5: 3451-3454.

[20]   A.S. Karpov, E. Merkul, F. Rominger and T.J.J. Muller. 2005. Concise syntheses of meridianins *via* carbonylative alkynylation and a novel four-component pyrimidine synthesis. Angew. Chem. Inter. Ed. 44: 6951-6956.

[21]   B. Willy and T.J.J. Müller. 2008. Consecutive multi-component syntheses of heterocycles *via* palladium-copper catalyzed generation of alkynones. ARKIVOC (i): 195-208.

[22]   E.M. Beccalli, G. Broggini, M. Martinelli, N. Masciocchi and S. Sottocornola. 2006. New 4-spiroannulated tetrahydroisoquinolines by a one-pot sequential procedure. Isolation and characterization of σ-alkylpalladium Heck intermediates. Org. Lett. 8: 4521-4524.

[23]   S. Nag and S. Batra. 2011. Applications of allylamines for the syntheses of aza-heterocycles. Tetrahedron 67: 8959-9061.

[24]   Y.-H. Zhang and J.-Q. Yu. 2009. Pd(II)-catalyzed hydroxylation of arenes with 1 atm of O_2 or air. J. Am. Chem. Soc. 131: 14654-14655.

[25]   M.-K. Zhu, J.-F. Zhao and T.-P. Loh. 2010. Palladium-catalyzed oxime assisted intramolecular dioxygenation of alkenes with 1 atm of air as the sole oxidant. J. Am. Chem. Soc. 132: 6284-6285.

[26]   Z. Shi, C. Zhang, C. Tanga and N. Jiao. 2012. Recent advances in transition-metal catalyzed reactions using molecular oxygen as the oxidant. Chem. Soc. Rev. 41: 3381-3430.

[27]   V.A. Schmidt and E.J. Alexanian. 2010. Metal-free, aerobic dioxygenation of alkenes using hydroxamic acids. Angew. Chem. Int. Ed. 49: 4491-4494.

[28]   B.C. Giglio, V.A. Schmidt and E.J. Alexanian. 2011. Metal-free, aerobic dioxygenation of alkenes using simple hydroxamic acid derivatives. J. Am. Chem. Soc. 133: 13320-13322.

[29]   S.E. Denmark and J.M. Kallemeyn. 2005. Synthesis of 3,4,5-trisubstituted isoxazoles *via* sequential [3+2] cycloaddition/ silicon-based cross-coupling reactions. J. Org. Chem. 70: 2839-2842.

[30]   Y. Yoshida, T. Kurahashi and S. Matsubara. 2011. Nickel-catalyzed heteroannulation of *o*-haloanilines with alkynes. Chem. Lett. 40: 1067-1068.

[31]   B.R. Rosen, J.E. Ney and J.P. Wolfe. 2010. Use of aryl chlorides as electrophiles in Pd-catalyzed alkene difunctionalization reactions. J. Org. Chem. 75: 2756-2759.

[32]   (a) N.M. Fedou, P.J. Parsons, E.M.E. Viseux and A.J. Whittle. 2005. Multicomponent cascade reactions: sequential [1+4] and [2+3] cycloadditions for the generation of heterocyclic ring systems. Org. Lett. 7: 3179-3182.
       (b) I.N.N. Namboothiri and N. Rastogi. 2008. Isoxazolines from nitro compounds: synthesis and applications. Synthesis of heterocycles *via* cycloadditions, A. Hassner, Ed., Springer-Verlag, Germany, Top. Heterocycl. Chem. 12: 1-44.

[33]   E. Abele and E. Lukevics. 2000. Recent advances in the synthesis of heterocycles from oximes. Heterocycles 53: 2285-2326.

[34]   K. Maeda, T. Hosokawa, S.-I. Murahashi and I. Moritani. 1973. The reaction of α,β-unsaturated ketoximes into isoxazoles with palladium complexes. Tetrahedron Lett. 14: 5075-5076.

[35]   L. Djakovitch and P. Rollet. 2004. Sonogashira cross-coupling reactions catalyzed by copper-free palladium zeolites. Adv. Synth. Catal. 346: 1782-1792.

[36]   E. Grochowski and J. Jurczak. 1976. A new synthesis of *O*-alkylhydroxylamines. Synthesis 10: 682-684.

[37]   N.I. Totah and S.L. Schreiber. 1991. Thermodynamic spiroketalization as an efficient method of stereochemical communication. J. Org. Chem. 56: 6255-6256.

[38]   H. Iwagami, M. Yatagai, M. Nakazawa, H. Orita, Y. Honda, T. Ohnuki and T. Yukawa. 1991. Synthesis of a chiral α-(aminooxy)arylacetic ester. A route through a chiral 2-hydroxy-2-phenylacetic acid derivative. Bull. Chem. Soc. Jpn. 64: 175-182.

[39]   R.W. Bates, J. Boonsombat, Y. Lu, J.A. Nemeth, K. Sa-Ei, P. Song, M.P. Cai, P.B. Cranwell and S. Winbush. 2008. *N,O*-Heterocycles as synthetic intermediates. Pure Appl. Chem. 80: 681-685.

[40]   R.W. Bates and K. Sa-Ei. 2002. *O*-Alkenyl hydroxylamines: a new concept for cyclofunctionalization. Org. Lett. 4: 4225-4227.

[41]   E.M. Beccalli, G. Broggini, M. Martinelli and S. Sottocornola. 2007. C-C, C-O, C-N Bond formation on sp^2 carbon by Pd(II)-catalyzed reactions involving oxidant agents. Chem. Rev. 107: 5318-5365.

[42]   A. Das, A. Kulkarni and B. Torok. 2012. Environmentally benign synthesis of heterocyclic compounds by combined microwave-assisted heterogeneous catalytic approaches. Green Chem. 14: 17-34.

[43]   P.M. Wovkulich, F. Barcelos, A.D. Batcho, J.F. Sereno, E.G. Baggiolini, B.M. Hennessy and M.R. Uskokovic. 1984. Stereoselective total synthesis of 1α,25S,26-trihydroxycholecalciferol. Tetrahedron 40: 2283-2296.

[44]   B.M. Trost, J. Dumas and M. Villa. 1992. New strategies for the synthesis of vitamin D metabolites *via* palladium-catalyzed reactions. J. Am. Chem. Soc. 114: 9836-9845.

[45]   E. Merkul and T.J.J. Müller. 2006. A new consecutive three-component oxazole synthesis by an amidation-coupling-cycloisomerization (ACCI) sequence. Chem. Commun. 46: 4817-4819.

[46]   N.R. Deprez and M.S. Sanford. 2007. Reactions of hypervalent iodine reagents with palladium: mechanisms and applications in organic synthesis. Inorg. Chem. 46: 1924-1935.

[47]   L.V. Desai, K.L. Hull and M.S. Sanford. 2004. Palladium-catalyzed oxygenation of unactivated sp^3 C-H bonds. J. Am. Chem. Soc. 126: 9542-9543.

[48]   D. Kalyani and M.S. Sanford. 2005. Regioselectivity in palladium-catalyzed C-H activation/oxygenation reactions. Org. Lett. 7: 4149-4152.

[49]   D. Kalyani, A.R. Dick, W.Q. Anani and M.S. Sanford. 2006. A simple catalytic method for the regioselective halogenation of arenes. Org. Lett. 8: 2523-2526.

[50]   D.-H. Wang, X.-S. Hao, D.-F. Wu and J.-Q. Yu. 2006. Palladium-catalyzed oxidation of Boc-protected N-methylamines with IOAc as the oxidant: a Boc-directed sp^3 C-H bond activation. Org. Lett. 8: 3387-3390.

[51]   L.L. Welbes, T.W. Lyons, K.A. Cychosz and M.S. Sanford. 2007. Synthesis of cyclopropanes *via* Pd(II/IV)-catalyzed reactions of enynes. J. Am. Chem. Soc. 129: 5836-5837.

[52]   L.V. Desai and M.S. Sanford. 2007. Construction of tetrahydrofurans by PdII/PdIV-catalyzed aminooxygenation of alkenes. Angew. Chem. Int. Ed. 46: 5737-5740.

[53]   G. Liu and S.S. Stahl. 2006. Highly regioselective Pd-catalyzed intermolecular aminoacetoxylation of alkenes and evidence for *cis*-aminopalladation and S$_N$2 C-O bond formation. J. Am. Chem. Soc. 128: 7179-7181.

[54]   J. Streuff, C.H. Hoevelmann, M. Nieger and K. Muniz. 2005. Palladium(II)-catalyzed intramolecular diamination of unfunctionalized alkenes. J. Am. Chem. Soc. 127: 14586-14587.

[55]   K. Muniz, C.H. Hoevelmann and J. Streuff. 2008. Oxidative diamination of alkenes with ureas as nitrogen sources: mechanistic pathways in the presence of a high oxidation state palladium catalyst. J. Am. Chem. Soc. 130: 763-773.

[56]   R. Giri, X. Chen and J.-Q. Yu. 2005. Palladium-catalyzed asymmetric iodination of unactivated C-H bonds under mild conditions. Angew. Chem. Int. Ed. 44: 2112-2115.

[57]   O. Daugulis and V.G. Zaitsev. 2005. Anilide o-arylation by using C-H activation methodology. Angew. Chem. Int. Ed. 44: 4046-4048.

[58]   A.R. Dick, K.L. Hull and M.S. Sanford. 2004. A highly selective catalytic method for the oxidative functionalization of C-H bonds. J. Am. Chem. Soc. 126: 2300-2301.

[59]   A.R. Dick, J.W. Kampf and M.S. Sanford. 2005. Unusually stable palladium(IV) complexes: detailed mechanistic investigation of C-O bond-forming reductive elimination. J. Am. Chem. Soc. 127: 12790-12791.

[60]   D. Kalyani and M.S. Sanford. 2008. Oxidatively intercepting Heck intermediates: Pd-catalyzed 1,2- and 1,1-arylhalogenation of alkenes. J. Am. Chem. Soc. 130: 2150-2151.

[61]   D. Kalyani, A.R. Dick, W.Q. Anani and M.S. Sanford. 2006. Scope and selectivity in palladium-catalyzed directed C-H bond halogenation reactions. Tetrahedron 62: 11483-11498.

[62]   (a) V.V. Zhdankin. 2009. Hypervalent iodine(III) reagents in organic synthesis. ARKIVOC (i): 1-62.
       (b) M.S. Yusubov, V.N. Nemykin and V.V. Zhdankin. 2010. Transition metal-mediated oxidations utilizing monomeric iodosyl- and iodylarene species. Tetrahedron 66: 5745-5752.

[63] E.J. Alexanian, C. Lee and E.J. Sorensen. 2005. Palladium-catalyzed ring-forming aminoacetoxylation of alkenes. J. Am. Chem. Soc. 127: 7690-7691.

[64] R. Moran-Ramallal, R. Liz and V. Gotor. 2008. Regioselective and stereospecific synthesis of enantiopure 1,3-oxazolidin-2-ones by intramolecular ring opening of 2-(Boc-aminomethyl)aziridines. Preparation of the anti-biotic linezolid. Org. Lett. 10: 1935-1938.

[65] K.J. Fraunhoffer and M.C. White. 2007. *syn*-1,2-Amino alcohols *via* diastereoselective allylic C-H amination. J. Am. Chem. Soc. 129: 7274-7276.

[66] R.C. Larock, T.R. Hightower, L.A. Hasvold and K.P. Peterson. 1996. Palladium(II)-catalyzed cyclization of olefinic tosylamides. J. Org. Chem. 61: 3584-3585.

[67] A. Rudi, L. Chill, M. Aknin and Y. Kashman. 2003. Didmolamide A and B, two new cyclic hexapeptides from the marine ascidian *Didemnum molle*. J. Nat. Prod. 66: 575-577.

[68] S.-L. You, H. Razavi and J.W. Kelly. 2003. A biomimetic synthesis of thiazolines using hexaphenyloxodiphosphonium trifluoromethanesulfonate. Angew. Chem. Int. Ed. 42: 83-85.

[69] S.L. You and J.W. Kelly. 2005. Total synthesis of didmolamides A and B. Tetrahedron Lett. 46: 2567-2570.

[70] Z. Moussa. 2012. The Hendrickson 'POP' reagent and analogues thereof: synthesis, structure, and application in organic synthesis. ARKIVOC (i): 432-490.

[71] C. Bolm and J.P. Hilderbrand. 2000. Palladium-catalyzed *N*-arylation of sulfoximine with aryl bromides and aryl iodides. J. Org. Chem. 65: 169-175.

[72] C. Bolm and J.P. Hildebrand. 1998. Palladium-catalyzed carbon-nitrogen bond formation: a novel, catalytic approach towards *N*-arylated sulfoximines. Tetrahedron Lett. 39: 5731-5734.

[73] R.D. Dghaym, R. Dhawan and B.A. Arndtsen. 2001. The use of carbon monoxide and imines as peptide derivative synthons: a facile palladium-catalyzed synthesis of α-amino acid derived imidazolines. Angew. Chem. Int. Ed. 40: 3228-3230.

[74] R. Dhawan, R.D. Dghaym and B.A. Arndtsen. 2003. The development of a catalytic synthesis of münchnones: a simple four-component coupling approach to α-amino acid derivatives. J. Am. Chem. Soc. 125: 1474-1475.

[75] R. Dhawan and B.A. Arndtsen. 2004. Palladium-catalyzed multicomponent coupling of alkynes, imines, and acid chlorides: a direct and modular approach to pyrrole synthesis. J. Am. Chem. Soc. 126: 468-469.

[76] B.A. Arndtsen. 2009. Metal-catalyzed one-step synthesis: towards direct alternatives to multistep heterocycle and amino acid derivative formation. Chem. Eur. J. 15: 302-313.

[77] C.A. Merlic, A. Baur and C.C. Aldrich. 2000. Acylamino chromium carbene complexes: direct carbonyl insertion, formation of münchnones and trapping with dipolarophiles. J. Am. Chem. Soc. 122: 7398-7399.

[78] H. Alper and M. Tanaka. 1979. Novel syntheses of mesoionic compounds and α-amino acid derivatives from acyltetracarbonylferrates. J. Am. Chem. Soc. 101: 4245-4249.

[79] D.M. D'Souza and T.J.J. Muller. 2007. Multi-component syntheses of heterocycles by transition-metal catalysis. Chem. Soc. Rev. 36: 1095-1108.

[80] B. Alcaide, P. Almendros, T. Martinez del Campo and R. Rodriguez-Acebes. 2007. Diversity-oriented preparation of enantiopure spirocyclic 2-azetidinones from α-oxo-β-lactams through Barbier-type reactions followed by metal-catalyzed cyclizations. Adv. Synth. Catal. 349: 749-758.

[81] C. Jonasson, A. Horvath and J.-E. Backvall. 2000. Intramolecular palladium(II)-catalyzed 1,2-addition to allenes. J. Am. Chem. Soc. 122: 9600-9609.

[82] B. Alcaide and P. Almendros. 2011. Allenyl-β-lactams: versatile scaffolds for the synthesis of heterocycles. Chem. Rec. 11: 311-330.

[83] L.B. Wolf, K.C.M.F. Tjen, H.T. Brink, R.H. Blaauw, H. Hiemstra, H.E. Schoemaker and F.P.J.T. Rutjes. 2002. Palladium-catalyzed cyclization reactions of acetylene-containing amino acids. Adv. Synth. Catal. 344: 70-83.

[84] D. Bouyssi, M. Cavicchioli and G. Balme. 1997. Palladium-catalyzed synthesis of stereodefined 4-arylidene-3 tosyloxazolidin-2-ones from 2-propynyl tosylcarbamates and unsaturated halides (or triflate). Synlett 8: 944-946.

[85] P.A. Jacobi and H. Liu. 1999. Synthesis of 1,2,3,7,8,9-hexahydrodipyrrins and secocorrins: important precursors for the construction of corrins. Org. Lett. 1: 341-344.

[86] P.A. Jacobi and H. Liu. 2000. On the mechanism of Pd0-initiated coupling-cyclization of γ-aminoalkynes. J. Org. Chem. 65: 7676-7681.

[87] W.F.J. Karstens, M. Stol, F.P.J.T. Rutjes, H. Kooijman, A.L. Spek and H. Hiemstra. 2001. Palladium catalyzed cyclization reactions of acetylenic lactams. J. Organomet. Chem. 624: 244-258.

[88] A. Lei and X. Lu. 2000. Palladium(II)-catalyzed tandem intramolecular aminopalladation of alkynes and conjugate addition. Synthesis of oxazolidinones, imidazolidinones, and lactams. Org. Lett. 2: 2699-2702.

[89] G. Liu and X. Lu. 2001. Palladium(II)-catalyzed tandem reaction of intramolecular aminopalladation of allenyl N-tosylcarbamates and conjugate addition. Org. Lett. 3: 3879-3882.

[90] I. Kadota, A. Shibuya, L.M. Lutete and Y. Yamamoto. 1999. Palladium/benzoic acid catalyzed hydroamination of alkynes. J. Org. Chem. 64: 4570-4571.

[91] T.E. Muller, M. Grosche, E. Herdtweck, A.-K. Pleier, E. Walter and Y.-K. Yan. 2000. Developing transition-metal catalysts for the intramolecular hydroamination of alkynes. Organometallics 19: 170-183.

[92] G.B. Bajracharya, Z. Huo and Y. Yamamoto. 2005. Intramolecular hydroamination of alkynes catalyzed by Pd(PPh₃)₄/triphenylphosphine under neutral conditions. J. Org. Chem. 70: 4883-4886.

[93] I.W. Davies, D.I.C. Scopes and T. Gallagher. 1993. Metal ion-mediated heteroatom cyclizations. Application of aryl/alkenyl palladium(II)-based electrophilic triggers. Synlett 1: 85-87.

[94] S.-K. Kang, T.-G. Baik and A.N. Kulak. 1999. Palladium(0)-catalyzed coupling cyclization of functionalized allenes with hypervalent iodonium salts. Synlett 3: 324-326.

[95] S.-K. Kang, T.-G. Baik and Y. Hur. 1999. Palladium(0)-catalyzed coupling of allenyl N-tosylcarbamates with hypervalent iodonium salts. Tetrahedron 55: 6863-6870.

[96] W.F.J. Karstens, M. Stol, F.P.J.T. Rutjes and H. Hiemstra. 1998. Palladium-catalyzed cyclization of enantiopure allenic lactams prepared from a pyroglutamic acid derived organozinc reagent. Synlett 10: 1126-1128.

[97] W.F.J. Karstens, F.P.J.T. Rutjes and H. Hiemstra. 1997. Palladium-catalyzed coupling/cyclization reactions of allene-substituted lactams. Tetrahedron Lett. 38: 6275-6278.

[98] R. Grigg, C. Kilner, E. Mariani and V. Sridharan. 2006. Palladium-catalyzed cyclization-anion capture processes: *in situ* 'zipper' generation *via* intramolecular nucleophilic capture of π-allylpalladium species. Synlett 18: 3021-3024.

[99] M. Kimura, K. Fugami, S. Tanaka and Y. Tamaru. 1992. Palladium-catalyzed regio- and stereo-selective allylamination of allenic alcohols. J. Org. Chem. 57: 6377-6379.

[100] W.F.J. Karstens, D. Klomp, F.P.J.T. Rutjes and H. Hiemstra. 2001. N-Acyliminium ion chemistry and palladium catalysis: a useful combination to obtain bicyclic heterocycles. Tetrahedron 57: 5123-5130.

[101] C. Hyland. 2005. Cyclizations of allylic substrates *via* palladium catalysis. Tetrahedron 61: 3457-3471.

[102] N.T. Patil and Y. Yamamoto. 2006. Palladium catalyzed cascade reactions involving π-allyl palladium chemistry. Top. Organomet. Chem. 19: 91-113.

[103] B.M. Trost and A.R. Sudhakar. 1987. *Cis* hydroxyamination equivalent. Application to the synthesis of (-)-acosamine. J. Am. Chem. Soc. 109: 3792-3794.

[104] B.M. Trost and R. Hurnaus. 1989. On the mechanism of Pd(O) catalyzed formation of oxazolidin-2-ones from vinyl epoxides. Tetrahedron Lett. 30: 3893-3896.

[105] J.-G. Shim and Y. Yamamoto. 1999. A novel and effective route to 1,3-oxazolidine derivatives. Palladium-catalyzed regioselective [3+2] cycloaddition of vinylic oxiranes with imines. Tetrahedron Lett. 40: 1053-1056.

[106] K. Takahashi, N. Haraguchi, J. Ishihara and S. Hatakeyama. 2008. Synthetic studies directed toward kaitocephalin: a highly stereocontrolled route to the right-hand pyrrolidine core. Synlett 5: 671-674.

[107] Y. Noguchi, H. Uchiro, T. Yamada and S. Kobayashi. 2001. Synthetic study of polyoxypeptin: stereoselective synthesis of (2S,3R)-3-hydroxy-3-methylproline. Tetrahedron Lett. 42: 5253-5256.

[108] B. Gabriele, G. Salerno, M. Costa and G.P. Chiusoli. 2003. Recent developments in the synthesis of heterocyclic derivatives by PdI$_2$-catalyzed oxidative carbonylation reactions. J. Organomet. Chem. 687: 219-228.

[109] I. Chiarotto and M. Feroci. 2001. Palladium-catalyzed electrochemical carbonylation of 2-amino-1-alkanols to oxazolidin-2-ones under very mild conditions. Tetrahedron Lett. 42: 3451-3453.

[110] F. Li and C. Xia. 2004. Synthesis of 2-oxazolidinone catalyzed by palladium on charcoal: a novel and highly effective heterogeneous catalytic system for oxidative cyclocarbonylation of β-aminoalcohols and 2-aminophenol. J. Catal. 227: 542-546.

[111] B. Gabriele, G. Salerno, R. Mancuso and M. Costa. 2004. Efficient synthesis of ureas by direct palladium-catalyzed oxidative carbonylation of amines. J. Org. Chem. 69: 4741-4750.

[112] B. Gabriele, P. Plastina, G. Salerno, R. Mancuso and M. Costa. 2007. An unprecedented Pd-catalyzed, water-promoted sequential oxidative aminocarbonylation-cyclocarbonylation process leading to 2-oxazolidinones. Org. Lett. 9: 3319-3322.

[113] M. Yoshida, Y. Ohsawa, K. Sugimoto, H. Tokuyama and M. Ihara. 2007. Synthesis of vinyl-oxazolidinones by palladium-catalyzed CO$_2$-recycling reaction of 4-(benzylamino)-2-butenyl carbonates. Tetrahedron Lett. 48: 8678-8682.

[114] D. Fujino, S. Hayashi, H. Yorimitsu and K. Oshima. 2009. Palladium-catalyzed arylative cyclization of N-allylacetamides with aryl halides yielding benzyl-substituted oxazolines. Chem. Commun. 38: 5754-5756.

[115] A. Bacchi, M. Costa, B. Gabriele, G. Pelizzi and G. Salerno. 2002. Efficient and general synthesis of 5-(alkoxycarbonyl)methylene-3-oxazolines by palladium-catalyzed oxidative carbonylation of prop-2-ynylamides. J. Org. Chem. 67: 4450-4457.

[116] B. Gabriele, G. Salerno, D. Brindisi, M. Costa and G.P. Chiusoli. 2000. Synthesis of 2-oxazolidinones by direct palladium-catalyzed oxidative carbonylation of 2-amino-1-alkanols. Org. Lett. 2: 625-627.

[117] B. Gabriele, R. Mancuso, G. Salerno and M. Costa. 2003. An improved procedure for the palladium-catalyzed oxidative carbonylation of β-amino alcohols to oxazolidin-2-ones. J. Org. Chem. 68: 601-604.

[118] B.M. Trost. 1989. Cyclizations *via* palladium-catalyzed allylic alkylation. Angew. Chem. Int. Ed. Engl. 28: 1173-1192.

[119] X.-F. Wu, H. Neumann and M. Beller. 2013. Synthesis of heterocycles *via* palladium-catalyzed carbonylations. Chem. Rev. 113: 1-35.

[120] K. Inamoto, C. Hasegawa, K. Hiroya and T. Doi. 2008. Palladium-catalyzed synthesis of 2-substituted benzothiazoles *via* a C-H functionalization/intramolecular C-S bond formation process. Org. Lett. 10: 5147-5150.

[121] C. Larksarp and H. Alper. 1997. Palladium(0)-catalyzed asymmetric cycloaddition of vinyloxiranes with heterocumulenes using chiral phosphine ligands: an effective route to highly enantioselective vinyloxazolidine derivatives. J. Am. Chem. Soc. 119: 3709-3715.

[122] C. Larksarp and H. Alper. 1999. Synthesis of 1,3-oxazine derivatives by palladium-catalyzed cycloaddition of vinyloxetanes with heterocumulenes. Completely stereoselective synthesis of bicyclic 1,3-oxazines. J. Org. Chem. 64: 4152-4158.

[123] D.C.D. Butler, G.A. Inman and H. Alper. 2000. Room temperature ring-opening cyclization reactions of 2-vinylaziridines with isocyanates, carbodiimides, and isothiocyanates catalyzed by [Pd(OAc)$_2$]/PPh$_3$. J. Org. Chem. 65: 5887-5890.

[124] B.M. Trost and D.R. Fandrick. 2003. Dynamic kinetic asymmetric cycloadditions of isocyanates to vinylaziridines. J. Am. Chem. Soc. 125: 11836-11837.

[125] J.-G. Shim and Y. Yamamoto. 2000. A new synthetic route to 1,3-oxazolidines *via* palladium-catalyzed regioselective [3+2] cycloaddition of vinylic oxiranes with imines. Heterocycles 52: 885-895.

[126] (a) M. Kimura, Y. Wakamiya, Y. Horino and Y. Tamaru. 1997. Efficient synthesis of 4-ethenylidene-2-oxazolidinones *via* palladium-catalyzed aminocyclization of 2-butyn-1,4-diol biscarbamates. Tetrahedron Lett. 38: 3963-3966.

(b) T. Lu, Z. Lu, Z.-X. Ma, Y. Zhang and R.P. Hsung. 2013. Allenamides: a powerful and versatile building block in organic synthesis. Chem. Rev. 113: 4862-4904.

[127] L.E. Overman and T.P. Remarchuk. 2002. Catalytic asymmetric intramolecular aminopalladation: enantioselective synthesis of vinyl-substituted 2-oxazolidinones, 2-imidazolidinones, and 2-pyrrolidinones. J. Am. Chem. Soc. 124: 12-13.

[128] C.T. Walsh and G. Wright. 2005. Introduction: anti-biotic resistance. Chem. Rev. 105: 391-394.

[129] G. Zou, K. Reddy and J.R. Falck. 2001. Ag(I)-promoted Suzuki-Miyaura cross-coupling of *n*-alkylboronic acids. Tetrahedron Lett. 42: 7213-7215.

[130] J.R. Falck, P.S. Kumar, Y.K. Reddy, G. Zou and J.H. Capdevila. 2001. Stereospecific synthesis of EET metabolites *via* Suzuki-Miyaura coupling. Tetrahedron Lett. 42: 7211-7212.

[131] X. Cattoen and M.A. Pericas. 2007. Suzuki cross-coupling on enantiomerically pure epoxides: efficient synthesis of diverse, modular amino alcohols from single enantiopure precursors. J. Org. Chem. 72: 3253-3258.

[132] R. Martin and S.L. Buchwald. 2008. Palladium-catalyzed Suzuki-Miyaura cross-coupling reactions employing dialkylbiaryl phosphine ligands. Acc. Chem. Res. 41: 1461-1473.

[133] J.E. Ney and J.P. Wolfe. 2004. Palladium-catalyzed synthesis of *N*-aryl pyrrolidines from γ-(*N*-arylamino) alkenes: evidence for chemoselective alkene insertion into Pd-N bonds. Angew. Chem. Int. Ed. 43: 3605-3608.

[134] M.B. Bertrand, J.D. Neukom and J.P. Wolfe. 2008. Mild conditions for Pd-catalyzed carboamination of *N*-protected hex-4-enylamines and 1-, 3-, and 4-substituted pent-4-enylamines. Scope, limitations, and mechanism of pyrrolidine formation. J. Org. Chem. 73: 8851-8860.

[135] G.S. Lemen and J.P. Wolfe. 2010. Pd-catalyzed carboamination of oxazolidin-2-ones: a stereoselective route to *trans*-2,5-disubstituted pyrrolidines. Org. Lett. 12: 2322-2325.

[136] N.C. Giampietro and J.P. Wolfe. 2008. Stereoselective synthesis of *cis*- or *trans*-3,5-disubstituted pyrazolidines *via* Pd-catalyzed carboamination reactions: use of allylic strain to control product stereochemistry through *N*-substituent manipulation. J. Am. Chem. Soc. 130: 12907-12911.

[137] G.S. Lemen, N.C. Giampietro, M.B. Hay and J.P. Wolfe. 2009. Influence of hydroxylamine conformation on stereocontrol in Pd-catalyzed isoxazolidine-forming reactions. J. Org. Chem. 74: 2533-2540.

[138] J.A. Fritz and J.P. Wolfe. 2008. Stereoselective synthesis of imidazolidin-2-ones *via* Pd-catalyzed alkene carboamination. Scope and limitations. Tetrahedron 64: 6838-6852.

[139] J.S. Nakhla, D.M. Schultz and J.P. Wolfe. 2009. Palladium-catalyzed alkene carboamination reactions for the synthesis of substituted piperazines. Tetrahedron 65: 6549-6570.

[140] M.L. Leathen, B.R. Rosen and J.P. Wolfe. 2009. New strategy for the synthesis of substituted morpholines. J. Org. Chem. 74: 5107-5110.

[141] J.P. Wolfe. 2008. Stereoselective synthesis of saturated heterocycles *via* Pd-catalyzed alkene carboetherification and carboamination reactions. Synlett 19: 2913-2937.

[142] S.R. Chemler. 2009. The enantioselective intramolecular aminative functionalization of unactivated alkenes, dienes, allenes and alkynes for the synthesis of chiral nitrogen heterocycles. Org. Biomol. Chem. 7: 3009-3019.

[143] G. Zhang, L. Cui, Y. Wang and L. Zhang. 2010. Homogeneous gold-catalyzed oxidative carboheterofunctionalization of alkenes. J. Am. Chem. Soc. 132: 1474-1475.

[144] C.F. Rosewall, P.A. Sibbald, D.V. Liskin and F.E. Michael. 2009. Palladium-catalyzed carboamination of alkenes promoted by *N*-fluorobenzenesulfonimide *via* C-H activation of arenes. J. Am. Chem. Soc. 131: 9488-9489.

[145] D.C. Leitch, P.R. Payne, C.R. Dunbar and L.L. Schafer. 2009. Broadening the scope of group 4 hydroamination catalysis using a tethered ureate ligand. J. Am. Chem. Soc. 131: 18246-18247.

[146] A.L. Reznichenko and K.C. Hultzsch. 2010. C_2-Symmetric zirconium bis(amidate) complexes with enhanced reactivity in aminoalkene hydroamination. Organometallics 29: 24-27.

[147] J.-G. Roveda, C. Clavette, A.D. Hunt, S.I. Gorelsky, C.J. Whipp and A.M. Beauchemin. 2009. Hydrazides as tunable reagents for alkene hydroamination and aminocarbonylation. J. Am. Chem. Soc. 131: 8740-8741.

[148] M.R. Gagne, C.L. Stern and T.J. Marks. 1992. Organolanthanide-catalyzed hydroamination. A kinetic, mechanistic, and diastereoselectivity study of the cyclization of *N*-unprotected amino olefins. J. Am. Chem. Soc. 114: 275-294.

[149] J.D. Neukom, A.S. Aquino and J.P. Wolfe. 2011. Synthesis of saturated 1,4-benzodiazepines *via* Pd-catalyzed carboamination reactions. Org. Lett. 13: 2196-2199.

[150] A.S. Kende, K. Kawamura and R.J. DeVita. 1990. Enantioselective total synthesis of neooxazolomycin. J. Am. Chem. Soc. 112: 4070-4072.

[151] N. Henaff and A. Whiting. 1999. A convergent stereoselective total synthesis of racemic phthoxazolin A. Org. Lett. 1: 1137-1139.

[152] Z.-W. An, M. Catellani and G.P. Chiusoli. 1990. Palladium-catalyzed synthesis of aurone from salicyloyl chloride and phenylacetylene. J. Organomet. Chem. 397: 371-373.

[153] C.M. Shafer and T.F.J. Molinsky. 1998. Monosubstituted oxazoles. Synthesis of 5-substituted oxazoles by directed alkylation. Org. Chem. 63: 551-555.

[154] J.P. Marino and H.N. Nguyen. 2003. Copper-mediated regioselective allylation and propargylation of 2-(alkylthio)oxazoles. Tetrahedron Lett. 44: 7395-7398.

[155] S. Hatakeyama. 2009. Indium-catalyzed Conia-ene reaction for alkaloid synthesis. Pure Appl. Chem. 81: 217-226.

[156] A.V. Gulevich, A.G. Zhdanko, R.V.A. Orru and V.G. Nenajdenko. 2010. Isocyanoacetate derivatives: synthesis, reactivity, and application. Chem. Rev. 110: 5235-5331.

[157] M. Kimura, N. Saeki, S. Uchida, H. Harayama, S. Tanaka, H. Fugami and Y. Tamaru. 1993. Pd^{2+}-catalyzed oxidative aminocarbonylation of *O*-2,3-butadienyl and *O*-3,4 pentadienyl *N*-tosylcarbamates. Tetrahedron Lett. 34: 7611-7614.

[158] M. Kimura, S. Tanaka and Y. Tamaru. 1995. Palladium-catalyzed stereoselective allylaminocyclization and 1,3-butadien-2-ylaminocyclization of allenyl tosylcarbamates. J. Org. Chem. 60: 3764-3772.

[159] S. Danishefsky and E. Taniyama. 1983. Cyclizations of mercury and palladium substituted acyrylanilides. Tetrahedron Lett. 24: 15-18.

[160] Y. Tamaru, M. Hojo, H. Higashimura and Z. Yoshida. 1988. Urea as the most reactive and versatile nitrogen nucleophile for the palladium(2+)-catalyzed cyclization of unsaturated amines. J. Am. Chem. Soc. 110: 3994-4002.

[161] Y. Tamaru, M. Hojo and Z. Yoshida. 1988. Palladium(2+)-catalyzed intramolecular aminocarbonylation of 3-hydroxy-4-pentenylamines and 4-hydroxy-5-hexenylamines. J. Org. Chem. 53: 5731-5741.

[162] Y. Tamaru, H. Tanigawa, S. Itoh, M. Kimura, S. Tanaka, K. Fugami, T. Sekiyama and Z. Yoshida. 1992. Palladium(II)-catalyzed oxidative aminocarbonylation of unsaturated carbamates. Tetrahedron Lett. 33: 631-634.

[163] H. Harayama, H. Okuno, Y. Takahashi, M. Kimura, K. Fugami, S. Tanaka and Y. Tamaru. 1996. Chemoselective intramolecular aminocarbonylation of unsaturated amides under Wacker-type conditions. Tetrahedron Lett. 37: 7287-7290.

[164] H. Harayama, A. Abe, T. Sakado, M. Kimura, K. Fugami, S. Tanaka and Y. Tamaru. 1997. Palladium(II)-catalyzed intramolecular aminocarbonylation of *endo*-carbamates under Wacker-type conditions. J. Org. Chem. 62: 2113-2122.

[165] R.A.T.M. van Benthem, H. Hiemstra and W.N. Speckamp. 1992. Synthesis of *N*-Boc-protected 1-amino-3-alken-2-ols from allylic carbamates *via* palladium(II)-catalyzed oxidative cyclization. J. Org. Chem. 57: 6083-6085.

[166] R.A.T.M. van Benthem, H. Hiemstra, J.J. Michels and W.N. Speckamp. 1994. Palladium(II)-catalyzed oxidation of allylic amines with molecular oxygen. J. Chem. Soc. Chem. Commun. 3: 357-359.

[167] R.A.T.M. van Benthem, H. Hiemstra, P.W.N.M. van Leeuwen, J.W. Geus and W.N. Speckamp. 1995. Sulfoxide-stabilized giant palladium clusters in catalyzed oxidations. Angew. Chem. Int. Ed. 34: 457-460.

[168] A. Lei, X. Lu and G. Liu. 2004. A novel highly regio- and diastereoselective haloamination of alkenes catalyzed by divalent palladium. Tetrahedron Lett. 45: 1785-1788.

[169] L.F. Tietze, H. Ila and H.P. Bell. 2004. Enantioselective palladium-catalyzed transformations. Chem. Rev. 104: 3453-3516.

[170] A.B. Dounay and L.E. Overman. 2003. The asymmetric intramolecular Heck reaction in natural product total synthesis. Chem. Rev. 103: 2945-2964.

[171] C. Bolm, J.P. Hildebrand, K. Muniz and N. Hermanns. 2001. Catalyzed asymmetric arylation reactions. Angew. Chem. Int. Ed. 40: 3284-3308.

[172] N.-Y. Zhu and D. Yang. 2007. Catalytic asymmetric diamination of conjugated dienes and triene. J. Am. Chem. Soc. 129: 11688-11689.

[173] E. Merkul, O. Grotkopp and T.J.J. Muller. 2009. 2-Oxazol-5-ylethanones by consecutive three-component amidation-coupling-cycloisomerization (ACCI) sequence. Synthesis 3: 502-507.

[174] H.F. Wang, Y.M. Li, L.L. Jiang, R. Zhang, K. Jin, D.F. Zhao and C.Y. Duan. 2011. Ready synthesis of free N-H 2-arylindoles *via* the copper-catalyzed amination of 2-bromo-arylacetylenes with aqueous ammonia and sequential intramolecular cyclization. Org. Biomol. Chem. 9: 4983-4986.

[175] A. Prakash, M. Dibakar, K. Selvakumar, K. Ruckmani and M. Sivakumar. 2011. Efficient indoles and anilines syntheses employing *tert*-butyl sulfinamide as ammonia surrogate. Tetrahedron Lett. 52: 5625-5628.

[176] P.Y. Yao, Y. Zhang, R.P. Hsung and K. Zhao. 2008. A sequential metal-catalyzed C-N bond formation in the synthesis of 2-amido-indoles. Org. Lett. 10: 4275-4278.

[177] C.J. Ball and M.C. Willis. 2013. Cascade palladium- and copper-catalyzed aromatic heterocycle synthesis: the emergence of general precursors. Eur. J. Org. Chem. 425-441.

[178] B.M. Trost and A.R. Sudhakar. 1988. A stereoselective contrasteric conversion of epoxides to *cis*-oxazolidin-2-ones. J. Am. Chem. Soc. 110: 7933-7935.

[179] X. Lu. 2005. Control of the β-hydride elimination making palladium-catalyzed coupling reactions more diversified. Top. Catal. 35: 73-86.

[180] A. Lei, G. Liu and X. Lu. 2002. Palladium(II)-catalyzed highly regio- and diastereoselective cyclization of difunctional allylic N-tosylcarbamates. A convenient synthesis of optically active 4-vinyl-2-oxazolidinones and total synthesis of 1,4-dideoxy-1,4-imino-L-xylitol. J. Org. Chem. 67: 974-980.

[181] Y. Hirai, J. Watanabe, T. Nozaki, H. Yokoyama and S. Yamaguchi. 1997. Transition metal-mediated stereocontrolled cyclization of urethanes leading to versatile fused piperidines and its application to the synthesis of (+)-prosopinine and (+)-palustrine. J. Org. Chem. 62: 776-777.

[182] Y. Kozawa and M. Mori. 2002. Synthesis of different ring-size heterocycles from the same propargyl alcohol derivative by ligand effect on Pd(0). Tetrahedron Lett. 43: 1499-1502.

[183] H. Yokoyama and Y. Hirai. 2008. Palladium(II)-catalyzed cyclization *via* N-alkylation of an allyl alcohol with a urethane and its application to the syntheses of natural products. Heterocycles 75: 2133-2153.

[184] S.F. Kirsch and L.E. Overman. 2005. Catalytic asymmetric intramolecular aminopalladation: improved palladium(II) catalysts. J. Org. Chem. 70: 2859-2861.

[185] D. Kadzimirsz, D. Hildebrandt, K. Merz and G. Dyker. 2006. Isoindoles and dihydroisoquinolines by gold-catalyzed intramolecular hydroamination of alkynes. Chem. Commun. 6: 661-662.

[186] C.F. Bender and R.A. Widenhoefer. 2005. Platinum-catalyzed intramolecular hydroamination of unactivated olefins with secondary alkylamines. J. Am. Chem. Soc. 127: 1070-1071.

[187] P.J. Boissarie, Z.E. Hamilton, S. Lang, J.A. Murphy and C.J. Suckling. 2011. A powerful palladium-catalyzed multicomponent process for the preparation of oxazolines and benzoxazoles. Org. Lett. 13: 6184-6187.

[188] R. Omar-Amrani, R. Schneider and Y. Fort. 2004. Novel synthetic strategy of N-arylated heterocycles *via* sequential palladium-catalyzed intra- and inter-arylamination reactions. Synthesis 15: 2527-2534.

[189] A. Fayol, Y.-Q. Fang and M. Lautens. 2006. Synthesis of 2-vinylic indoles and derivatives *via* a Pd-catalyzed tandem coupling reaction. Org. Lett. 8: 4203-4206.

[190] T.O. Viera, L.A. Meaney, Y.-L. Shi and H. Alper. 2008. Tandem palladium-catalyzed N,C-coupling/carbonylation sequence for the synthesis of 2-carboxyindoles. Org. Lett. 10: 4899-4901.

[191] M. Nagamochi, Y.Q. Fang and M. Lautens. 2007. A general and practical method of alkynyl indole and benzofuran synthesis *via* tandem Cu- and Pd-catalyzed cross-couplings. Org. Lett. 9: 2955-2958.

[192] M. Arthuis, R. Pontikis and J.-C. Florent. 2009. Palladium-catalyzed domino C,N-coupling/carbonylation/Suzuki coupling reaction: an efficient synthesis of 2-aroyl-/heteroaroylindoles. Org. Lett. 11: 4608-4611.

[193] W. Chen, M. Wang, P. Li and L. Wang. 2011. Highly efficient copper/palladium-catalyzed tandem Ullman reaction/arylation of azoles *via* C-H activation: synthesis of benzofuranyl and indolyl azoles from 2-(*gem*-dibromovinyl)phenols(anilines) with azoles. Tetrahedron 67: 5913-5919.

[194] J. Cho, Y.M. Lee, D. Kim and S. Kim. 2009. Design and synthesis of piperidine-containing sphingoid base analogues. J. Org. Chem. 74: 3900-3904.

[195] Y. Nagahara, T. Shinomiya, S. Kuroda, N. Kaneko, R. Nishio and M. Ikekita. 2005. Phytosphingosine induced mitochondria-involved apoptosis. Cancer Sci. 96: 83-92.

[196] M. Akazome, T. Kondo and Y. Watanabe. 1994. Palladium complex-catalyzed reductive *N*-heterocyclization of nitroarenes: novel synthesis of indole and 2*H*-indazole derivatives. J. Org. Chem. 59: 3375-3380.

[197] M. Akazome, T. Kondo and Y. Watanabe. 1991. Palladium complex-catalyzed reductive *N*-hetero-cyclization of *N*-(2-nitrobenzylidene)amines into 2*H*-indazole derivatives. J. Chem. Soc. Chem. Commun. 20: 1466-1467.

[198] F. Ragaini, P. Sportiello and S. Cenini. 1999. Investigation of the possible role of arylamine formation in the *o*-substituted nitroarenes reductive cyclization reactions to afford heterocycles. J. Organomet. Chem. 577: 283-291.

[199] S. Cenini, S. Console, C. Crotti and S. Tolari. 1993. Metal catalyzed deoxygenation by carbon monoxide of *o*-substituted nitrobenzenes. Synthesis of 1,4-dihydro-2*H*-3,1-benzoxazin-2-one derivatives. J. Organomet. Chem. 451: 157-162.

[200] M. Akazome, T. Kondo and Y. Watanabe. 1992. Novel synthesis of indoles *via* palladium-catalyzed reductive *N*-heterocyclization of *o*-nitrostyrene derivatives. Chem. Lett. 5: 769-772.

[201] R. Han, S. Chen, S.J. Lee, F. Qi, X. Wu and B.H. Kim. 2006. Indium-mediated reductive cyclization of 2-nitrochalcones to quinolines. Heterocycles 68: 1675-1684.

[202] C. Crotti, S. Cenini, A. Bossoli, B. Rindone and F. Demartin. 1991. Synthesis of carbazole by $Ru_3(CO)_{12}$-catalyzed reductive carbonylation of 2-nitrobiphenyl: the crystal and molecular structure of $Ru_3(\mu_3-NC_6H_4-o-C_6H_5)_2(CO)_9$. J. Mol. Catal. 70: 175-187.

[203] M. Pizzotti, S. Cenini, S. Quici and S. Tollari. 1994. Role of alkali halides in the synthesis of nitrogen containing heterocycles by reductive carbonylation of aromatic nitro-derivatives catalyzed by $Ru_3(CO)_{12}$. J. Chem. Soc. Perkin Trans. 2 4: 913-917.

[204] J.H. Smitrovich and I.W. Davies. 2004. Catalytic C-H functionalization driven by CO as a stoichiometric reductant: application to carbazole synthesis. Org. Lett. 6: 533-535.

[205] J.E. Kmiecik. 1965. Reduction of organic compounds by carbon monoxide. The reductive coupling of aromatic nitro compounds. J. Org. Chem. 30: 2014-2020.

[206] P. Braunstein, J. Kervennal and J.L. Richert. 1985. Reductive carbonylation of *o*-nitrophenol with a Fe-Pd cluster derived heterogeneous catalyst; CO migration in $[FePdPt(CO)_4(Ph_2PCH_2PPh_2)_2]$. Angew. Chem. Int. Ed. 24: 768-770.

[207] N. Saroja, E. Laxminarayana, K.R.S. Prasad and J.V.S. Kumar. 2012. Microwave assisted synthesis of 2-(7-(3-hydroxydiphenylamino)-9,9-diethyl-2-fluorenyl)benzothiazole and 2-(7-(3-hydroxydiphenyl-amino)-9,9-diethyl-2-fluorenyl)benzoxazoles. Der Pharm. Chem. 4: 690-693.

[208] M.D. Surman, M.J. Mulvihill and M.J. Miller. 2002. Novel 1,4-benzodiazepines from acylnitroso-derived hetero-Diels-Alder cycloadducts. Org. Lett. 4: 139-141.

[209] P.N. Confalone and E.M. Huie. 1988. The [3+2] nitrone-olefin cycloaddition reaction. Org. React. 36: 1-173.

[210] K.V. Gothelf and K.A. Jorgensen. 2000. Catalytic enantioselective 1,3-dipolar cycloaddition reactions of nitrones. Chem. Commun. 16: 1449-1458.

[211] S. Kanemasa. 2002. Metal-assisted stereocontrol of 1,3-dipolar cycloaddition reactions. Synlett 9: 1371-1387.

[212] J.P. Wolfe. 2006. Stereoselective synthesis of saturated heterocycles *via* Pd-catalyzed alkene carboetherification and carboamination reactions. Synlett 4: 571-582.

[213] C. Wolf and H. Xu. 2011. Asymmetric catalysis with chiral oxazolidine ligands. Chem. Commun. 47: 3339-3350.

[214] S. Gandhi, A. Bisai, B.A. Bhanu Prasad and V.K. Singh. 2007. Studies on the reaction of aziridines with nitriles and carbonyls: synthesis of imidazolines and oxazolidines. J. Org. Chem. 72: 2133-2142.

[215] S. Fioravanti, F. Marchetti, L. Pellacani, L. Ranieri and P.A. Tardella. 2008. Stereoselective aza-MIRC reactions on optically active (*E*)-nitro alkenes. Tetrahedron: Asymmetry 19: 231-236.

[216] W. Adam, T. Wirth, A. Pastor and K. Peters. 1998. Dramatic diastereoselectivity differences in the asymmetric ene reactions of triazolinediones and singlet oxygen with chiral 2,2-dimethyloxazolidine derivatives of tiglic acid. Eur. J. Org. Chem. 3: 501-506.

[217] F.E. Michael, P.A. Sibbald and B.M. Cochran. 2008. Palladium-catalyzed intramolecular chloroamination of alkenes. Org. Lett. 10: 793-796.

Chapter 7

Six-Membered N-Heterocycles

7.1 Introduction

Heterocycles and implicit nitrogen-containing heterocycles are becoming very important in all aspects of applied and pure chemistry. Development of new synthetic methodology, isolation from natural sources, finding modern applications of various heterocycles in pharmaceutical field, in chemistry, industry or medicine are the subjects which are intensively described and studied by biologists, chemists, and researchers [1a-d]. Heterocycles are not only important due to their abundance in organic chemistry but they are also very important for their biological, chemical, and technological applications. For many decades, N-heterocycles are utilized as medicinal compounds, and form the basis for various drugs like captopril (hypertension), morphine (analgesic), and vincristine (cancer chemotherapy) [2-4].

The six-membered heterocyclic compounds are pharmaceutical actives. Six-membered heterocycles like substituted pyridines possess a wide range of pharmacological activity. They are utilized to modulate anginapectoris, hypertension, anti-diabetic, act as Ca^{2+} channel blockers, anti-tumor, and heptaprotective properties. In addition, pyridine derivatives are also utilized as organocatalysts and organic bases in organic synthesis. The fused quinoline functionality is also present in a number of biologically active and naturally occurring compounds [5-16].

In this chapter, I have focused on applications of palladium for the generation of many six-membered N-heterocycles. Palladium-mediated synthesis of different heterocycles is classified into following categories based on the type of rings.

7.2 Palladium assisted synthesis of six-membered heterocycles with nitrogen heteroatom

7.3 Synthesis of six-membered nitrogen-containing heterocycles

Substituted pyridines were prepared *via* one-pot domino cyclization-oxidative aromatization in the presence of bifunctional noble metal-solid acid catalyst, palladium/carbon/K-10 montmorillonite under MWI. The cyclization occurred readily with strong solid acid while Pd dehydrogenated the dihydropyridine intermediate (**Scheme 1**) [17].

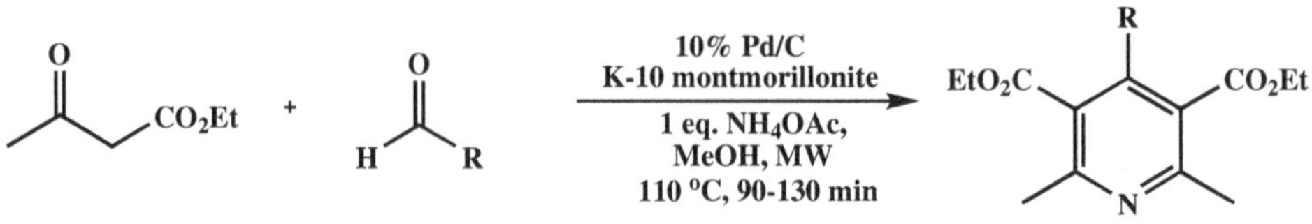

Scheme-1

Harrity [18] used chiral aziridines and TMM for the preparation of chiral piperidines *via* a novel [3+3]-cycloaddition reaction **(Scheme 2)**. Enantiopure piperidines were obtained stereoselectively in good yield *via* Pd-catalyzed cycloaddition. Enantiopure piperidines act as precursors in the short natural product synthesis of (-)-pseudoconhydrine.

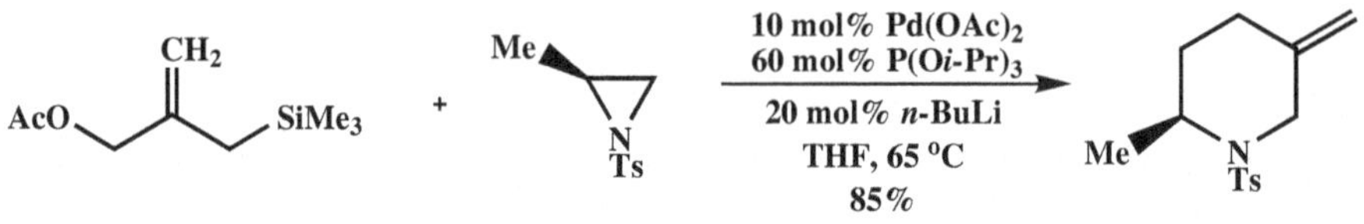

Scheme-2

The stereogenic centre of product arises from L-serine-derived organozinc reagent [19]. Pd-mediated coupling of organozincate with acryloyl chloride generated the terminal enone directly **(Scheme 3)**. The exposure of enone containing α-amino acid to anhydrous, acidic conditions promoted the 6-*endo-trig* cyclization to give 4-oxopipecolic acid benzyl ester in quantitative yield.

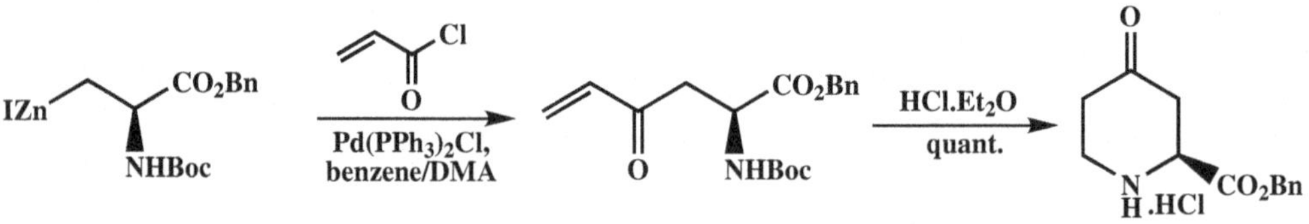

Scheme-3

An organopalladium(II) intermediate was produced upon oxidative addition of palladium(0) catalyst to the starting species (triflate, halide, acetate etc). During the synthesis of one ring this intermediate successively engaged the anion capture agent and the terminating species. Before passing to the terminating phase and then anion capture the initial organopalladium(II) intermediate engaged one or more relay species in polycyclization processes. This was illustrated for biscyclization of an aryl starter species in **Scheme 4**. The *exo*-cyclization to generate the smallest ring was invariably preferred over *endo*-cyclization [20].

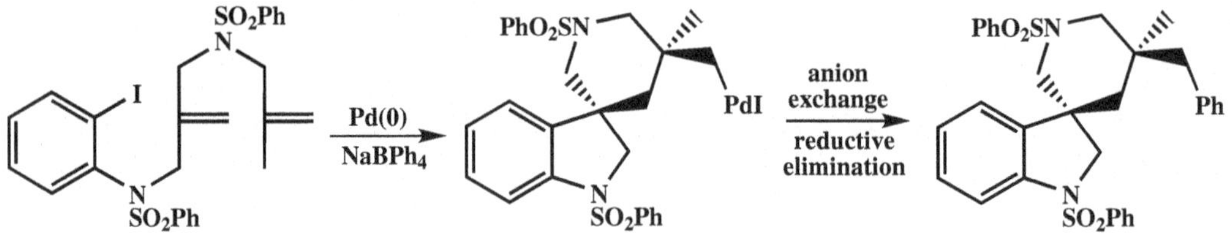

Scheme-4

The sedamine was generated as shown in **Scheme 5** [21-22]. Isoxazolidine was prepared in optically active fashion by asymmetric allylation of benzaldehyde with isoxazolidine and the additional carbon atoms were installed by a reduction-Wittig sequence. A hydroxy lactam was obtained as a single isomer by a tandem double hydrogenation-lactamization. The hydroxy lactam then formed sedamine utilizing simple manipulations [23-26].

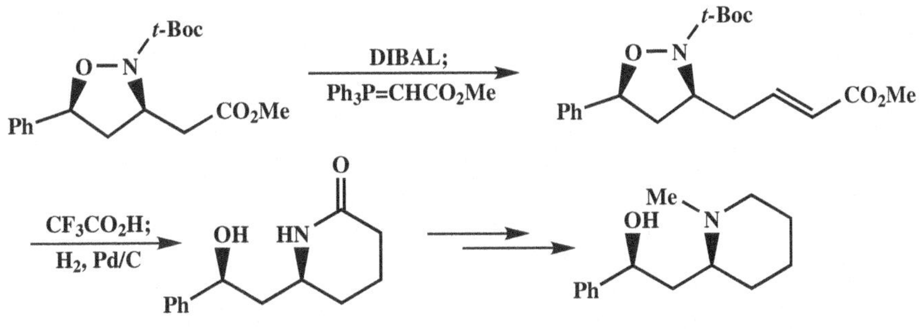

Scheme-5

Eriksson and co-workers [27] used carbamate for the synthesis of hydroxylamine derivative; in turn carbamate was prepared from allyl carbamate. The 2-methyl tetrahydropyridine-*N*-oxide was formed by an acid-catalyzed intramolecular condensation with masked aldehyde, then the 2-methyl tetrahydropyridine-*N*-oxide was converted into naturally occurring alkaloids dihydropinidine, potential anti-feedants against the pine weevil, *Hylobius abietis* (**Scheme 6**) [28].

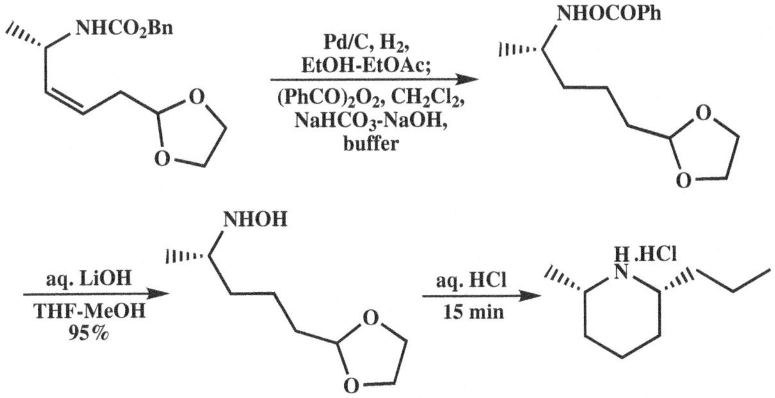

Scheme-6

Kim et al. [29] synthesized tetrahydropyridines in moderate yields (in addition to isoquinolines) from cyclization of amides in the presence of palladium catalyst (**Scheme 7**) [28].

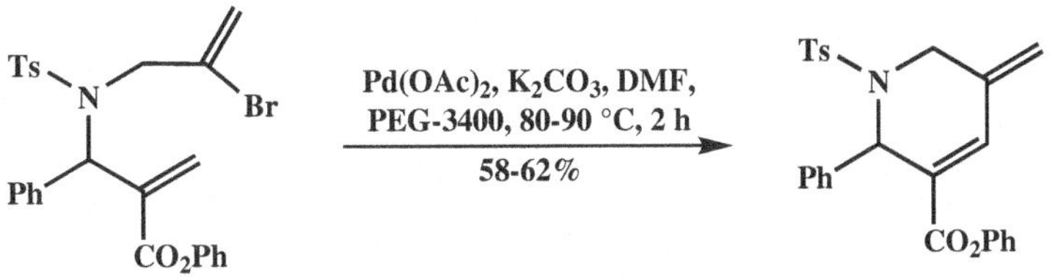

Scheme-7

Bukovec and Kazmaier [30] reported Stille coupling of stannylated allylamine with iodoacrylate for the synthesis of a six-membered lactam in the presence of [Pd(allyl)Cl]$_2$PPh$_3$ catalyst (**Scheme 8**) [28].

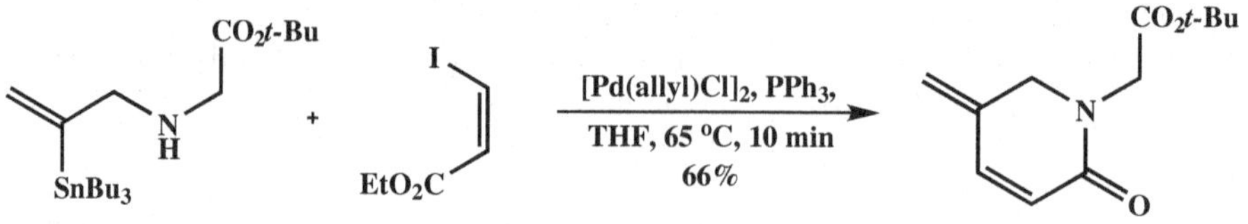

Scheme-8

Gabriele and co-workers [31] synthesized carbonyl derivatives, like (pyridine-2-one)-3-acetic amides *via* palladium iodide-potassium iodide-catalyzed oxidative carbonylation of (Z)-(2-ene-4-ynyl)amines, on the basis of reaction conditions and substituents present on substrate **(Scheme 9)**. In most of the cases, the use of an excess of carbon dioxide was beneficial to product selectivity as well as reaction rate [28].

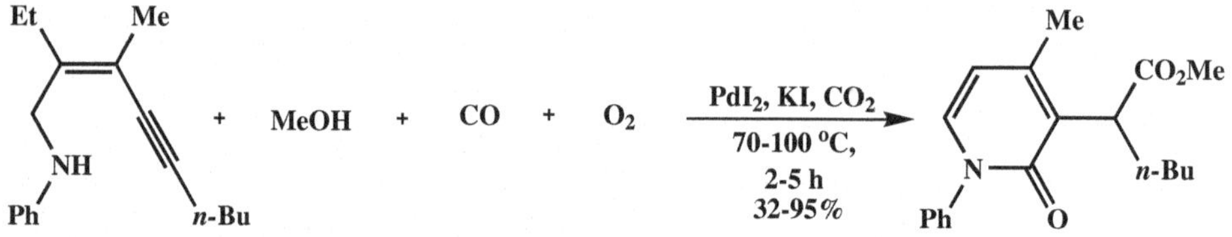

Scheme-9

Webber and Krische [32] modified the protocol with enoneallyl carbonates for easy synthesis of *N*-protected piperidines **(Scheme 10)**. The electrophilic features of TsujieTrost reaction and nucleophilic features of Morita-Baylis-Hillman reaction were combined in this palladium(0)-catalyzed enone cycloallylation reaction [28].

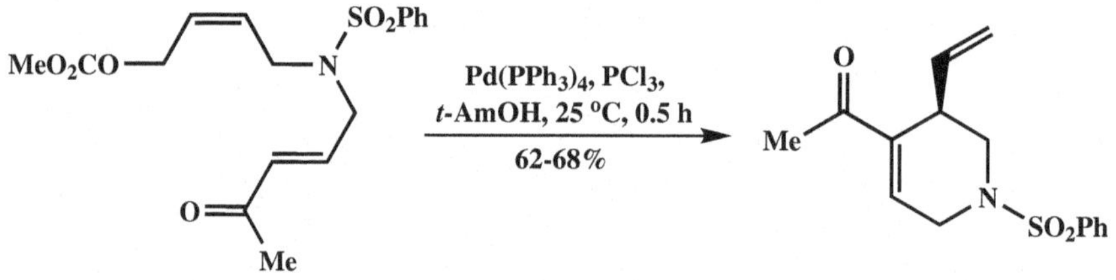

Scheme-10

Guillot [33] synthesized azabicyclo[3.1.0]hexan-1-ols *via* Kulinkovich cyclopropanation reaction from many unnatural and natural β-amino acid derivatives. The ring cleavage and subsequent rearrangement of azabicyclo[3.1.0]hexan-1-ols formed diverse intermediates like piperidinones, pyrrolidinones, dihydropiperidinones, pyridines, and tricyclic piperidinones **(Scheme 11)**. These diverse intermediates were used in pharmaceuticals [28].

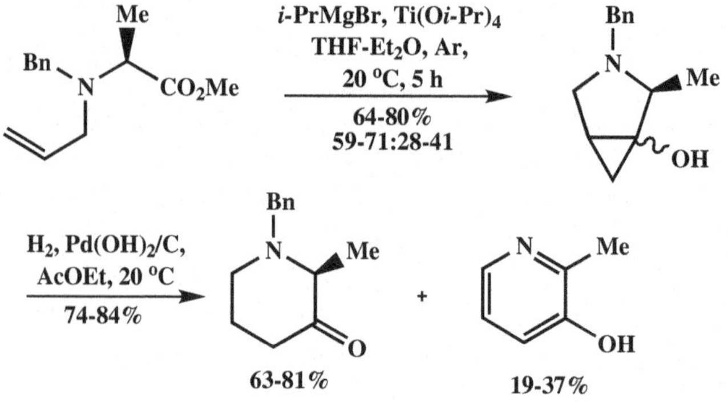

Scheme-11

The chalcones provided an excellent pathway to novel syntheses of heterocyclic compounds in one-pot synthetic protocols. As heterodienes, chalcones were synthesized by a subsequent Diels-Alder reaction with inverse electron demand to afford cycloadduct which upon hydrolyses provided 1,5-diketones. However, upon addition of CH_3COOH and ammonium chloride the same cycloadduct acted as a key intermediate in consecutive CIR-cycloaddition-cyclocondensation sequence for the preparation of highly annelated or substituted pyridines **(Scheme 12)** [34-36].

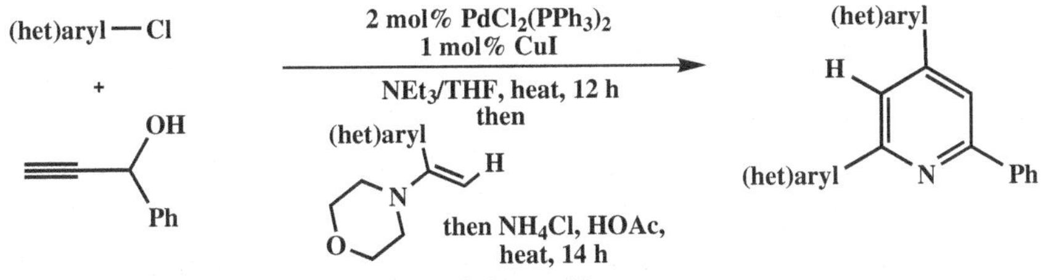

Scheme-12

Fluorination of alkenes was carried out with Pd catalysts. Liu et al. [37-39] reported an oxidative fluoroamination of alkenes with Pd catalyst (mechanistically similar to oxidative chlorination of alkenes) [40-41]. Various fluorinated piperidine derivatives were formed with high regio-selectivity. The reaction involved (1) *trans*-aminopalladation of alkenes, (2) oxidation of Csp^3-palladium(II) intermediate to Csp^3-palladium(IV)(F), and (3) reductive elimination of Csp^3-palladium(IV)(F) intermediate. The final C-F bond was formed through a direct reductive elimination strategy **(Scheme 13)**. The C-F bond formed with F^+ reagent and the reaction occurred by oxidative fluorination of carbon-palladium bond with inorganic fluoride salt and oxidant. For this conversion both hypervalent iodide reagent and AgF were crucial. The fluorination product was not afforded when *N*-aryl acryamide was reacted at slightly higher temperatures in the presence of $AgF/PhI(OPiv)_2$ catalytic system. Instead, carbon-hydrogen bond activation of CH_3CN was reported, and AgF played the role of Lewis acid as well as base [42].

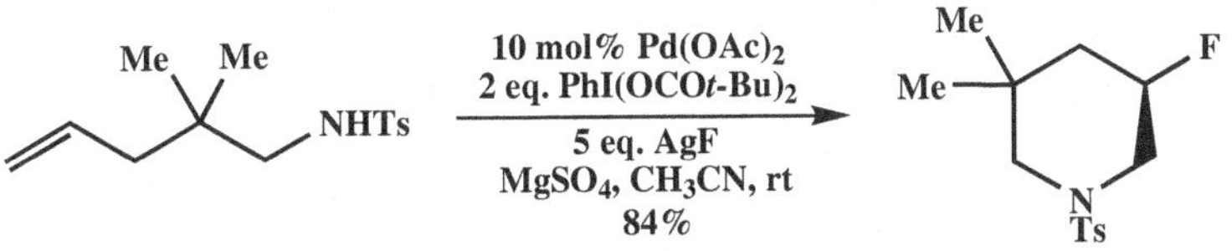

Scheme-13

Alkenes were utilized as precursors for the synthesis of 1,4-DHPs. Jiang and co-workers [43] in 2011 used amines, aldehydes, and electron deficient alkenes for multi-component preparation of 1,4-dihydropyridines directly in the presence of Pd(II) catalyst under oxygen atmosphere. The 1,4-dihydropyridines were observed in moderate to good yields. In contrast to benzaldehyde derivatives, heteroaromatic aldehydes did not work well and afforded the products in lower yields **(Scheme 14)** [44].

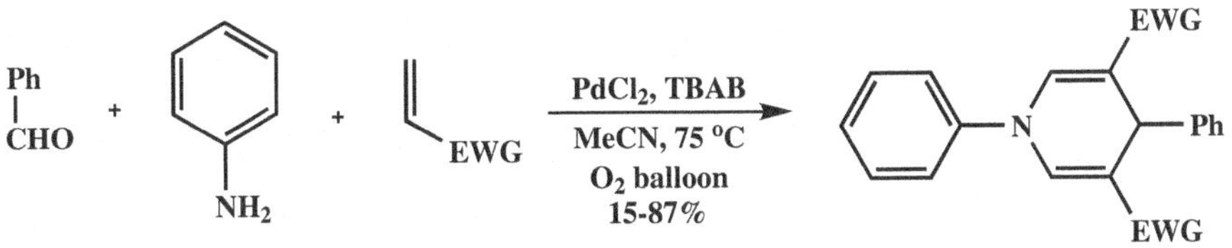

Scheme-14

Electron rich alkenes produced enaminone intermediates which synthesized 2,6-unsubstituted 1,4-dihydropyridines. Fair to good yields of 1,4-dihydropyridines were provided in the presence of Lewis acid Sc(OTf)$_3$. However, the main drawbacks of this protocol were reaction time (2-19 d), presence of enaminone intermediates and other side products **(Scheme 15)** [44-45].

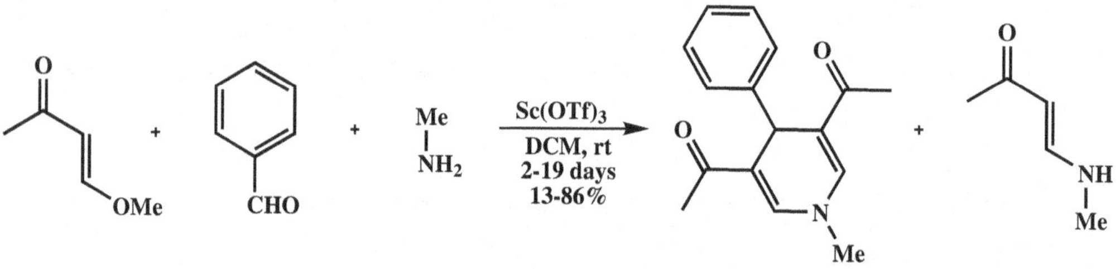

Scheme-15

Unsaturated α-ketoesters and α-ketoamides underwent intramolecular oxidative cyclization under aerobic condition in the presence of Pd catalyst and Yb(OTf)$_3$ [46-47]. The Yb(OTf)$_3$ acted as a Lewis acid to enhance the nucleophilicity of substrate toward palladium(II)-activated olefin and to promote the enolization of substrate **(Scheme 16)**. A number of six-, seven-, and eight-membered nitrogen and oxygen heterocycles were synthesized regioselectively in good yields under very mild conditions [48].

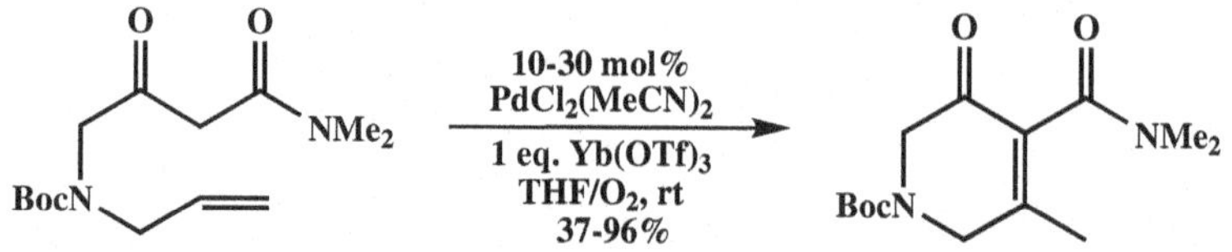

Scheme-16

The cyclization of hex-5-enylamine under Wacker-type conditions afforded nitrogenated heterocyclic compounds **(Scheme 17)**. The cyclic imines were obtained from other alkenes containing a primary or secondary amino group, while aminoketones were products of tertiary aminoalkenes [48-49].

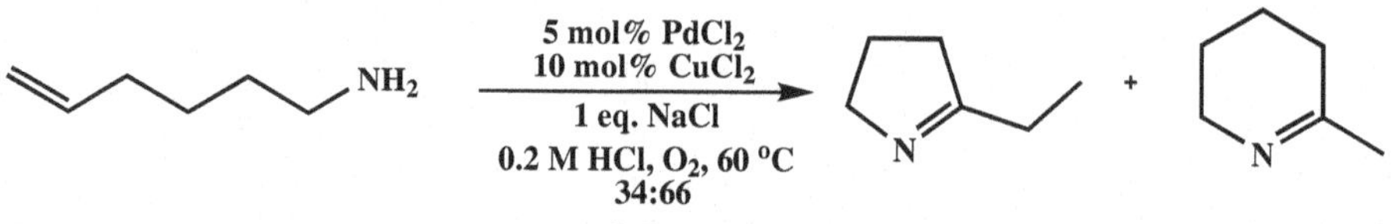

Scheme-17

The isoxazolidine-5-spirocyclopropanes were rearranged to dihydro- or tetrahydropyridones. The reaction occurred by reductive opening of isoxazolidine ring to form the aminocyclopropanol followed by subsequent domino ring-opening/cyclization/oxidation in the presence of palladium(II) catalyst **(Scheme 18)** [50]. Moreover, by a mere change of catalyst the oxidation level of products can be controlled [48].

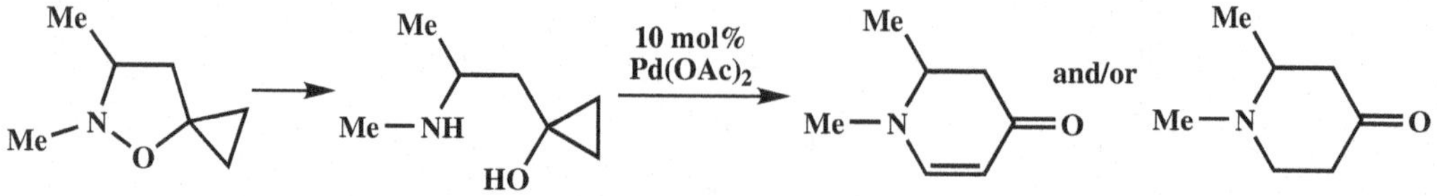

Scheme-18

Depending on the nature of arylating agent either the open-chain products or 2-arylpiperidines were afforded by regiospecific arylation-amination of *N*-tosylated alkenyl amines in PhSnBu$_3$ **(Scheme 19)** [48, 51].

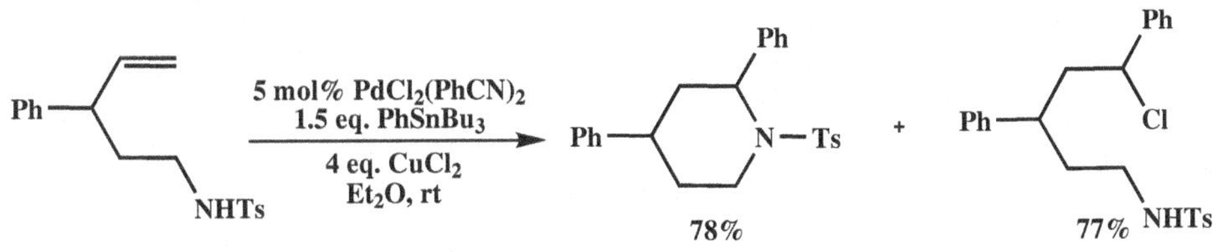

Scheme-19

The double cyclization of 6-(benzyloxycarbonylamino)-hex-1-en-3-ol afforded bridged-ring skeleton in the presence of palladium(II) catalyst **(Scheme 20)** [52-53]. The chemoselectivity was affected with the change of a solvent. Besides bicyclic derivative the epimeric C-1 chlorinated azasugars were obtained employing dimethylformamide or tetrahydrofuran as solvent [48].

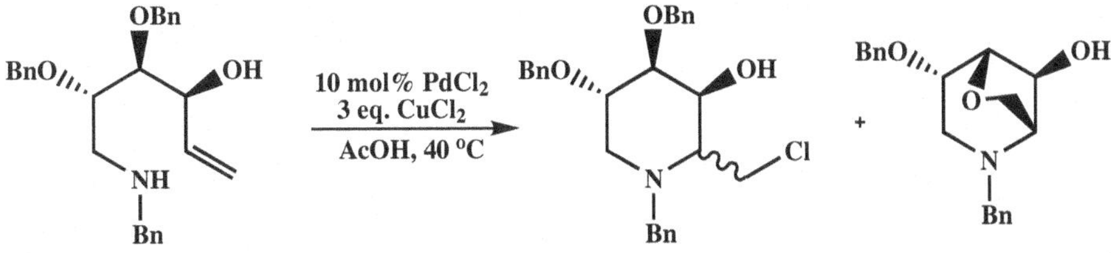

Scheme-20

Yokoyama and co-workers [54] described the cyclization of carbamate to afford piperidine in the presence of Pd catalyst, the formed piperidine was transformed into 1-deoxymannojirimycin, with excellent diastereoselectivity **(Scheme 21)**.

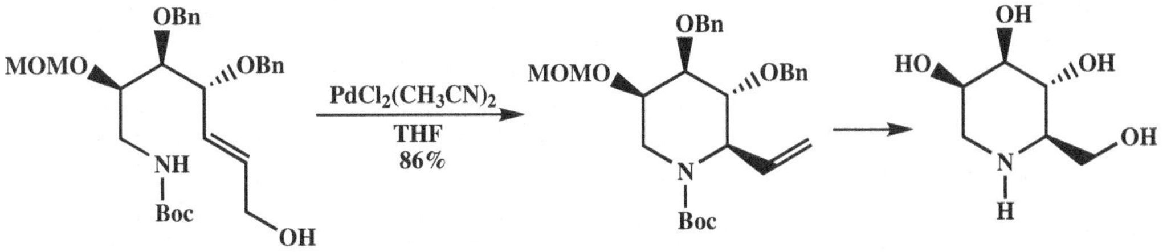

Scheme-21

Knight and co-workers [55] synthesized α-lactams, 3,6-dihydro-1*H*-pyridin-2-ones, in good to high yields by decarboxylative carbonylation of amino acid-derived 5-vinyloxolidin-2-ones with Pd catalyst **(Scheme 22)**. The reaction occurred with elimination of carbon dioxide to produce the allylpalladium intermediate, followed by insertion of carbon monoxide.

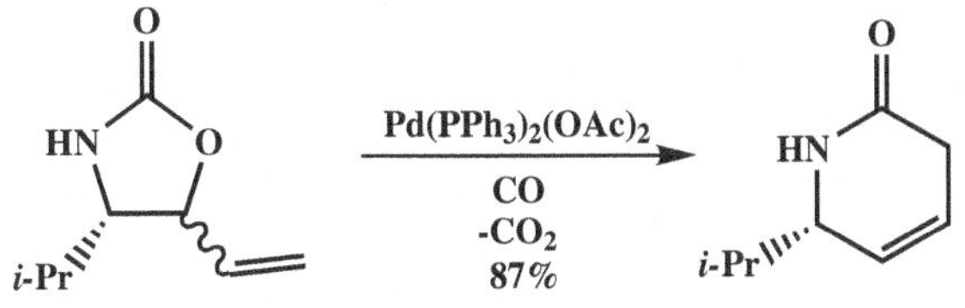

Scheme-22

Shim [56] prepared heterocycles by catalytic amphiphilic bis-allylation in intramolecular fashion. The divinylpiperidones were synthesized from the reaction of allyl stannane-allyl chloride with isocyanates using a Pd catalyst **(Scheme 23)]**.

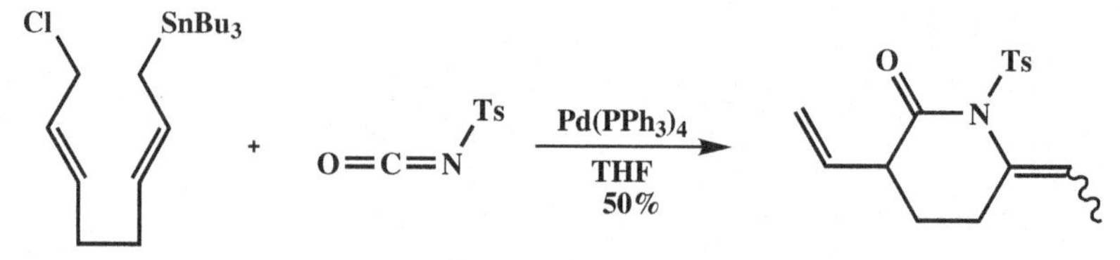

Scheme-23

Takasu [57] carried out intermolecular aza double Michael reaction under catalytic reaction conditions. The α,β-unsaturated carbonyl compounds and α,β-unsaturated amides were reacted for the preparation of piperidin-2-ones in two steps. The conjugate addition reaction of amides with enones to form β-amideketones was promoted in the presence of catalytic amounts of Pd(PhCN)$_2$Cl$_2$. The β-amideketones were then cyclized under basic conditions to afford piperidin-2-ones **(Scheme 24-25)** [58].

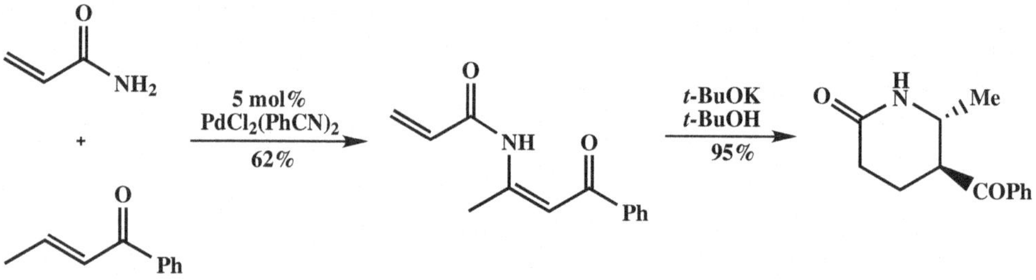

Scheme-24

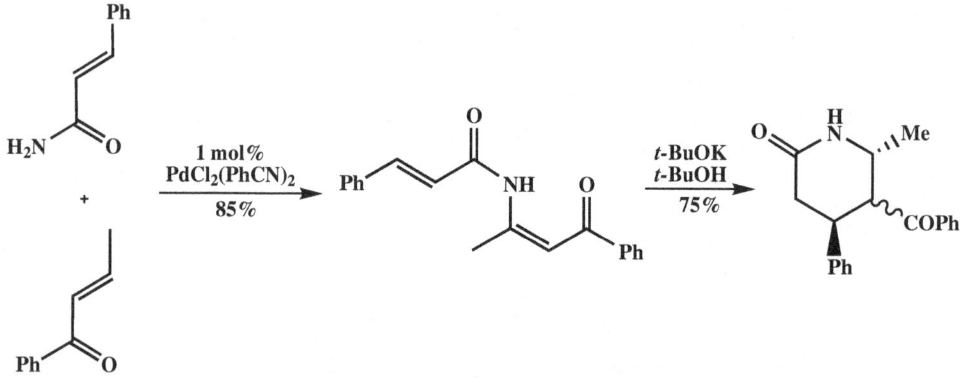

Scheme-25

The reaction has been successfully applied for the synthesis of pyrroles and pyridines from unsaturated *O*-pentafluorobenzoyl oxime [59-61]. Pyrrole was obtained as major product when the reaction was carried out under optimum conditions, and treatment of crude reaction mixture with pyrollidine **(Scheme 26)**. However, carrying out the reaction in the presence of 5 eq. (*n*-Bu)$_4$NCl as an additive, and further treatment of crude reaction mixture with pyrrolidine gave pyridine as major product [62-64].

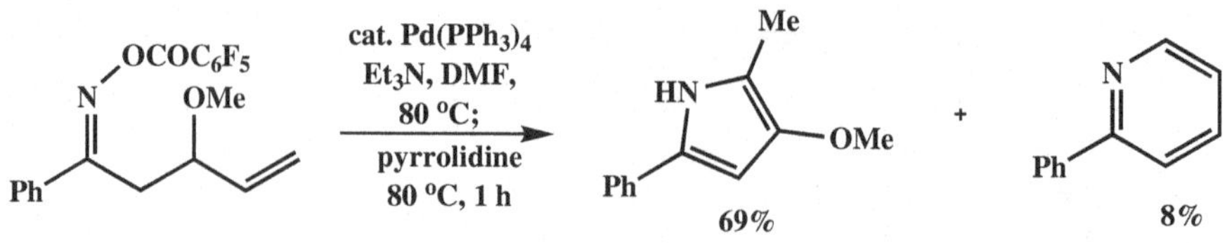

Scheme-26

This reaction worked effectively with conjugated oxime substrate to give pyridine in good yield **(Scheme 27)** [65].

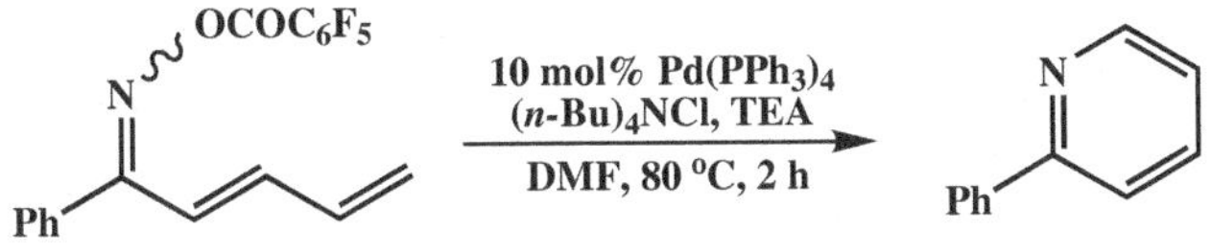

Scheme-27

Larock, Weinreb and coworkers [66] reported the synthesis of vinyl piperidines from *N*-tosyl amino olefins and vinyl halides in the presence of a palladium catalyst. Nucleophilic attack of allyl Pd intermediate afforded the piperidine pendant sulfonamide on vinyl piperidines product **(Scheme 28)**.

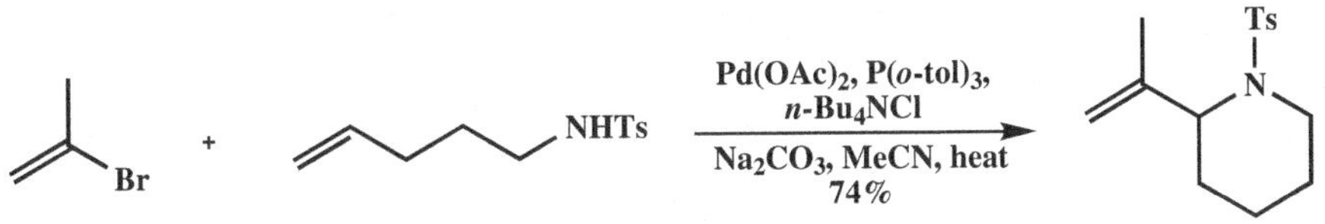

Scheme-28

Michael et al. [67] reported a hydroamination reaction of amino olefin substrates to provide piperidines. For example, amino olefin was converted to methyl substituted piperidine in the presence of tridentate palladium catalyst and $AgBF_4$. These reactions presumably proceeded through nucleophilic attack of amine on palladium activated olefin. Upon protonolysis, the piperidine product was generated **(Scheme 29)**.

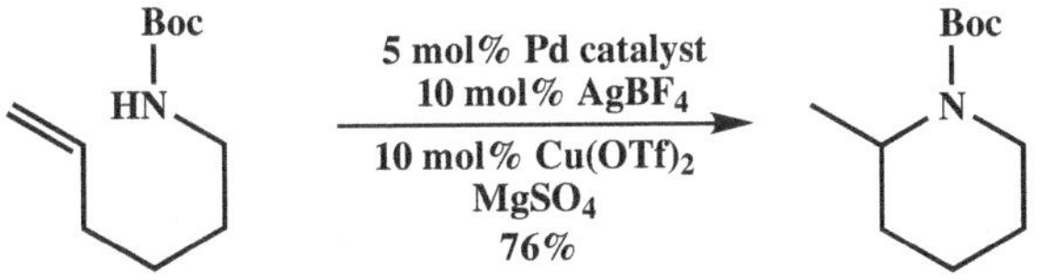

Scheme-29

The synthesis of piperidines *via* palladium-catalyzed carboamination reactions was carried out to: 1) examine and identify suitable reaction conditions for the transformation by screening various ligands, which have been shown to have largest impact on chemical yield of analogous five-membered ring transformations; and 2) examine the diastereoselectivity of reactions involving amino alkenes, which would provide disubstituted piperidines **(Scheme 30)** [67].

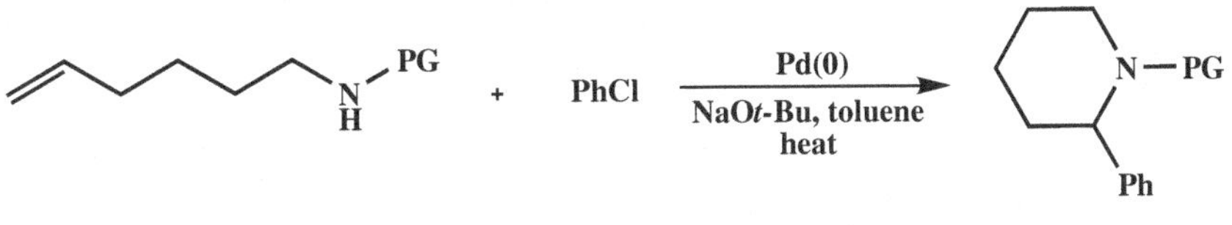

Scheme-30

The synthesis of piperidines *via* palladium-catalyzed carboamination reactions demonstrated the feasibility of preparing six-membered rings with this method. However, in most cases, modest yields were obtained due to competing side reactions, and formation of 2,6-disubstituted products was very difficult **(Scheme 31)** [68].

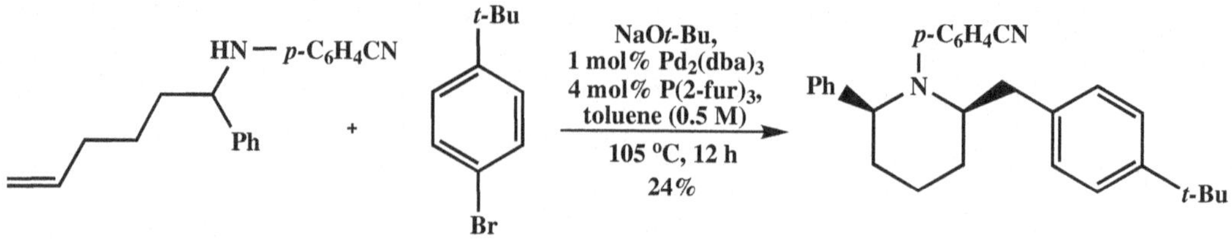

Scheme-31

The conjugate addition of a homochiral lithium amide to an α,β-unsaturated ester with a second α,β-unsaturated acceptor resulted in an intermolecular version of trapping of enolate for the synthesis of polysubstituted piperidones. Amino polyesters with high levels of 2,3-*anti* stereoselectivity were formed upon conjugate addition of lithium (*S*)-*N*-benzyl-*N*-(*R*-methylbenzyl) amide to acrylates and further coupling of formed enolate with alkylidene malonates. The piperidones were produced by hydrogenolysis of amino polyesters and concomitant cyclization. With aryl substituents in both malonate and ester components higher yields and diastereoselectivities were reported, although the reaction tolerated both alkenyl and alkyl moieties (**Scheme 32**) [69-70].

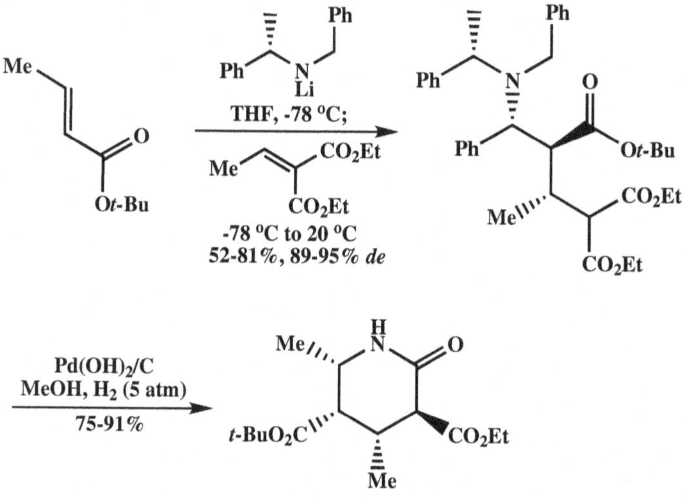

Scheme-32

Tsukamato [71] synthesized 1,4-disubstituted-1,2,3,6-tetrahydropyridines by cyclization of allenyl- and alkynyliminiums. Based on the nature of heteroaryl- or arylboronic acids two different catalytic systems were developed for alkynyliminiums. Pd(PPh$_3$)$_4$ catalyst provided excellent results for electron-rich or neutral acids, whereas for acids containing electron-withdrawing groups it was necessary to use PdCp(η^3-C$_3$H$_5$) and PPh(c-C$_6$H$_{11}$)$_2$ as a ligand (**Scheme 33**) [72].

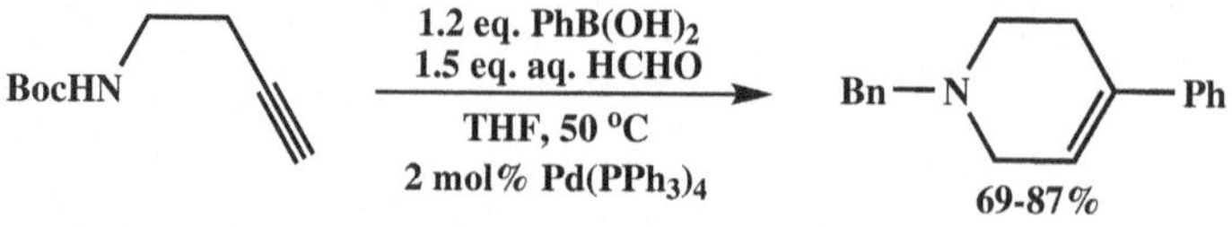

Scheme-33

The palladium(0) was added onto triple bond, followed by nucleophilic attack on *in situ* produced iminium. The formed vinylpalladium species was reacted with boron or alkynyl compound. More substituted tetrahydropyridines were obtained in good to excellent yields from allenylamines which were also compatible with this *anti*-Wacker process (**Scheme 34**) [72-73].

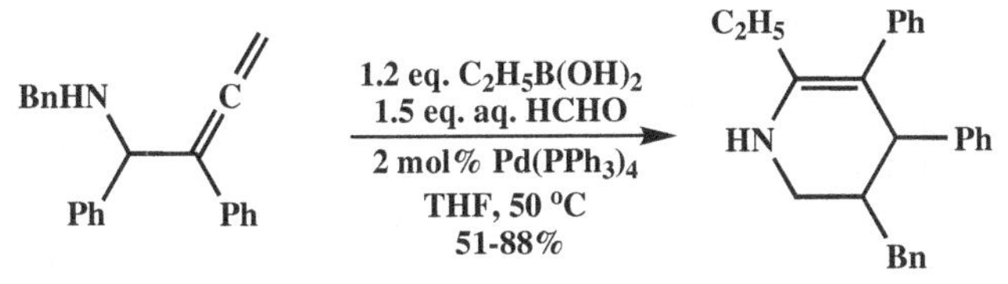

Scheme-34

Katsumura et al. [73] reported the synthesis of pyridines. A one-pot imine synthesis, Stille coupling, 6π-azaelectrocyclization and aminoacetal formation were involved in the synthesis of chiral 2,4-disubstituted 1,2,5,6-tetrahydropyridines **(Scheme 35)** [72].

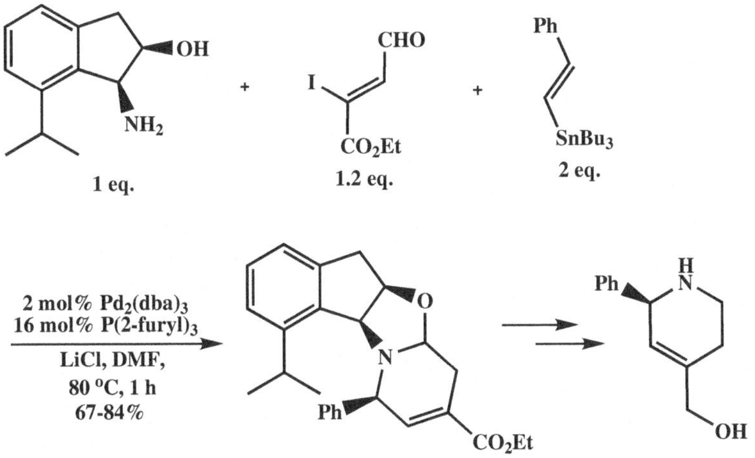

Scheme-35

There were only few reports on the synthesis of isoquinolines, before Larock's [74] studies, in the presence of Pd catalyst. These methods suffer from major disadvantage that they were stoichiometric with respect to Pd. Roesch and Larock [74] reported a catalytic version of these syntheses. A number of *N*-heterocycles such as isoquinoline and pyridine were produced by a Pd-catalyzed iminoannulation of internal alkynes. The *tert*-butylimines underwent iminoannulation while *i*-Pr-, Me-, allyl- and benzylimines did not form desired products. In most of the cases vinylic and aryl imines yielded pyridine derivatives with high regioselectivity **(Scheme 36)** [75].

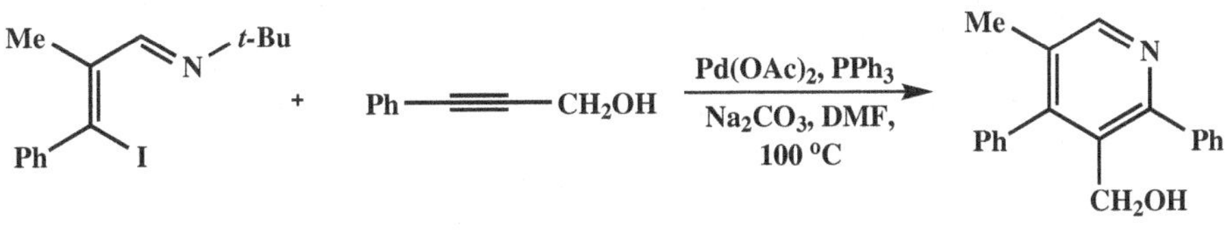

Scheme-36

Alkenes underwent a Wacker-type aerobic oxidative cyclization in the presence of a base-free $Pd(DMSO)_2(TFA)_2$ catalyst for the preparation of six-membered *N*-heterocycles. Many heterocyclic compounds, such as piperidines, morpholines, piperazinones, and piperazines were accessible by this protocol **(Scheme 37)** [76].

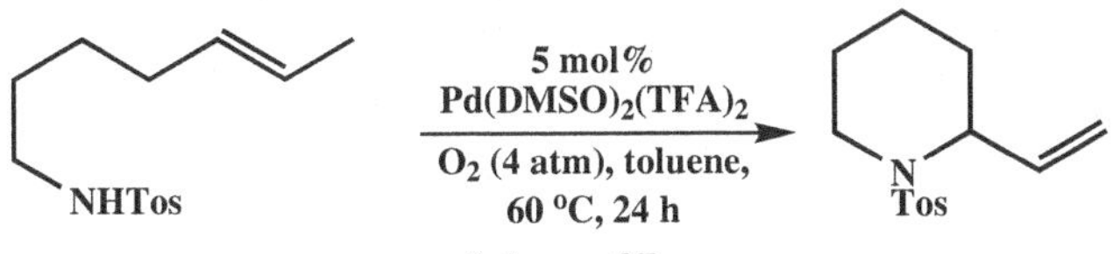

Scheme-37

The azetidine, indoline, and pyrrolidine compounds were synthesized by intramolecular amination of unactivated carbon-hydrogen bonds at γ and δ positions of picolinamide (PA) protected amine substrates in the presence of Pd catalyst. This protocol enjoyed inexpensive reagents, low catalyst loading, predictable selectivities and convenient operating conditions **(Scheme 38)** [77].

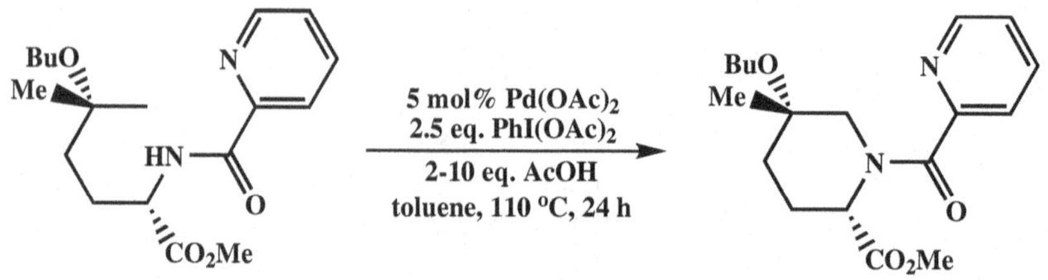

Scheme-38

Zard and co-workers [78] synthesized 3-arylpyridines involving radical 1,4-aryl migrations. The 1,4-aryl transfer product was formed *via* a xanthate addition to *N*-allylarylsulfonamide, followed by acetylation and treatment with DLP. Following acidic hydrolysis the 1,4-aryl transfer product was transformed into desired piperidine **(Scheme 39)** [28].

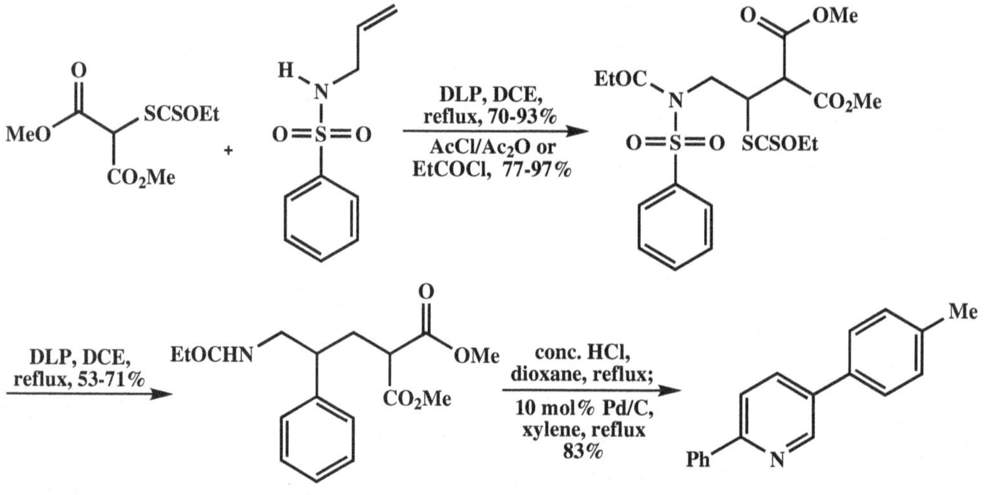

Scheme-39

Qing and co-workers [79] used allylamine for the production of *gem*-4,4-difluoromethylenated iminosugars **(Scheme 40)** and their biological activity was evaluated as glycosidase inhibitors at different *p*H values. Simultaneously, the effect of fluorine substituent on bioactivity was also studied [28].

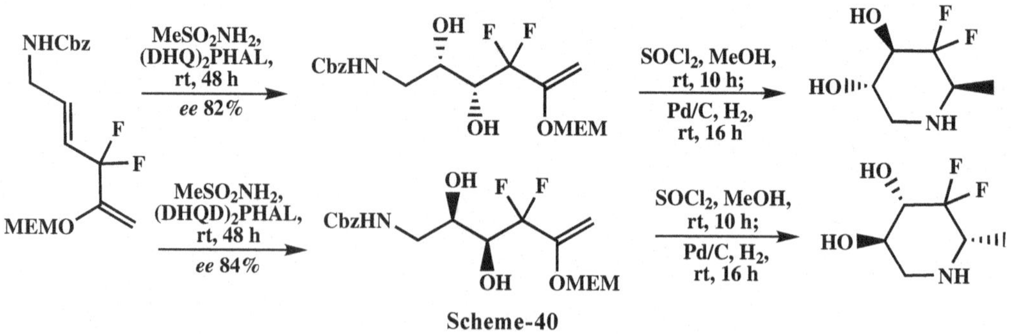

Scheme-40

The nitrogen-containing heterocycles were produced diastereo- and enantioselectively by a one-pot Ru-catalyzed enyne coupling of starting substrate followed by asymmetric carbon-nitrogen bond formation in the presence of Pd catalyst **(Scheme 41)** [80]. The enyne coupling occurred through the formation of ruthenacycle followed by elimination-reductive elimination.

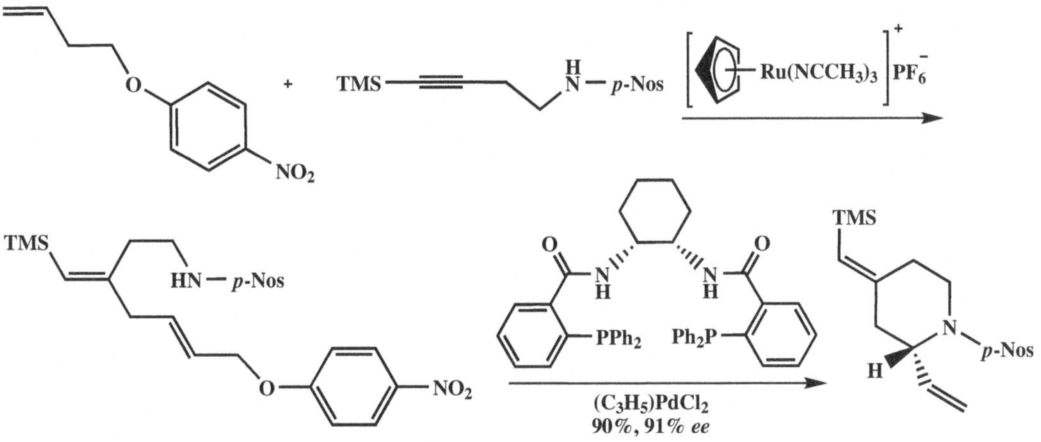

Scheme-41

In a paper by Schreiber et al. [81], a B/C/P strategy that relies on an organocatalyzed *syn*-diastereoselective Mannich reaction, as the couple phase, was described. According to their work several different skeletons can be achieved in 3-4 steps starting from commercially available reagents **(Scheme 42)**. During the couple phase, commercially available building blocks were coupled *via* a Mannich reaction to form *syn*-diastereomeric aminoaldehyde. Derivatization of aldehyde functionality in aminoaldehyde *via* a Wittig reaction afforded *syn* product. Following alkylation reactions yielded densely functionalized templates, poised for subsequent intramolecular functional group pairing reactions.

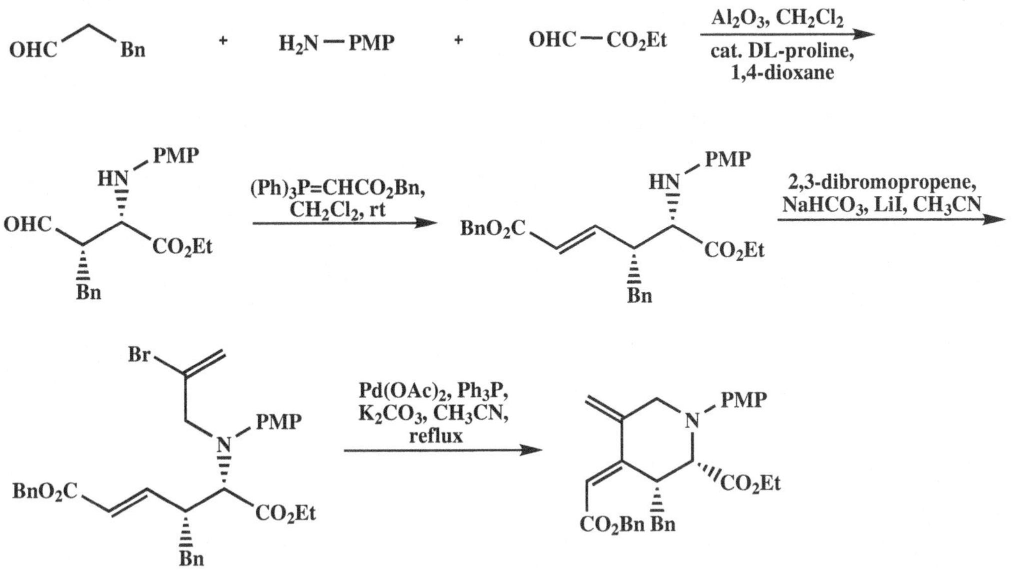

Scheme-42

Battistini and co-workers [82] reported the synthesis of six-membered lactam using a vinylogous version of Mannich type addition as a key reaction in their synthesis **(Scheme 43)**. This synthetic target, again lacks the PI′ substituent and was formed after a tedious multistep synthesis.

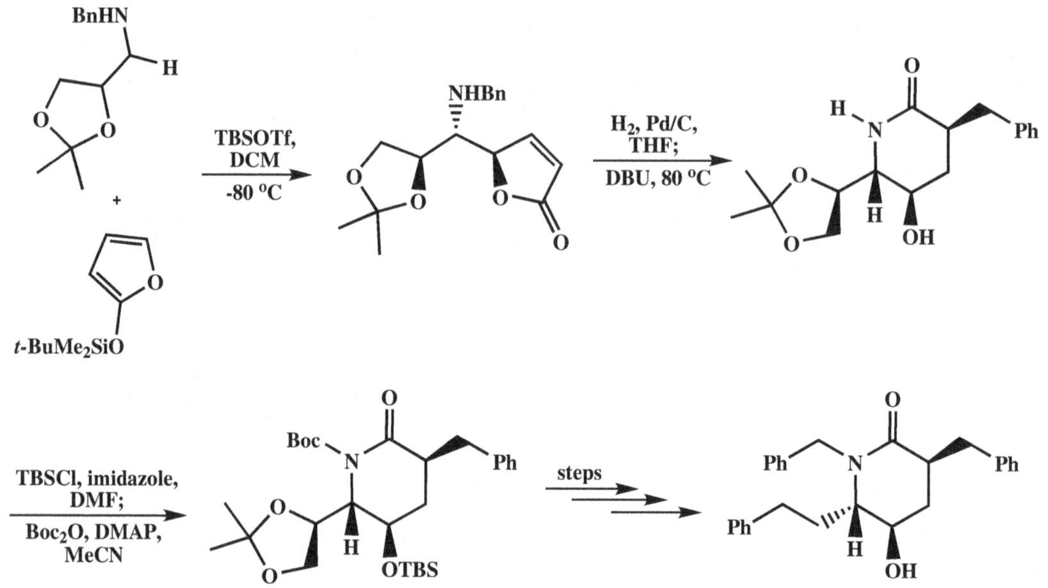

Scheme-43

Access to 4-oxo-, *cis*-4-hydroxy- and *trans*-4-hydroxypipecolic acid was possible with a route developed by Burger et al. [83] which employed an intramolecular aza-conjugate addition as key step to construct the heterocycle. L-Aspartic acid was enantiopure synthetic precursor for the approach, which was reacted with hexafluoroacetone to give protected oxazolidinone **(Scheme 44)**. Intermediate oxazolidinone was converted to acid chloride and then subjected to standard Stille coupling conditions with vinyltrimethyltin as corresponding partner to produce unsaturated amino acid derivative. Subsequent Lewis acid-induced 6-*endo-trig* conjugate addition generated saturated *N*-heterocycle in 60% yield. Finally de-protection yielded 4-oxopipecolic acid quantitatively.

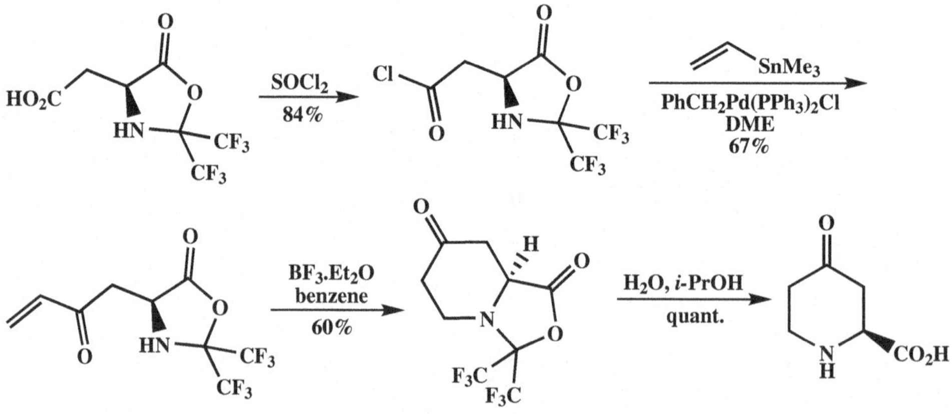

Scheme-44

The bromomethyl vinyl ketone equivalent was synthesized in three steps from allyl iodide **(Scheme 45)**. A Prins reaction with allyl iodide and paraformaldehyde followed by elimination under reduced pressure produced methylene-1,3-dioxane. Bromination of methylene-1,3-dioxane in the presence of base generated bromomethyl vinyl ketone equivalent in 57% yield over three steps. Williams' lactone [84] was alkylated stereoselectively with allylic bromide to produce enol ether. The enone moiety was then unveiled under thermal conditions *via* fragmentation and Boc protecting group was removed to yield intermediate. A concomitant 6-*endo-trig* conjugate addition reaction occurred to generate the pipecolic acid core. Stereoselective reduction of ketone installed the 4-hydroxy substituent as a single diastereomer and then hydrogenolysis liberated carboxylic acid side-chain to give the natural stereoisomer, (2S,4R)-4-hydroxypipecolic acid in excellent yield.

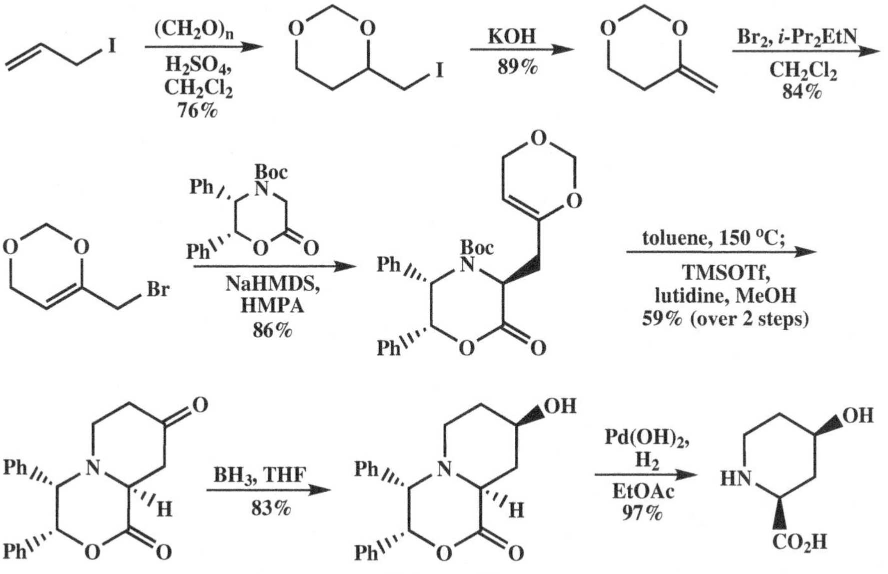

Scheme-45

This synthetic route involved the formation of oxazolidine from trifluoroacetaldehyde methyl hemiacetal and (R)-phenylglycinol **(Scheme 46)**. It produced a 2:1 mixture of diastereomers in 98% yield. Subsequently, the diastereomeric mixture was treated with silyl enol ether to give β-amino ketone with high diastereoselectivity. The high level of diastereoselectivity was accounted by the formation of a chiral imine which resulted from ring-opening of oxazolidine. It produced a rigid, ordered intermediate with phenyl group blocking one face and therefore, selective attack occurred from the opposing face [85]. Protection of carbonyl as ketal, followed by hydrogenolysis generated substrate for the intramolecular Mannich reaction. Formation of pipecolic acid core was achieved using ethyl glyoxylate to give an imine. Under acidic conditions, the ketal ring opened to give corresponding enol ether, which cyclized onto imine to produce desired N-heterocycle and regeneration of the ketal protecting group occurred *in situ*. *Cis*-trifluoromethyl pipecolic acid was major diastereomer obtained in 85:15 *cis:trans* ratio as a result of intramolecular Mannich reaction.

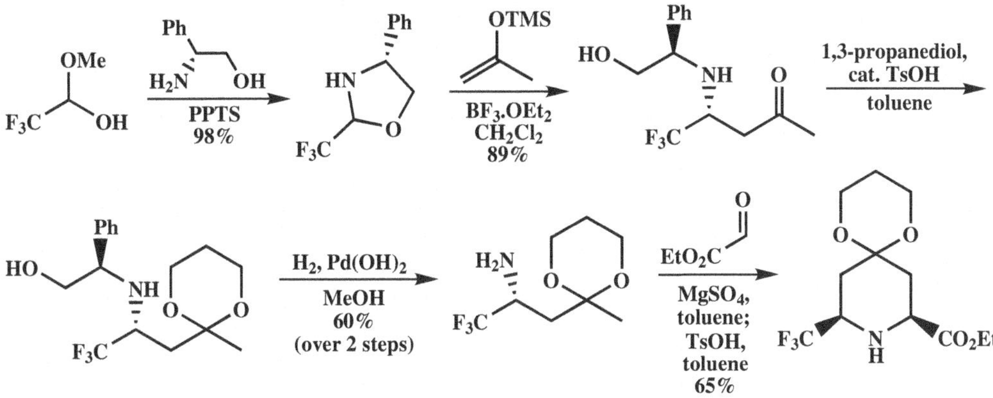

Scheme-46

The synthesis employed a Sonogashira cross-coupling reaction using 3-bromopropargyl alcohol and silyl-protected acetylene to give diyne (**Scheme 47**). LAH selectively reduced the alkyne with pendant hydroxyl group to yield the *E*-isomer of allylic alcohol in excellent yield. Allylic alcohol was subjected to Sharpless asymmetric epoxidation conditions with (-)-diethyl tartrate to produce epoxy alcohol in good yield with good enantiomeric excess. Epoxy alcohol was reacted with allyl isocyanate to generate allyl carbamate. Regioselective intramolecular ring-opening of epoxide produced oxazolidinone in excellent yield. Removal of silyl protecting group, followed by acetylation of free hydroxyl generated the substrate for tandem ring-closing metathesis and subsequent cross-metathesis reaction. Enyne was subjected to metathesis conditions using Grubbs second-generation catalyst in the presence of 1-tetradecene to afford diene in good yield and with complete *E*-selectivity of external alkene. Completion of the

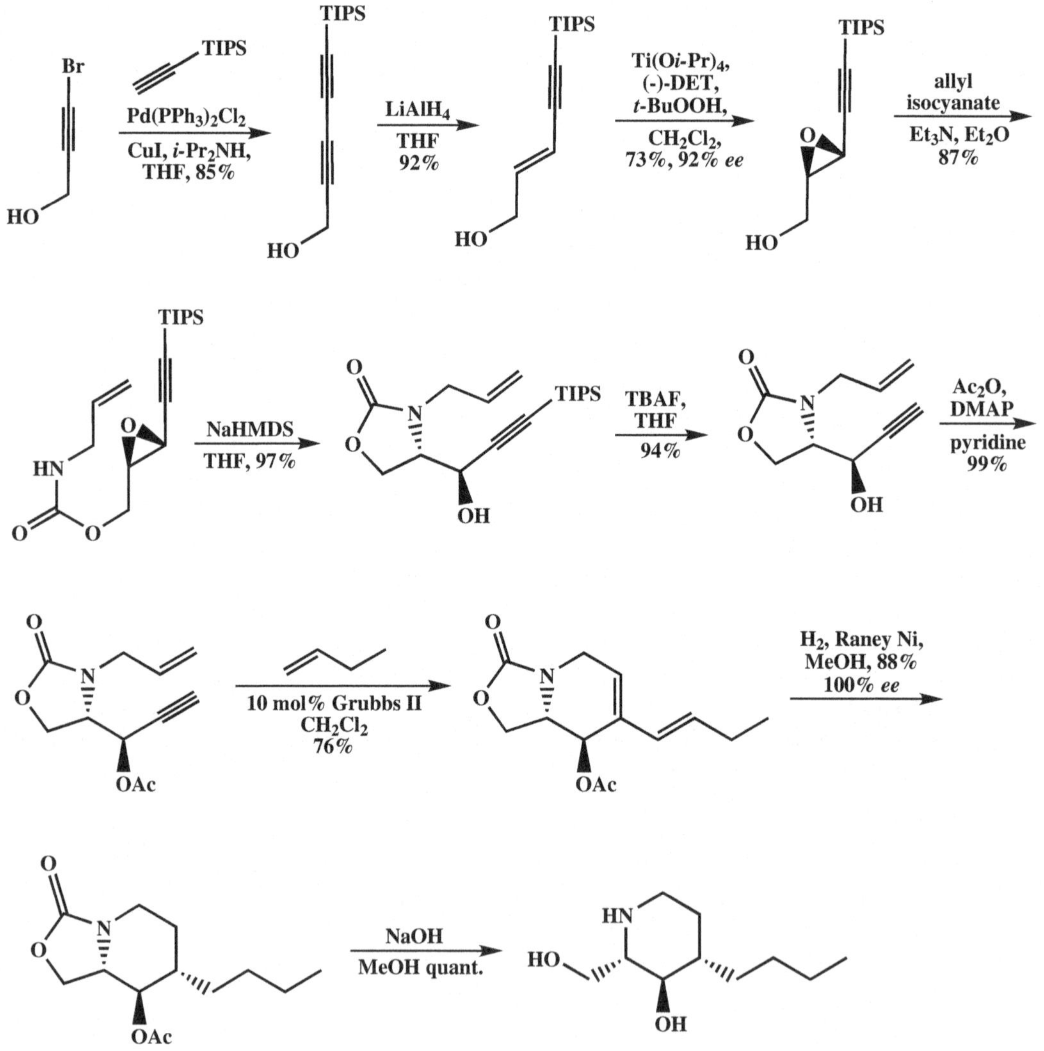

Scheme-47

synthesis involved hydrogenation of diene using Raney Ni, which proceeded with complete facial selectivity. Finally, hydrolysis of oxazolidinone ring and acetate group produced (2*S*,3*R*,4*S*)-trisubsituted piperidine in 10 linear steps in 30% overall yield. The chirality was achieved using asymmetric catalysis and therefore it would be feasible to use opposite enantiomer of diethyl tartrate to obtain *ent*-trisubstituted piperidine. The highly functionalized diene intermediate may also allow variations to piperidine template making this a versatile synthetic route [86-88].

7.4 Synthesis of six-membered nitrogen-containing heterocycles fused with aromatics

The Pd-catalyzed iminoannulation of allenes formed isoquinolines and pyridines. Fruhauf and co-workers [89] used 1,1-dimethylallene and cyclopalladated α-tetralone ketimines for the synthesis of nitrogen heterocycles using stoichiometric Pd. Isoquinolines and pyridines were formed when *ortho*-halide substituted imines were reacted with monosubstituted allenes in the presence of Pd catalyst [90]. *t*-Bu substituted imines resulted in exclusive attack at less substituted end but this group was difficult to remove sometimes so moderate yields were observed. Higher yields but lower regioselectivity was obtained from 3-aminopropionitrile imines **(Scheme 48-49)** [75].

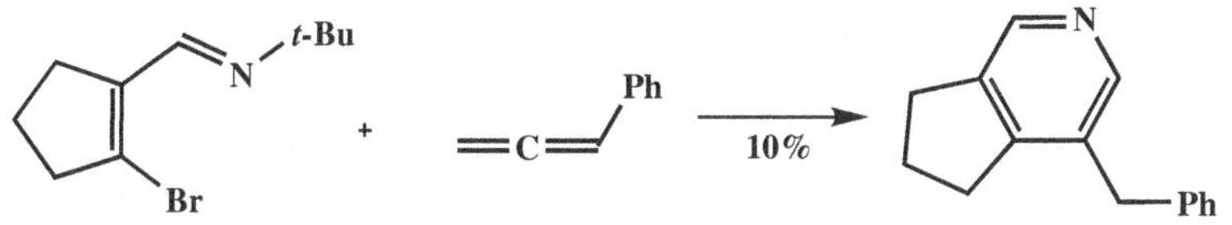

Scheme-48

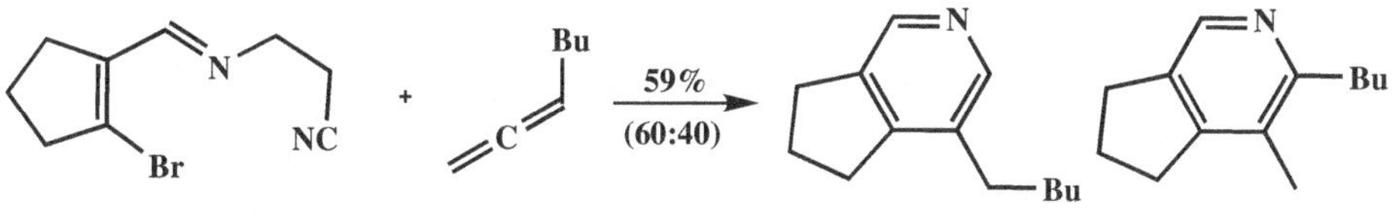

Scheme-49

The commercial available 6-bromopiperonal synthesized natural product trisphaeridine in three steps through formyl and oxime ether derivatives. The trisphaeridine was formed in 70% yield from oxime ether under MWI in *t*-BuPh. Previously, the trisphaeridine was generated *via* cyclization of *N*-(2-bromobenzyl)aniline induced by TBTH [91], *via* internal palladium-catalyzed aryl-aryl coupling reaction of methoxymethyl ether protected halo amides, followed by reduction with lithium aluminium hydride and treatment with hydrochloric acid [92], and by palladium(0)-mediated Ullmann cross-coupling of 1-bromo-2-nitrobenzene with 6-bromopiperonal [93]. This method was simply extended for the synthesis of benzo[*c*][1,7]naphthiridine derivatives. The formyl derivative was formed with palladium-catalyzed coupling of 6-bromopiperonal and pyridin-4-ylboronic acid. Then, formyl derivative was converted into *O*-phenyl oxime ether in good yield. However, when *O*-phenyl oxime ether reacted under MWI, the benzonaphthiridine was not produced. Instead, a mixture of imine and its hydrolysis product formyl derivative was obtained. Results have suggested that there was a slow ring closure of intermediate iminyl radical onto pyridine ring as compared to cyclization onto phenyl ring and unable to compete with H-atom abstraction from other reaction components. There are comparatively rare reports on ring closures of C-centered radicals onto pyridine rings [94] and in comparison to ring closure onto pyridinium salts the reaction was usually low-yielding [95-96]. In comparison to C-centered radicals, the iminyl radicals were expected to be electrophilic, and therefore their even slower cyclization onto pyridine, due to an unfavorable polar effect with the ring *N*-atom, makes reasonable sense **(Scheme 50)** [97].

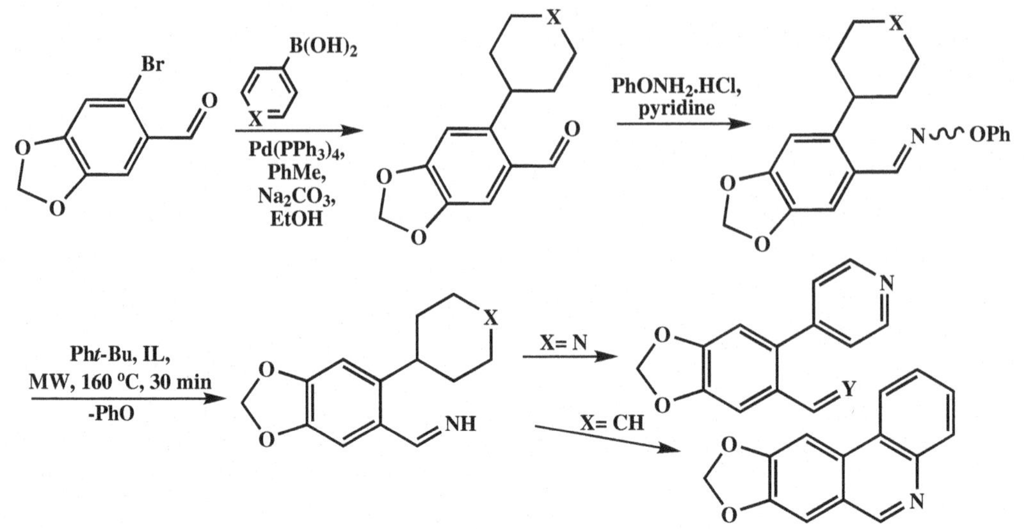

Scheme-50

Ishibashi et al. [98] generated a tricyclic framework and diaryl quaternary centre of indenotetrahydropyridine unit of a cytotoxic alkaloid, haouamine A *via* an intramolecular cascade Mizorokie Heck reaction of allyl carbamate **(Scheme 51)** [28].

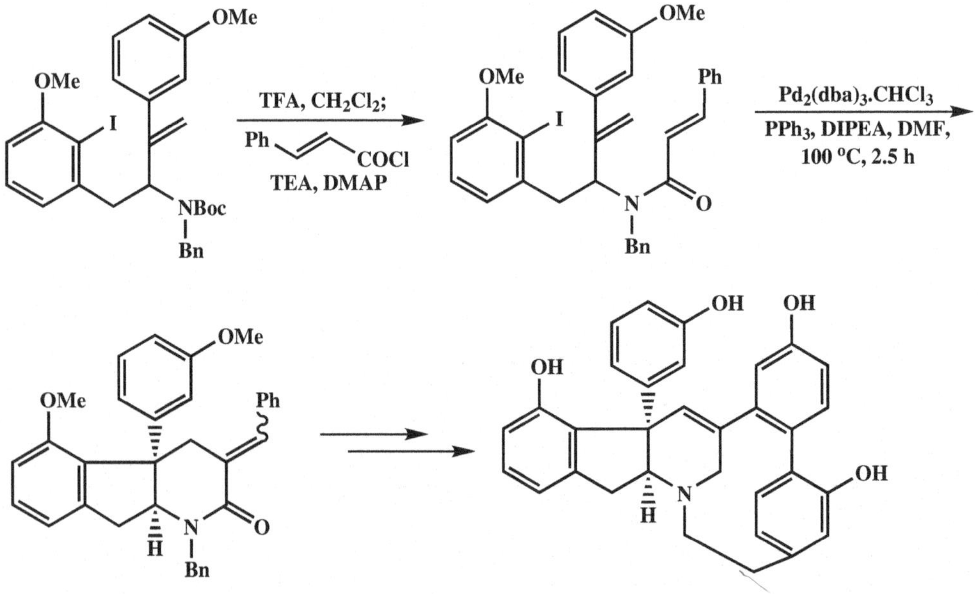

Scheme-51

7.5 Synthesis of six-membered nitrogen-containing heterocycles fused with other heterocycles

An intramolecular Mannich-type reaction was also investigated by Aitken et al. [99] for the synthesis of 4-oxopipecolic acid. Enantiomerically pure oxazolidine was deprotonated with LDA and subsequent nucleophilic attack on methoxymethyl ether-protected allyl chloride gave intermediate as major diastereomer (**Scheme 52**). The key cyclization step took place under Lewis acid catalyzed conditions to form the *N*-heterocyclic core with two possible products.

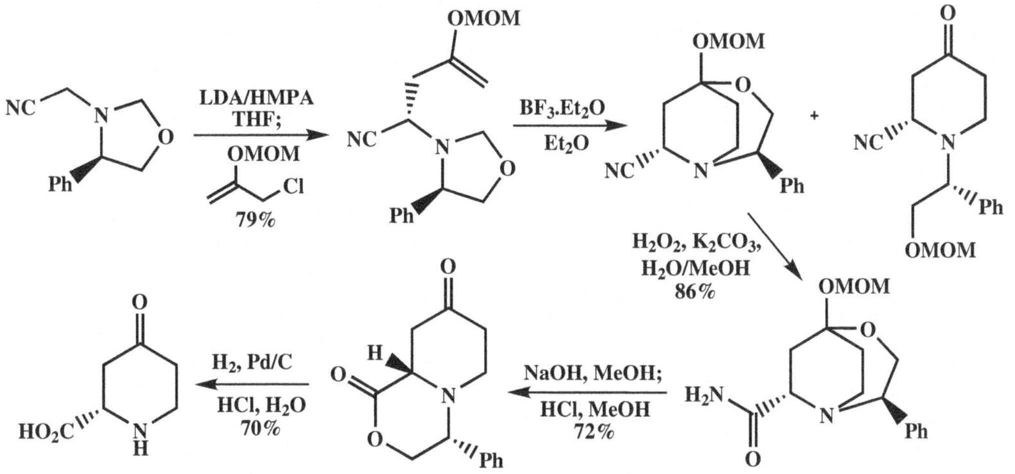

Scheme-52

The bicyclic and tricyclic heterocycles were produced by Okano and co-workers [100] in this novel pathway. The nucleophilic moiety containing allenic bromoalkenes underwent a 'zipper mode' cascade cyclization in the presence of tetrabutylammonium fluoride or cesium carbonate in acetonitrile with catalytic amount of palladium(0) (**Scheme 53**) [28].

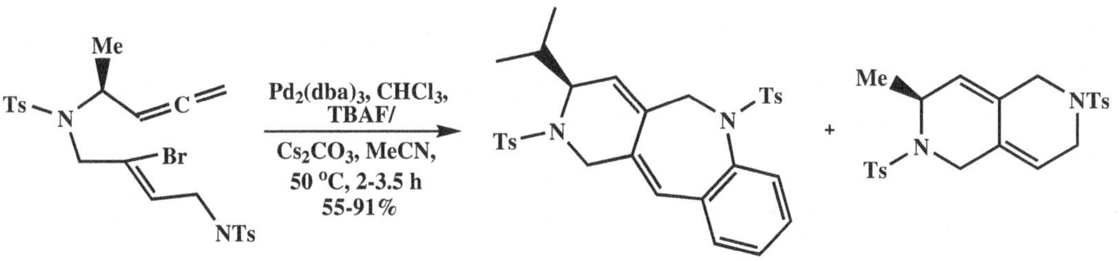

Scheme-53

A palladium-catalyzed tandem cyclization-cross-coupling method was explained by Ishikura and co-workers [101] for the synthesis of allylamine derivative and 1*H*-indol-2-yltrialkylborane. The 2-(4-piperidylmethyl)indole was formed from allylamine derivative and 1*H*-indol-2-yltrialkylborane. The 2-(4-piperidylmethyl)indole was employed as a precursor for the construction of tubifoline (**Scheme 54**). Minor yield of side product was reported in this reaction [28].

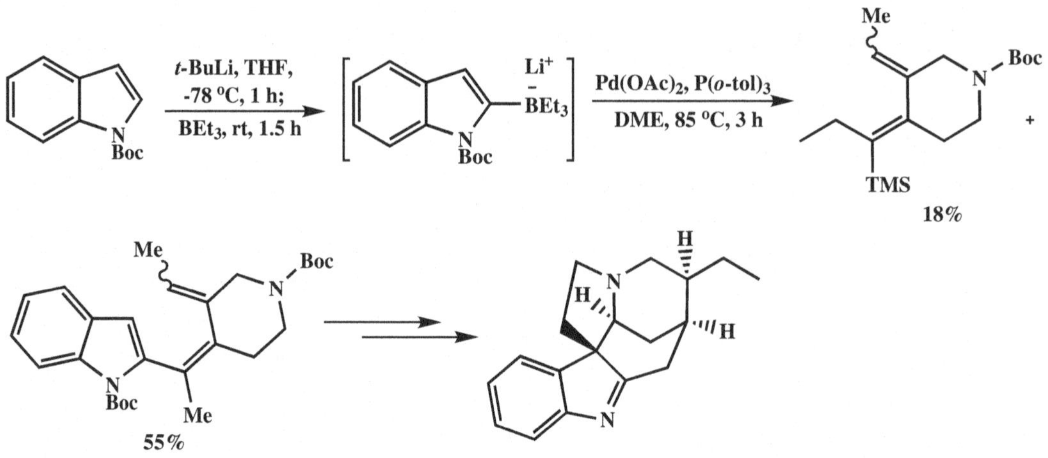

Scheme-54

Thienopyridines and furopyridines were synthesized from 3-bromothiophene-2-carbaldehydes and 3-bromofuran-2-carbaldehydes respectively. Commercially available 2-bromoarylaldehydes, terminal acetylenes, and ammonium acetate were reacted in the presence of a Pd catalyst under MWI for the preparation of thienopyridine and furopyridine derivatives. The imination reagent NH_4OAc afforded superior results than aqueous NH_3 counterpart. Cu catalyst was not necessary in this method (**Scheme 55**) [102-103].

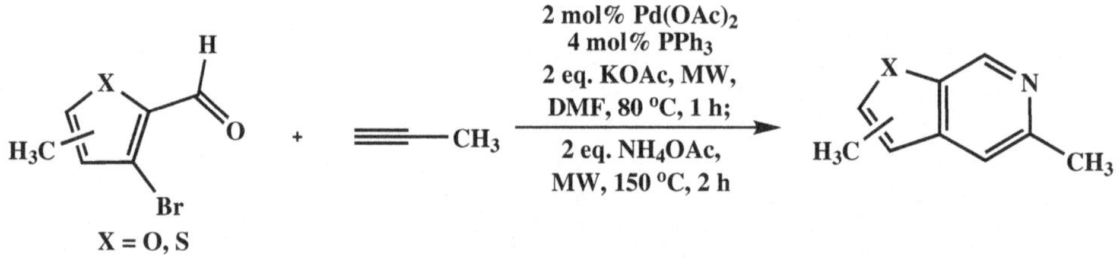

Scheme-55

The tryptamines and carbonyl compounds like aromatic glyoxals and benzaldehyhdes were reacted in a one-step for the synthesis of β-carbolines with bifunctional palladium/carbon/K-10 catalyst [104] (**Scheme 56**). A one-pot, three-step domino sequence produced the final products. An imine was formed in the first step upon condensation of aldehyde/glyoxal with the primary amino group of tryptamine. The imine underwent Pictet-Spengler cyclization reaction in the presence of a K-10 catalyst in second step. In third and final step, β-carbolines were synthesized in good to excellent yields from tetrahydro-β-carboline intermediate in the presence of a palladium/carbon catalyst.

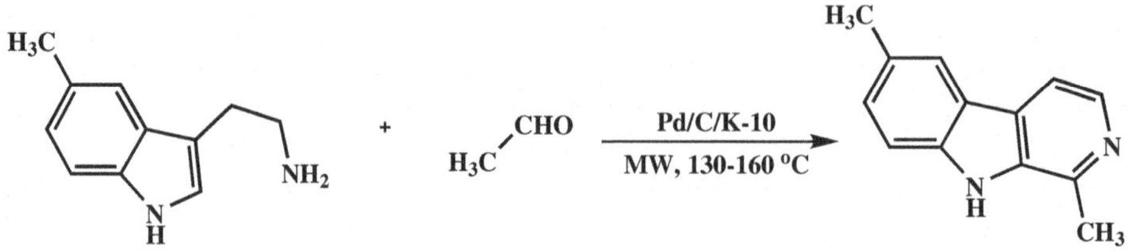

Scheme-56

The tetrahydroindolizine moiety was first prepared by using an oxidative Heck cyclization of pyrrole. This Pd(II) oxidation process was carried out in the presence of Pd diacetate and *tert*-butylhydroperoxide as oxidant to give tetrahydroindolizine in 75% yield. A palladation at C2 occurred *via* intermediate formation followed by rearomatization with the loss of CH_3COOH and a Heck-type reaction to yield the tetrahydroindolizine. The iodopyrrole, obtained in few steps from azafulvene, was submitted to modify Jeffery conditions to form the final product in good yield. After few steps the tetrahydroindolizine was converted into iodoaryl cylization's precursor, the intramolecular carbon-hydrogen arylation was then engaged to produce biaryl derivative under previously established reaction conditions **(Scheme 57)** [105-107].

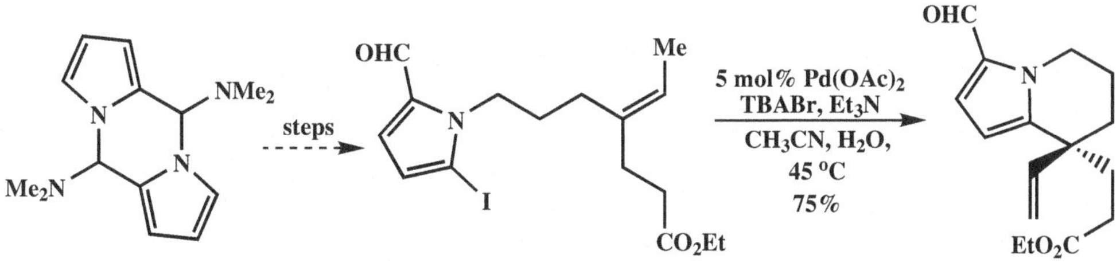

Scheme-57

The strategy to functionalize the pyrrole ring has been established, the total synthesis of racemic rhazinicine was engaged as follows. The *N*-Boc protected 2-trimethylsilyl pyrrole was used as starting material and submitted to sequential one-pot irridium/palladium catalytic

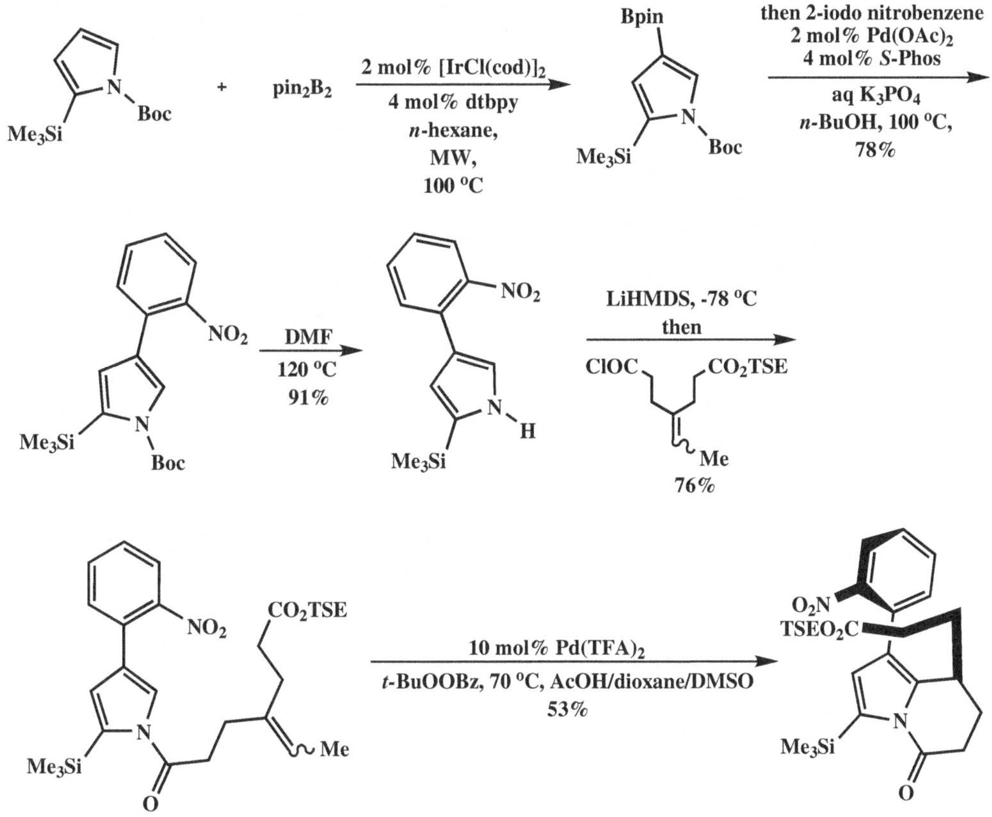

Scheme-58

reaction to furnish good yields of expected cross-coupling product as single isomer. This reaction probably took place as follows. The aromatic carbon-hydrogen bond cleavage occurred either through an oxidative addition or sigma bond metathesis to form the iridium hydride complex followed by a reductive elimination to form the pyrrol boronic acid. After the removal of Boc group, the pyrrole was converted into compound ready to be submitted to reaction conditions to perform the intramolecular oxidative Heck cyclization. Treatment of formed compound with 10 mol% of Pd(TFA)$_2$ and *tert*-BuOOBz as oxidant give final compound. Last steps to obtain the target compound consist first to reduce the C-C double bond into ethyl group and the nitro into aniline under hydrogen followed by a cleavage of trimethylsilyl and 2-trimethylsilylethyl protecting groups in the presence of aluminium(III) chloride and then a macrolactamization using Mukaiyama's reagent **(Scheme 58)** [107].

The *N*-alkylated pyrrole was obtained by nucleophilic substitution of tosyate group with potassium salt of pyrrole **(Scheme 59)**. The clean synthesis of tetrahydroindolizine was reported with requisite quaternary stereocenter in 69% yield in the presence of 10 mol% of palladium acetate and TBHP. A single regioisomer of aldehyde was formed from tetrahydroindolizine under Vilsmeier-Haack formylation [108-109].

The azafulvene was quenched with molecular iodine and C-metalated with *tert*-BuLi. The hydrolysis of azafulvene with NaOAc afforded 5-iodo-2-pyrrole carbaldehyde in refluxing tetrahydrofuran. The *N*-alkylated pyrrole was formed in high yields from nucleophilic substitution of tosylate with potassium salt of pyrrole. The annulated pyrrole was obtained in good yield by Heck reaction of pyrrole under modified Jeffery conditions **(Scheme 60)** [110-111].

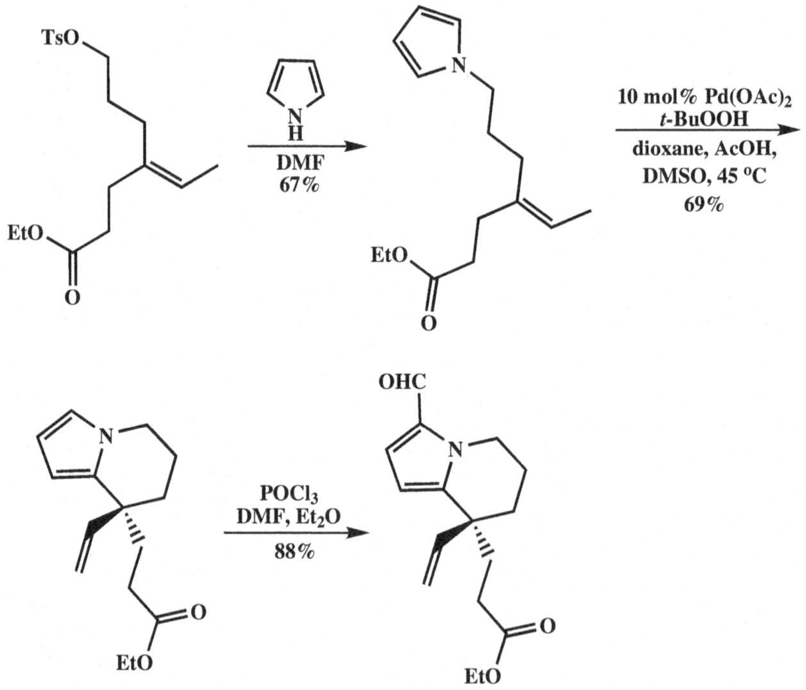

Scheme-59

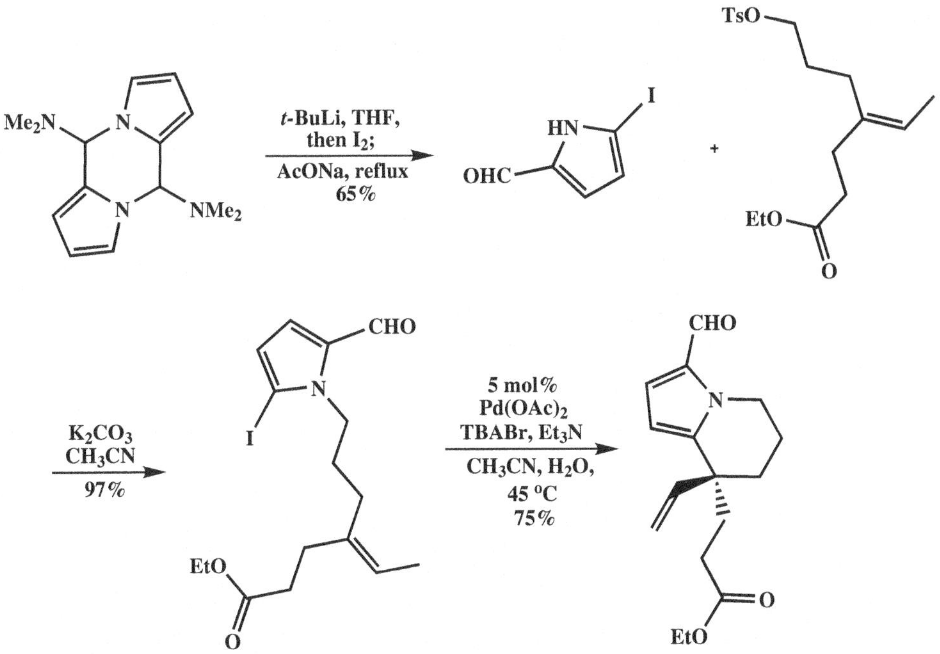

Scheme-60

A mixture of highly polar compounds (not characterized) was obtained on exposure of aldol adduct to triphenylphosphine-water reductive system. The little cyclization product was synthesized on hydrogenation reaction of azidoaldol carried out in Boc₂O, while the side-products were obtained in major amounts in mixture. Then, the reduction of azide and *in situ* cyclization and protection of resultant secondary amine was conducted. Interestingly, the 4-hydroxypipecolic acid analogue with a bicyclic β-lactam structure was afforded on exposure of azidoaldol to hydrogen (1 atm) at rt in ethyl acetate and a catalytic amount of palladium (10% on C) followed by addition of benzyl chloroformate **(Scheme 61)** [112].

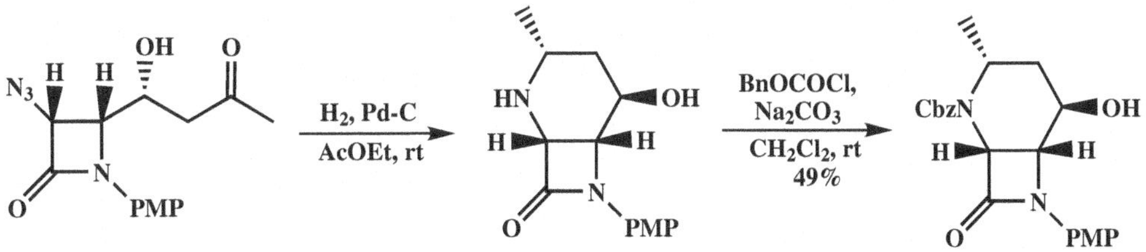

Scheme-61

The trihalopyridine was used for the synthesis of drug intermediate *via* a regioselective tandem Heck-lactamization **(Scheme 62)** [113-114].

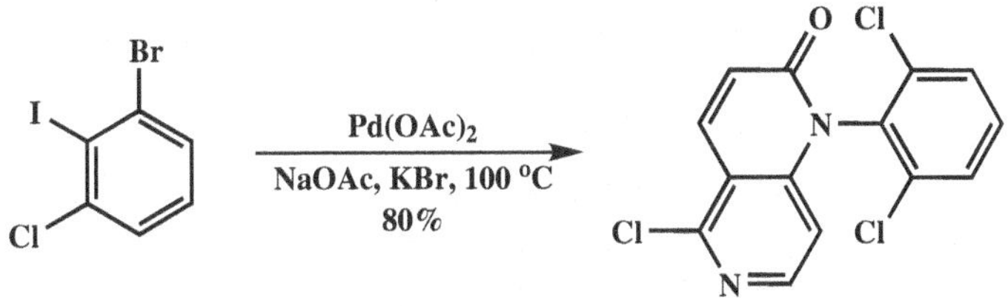

Scheme-62

The (+)-halichlorine acts as an immunoglobulin inhibitor. Danishefsky et al. [115a] in 1999 described the preparation of (+)-halichlorine by β-alkylated SM cross-coupling of Z-iodoacrylate in the presence of borane, de-protection and intramolecular Michael addition **(Scheme 63)** [115b].

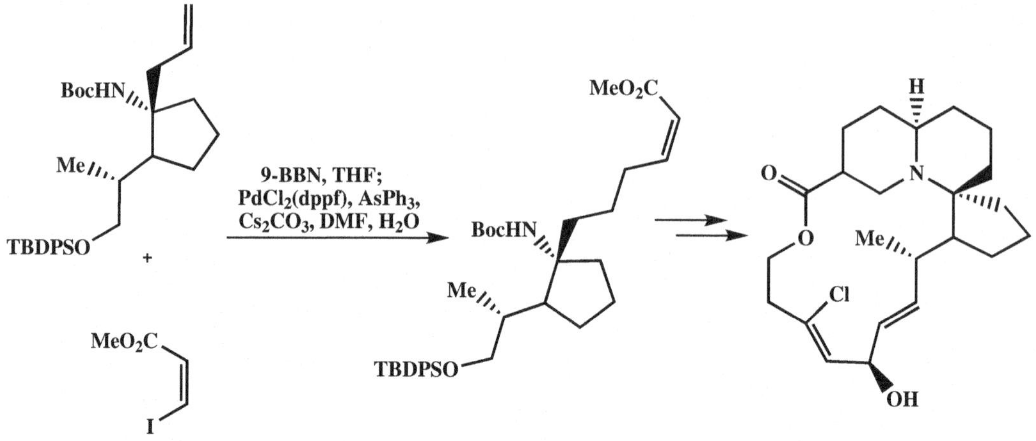

Scheme-63

The indole alkaloids of vallesiachotamine type were synthesized by this procedure. Naturally these indole alkaloids were produced by condensation of N-4 with C-17 in intermediate strictosidine. An aldehyde functionality and intermediate compound possessing a lactam were formed from secondary amine after de-protection by hydrogenolysis and attack on lactone moiety. The indole alkaloid dihydroantirhin was formed by reduction of intermediate with LiAlH$_4$ [116-117]; 10% of 20-epimer was reported in obtained product **(Scheme 64)** [118-119].

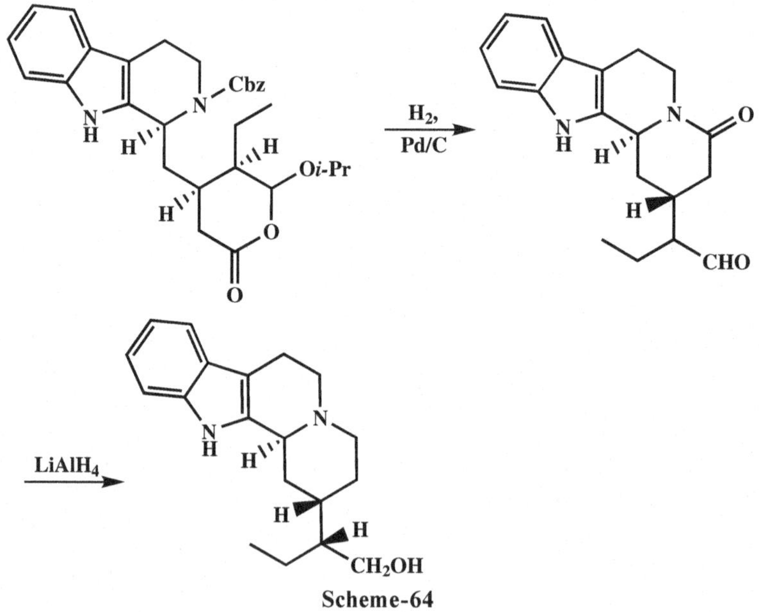

Scheme-64

The 1-vinyl-1,2,3,4-tetrahydro-γ-carbolines and 4-vinyl-1,2,3,4-tetrahydro-β-carbolines were formed by conventional Friedel-Crafts pathway. The regioselective intramolecular allylic alkylation of allylamines present at the 2-position of indole was carried out in the presence of palladium catalyst **(Scheme 65-66)** [28, 120].

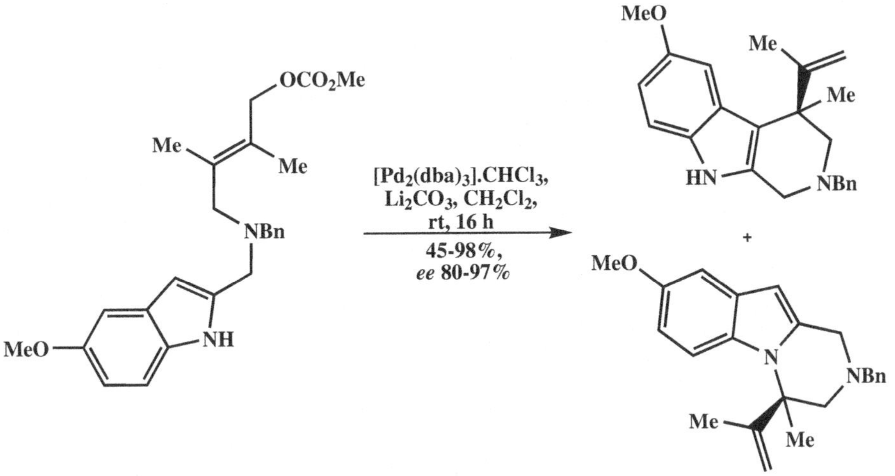

Scheme-65

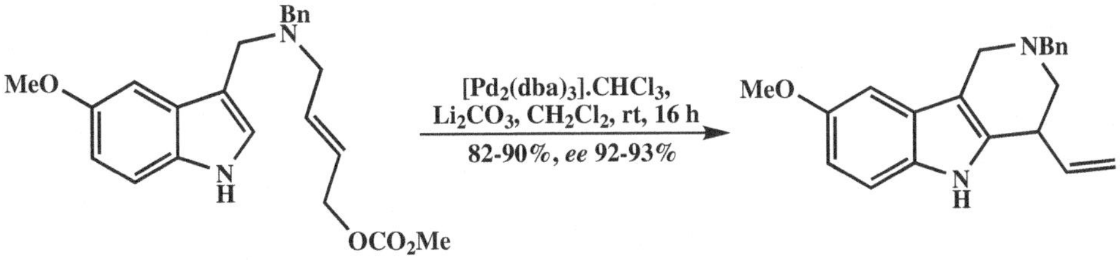

Scheme-66

Liu and Widenhoefer [121] used substituted allylamide and stoichiometric cupric chloride as a terminal oxidant for the preparation of a tetrahydro-β-carbolinone derivative *via* palladium-catalyzed carboalkoxylation of unactivated olefin **(Scheme 67)** [28].

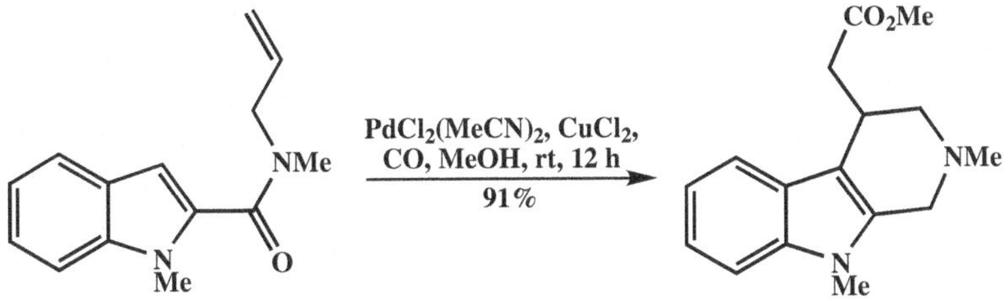

Scheme-67

Ohta and co-workers [122] generated polycyclic indole skeletons. The domino three-component coupling cyclization of 2-ethynylanilines with paraformaldehyde and *N*-butyl allylamine formed 2-(aminomethyl)indoles in the presence of copper catalyst. The final products were synthesized *via* palladium-catalyzed carbon-hydrogen functionalization of C-3 position of 2-(aminomethyl)indoles **(Scheme 68)** [28].

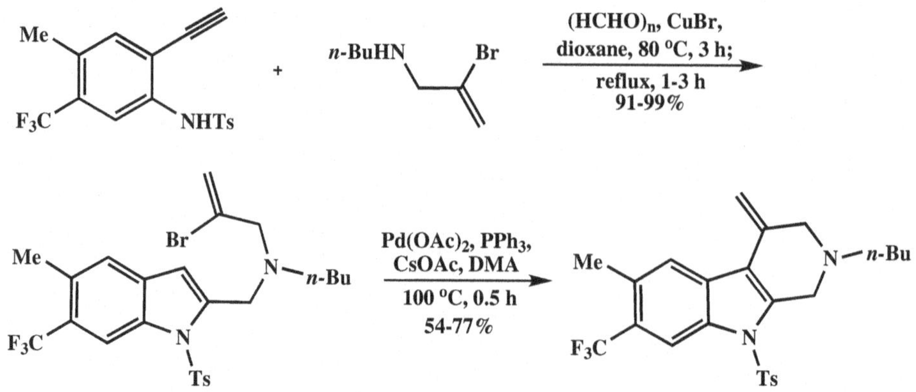

Scheme-68

The opioid agonistic alkaloid mitragynine was generated by Cook and co-workers [123-124]. The reaction proceeded through the formation of allylamine intermediate. This intermediate was synthesized *via* an asymmetric Pictete Spengler reaction and a Ni(cod)$_2$-mediated cyclization **(Scheme 69)** [28, 125].

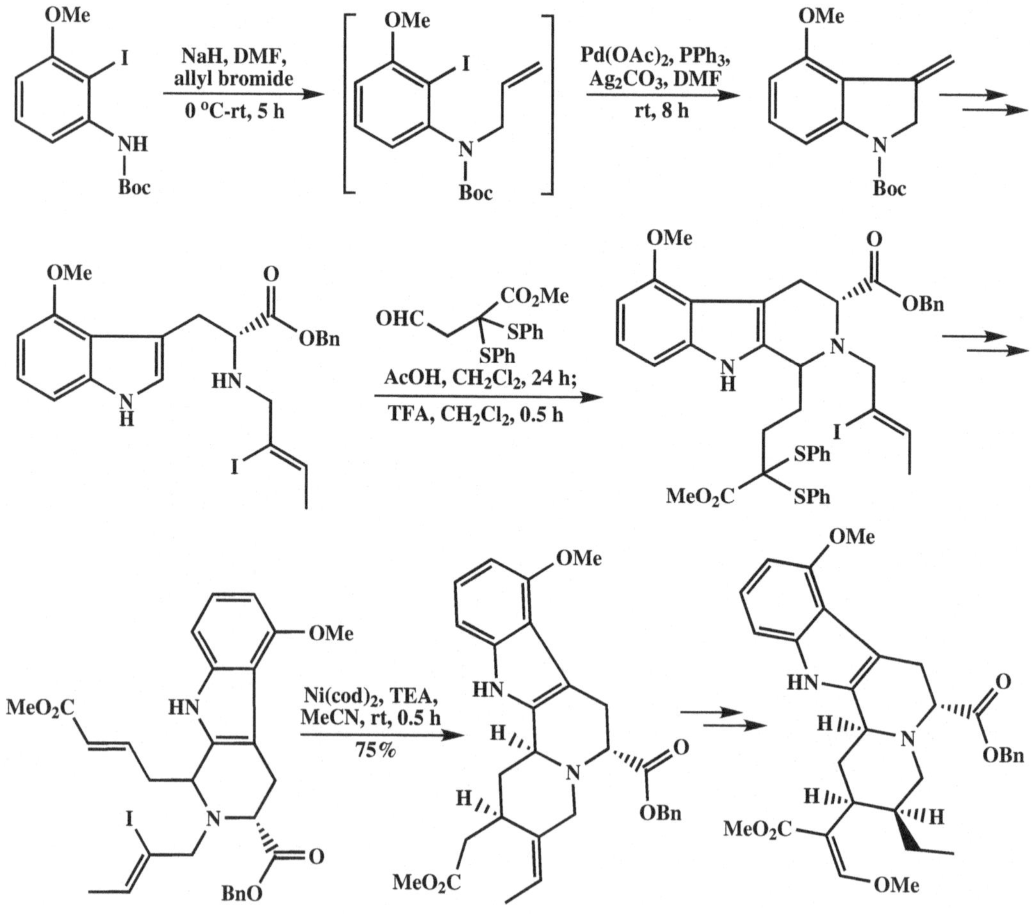

Scheme-69

The sulfonamide was obtained in quantitative yields by tosyl protection of primary amine within tryptamine. Similarly, excellent yields (90%) of 2-bromoindole were obtained in bromination of C2 position. The precursor was treated with Pd(PPh$_3$)$_4$, butyl acrylate and potassium carbonate to afford tetrahydro-β-carboline in a promising yield of 30% **(Scheme 70)**. Moderate yield (27%) of carboline was obtained from tryptamine in three steps. This result has suggested that this particular ring system can be generated with the application of domino Heck-aza-Michael reaction. Three characters of domino Heck-aza-Michael reaction for the optimization of reaction (to improve the yield) were: the nucleophilicity of sulfonamide, the Heck reaction, and the degree of electron deficiency of Michael acceptor. The initial step of this domino process *i.e.* Heck reaction, was optimized first in terms of base, Pd catalyst, and solvent [126-129].

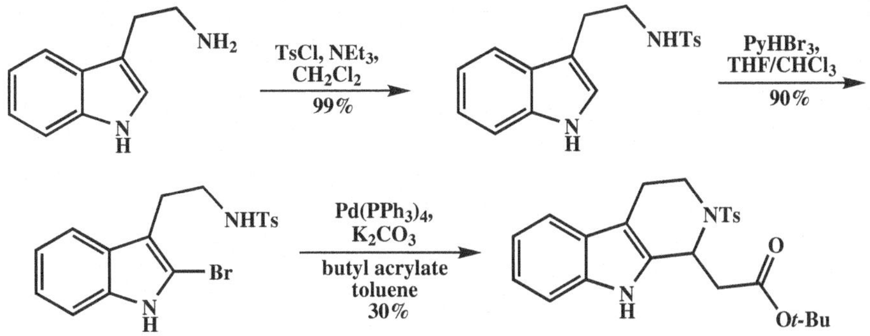

Scheme-70

Bates and Lu [130] reported sequential cross metathesis and hydrogenation of allylamine for the synthesis of 1,3-amino alcohol. The preparation of porantheridine A was performed in this formal synthesis **(Scheme 71)** [28].

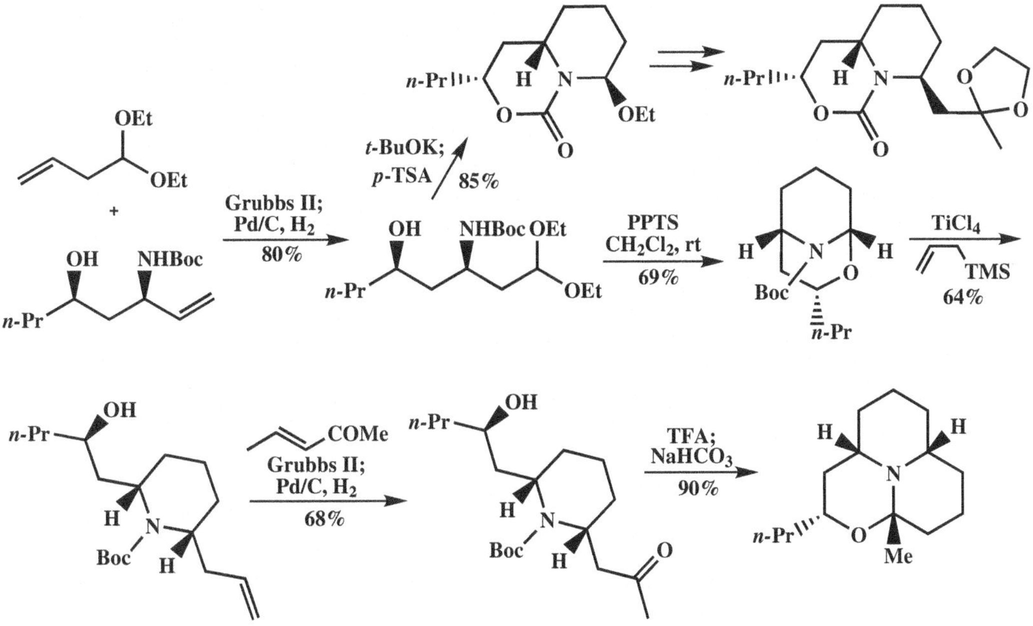

Scheme-71

The β-enaminones are very important building blocks in heterocyclic chemistry. The β-enaminones were formed by the reaction of ynones with primary and secondary amines, besides the reaction with difunctional substrates. Muller et al. [131-134] reported moderate to good yields of tetrahydrocarbolines in four-component reaction which involved α,β-unsaturated acid chlorides as fourth component due to unique ambiphilic reactivity and enormous synthetic potential of β-enaminones **(Scheme 72)**. An acyliminium ion was formed in final step of an aza-annulation reaction which concluded in a Pictet-Spengler cyclization [36].

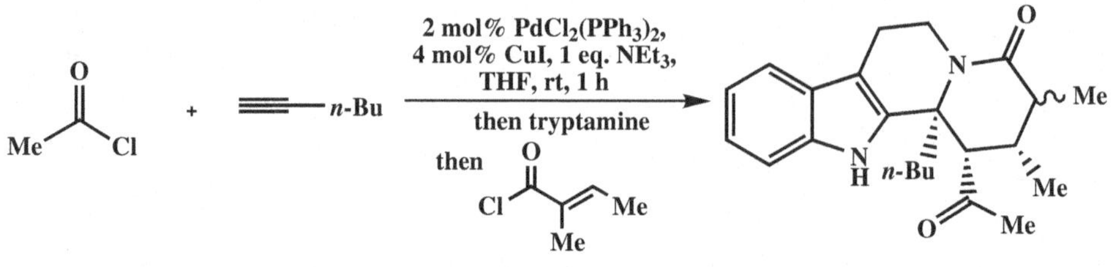

Scheme-72

The *N*-tosyl enimines were more reactive than enones. Annelated pyridines were obtained when *N*-tosyl enimines were treated with very electron rich dienophiles like *N,S*-ketene acetals in a CIR-[4+2]-cycloaddition-aromatization sequence **(Scheme 73)** [135]. Moderate to good yields with excellent regioselectivities of highly fluorescent [1,8]naphthyridines, pyrrolo[2,3-*b*] pyridines, and pyrido[2,3-*b*]azepines were observed by this three-component reaction [36].

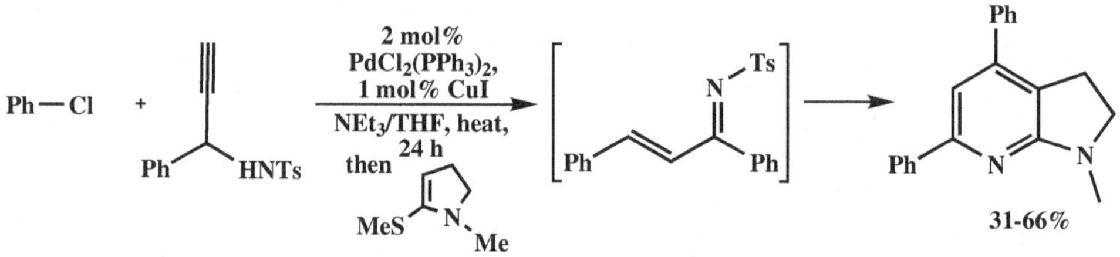

Scheme-73

The configurationally stable ketone was afforded by the reaction of epoxyalcohol with DMP (Dess-Martin periodinane) (or with IBX; 88% yield). Excellent yields without any loss of stereochemical information (>98% *ee*) were obtained in subsequent Grignard addition and S_N2-substitution of tertiary alcohol to allene. Alternatively, the substrate was first treated with methylmagnesium cuprate and then with excess of MeMgX in a one-pot procedure for the transformation of ketone into allene *via* a tandem S_N2-substitution-1,2-addition. The allenic diol was also provided in 93% yield with excellent stereocontrol (>98% *ee*) by this process. The key intermediate was obtained with high stereochemical purity (96% *de*, >98% *ee*) in excellent yield (97%) by subsequent axis-to-center chirality transfer by Au-catalyzed cycloisomerization (0.05 mol% of AuCl$_3$ in tetrahydrofuran) **(Scheme 74)** [136-138].

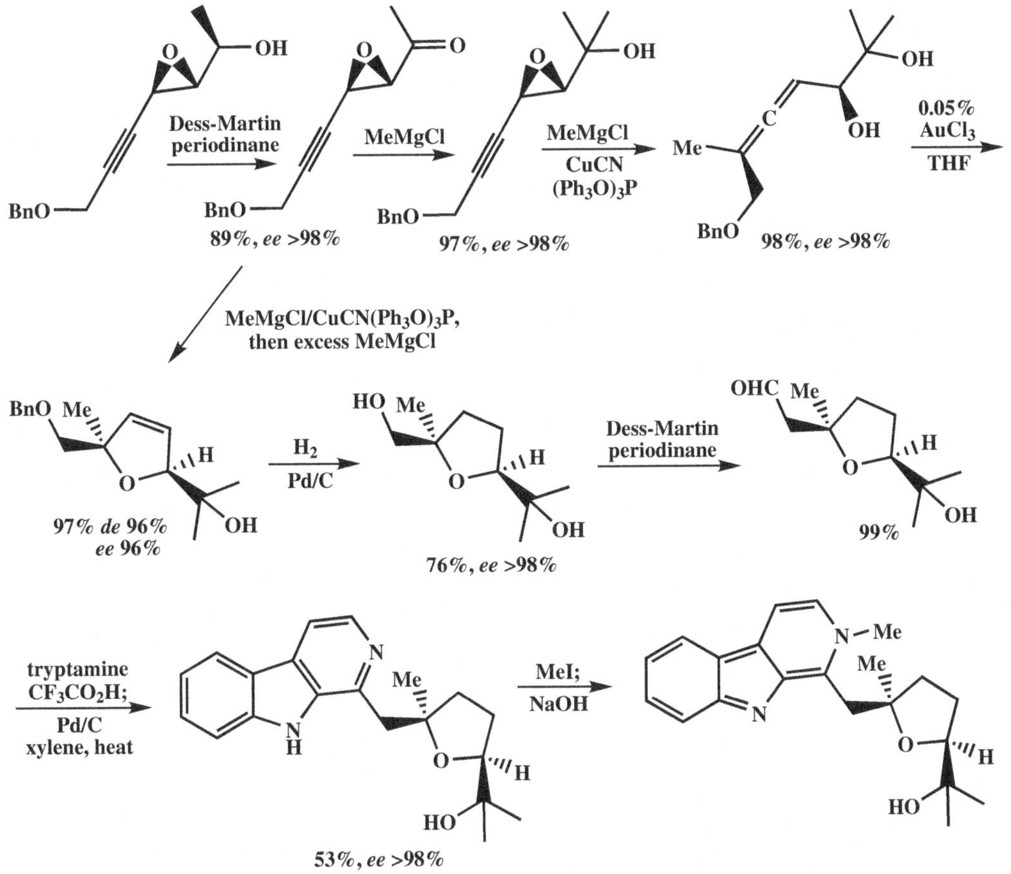

Scheme-74

The coupling cyclization reaction of *N*-allylpyrrole-2-carboxamide derivatives afforded a mixture of two isomeric pyrrolopyridines **(Scheme 75)** [139]. A cationic spiro-palladium intermediate was formed with PdCl$_2$-(MeCN)$_2$/benzoquinone catalytic system at 100 °C in dimethylformamide/tetrahydrofuran. The formed intermediate *via* an anionotropic shift and subsequent loss of a proton afforded two different skeleton types [48].

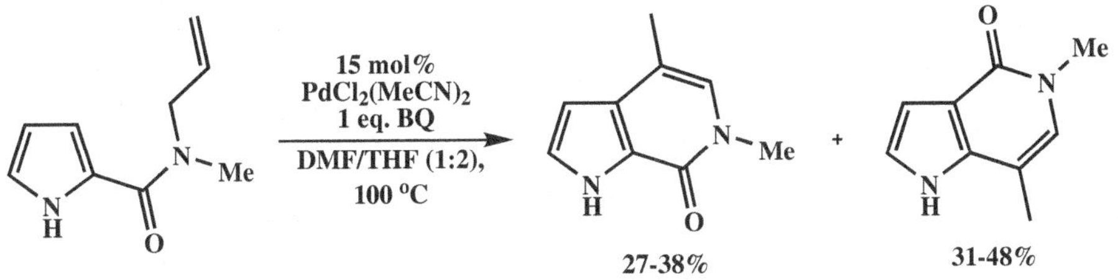

Scheme-75

The *N*-allylindole-2-carboxamide derivatives formed the α-carbolinones in excellent yields *via* oxidative coupling step in the presence of benzoquinone and PdCl$_2$(MeCN)$_2$ in dimethylformamide/tetrahydrofuran **(Scheme 76)** [48, 140-141].

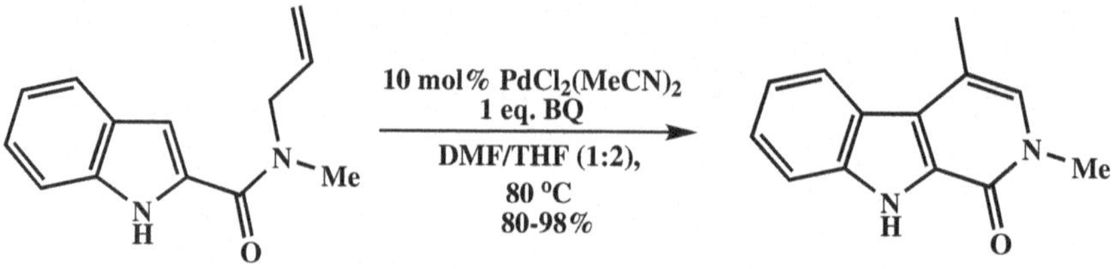

Scheme-76

Optimal results were observed with 10 mol% of triphenylphosphine along with 5 mol% of PdCl₂(MeCN)₂ catalyst system. The product was formed at 100 °C after 6 h in 92% yield. With a carbocycle containing an alkyl protecting group as well as with *N*- and *O*-possessing heterocycles on triazole afforded high to quantitative yields. Many *N*-aryl triazoles also reacted. Moderate yield was observed from electron-poor substrate containing a NO₂ group whereas both electron neutral and rich Heck products were produced efficiently. Finally, quantitative yield of annulation onto *N*-tether of triazole was obtained **(Scheme 77)** [142-143].

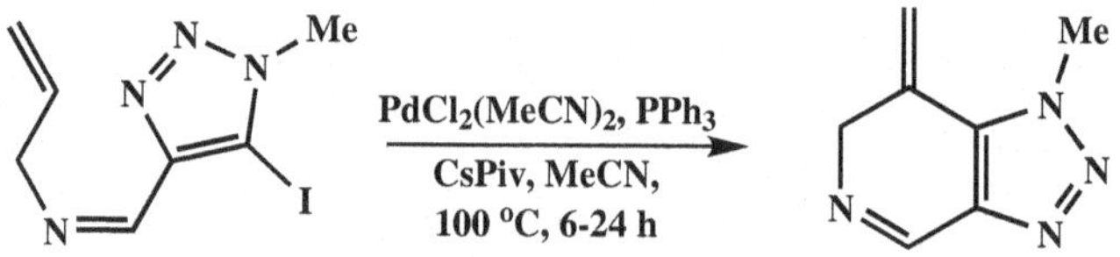

Scheme-77

Moderate yields of 5-annulated pyrrole were reported when pyrrole possess electron-withdrawing ester functionalities at 2-position. The iodouracils were used instead of iodoarenes and provided modest yields **(Scheme 78)** [144].

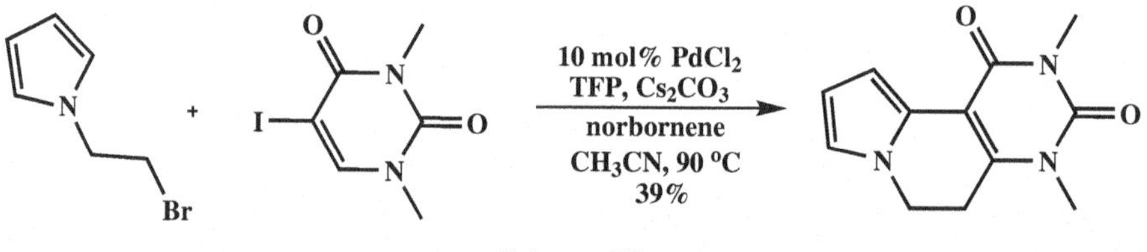

Scheme-78

An efficient way to a furan ring assembled with an indolizinone core was afforded when classical Wacker-type oxidation conditions (*i.e.*, cupric chloride, palladium chloride, and oxygen in dimethylformamide-H₂O) were applied **(Scheme 79)**. The 2-pyrrolidinone and methyl acrylate reacted to form the starting bicyclic system *via* a rhodium(II)-catalyzed 1,3-dipolar cycloaddition [48, 145].

Lactones were provided from *N*-(3-hydroxy-4-pentenyl)-substituted tosylamides, ureas, and carbamates by aminocarbonylation in palladium chloride/cupric chloride and acetic acid [146-147]. In case of ureas a similar cyclization was reported. On the basis of different catalytic conditions substituted benzylamine afforded a different stereoselective outcome **(Scheme 80)** [48, 148].

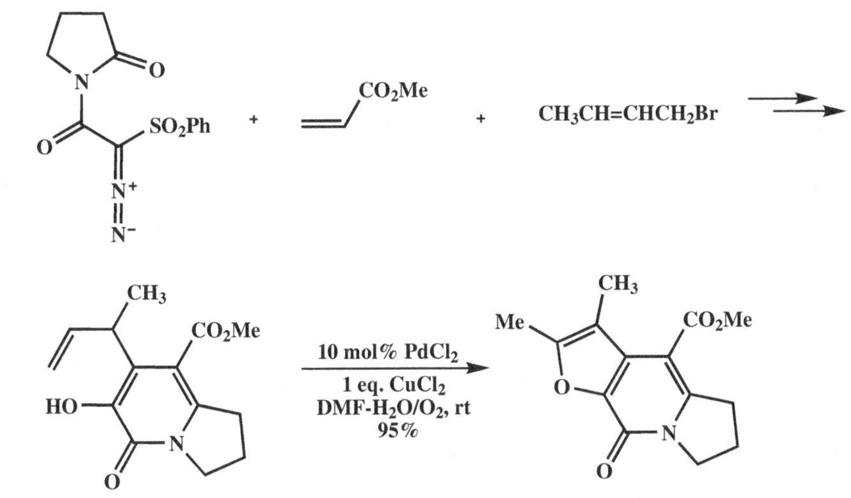

Scheme-79

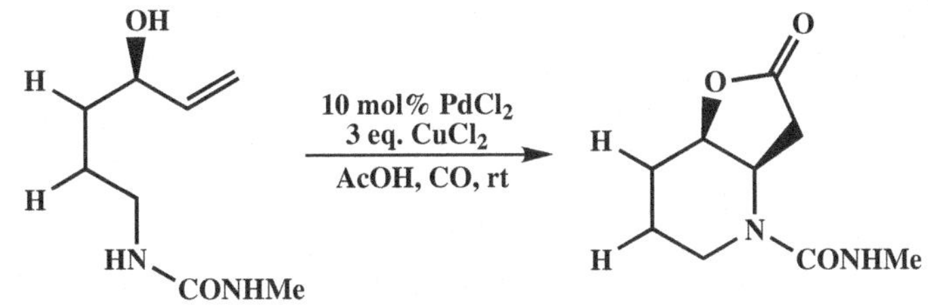

Scheme-80

The annulated carbolines were synthesized by this type of reaction as shown in **Scheme 81** [149].

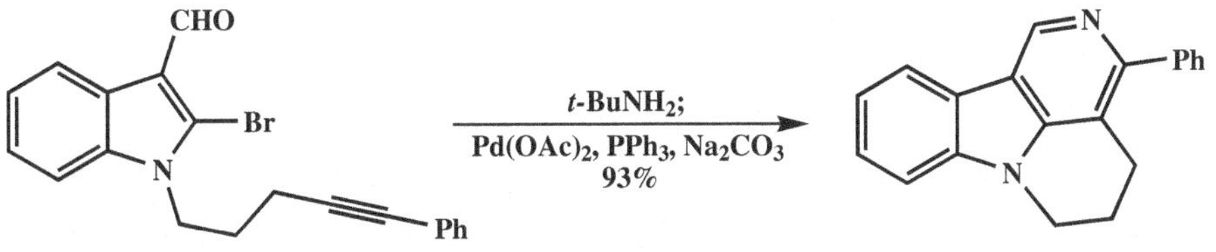

Scheme-81

Mori [150-152] produced enamide or allenamide in a selective manner on the basis of ligand used by aminocyclization of β-lactam possessing propargyl benzoate **(Scheme 82)**. Through the Pd intermediate an allenamide with a carbapenam skeleton was obtained as major product in the presence of a monodentate ligand like P(*o*-tolyl)$_3$. However, the sole elimination product enamide was formed from Pd π-allyl complex when bidentate ligand 1,1′-bis(diphenylphosphino) ferrocene was utilized [1c].

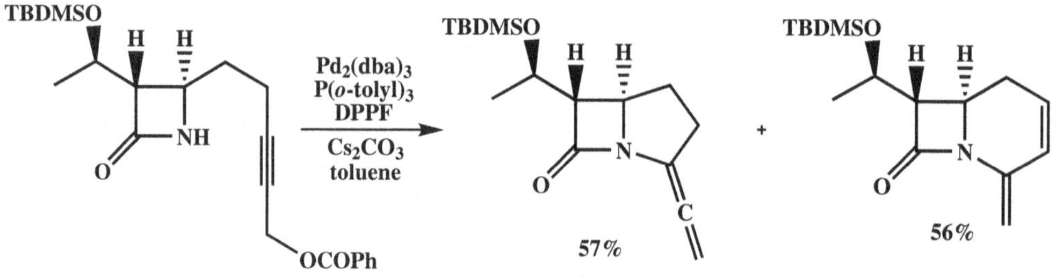

Scheme-82

Hesse and Kirsch [153] reported the reactivity of imines of β-chloroacroleins. The pyridine-fused ring systems were formed when chloro compounds were reacted in one-pot method **(Scheme 83)** [75]. Chloro compounds were less reactive than their bromo- and iodo-parts.

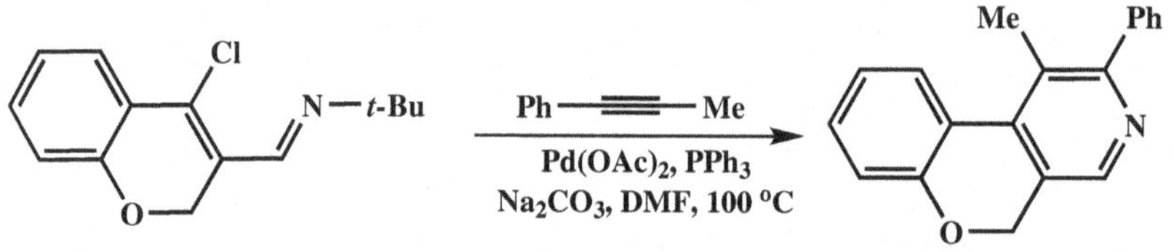

Scheme-83

Metal-catalyzed methods have also been developed. Hirai [154] reported the stereoselective synthesis of vinyl piperidine from oxazolidinone in the presence of a palladium catalyst. Activation of alkene by palladium(II) followed by nucleophilic attack occurred *via* transition state to afford vinyl piperidine alkoxide elimination **(Scheme 84)**.

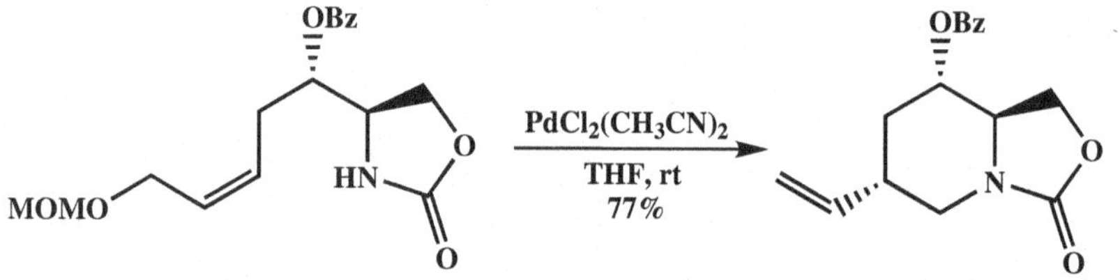

Scheme-84

The first system examined was *tert*-butoxycarbonyl (Boc) protected 2-bromotryptamine. The requisite functionalized tryptamine was prepared by Boc-protection at *N*10-amine, followed by bromination of indole-2-position using pyridinium tribromide. This substrate was then subjected to previously identified conditions for the intermolecular Heck reaction with butyl acrylate **(Scheme 85)**. This reaction exclusively formed Heck adduct with none of the domino product identified *via* initial analysis of crude reaction mixture by 1H NMR spectroscopy. Although the *N*10-amine was sufficiently protected to allow Heck reaction to occur, the carbamate was not nucleophilic enough to undergo aza-Michael addition. As such, the Boc protecting group was not considered ideal for domino process [155-156].

Alkyl-sulfonamides have been shown to be readily functionalized using a range of methods including allylation, Mitsunobu reactions and more importantly aza-Michael addition [157-160]. Due to its ready availability, the *p*-toluenesulfonyl (tosyl) protecting group was investigated for *N*10-amine of tryptamine. To investigate the likelihood of a domino process occurring with sulfonamide system, 2-bromosulfonamide and butyl acrylate (1.2 eq.) was subjected to conditions previously identified for Heck reaction at indole-2-position **(Scheme 86)**. The first reaction attempted with this tosyl-2-bromosulfonamide afforded domino Heck-aza-Michael adduct as major product in 44% yield [161].

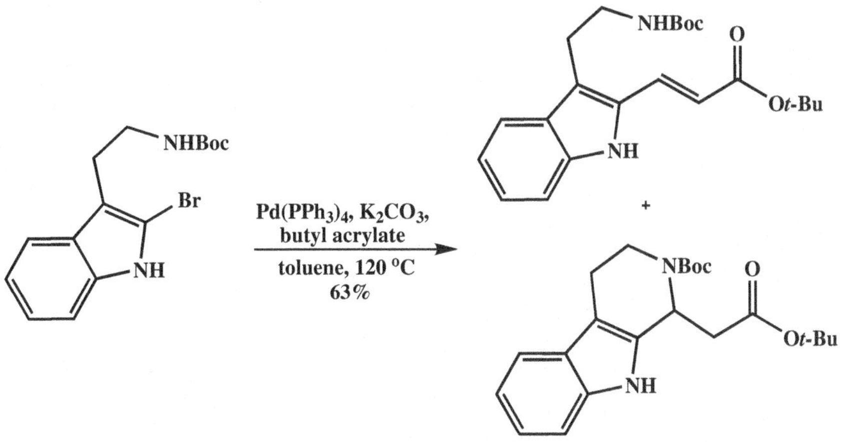

Scheme-85

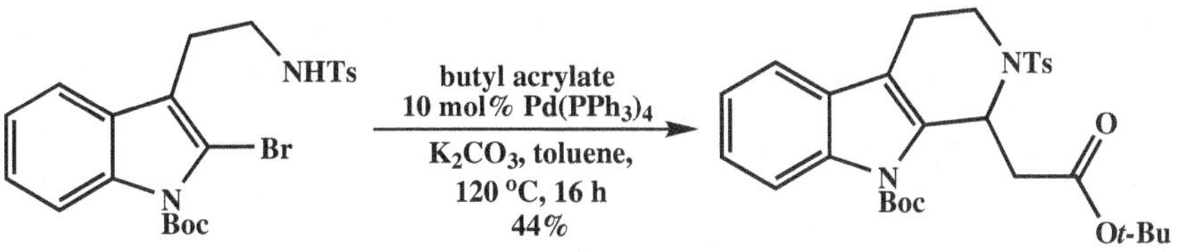

Scheme-86

Predominantly, the use of stronger bases and more polar solvents resulted in aza-Michael addition occurring at sulfonamide or indole nitrogen before Heck reaction had taken place at indole-2-position. This often resulted in a complex mixture of inseparable compounds (including desired compound and several by-products). To minimize side reactions, the domino Heck-aza-Michael process for this *N*-sulfonyl-2-bromotryptamine system was confined to the use of mild bases and relatively non-polar solvents, allowing sufficient time for Heck reaction to take place before aza-Michael addition occurred **(Scheme 87)** [162].

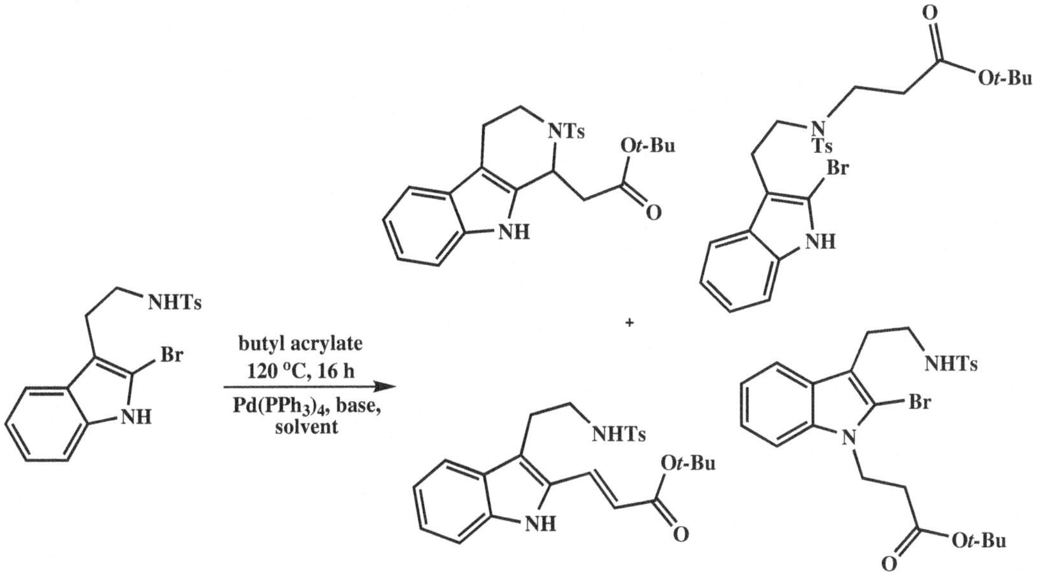

Scheme-87

The domino reaction was performed using catalytic conditions that produced highest yields of analogous tetrahydro-β-carboline (**Scheme 88**). Following analysis of crude reaction mixture, the major product identified from this attempted domino reaction was intermolecular aza-Michael product along with desired product. This result confirmed that domino reaction was indeed a plausible pathway to access benzothiophene-based *N*-heterocycles, however a much more efficient synthesis of domino precursor was required before further optimization of this reaction sequence can be carried out [163].

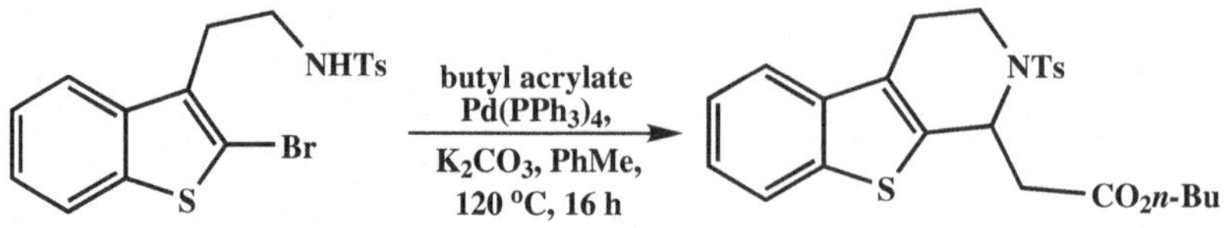

Scheme-88

The first system investigated for multi-component domino Heck-aza-Michael process was tetrahydro-β-carbolines. The requisite domino precursor was prepared in three steps from tryptamine as previously described. Initial investigations employed acryloyl chloride and benzylamine to afford *N*-benzylacrylamide needed for the Heck reaction. The first reaction was carried out by adding acryloyl chloride to a solution containing benzylamine and potassium carbonate in PhMe. After stirring for one hr to allow sufficient time for acrylamide formation, the tosyl-2-bromotryptamine and Pd(PPh$_3$)$_4$ were added and the reaction mixture was heated to 120 °C for 16 h (**Scheme 89**). As the Heck reaction was taking place in a good yield, it was known that acrylamide formation was successful [164].

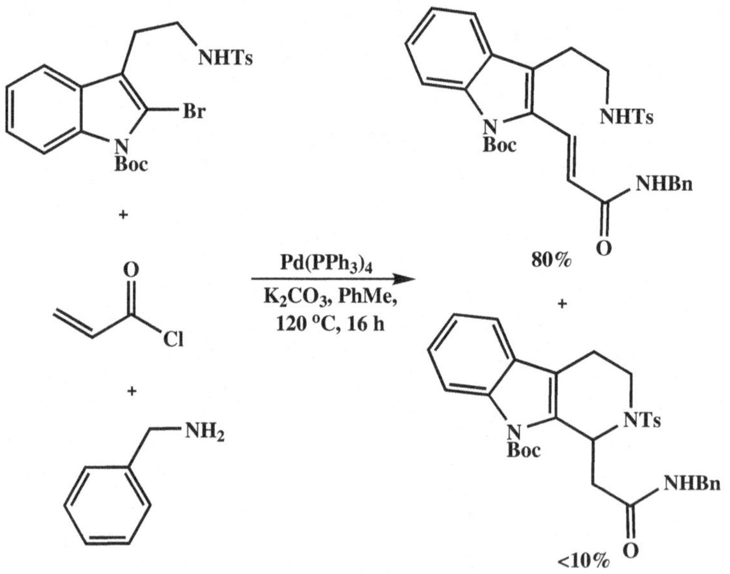

Scheme-89

The asymmetric domino reaction was performed from modified domino substrate silyl ether in the presence of 3-buten-2-one (**Scheme 90**). The crude product was purified by column chromatography after a simple work-up to provide tetrahydro-β-carboline ketone derivative in 81% yield as an inseparable mixture of diastereomers. Following analysis with chiral HPLC (60% *de*) the diastereomeric ratio of product was confirmed [165-166a, b].

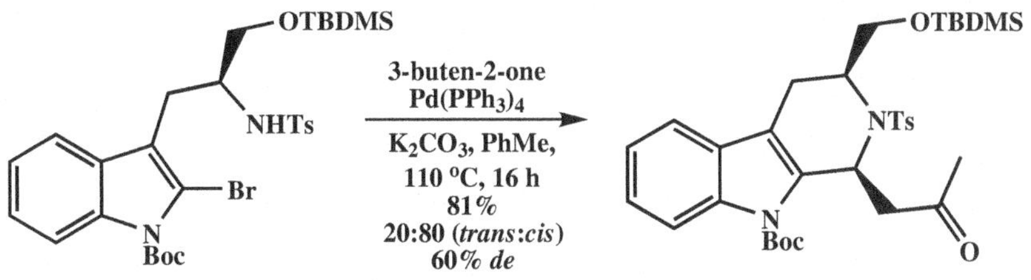

Scheme-90

The application of domino Heck-aza-Michael methodology in total synthesis could also be investigated. Utilizing asymmetric variant, it was envisaged that access to intermediates in a proposed total synthesis of both elaeocarpidine and ajmalicine would be available **(Scheme 91)** [167-169].

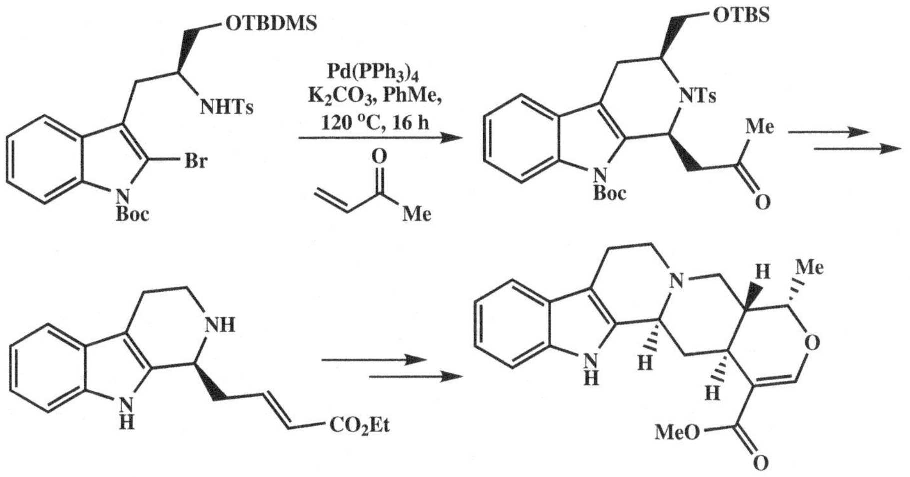

Scheme-91

REFERENCES

[1] (a) N. Kaur. 2015. Palladium catalysts: synthesis of five-membered *N*-heterocycles fused with other heterocycles. Catal. Rev. 57: 1-78.

(b) N. Kaur and D. Kishore. 2014. Microwave-assisted synthesis of six-membered *O,O*-heterocycles. Synth. Commun. 44: 3082-3111.

(c) N. Kaur and D. Kishore. 2014. Microwave-assisted synthesis of six-membered *O*-heterocycles. Synth. Commun. 44: 3047-3081.

(d) Y.Y. Nakamura. 2004. Transition-metal-catalyzed reactions in heterocyclic synthesis. Chem. Rev. 104: 2127-2198.

[2] A.A. Patel and G.A. Mehta. 2010. Synthesis of novel heterocyclic compounds and their biological evaluation. Der Pharma Chemica 2: 215-223.

[3] V.S. Dinakaran, B. Bomma and K.K. Srinivasan. 2012. Fused pyrimidines: the heterocycle of diverse biological and pharmacological significance. Der Pharma Chemica 4: 255-265.

[4] J.D. Sunderhaus, C. Dockendorff and S.F. Martin. 2009. Synthesis of diverse heterocyclic scaffolds *via* tandem additions to imine derivatives and ring-forming reactions. Tetrahedron 65: 6454-6469.

[5] M.C. Bagley, D.D. Hughes, H.M. Sabo, P.H. Taylor and X. Xiong. 2003. One-pot synthesis of pyridines or pyrimidines by tandem oxidation-heteroannulation of propargylic alcohols. Synlett 10: 1443-1446.

[6]   A. Gonzalez-Gomez, G. Dominguez and J. Perez-Castells. 2005. Enyne and dienyne metathesis reactions in β-carbolines. Tetrahedron Lett. 46: 7267-7270.

[7]   S. Murugesan, F. Jiang, M. Achard, C. Bruneau and S. Derien. 2012. Regio- and stereoselective syntheses of piperidine derivatives *via* ruthenium-catalyzed coupling of propargylic amides and allylic alcohols. Chem. Commun. 48: 6589-6591.

[8]   W.-H. Chiou, G.-H. Lin and C.-W. Liang. 2010. Facile syntheses of enantiopure 3-hydroxypiperidine derivatives and 3-hydroxypipecolic acids. J. Org. Chem. 75: 1748-1751.

[9]   M. Motamed, E.M. Bunnelle, S.W. Singaram and R. Sarpong. 2007. Pt(II)-catalyzed synthesis of 1,2-dihydropyridines from aziridinyl propargylic esters. Org Lett. 9: 2167-2170.

[10]   T.K. Hyster and T. Rovis. 2011. Pyridine synthesis from oximes and alkynes *via* rhodium(III) catalysis: Cp* and Cpt provide complementary selectivity. Chem. Commun. 47: 11846-11848.

[11]   Y. Nakao. 2011. Transition-metal-catalyzed C-H functionalization for the synthesis of substituted pyridines. Synthesis 20: 3209-3219.

[12]   N.A. Markina, R. Mancuso, B. Neuenswander, G.H. Lushington and R.C. Larock. 2011. Solution-phase parallel synthesis of a diverse library of 1,2-dihydroisoquinolines. ACS Comb. Sci. 13: 265-271.

[13]   V.S.P.R. Lingam, A. Thomas, K. Mukkanti and B. Gopalan. 2011. Simple and convenient approach for synthesis of tetrahydroquinoline derivatives and studies on aza-Cope rearrangement. Synth. Commun. 41: 1809-1828.

[14]   X.-S. Wang, Z.-S. Zeng, D.-Q. Shi, X.-Y. Wei and Z.-M. Zong. 2004. One-step synthesis of 2-amino-3-cyano-4-aryl-1,4,5,6-tetrahydropyrano-[3,2-*c*]quinolin-5-one derivatives using KF-Al$_2$O$_3$ as catalyst. Synth. Commun. 34: 3021-3027.

[15]   R. Hiessbock, C. Wolf, E. Richter, M. Hitzler, P. Chiba, M. Kratzel and G. Ecker. 1999. Synthesis and *in vitro* multidrug resistance modulating activity of a series of dihydrobenzopyrans and tetrahydroquinolines. J. Med. Chem. 42: 1921-1926.

[16]   C. Gronnier, Y. Odabachian and F. Gagosz. 2011. Gold(I)-catalyzed formation of dihydroquinolines and indoles from *N*-aminophenyl propargyl malonates. Chem. Commun. 47: 218-220.

[17]   O. De Paolis, J. Baffoe, S.M. Landge and B. Torok. 2008. Multicomponent domino cyclization-oxidative aromatization on a bifunctional Pd/C/K-10 catalyst: an environmentally benign approach toward the synthesis of pyridines. Synthesis 21: 3423-3428.

[18]   S.J. Hedley, W.J. Moran, A.H.G.P. Prenzel, D.A. Price and J.P.A. Harrity. 2001. Synthesis of functionalized piperidines through a [3+3] cycloaddition strategy. Synlett 10: 1596-1598.

[19]   R.F.W. Jackson, N. Wishart, A. Wood, K. James and M.J. Wythes. 1992. Preparation of enantiomerically pure protected 4-oxo α-amino acids and 3-aryl α-amino acids from serine. J. Org. Chem. 57: 3397-3404.

[20]   R. Grigg and V. Sridharan. 1998. Heterocycles *via* Pd catalyzed molecular queuing processes. Relay switches and the maximization of molecular complexity. Pure Appl. Chem. 70: 1047-1057.

[21]   R.W. Bates and J. Boonsombat. 2005. Synthesis of sedamine by tethered cyclofunctionalization. Org. Biomol. Chem. 3: 520-523.

[22]   R.W. Bates and K. Sa-Ei. 2002. Syntheses of the sedum and related alkaloids. Tetrahedron 58: 5957-5978.

[23]   R.W. Bates, J. Boonsombat, Y. Lu, J.A. Nemeth, K. Sa-Ei, P. Song, M.P. Cai, P.B. Cranwell and S. Winbush. 2008. *N,O*-heterocycles as synthetic intermediates. Pure Appl. Chem. 80: 681-685.

[24]   L.T. Kaspar and L. Ackermann. 2005. Three-component indole synthesis using *o*-dihaloarenes. Tetrahedron 61: 11311-11316.

[25]   X.-H. Duan, X.-Y. Li, L.-N. Guo, M.-C. Liao, W.-M. Liu and Y.-M. Liang. 2005. Palladium-catalyzed one-pot synthesis of highly substituted furans by a three-component annulation reaction. J. Org. Chem. 70: 6980-6983.

[26]   M. Syamala. 2009. Recent progress in three-component reactions: an update. Org. Prep. Proced. Int. 41: 1-68.

[27]   C. Eriksson, K. Sjoedin, F. Schlyter and H.-E. Hoegberg. 2006. Synthesis of (+)- and (-)-dihydropinidine by diastereoselective dimethylzinc promoted allylation of 2-methyltetrahydropyridine-*N*-oxide with an allylboronic ester. Tetrahedron: Asymmetry 17: 1074-1080.

[28] S. Nag and S. Batra. 2011. Applications of allylamines for the syntheses of aza-heterocycles. Tetrahedron 67: 8959-9061.

[29] S. Gowrisankar, H.S. Lee, J.M. Kim and J.N. Kim. 2008. Pd-mediated synthesis of 2-arylquinolines and tetrahydropyridines from modified Baylis-Hillman adducts. Tetrahedron Lett. 49: 1670-1673.

[30] C. Bukovec and U. Kazmaier. 2009. A straightforward protocol for one-pot allylic aminations/Stille couplings. Org. Lett. 11: 3518-3521.

[31] B. Gabriele, G. Salerno, A. Fazio and L. Veltri. 2006. Versatile synthesis of pyrrole-2-acetic esters and (pyridine-2-one)-3-acetic amides by palladium-catalyzed, carbon dioxide-promoted oxidative carbonylation of (Z)-(2-en-4-ynyl)amines. Adv. Synth. Catal. 348: 2212-2222.

[32] P. Webber and M.J. Krische. 2008. Concise stereocontrolled formal synthesis of (+/-)-quinine and total synthesis of (+/-)-7- hydroxyquinine *via* merged Morita-Baylis-Hillman-Tsuji-Trost cyclization. J. Org. Chem. 73: 9379-9387.

[33] M. Jida, R. Guillot and J. Ollivier. 2007. Azabicyclo[3.1.0]hexane-1-ols as frameworks for the asymmetric synthesis of biologically active compounds. Tetrahedron Lett. 48: 8765-8767.

[34] N.A.M. Yehia, K. Polborn and T.J.J. Muller. 2002. A novel four component one-pot access to pyridines and tetrahydroquinolines based upon a coupling-isomerization sequence. Tetrahedron Lett. 43: 6907-6910.

[35] O.G. Dediu, N.A.M. Yehia, T. Oeser, K. Polborn and T.J.J. Muller. 2005. Coupling-isomerization-enamine addition-cyclocondensation sequences: a multicomponent approach to substituted and annelated pyridines. Eur. J. Org. Chem. 9: 1834-1848.

[36] D.M. D'Souza and T.J.J. Muller. 2007. Multi-component syntheses of heterocycles by transition-metal catalysis. Chem. Soc. Rev. 36: 1095-1108.

[37] T. Wu, G. Yin and G. Liu. 2009. Palladium-catalyzed intramolecular aminofluorination of unactivated alkenes. J. Am. Chem. Soc. 131: 16354-16355.

[38] G. Yin and G. Liu. 2008. Palladium-catalyzed oxidative cyclization of enynes with hydrogen peroxide as the oxidant. Angew. Chem. Int. Ed. 47: 5442-5445.

[39] G. Yin, T. Wu and G. Liu. 2012. Highly selective palladium-catalyzed intramolecular chloroamination of unactivated alkenes by using hydrogen peroxide as an oxidant. Chem. Eur. J. 18: 451-455.

[40] W. Oloo, P.Y. Zavalij, J. Zhang, E. Khaskin and A.N.J. Vedernikov. 2010. Preparation and C-X reductive elimination reactivity of monoaryl Pd(IV)-X complexes in water (X = OH, OH$_2$, Cl, Br). J. Am. Chem. Soc. 132: 14400-14402.

[41] T. Wu, X. Mu and G. Liu. 2011. Palladium-catalyzed oxidative arylalkylation of activated alkenes: dual C-H bond cleavage of an arene and acetonitrile. Angew. Chem. Int. Ed. 50: 12578-12581.

[42] Liu, G. 2012. Transition metal-catalyzed fluorination of multi carbon-carbon bonds: new strategies for fluorinated heterocycles. Org. Biomol. Chem. 10: 6243-6248.

[43] H. Jiang, X. Ji, X. Li, Z. Chen and A. Wang. 2011. Palladium-assisted multicomponent cyclization of aromatic aldehydes, arylamines and terminal olefins under molecular oxygen: an assembly of 1,4-dihydropyridines. Org. Biomol. Chem. 9: 5358-5361.

[44] J.-P. Wan and Y. Liu. 2012. Recent advances in new multicomponent synthesis of structurally diversified 1,4-dihydropyridines. RSC Adv. 2: 9763-9777.

[45] P.R. Girling, A.S. Batsanov, H.C. Shen and A. Whiting. 2012. A multicomponent formal [1+2+1+2]-cycloaddition for the synthesis of dihydropyridines. Chem. Commun. 48: 4893-4895.

[46] D. Yang, J.-H. Li, Q. Gao and Y.-L. Yan. 2003. Lanthanide triflate-promoted palladium-catalyzed cyclization of alkenyl β-keto esters and amides. Org. Lett. 5: 2869-2871.

[47] K.-T. Yip, J.-H. Li, O.-Y. Lee and D. Yang. 2005. Aerobic oxidative cyclization under Pd(II) catalysis: a regioselective approach to heterocycles. Org. Lett. 7: 5717-5719.

[48] E.M. Beccalli, G. Broggini, M. Martinelli and S. Sottocornola. 2007. C-C, C-O, C-N Bond formation on sp^2 carbon by Pd(II)-catalyzed reactions involving oxidant agents. Chem. Rev. 107: 5318-5365.

[49] B. Pugin and L.M. Venanzi. 1983. Palladium-catalyzed oxidation of amino alkenes to cyclic imines or enamines and amino ketones. J. Am. Chem. Soc. 105: 6877-6881.

[50] J. Revuelta, S. Cicchi and A. Brandi. 2005. Two-step metal-mediated transformation of isoxazolidine-5-spirocyclopropanes into pyridone derivatives. J. Org. Chem. 70: 5636-5642.

[51]   Y. Tamaru, M. Hojo, S.-I. Kawamura and Z.-I. Yoshida. 1986. Synthesis of five- and six-membered nitrogen heterocycles *via* palladium(II)-catalyzed cyclization of unsaturated amides. J. Org. Chem. 51: 4089-4090.

[52]   P. Szolcsanyi and T. Gracza. 2005. Novel Pd(II)-catalyzed *N,O*-bicyclization as an efficient route to the 6-oxa-2-azabicyclo[3.2.1]octane skeleton. Chem. Commun. 31: 3948-3950.

[53]   P. Szolcsanyi and T. Gracza. 2006. PdCl$_2$/CuCl$_2$-catalyzed chlorocyclization of sugar-derived aminoalkenitols in the synthesis of new iminohexitols. Tetrahedron 62: 8498-8502.

[54]   H. Yokoyama, K. Otaya, H. Kobayashi, M. Miyazawa, S. Yamaguchi and Y. Hirai. 2000. Palladium(II)-catalyzed cyclization of urethanes and total synthesis of 1-deoxymannojirimycin. Org. Lett. 2: 2427-2429.

[55]   J.G. Knight, S.W. Ainge, A.M. Harm, S.J. Harwood, H.I. Maughan, D.R. Armour, D.M. Hollinshead and A.A. Jaxa-Chamiec. 2000. Enantioselective synthesis of 3,6-dihydro-1*H*-pyridin-2 ones: unexpected regioselectivity in the palladium-catalyzed decarboxylative carbonylation of 5-vinyloxazolidin-2-ones. J. Am. Chem. Soc. 122: 2944-2945.

[56]   H. Nakamura, K. Aoyagi, J.-G. Shim and Y. Yamamoto. 2001. Catalytic amphiphilic allylation *via* bis-π-allylpalladium complexes and its application to the synthesis of medium-sized carbocycles. J. Am. Chem. Soc. 123: 372-377.

[57]   K. Takasu, N. Nishida and M. Ihara. 2004. Palladium-catalyzed hydroamidation of enones. Synlett 10: 1844-1846.

[58]   M. Ihara. 2006. Cascade reactions for syntheses of heterocycles. ARKIVOC (vii): 416-438.

[59]   H. Tsutsui and K. Narasaka. 1999. Synthesis of pyrrole derivatives by the Heck-type cyclization of γ,δ-unsaturated ketone *O*-(pentafluorobenzoyl)oximes. Chem. Lett. 1: 45-46.

[60]   M. Kitamura and K. Narasaka. 2002. Synthesis of aza-heterocycles from oximes by amino-Heck reaction. Chem. Rec. 2: 268-277.

[61]   H. Tsutsui, M. Kitamura and K. Narasaka. 2002. Synthesis of pyrrole derivatives by palladium-catalyzed cyclization of γ,δ-unsaturated ketone *O*-pentafluorobenzoyloximes. Bull. Chem. Soc. Jpn. 75: 1451-1460.

[62]   R. Grigg, V. Sridharan, P. Stevenson and T. Worakun. 1986. Palladium(II) catalyzed construction of tetrasubstituted carbon centres, and spiro and bridged-ring compounds from enamides of 2-Iodobenzoic acids. Chem. Commun. 23: 1697-1699.

[63]   L.S. Hegedus, M.R. Sestrick, E.T. Michaelson and P.J. Harrington. 1989. Palladium-catalyzed reactions in the synthesis of 3- and 4-substituted indoles. J. Org. Chem. 54: 4141-4146.

[64]   M. Kitamura, D. Kudo and K. Narasaka. 2006. Palladium(0)-catalyzed synthesis of pyridines from β-acetoxy-γ,δ-unsaturated ketone oximes. ARKIVOC (iii): 148-162.

[65]   H. Tsutsui and K. Narasaka. 2001. Synthesis of pyridine and isoquinoline derivatives by the palladium-catalyzed cyclization of olefinic ketone *O*-pentafluorobenzoyloximes. Chem. Lett. 30: 526-527.

[66]   R.C. Larock, H. Yang, S.M. Weinreb and R.J. Herr. 1994. Synthesis of pyrrolidines and piperidines *via* palladium-catalyzed coupling of vinylic halides and olefinic sulfonamides. J. Org. Chem. 59: 4172-4178.

[67]   F.E. Michael and B.M. Cochran. 2006. Room temperature palladium-catalyzed intramolecular hydroamination of unactivated alkenes. J. Am. Chem. Soc. 128: 4246-4247.

[68]   M. Mouhtaram, L. Jung and J.F. Stambach. 1993. Novel synthesis of substituted phenylpiperazines by addition of benzylamine or methylamine to β-nitrostyrene. Tetrahedron 49: 1391-1400.

[69]   S.G. Davies, P.M. Roberts and A.D. Smith. 2007. Asymmetric three- and [2+1]-component conjugate addition reactions for the stereoselective synthesis of polysubstituted piperidinones. Org. Biomol. Chem. 5: 1405-1415.

[70]   T.E. Muller, K.C. Hultzsch, M. Yus, F. Foubelo and M. Tada. 2008. Hydroamination: direct addition of amines to alkenes and alkynes. Chem. Rev. 108: 3795-3892.

[71]   H. Tsukamoto and Y. Kondo. 2008. Palladium(0)-catalyzed alkynyl and allenyl iminium ion cyclizations leading to 1,4-disubstituted 1,2,3,6-tetrahydropyridines. Angew. Chem. Int. Ed. 47: 4851-4854.

[72]   D. Bouyssi, N. Monteiro and G. Balme. 2011. Amines as key building blocks in Pd-assisted multicomponent processes. Beilstein J. Org. Chem. 7: 1387-1406.

[73] T. Kobayashi, M. Nakashima, T. Hakogi, K. Tanaka and S. Katsumura. 2006. Development of a one-pot asymmetric azaelectrocyclization protocol: synthesis of chiral 2,4-disubstituted 1,2,5,6-tetrahydropyridines. Org. Lett. 8: 3809-3812.

[74] K.R. Roesch and R.C. Larock. 1998. Synthesis of isoquinolines and pyridines *via* palladium-catalyzed iminoannulation of internal acetylenes. J. Org. Chem. 63: 5306-5307.

[75] G. Kirsch, S. Hesse and A. Comel. 2004. Synthesis of five- and six-membered heterocycles through palladium-catalyzed reactions. Curr. Org. Synth. 1: 47-63.

[76] Z. Lu and S.S. Stahl. 2012. Intramolecular Pd(II)-catalyzed aerobic oxidative amination of alkenes: synthesis of six-membered *N*-heterocycles. Org. Lett. 14: 1234-1237.

[77] G. He, Y. Zhao, S. Zhang, C. Lu and G. Chen. 2012. Highly efficient syntheses of azetidines, pyrrolidines, and indolines *via* palladium catalyzed intramolecular amination of C(sp^3)-H and C(sp^2)-H bonds at γ and δ positions. J. Am. Chem. Soc. 134: 3-6.

[78] A. Gheorghe, B. Quiclet-Sire, X. Vila and S.Z. Zard. 2007. Synthesis of substituted 3-arylpiperidines and 3-arylpyrrolidines by radical 1,4 and 1,2-aryl migrations. Tetrahedron 63: 7187-7212.

[79] R.-W. Wang, X.-L. Qiu, M. Bols, F. Ortega-Caballero and F.-L. Qing. 2006. Synthesis and biological evaluation of glycosidase inhibitors: *gem*-Difluoromethylenated nojirimycin analogues. J. Med. Chem. 49: 2989-2997.

[80] B.M. Trost and M.R. Machacek. 2002. An efficient one-pot enantio- and diastereoselective synthesis of heterocycles. Angew. Chem. Int. Ed. 41: 4693-4697.

[81] T. Uchida, M. Rodriquez and S.L. Shreiber. 2009. Skeletally diverse small molecules using a build/couple/pair strategy. Org. Lett. 11: 1559-1562.

[82] L. Battisini, G. Rassu, L. Pinna, F. Zanardi and G. Casiraghi. 1999. Diastereoselective synthesis of a novel lactam peptidomimetic exploiting vinylogous Mannich addition of 2-silyloxyfuran reagents. Tetrahedron: Asyrnmetry 10: 765-773.

[83] A. Golubev, N. Sewald and K. Burger. 1995. An efficient approach to the family of 4-substituted pipecolic acids. Syntheses of 4-oxo, *cis*-4-hydroxy-, and *trans*-4-hydroxy-L-pipecolic acids from L-aspartic acid. Tetrahedron Lett. 36: 2037-2040.

[84] R.M. Williams, P.J. Sinclair, D. Zhai and D. Chen. 1988. Practical asymmetric syntheses of α-amino acids through carbon-carbon bond constructions on electrophilic glycine templates. J. Am. Chem. Soc. 110: 1547-1557.

[85] F. Huguenot and T. Brigaud. 2006. Convenient asymmetric synthesis of β-trifluoromethyl-β-amino acid, β-amino ketones, and γ-amino alcohols *via* Reformatsky and Mannich-type reactions from 2-trifluoromethyl-1,3-oxazolidines. J. Org. Chem. 71: 2159-2162.

[86] J. Cho, Y.M. Lee, D. Kim and S. Kim. 2009. Design and synthesis of piperidine-containing sphingoid base analogues. J. Org. Chem. 74: 3900-3904.

[87] Y. Nagahara, T. Shinomiya, S. Kuroda, N. Kaneko, R. Nishio and M. Ikekita. 2005. Phytosphingosine induced mitochondria-involved apoptosis. Cancer Sci. 96: 83-92.

[88] G. Abbiati, E. Beccalli, A. Marchesini and E. Rossi. 2001. Synthesis of β-carbolines from 2-acyl-1-benzenesulfonyl-3-iodo-1*H*-indoles. Synthesis 16: 2477-2483.

[89] J.H. Diederen, M. Pfeffer, H.-W. Fruhauf, H. Hiemstra and K. Vrieze. 1998. Synthesis of new *N*-heterocycles; intramolecular ring closure with imines. Tetrahedron Lett. 39: 4111-4114.

[90] S. Rousset, M. Abarbi, J. Thibonnet, A. Duchêne and J.-L. Parrain. 2000. Palladium-catalyzed annulation reaction of allenyltins with β-iodo vinylic acids: selective synthesis of α-pyrones. Chem. Commun. 20: 1987-1988.

[91] T. Harayama, H. Akamatsu, K. Okamura, T. Miyagoe, T. Akiyama, H. Abe and Y. Takeuchi. 2001. Synthesis of trisphaeridine and norchelerythrine through palladium-catalyzed aryl-aryl coupling reactions. J. Chem. Soc. Perkin Trans. 1 5: 523-528.

[92] M.G. Banwell, D.W. Lupton, X. Ma, J. Renner and M.O. Sydnes. 2004. Synthesis of quinolines, 2-quinolones, phenanthridines, and 6(5*H*)-phenanthridinones *via* palladium[0]-mediated Ullmann cross-coupling of 1-bromo-2-nitroarenes with β-halo-enals, -enones, or -esters. Org. Lett. 6: 2741-2744.

[93]   E. Bacque, M.E. Qacemi and S.Z. Zard. 2004. Tin-free radical cyclizations for the synthesis of 7-azaoxindoles, 7-azaindolines, tetrahydro[1,8]naphthyridines, and tetrahydro-5*H*-pyrido[2,3-*b*] azepin-8-ones. Org. Lett. 6: 3671-3674.

[94]   D.H.R. Barton, B. Garcia, H. Togo and S.Z. Zard. 1986. Radical decarboxylative addition onto protonated heteroaromatic (and related) compounds. Tetrahedron Lett. 27: 1327-1330.

[95]   F. Minisci, E. Vismara and F. Fontana. 1989. Recent developments of free-radical substitutions of heteroaromatic bases. Heterocycles 28: 489-519.

[96]   R.U. Islam, M.J. Witcomb, E. van der Lingen, M.S. Scurrell and W. van Otterlo. 2011. *In situ* synthesis of a palladium-polyaniline hybrid catalyst for a Suzuki coupling reaction. J. Organomet. Chem. 696: 2206-2210.

[97]   L.L. Joyce, G. Evindar and R.A. Batey 2004. Copper- and palladium-catalyzed intramolecular C-S bond formation: a convenient synthesis of 2-aminobenzothiazoles. Chem. Commun. 4: 446-447.

[98]   T. Taniguchi, H. Zaimoku and H. Ishibashi. 2009. Formal total synthesis of haouamine A. J. Org. Chem. 74: 2624-2626.

[99]   K. Partogyan-Halim, L. Besson, D.J. Aitken and H.-P. Husson. 2003. Asymmetric synthesis of (*S*)-4-oxopipecolic acid by a 3+3 atom-unit assembly strategy. Eur. J. Org. Chem. 2: 268-273.

[100]   A. Okano, T. Mizutani, S. Oishi, T. Tanaka, H. Ohno and N. Fujii. 2008. Palladium-catalyzed biscyclization of allenic bromoalkenes through a zipper-mode cascade. Chem. Commun. 39: 3534-3536.

[101]   M. Ishikura, N. Takahashi, K. Yamada and T. Abe. 2008. A concise approach to (±)-tubifoline based on the palladium-catalyzed cross-coupling reaction of indolylborate. Heterocycles 75: 107-118.

[102]   M. Dell'Acqua, G. Abbiati and E. Rossi. 2010. Palladium-catalyzed, microwave-enhanced three-component synthesis of isoquinolines with aqueous ammonia. Synlett 17: 2672-2676.

[103]   D. Yang, S. Burugupalli, D. Daniel and Y. Chen. 2012. Microwave-assisted one-pot synthesis of isoquinolines, furopyridines, and thienopyridines by palladium-catalyzed sequential coupling-imination-annulation of 2-bromoarylaldehydes with terminal acetylenes and ammonium acetate. J. Org. Chem. 77: 4466-4472.

[104]   A. Das, A. Kulkarni and B. Torok. 2012. Environmentally benign synthesis of heterocyclic compounds by combined microwave-assisted heterogeneous catalytic approaches. Green Chem. 14: 17-34.

[105]   E.M. Beck, N.P. Grimster, R. Hatley and M.J. Gaunt. 2006. Mild aerobic oxidative palladium (II) catalyzed C-H bond functionalization: regioselective and switchable C-H alkenylation and annulation of pyrroles. J. Am. Chem. Soc. 128: 2528-2529.

[106]   E.M. Beck, R. Hatley and M.J. Gaunt. 2008. Synthesis of rhazinicine by a metal-catalyzed C-H bond functionalization strategy. Angew. Chem. Int. Ed. 47: 3004-3007.

[107]   D.L. Floc'h, N. Gouault, M. David and P. Wegheb. 2010. Three different approaches to C-H bond functionalization in the synthesis of anti-tumor alkaloids rhazinilam, rhazinal and rhazinicine. ARKIVOC (i): 247-259.

[108]   F. Freeman, D.S.H.L. Kim and E. Rodriguez. 1992. Preparation of 1,4-diketones and their reactions with bis(trialkyltin) or bis(triphenyltin) sulfide-boron trichloride. J. Org. Chem. 57: 1722-1727.

[109]   A. Erkkila and P. Pihko. 2006. Mild organocatalytic α-methylenation of aldehydes. J. Org. Chem. 71: 2538-2541.

[110]   F. Denat, H. Gaspard-Iloughmane and J. Dubac. 1992. Pyrrolyl compounds of main group elements. Synthesis of group 14 5-metallated pyrrole-2-carbaldehydes. J. Organomet. Chem. 423: 173-182.

[111]   S.N. Gradl, J.J. Kennedy-Smith, J. Kim and D. Trauner. 2002. A practical variant of the Claisen-Eschenmoser rearrangement: synthesis of unsaturated morpholine amides a practical variant of the Claisen-Eschenmoser rearrangement. Synlett 1437-2096.

[112]   B. Alcaide, P. Almendros, A. Luna and T. Martinez del Campo. 2008. Synthesis of novel enantiopure 4-hydroxypipecolic acid derivatives with a bicyclic β-lactam structure from a common 3-azido-4-oxoazetidine-2-carbaldehyde precursor. J. Org. Chem. 73: 1635-1638.

[113]   J.Y.L. Chung, R.J. Cvetovich, M. McLaughlin, J. Amato, F.-R. Tsay, M. Jensen, S. Weissman and D. Zewge. 2006. Synthesis of a naphthyridone p38 MAP kinase inhibitor. J. Org. Chem. 71: 8602-8609.

[114] F. Gosselin and W.D. Lubell. 1998. An olefination entry for the synthesis of enantiopure α,ω-diaminodicarboxylates and azabicyclo[X.Y.0]alkane amino acids. J. Org. Chem. 63: 7463-7471.

[115] (a) D. Trauner, J.B. Schwarz and S.J. Danishefsky. 1999. Total synthesis of (+)-halichlorine: an inhibitor of VCAM-1 expression. Angew. Chem. Int. Ed. 38: 3542-3545.
(b) S. Kotha, K. Lahiri and D. Kashinath. 2002. Recent applications of the Suzuki-Miyaura cross-coupling reaction in organic synthesis. Tetrahedron 58: 9633-9695.

[116] T. Kametani, T. Suzuki, E. Sato, M. Nishimura and K. Unno. 1982. Enantioselective synthesis of (+)-dihydroantirhine. J. Chem. Soc. Chem. Comm. 20: 1201-1203.

[117] G. Massiot, P. Thepenier, M.J. Jacquier, L. Le Men-Olivier and C. Delaude. 1992. Alkaloids from roots of *Strychnos potatorum*. Phytochemistry 31: 2873-2876.

[118] L.F. Tietze, J. Bachmann, J. Wichmann, Y. Zhou and T. Raschke. 1997. Efficient biomimetic synthesis of indole alkaloids of the vallesiachotamine group by a domino Knoevenagel hetero-Diels-Alder hydrogenation sequence. Liebigs Ann./Recueil 5: 881-886.

[119] L.F. Tietze and N. Rackelmann. 2004. Domino reactions in the synthesis of heterocyclic natural products and analogs. Pure Appl. Chem. 76: 1967-1983.

[120] M. Bandini, A. Melloni, F. Piccinelli, R. Sinisi, S. Tommasi and A. Umani-Ronchi. 2006. Highly enantioselective synthesis of tetrahydro-β-carbolines and tetrahydro-γ-carbolines *via* Pd-catalyzed intramolecular allylic alkylation. J. Am. Chem. Soc. 128: 1424-1425.

[121] C. Liu and R.A. Widenhoefer. 2006. Scope and mechanism of the Pd[II]-catalyzed arylation/carboalkoxylation of unactivated olefins with indoles. Chem. Eur. J. 12: 2371-2382.

[122] Y. Ohta, H. Chiba, S. Oishi, N. Fujii and H. Ohno. 2009. Construction of nitrogen heterocycles bearing an aminomethyl group by copper-catalyzed domino three-component coupling-cyclization. J. Org. Chem. 74: 7052-7058.

[123] J. Ma, W. Yin, H. Zhou and J.M. Cook. 2007. Total synthesis of the opioid agonistic indole alkaloid mitragynine and the first total syntheses of 9-methoxygeissoschizol and 9-methoxy-N_b-methylgeissoschizol. Org. Lett. 9: 3491-3494.

[124] J. Ma, W. Yin, H. Zhou, X. Liao and J.M. Cook. 2009. General approach to the total synthesis of 9-methoxy-substituted indole alkaloids: synthesis of mitragynine, as well as 9-methoxygeissoschizol and 9-methoxy-N_b-methylgeissoschizol. J. Org. Chem. 74: 264-273.

[125] S.G. Stewart, C.H. Heath and E.L. Ghisalberti. 2009. Domino or single-step Tsuji-Trost/Heck reactions and their application in the synthesis of 3-benzazepines and azepino[4,5-*b*]indole ring systems. Eur. J. Org. Chem. 12: 1934-1943.

[126] A.F. Littke and G.C. Fu. 2001. A versatile catalyst for Heck reactions of aryl chlorides and aryl bromides under mild conditions. J. Am. Chem. Soc. 123: 6989-7000.

[127] D.L. Priebbenow, L.C. Henderson, F.M. Pfeffer and S.G. Stewart. 2010. Domino Heck-Aza-Michael reactions: efficient access to 1-substituted tetrahydro-β-carbolines. J. Org. Chem. 75: 1787-1790.

[128] S. Luo, C.A. Zificsak and R.P. Hsung. 2003. Intramolecular formal aza-[3+3] cycloaddition approach to indoloquinolizidine alkaloids. A stereoselective total synthesis of ($\pm$)-tangutorine. Org. Lett. 5: 4709-4712.

[129] T. Uno, E. Beausoleil, R.A. Goldsmith, B.H. Levine and R.N. Zuckermann. 1999. New submonomers for poly *N*-substituted glycines (peptoids). Tetrahedron Lett. 40: 1475-1478.

[130] R.W. Bates and Y. Lu. 2009. A formal synthesis of porantheridine and an epimer. J. Org. Chem. 74: 9460-9465.

[131] A.S. Karpov and T.J.J. Muller. 2003. Straightforward novel one-pot enaminone and pyrimidine syntheses by coupling-addition-cyclocondensation sequences. Synthesis 18: 2815-2826.

[132] A.S. Karpov and T.J.J. Muller. 2003. New entry to a three-component pyrimidine synthesis by TMS-ynones *via* Sonogashira coupling. Org. Lett. 5: 3451-3454.

[133] A.S. Karpov, F. Rominger and T.J.J. Muller. 2005. A diversity oriented four-component approach to tetrahydro-β-carbolines initiated by Sonogashira coupling. Org. Biomol. Chem. 3: 4382-4391.

[134] A.S. Karpov, T. Oeser and T.J.J. Muller. 2004. A novel one-pot four-component access to tetrahydro-β-carbolines by a coupling-amination-aza-annulation-Pictet-Spengler sequence (CAAPS). Chem. Commun. 13: 1502-1503.

[135] O.G. Schramm, T. Oeser and T.J.J. Muller. 2006. Coupling-isomerization-*N,S*-ketene acetal-addition sequences- a three-component approach to highly fluorescent pyrrolo[2,3-*b*]pyridines, [1,8]naphthyridines, and pyrido[2,3-*b*]azepines. J. Org. Chem. 71: 3494-3500.

[136] D.B. Dess and J.C. Martin. 1983. Readily accessible 12-I-5 oxidant for the conversion of primary and secondary alcohols to aldehydes and ketones. J. Org. Chem. 48: 4155-4156.

[137] R.K. Boeckman, P. Shao and J.J. Mullins. 2000. The Dess-Martin periodinane: 1,1,1-triacetoxy-1,1-dihydro-1,2-benziodoxol-3(1*H*)-one. Org. Synth. 77: 141-152.

[138] F. Volz and N. Krause. 2007. Golden opportunities in natural product synthesis: first total synthesis of (-)-isocyclocapitelline and (-)-isochrysotricine by gold-catalyzed allene cycloisomerization. Org. Biomol. Chem. 5: 1519-1521.

[139] E.M. Beccalli, G. Broggini, M. Martinelli and G. Paladino. 2005. Pd-catalyzed intramolecular cyclization of pyrrolo-2-carboxamides: regiodivergent routes to pyrrolo-pyrazines and pyrrolo-pyridines. Tetrahedron 61: 1077-1082.

[140] E.M. Beccalli and G. Broggini. 2003. Uncommon intramolecular palladium-catalyzed cyclization of indole derivatives. Tetrahedron Lett. 44: 1919-1921.

[141] G. Abbiati, E.M. Beccalli, G. Broggini and C. Zoni. 2003. Regioselectivity on the palladium-catalyzed intramolecular cyclization of indole derivatives. J. Org. Chem. 68: 7625-7628.

[142] M. Lafrance, D. Lapointe and K. Fagnou. 2008. Mild and efficient palladium-catalyzed intramolecular direct arylation reactions. Tetrahedron 64: 6015-6020.

[143] J.M. Schulman, A.A. Friedman, J. Panteleev and M. Lautens. 2012. Synthesis of 1,2,3-triazole-fused heterocycles *via* Pd-catalyzed cyclization of 5-iodotriazoles. Chem. Commun. 48: 55-57.

[144] T.H.M. Jonckers, B.U.W. Maes, G.L.F. Lemiere, G. Rombouts, L. Pieters, A. Haemers and R.A. Dommisse. 2003. Synthesis of isocryptolepine *via* a Pd-catalyzed 'amination-arylation' approach. Synlett 5: 615-618.

[145] E.M. Mmutlame, J.M. Harris and A. Padwa. 2005. 1,3-Dipolar cycloaddition chemistry for the preparation of novel indolizinone-based compounds. J. Org. Chem. 70: 8055-8063.

[146] P. Szolcsanyi, T. Gracza, M. Koman, N. Pronayova and T. Liptaj. 2000. Total synthesis of new C-6 homologues of 1-deoxynojirimycin and 1-deoxy-L-idonojirimycin. Chem. Commun. 6: 471-472.

[147] P. Szolcsanyi, T. Gracza, M. Koman, N. Pronayova and T. Liptaj. 2000. Pd(II)-catalyzed aminocarbonylation as a key step in the total synthesis of new C-6 homologues of 1-deoxynojirimycin and 1-deoxy-L-idonojirimycin. Tetrahedron: Asymmetry 11: 2579- 2597.

[148] M. Babjak and P. Zalupsky. 2005. Regiocontrol in the palladium(II)-catalyzed oxycarbonylation of unsaturated polyols. ARKIVOC (v): 45-57.

[149] H. Zhang and R.C. Larock. 2002. Synthesis of annulated γ-carbolines by palladium-catalyzed intramolecular iminoannulation. Org. Lett. 4: 3035-3038.

[150] Y. Kozawa and M. Mori. 2001. Construction of a carbapenam skeleton using palladium-catalyzed cyclization. Tetrahedron Lett. 42: 4869-4873.

[151] Y. Kozawa and M. Mori. 2002. Synthesis of different ring-size heterocycles from the same propargyl alcohol derivative by ligand effect on Pd(0). Tetrahedron Lett. 43: 1499-1502.

[152] Y. Kozawa and M. Mori. 2003. Novel synthesis of carbapenam by intramolecular attack of lactam nitrogen toward η^1-allenyl and η^3-propargylpalladium complex. J. Org. Chem. 68: 8068-8074.

[153] S. Hesse and G. Kirsch. 2003. Synthesis of pyridine-fused ring systems from β-chloroacroleins: a comparison of three different pathways. Synthesis 5: 717-722.

[154] Y. Hirai, J. Watanabe, T. Nozaki, H. Yokoyama and S. Yamaguchi. 1997. Transition metal-mediated stereocontrolled cyclization of urethanes leading to versatile fused piperidines and its application to the synthesis of (+)-prosopinine and (+)-palustrine. J. Org. Chem. 62: 776-777.

[155] D.E. Davies, P.M. Doyle, R.D. Farrant, R.D. Hill, P.B. Hitchcock, P.N. Sanderson and D.W. Young. 2003. Synthesis of an external β-turn based on the GLDV motif of cell adhesion proteins. Tetrahedron Lett. 44: 8887-8891.

[156] A. Blum, J. Bottcher, B. Sammet, T. Luksch, A. Heine, G. Klebe and W.E. Diederich. 2008. Achiral oligoamines as versatile tool for the development of aspartic protease inhibitors. Bioorg. Med. Chem. 16: 8574-8586.

[157] D.K. Bates, X. Li and P.V. Jog. 2004. Simple thiazocine-2-acetic acid derivatives *via* ring-closing metathesis. J. Org. Chem. 69: 2750-2754.

[158] V. De Matteis, O. Dufay, D.C.J. Waalboer, F.L. van Delft, J. Tiebes and F.P.J.T. Rutjes. 2007. An improved ring-closing metathesis approach to fluorinated and trifluoromethylated nitrogen heterocycles. Eur. J. Org. Chem. 16: 2667-2675.

[159] D.K. Rayabarapu, A. Zhou, K.O. Jeon, T. Samarakoon, A. Rolfe, H. Siddiqui and P.R. Hanson 2009. α-Haloarylsulfonamides: multiple cyclization pathways to skeletally diverse benzofused sultams. Tetrahedron 65: 3180-3188.

[160] O. Miyata, A. Shirai, S. Yoshino, T. Nakabayashi, Y. Takeda, T. Kiguchi, D. Fukumoto, M. Ueda and T. Naito. 2007. Development of radical addition-cyclization-elimination reaction of oxime ether and its application to formal synthesis of ($\pm$)-martinelline. Tetrahedron 63: 10092-10117.

[161] Z.J. Han, C.S. Da, L. Qiu, M. Ni, Y.F. Zhou and R. Wang. 2006. The natural amino acid derived chiral sulfonamide ligands in the catalytic asymmetric addition of phenylacetylene to aldehydes. Lett. Org. Chem. 3: 143-148.

[162] S.S. Kinderman, M.M.T. Wekking, J.H. van Maarseveen, H.E. Schoemaker, H. Hiemstra and F. Rutjes. 2005. Catalytic *N*-sulfonyliminium ion-mediated cyclizations to α-vinyl-substituted isoquinolines and β-carbolines and applications in metathesis. J. Org. Chem. 70: 5519-5527.

[163] A.J. Catino, J.M. Nichols, R.E. Forslund and M.P. Doyle. 2005. Efficient aziridination of olefins catalyzed by mixed-valent dirhodium(II,III) caprolactamate. Org. Lett. 7: 2787-2790.

[164] X.L. Wu, J.J. Xia and G.W. Wang. 2008. Aminobromination of olefins with TsNH$_2$ and NBS as the nitrogen and bromine sources mediated by hypervalent iodine in a ball mill. Org. Biomol. Chem. 6: 548-553.

[165] E.J. Corey and A. Venkates. 1972. Protection of hydroxyl groups as *tert*-butyldimethylsilyl derivatives. J. Am. Chem. Soc. 94: 6190-6191.

[166] (a) L.B. Wolf, K.C.M.F. Tjen, H.T. Brink, R.H. Blaauw, H. Hiemstra, H.E. Schoemaker and F.P.J.T. Rutjes. 2002. Palladium-catalyzed cyclization reactions of acetylene-containing amino acids. Adv. Synth. Catal. 344: 70-83.
(b) D.L. Priebbenow, S.G. Stewart and F.M. Pfeffer. 2012. Asymmetric induction in domino Heck-aza-Michael reactions. Tetrahedron Lett. 53: 1468-1471.

[167] G. Massiot and T. Mulamba. 1984. Synthesis of (-)-ajmalicine from (-)-tryptophan. J. Chem. Soc. Chem. Commun. 11: 715-716.

[168] A. Boumendjel, J.-M. Nuzillard and G. Massiot. 1999. Synthesis of ajmalicine derivatives using Wittig-Horner and Knoevenagel reactions. Tetrahedron Lett. 40: 9033-9036.

[169] K. Diker, K. El Biach, M. Doe de Maindreville and J. Levy. 1997. Reductive Pictet-Spengler cyclization of nitriles in the presence of tryptamine: synthesis of indolo[2,3-*a*]quinolizidine, nazlinine, and elaeocarpidine. J. Nat. Prod. 60: 791-793.

CHAPTER 8

Six-Membered N-Polyheterocycles

8.1 Introduction

Diverse compounds such as anti-biotics, alkaloids, vitamins, essential amino acids, hormones, hemoglobin, and various dyes and synthetic drugs contain heterocycles as core skeletons. The ability of heterocyclic nuclei to act both as reactive pharmacophores and biomimetics has largely contributed to their unique value as traditional key elements of many drugs constituting the main structure within a number of natural products and exhibit a wide range of biological activities [1-3]. Due to their importance in biological area, the development of synthetic methods for nitrogen heterocyclic compounds and their fused scaffolds possessing a high degree of diversity has become a leading focus in modern drug discovery and design [4a-f].

This chapter covers the preparation of many quinoxalines and quinolines due to immense biological properties associated with them. Quinolines are valuable building blocks in pharmaceuticals and are known for exhibiting many biological properties like anti-inflammatory, anti-microbial, anti-oxidants, anti-asthmatic, anti-HIV, anti-cancer, anti-tuberculosis, and anti-leishmanial. Synthetic chloroquine as well as natural quinine and their analogues are some of the quinoline-based anti-malarials which are utilized for the treatment of malaria. They act by interfering haemoglobin digestion in the blood stages of malaria parasite's life cycle. Ciprofloxacin, norfloxacin, and levofloxacin are some of important anti-biotics which are based on a quinoline based anti-oxidant used as a pesticide as well as food preservative (E324) and is sold under fluoroquinolones. Oxamniquine is a tetrahydroquinoline based drug which is effective anthelmintic with schistosomicidal activity against *Schistosoma mansoni*. Martinellic acid and martinelline alkaloids possessing fused tetrahydroquinoline are isolated from the roots of *Martinella iquitosensis* which are used as an eye medication in South America. L-689560 serves as a very potent *N*-methyl-D-aspartate (NDMA) antagonist. To prevent the rancidification of fats in pet foods ethoxyquin is used as a preservative. It is also used as a rubber stabilizer. Some substituted quinolines exhibit potent anti-breast cancer activity. 4-Carboxyl quinoline derivative acts as a selective cyclooxygenase (COX 2) inhibitor with greater potency than reference drug celecoxib. The hydrazones based on quinoline shows excellent anti-tuberculosis and anti-bacterial activities [5-16].

8.2 Synthesis of quinolines

Buchwald et al. [17] synthesized a number of aza-heterocycles *via* Pd-catalyzed intramolecular coupling reaction (**Scheme 1**).

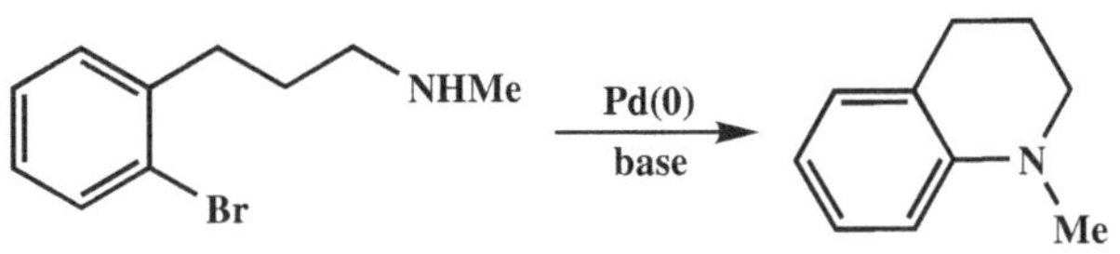

Scheme-1

Wang and Huang [18] reported this synthetic strategy for tetrahydroquinolines. Iodination of 4-aminobenzoic acid afforded 4-amino-3-iodobenzoic acid and was coupled to Rink resin. The annelation of solid-phase linked *o*-iodoanilines with 1,4-dienes occurred in the presence of Pd catalyst after tosylation. The tetrahydroquinolines were obtained in good purities (81%) and high yield (88%) upon cleavage from solid support **(Scheme 2)**.

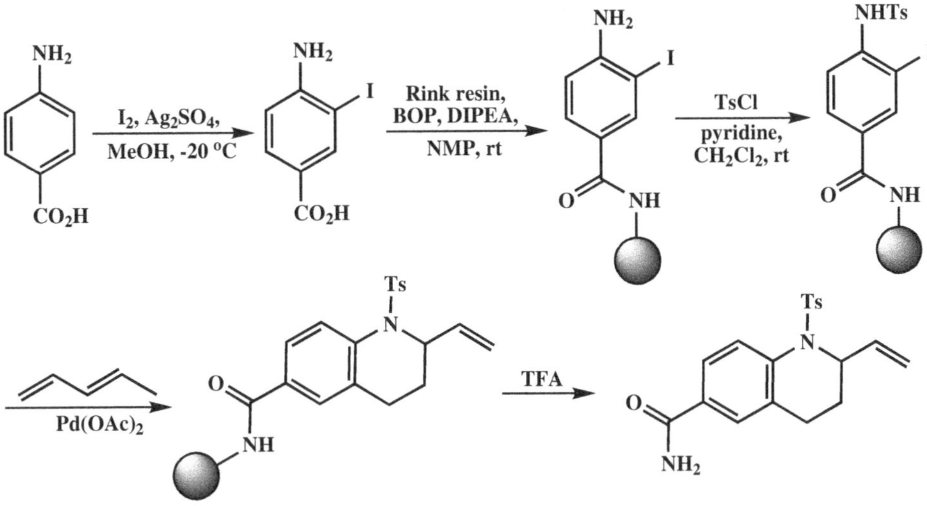

Scheme-2

The 2-arylquinolines were formed from (*o*-aminophenyl)-ynones *via* Pd-catalyzed transfer hydrogenation/heterocyclization. The reaction conditions employed 10 mol% of palladium/carbon in methanol and 3 eq. of ammonium formate **(Scheme 3)** [18].

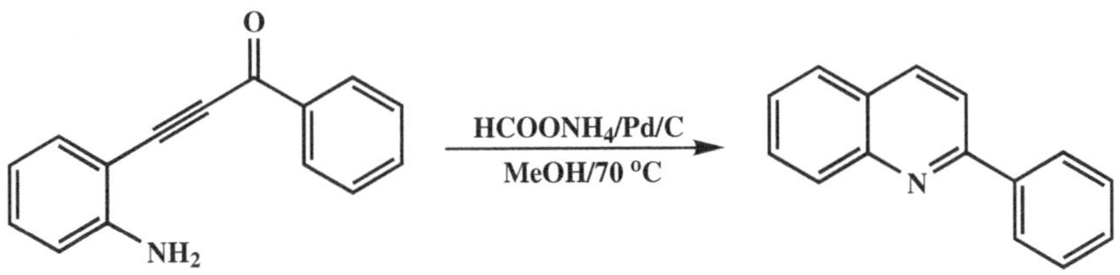

Scheme-3

Willis et al. [19] described a carbonylation method to synthesize quinolone. The alkenyl aminocarbonylation/intramolecular aryl amidation reactions were facilitated in the presence of a catalytic system with bidentate ligand 1,3-bis(diphenylphosphino)propane **(Scheme 4)**. Good yields of *N*-substituted products were observed. The regioisomeric isoquinolone products were formed by conducting the reaction in two stages and delaying the incorporation of CO. Florent et al. [20] subsequently observed the preparation of 3-substituted isoquinolones [21].

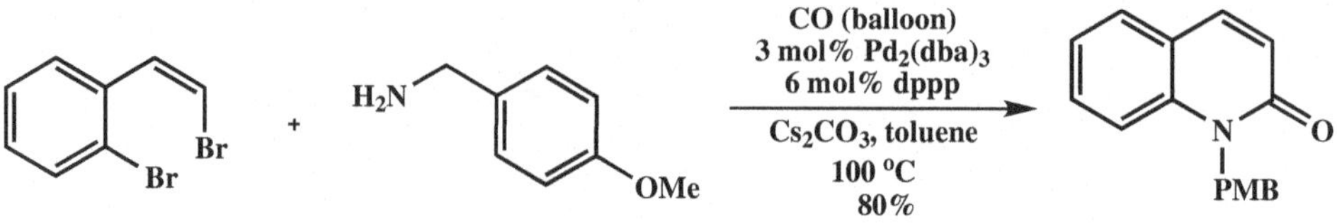

Scheme-4

Bulky alkyl substituents (*t*-Bu and cyclohexyl) possessing analogues were produced in lower yields because of unexpected formation of indolines in 38% **(Scheme 5)** and 15% yield, respectively **(Scheme 6)** [22]. This unexpected indoline formation presumably arises from the steric influences of these large groups giving the intermediates a favorable conformation for indoline formation, such that they were able to overcome the lower reactivity of amide nitrogen. The 10 mol% Pd(PPh$_3$)$_4$ was required to achieve a good yield of cyclohexyl tetrahydroquinoline analogue due to instability of diamine under reaction conditions [23a-b].

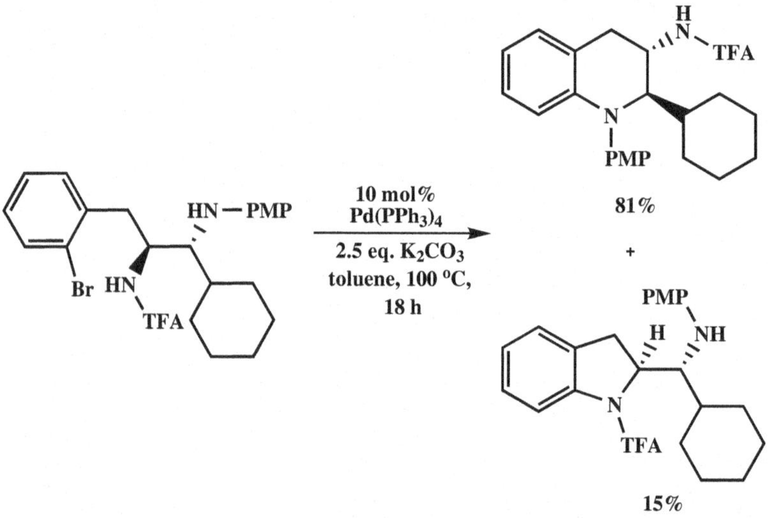

Scheme-5

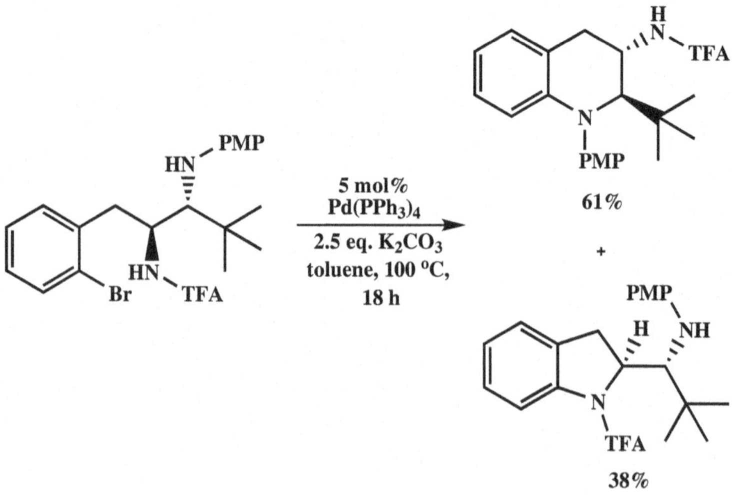

Scheme-6

Peat and Buchwald [24] developed catalyst system for the synthesis of simple tetrahydroquinolines and indolines. The indoline was formed in 54% yield by heating diamine with Pd(PPh$_3$)$_4$, potassium carbonate, and sodium *tert*-butoxide at 90 °C in PhMe for 3 h. Because of slight instability of indoline to oxidative cleavage under reaction conditions, trace amounts of indole and imine were produced along with product. The yield of indoline was increased to 91% by degassing of solvent, rigorous drying of bases, and carrying out the reaction at 100 °C. Many other catalyst systems were also investigated. Jackson [25] and Buchwald [26] previously employed Pd$_2$(dba)$_3$, cesium carbonate, and P(*o*-tol)$_3$ conditions for the preparation of 2-substituted indulines in poor yields. Moderate to good yields of indoline were observed with Pd$_2$(dba)$_3$/2,2-bis(diphenyl-phosphanyl)-1,1-binaphthyl and Pd(dppf)Cl$_2$/1,1'-bis(diphenylphosphino)ferrocene catalyst systems. Small amounts of tetrahydroquinoline were also reported under these conditions. The Pd(PPh$_3$)$_4$-catalyzed cyclization was also carried out with only sodium *tert*-butoxide base, however, the reaction did not occur cleanly as those conducted with two bases resulting in a lower yield of 77%. These results were in agreement with those observations made by Buchwald and co-workers [26]. The rate of reaction reduced and resulted in increased transformation to tetrahydroquinoline when only weaker base potassium carbonate was utilized **(Scheme 7)** [23b, 27].

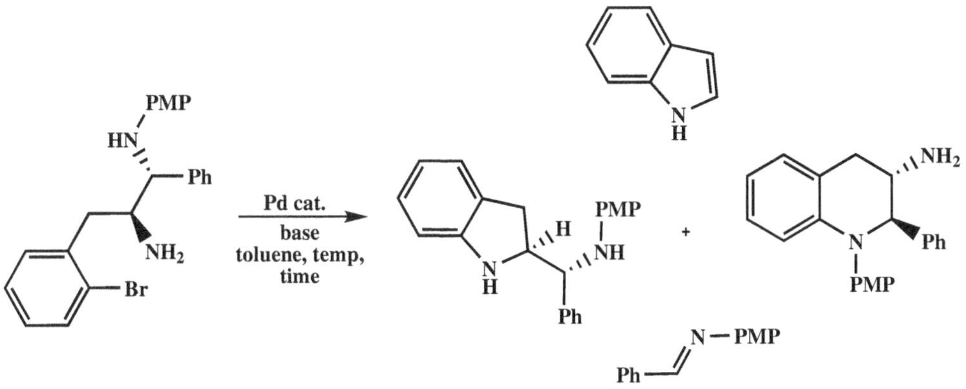

Scheme-7

In this synthetic pathway, the 2-arylquinolines **(Scheme 8)** were synthesized from allylamines *via* sequential Heck-type cyclization and aerobic oxidation [28-29].

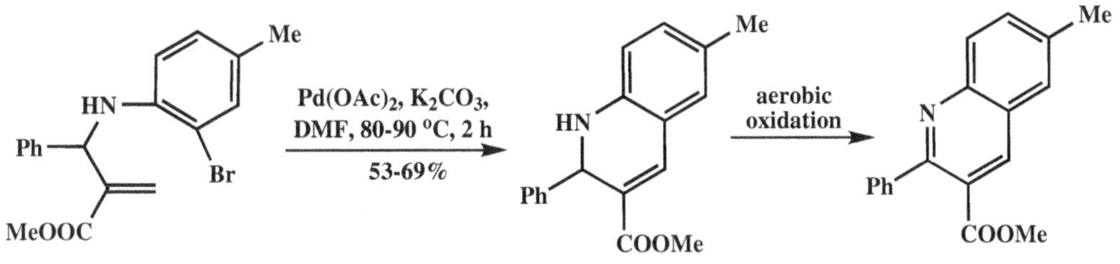

Scheme-8

Park and co-workers [30] reported the preparation of dihydroquinoline from allylamine substrate through an intramolecular carbon-nitrogen coupling reaction in the presence of palladium catalyst **(Scheme 9)** [29].

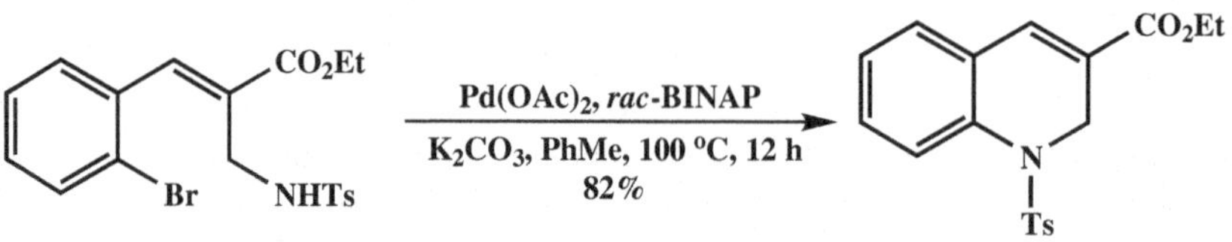

Scheme-9

Chen and co-workers [31] reported that allylamine derivative underwent a palladium-catalyzed intramolecular amination for the formation of 2-Z-alkenyl tetrahydroquinoline **(Scheme 10)** [29].

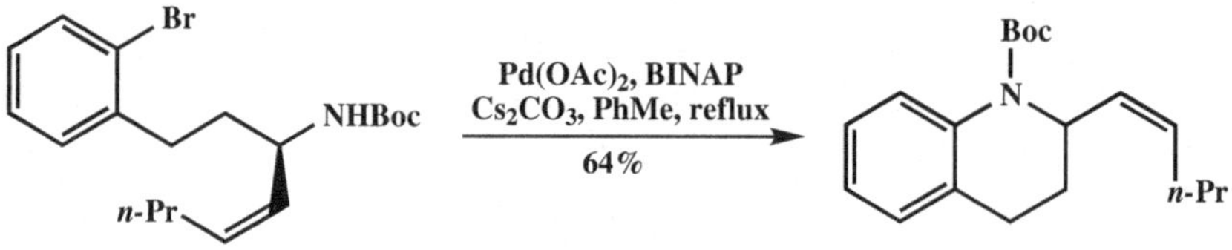

Scheme-10

The 2-methylquinolines were yielded *via* palladium-catalyzed aza-Wacker oxidative cyclization. The reaction afforded good yields at ambient temperature. Wang et al. [32] in 2008 described the preparation of 2-methylquinolines *via* Pd-catalyzed intramolecular aminopalladation of amine derivatives under mild conditions. As reported previously, the unusual 1,5-hydride alkyl to Pd migration was not reported in this aza-Wacker reaction, but dehydration was involved and produced quinolines. A number of 2-methylquinolines were delivered in good yields by virtue of this new protocol **(Scheme 11)** [33].

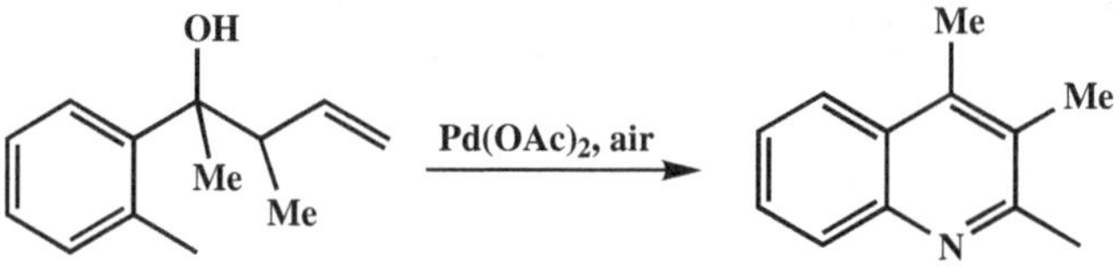

Scheme-11

Larock *et al.* [34-36] described a Pd-catalyzed cross-coupling of unsaturated anilide derivatives and vinyl halides or triflates for the synthesis of a number of dihydroquinoline as shown in **Scheme 12**. The intermediates π-allylpalladium complexes were reported in this process [14].

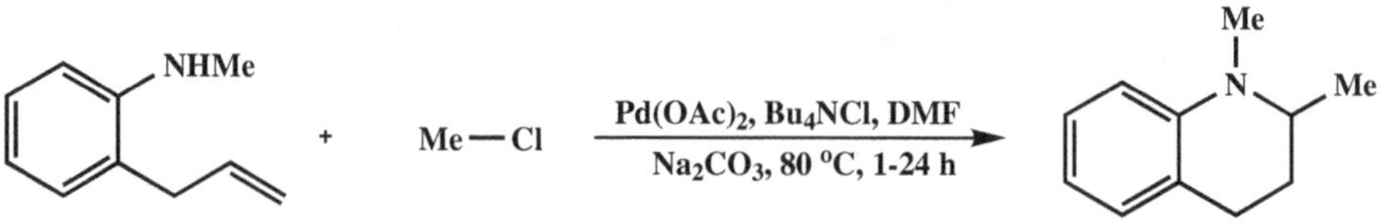

Scheme-12

Ligands used for the metal in this reaction were TMP and bis(*p*-tolylimino)acenaphthalene. The Pd bis-(2,4,6-trimethylbenzoate) was used as a catalyst with CO for the synthesis of quinoline alkaloid graveoline. An appreciative yield of 2,3-dihydro derivative was also observed along with graveoline [37]. Cenini and co-workers [38] have shown that initial reduction of NO_2 group to amino group may not be involved during the synthesis of 4-(1H)-quinolinones **(Scheme 13)**.

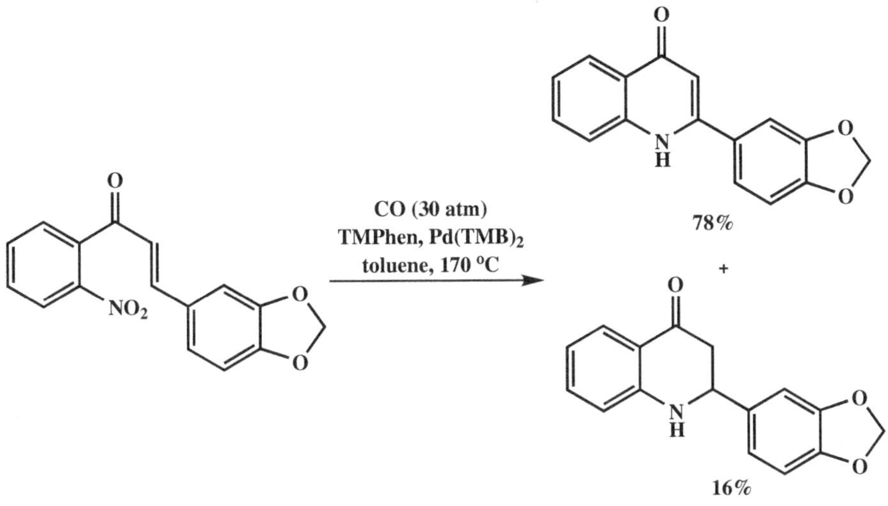

Scheme-13

The Pd-catalyzed creation of carbon-nitrogen bonds could be used to generate benzodiazepines. However, employing *o*-amidobenzoximes as precursors produced 2-quinolinones as sole product in the presence of a Pd catalyst **(Scheme 14)** [39].

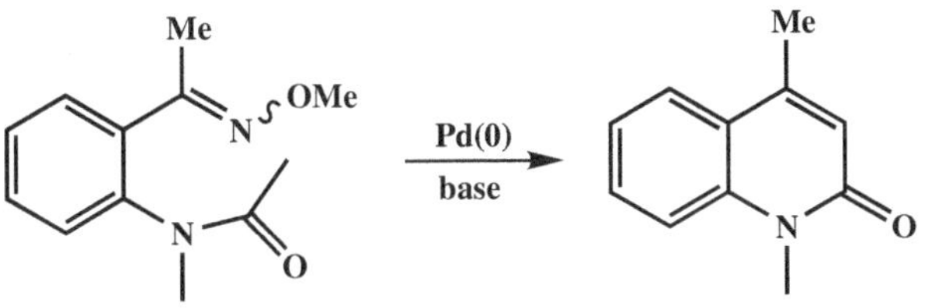

Scheme-14

Pd was broadly used as a catalyst for the construction of quinoline skeletons. Hegedus et al. [40] reported a palladium-catalyzed cyclization reaction of diaminoquinone, affording a mixture of indole and quinoline, as shown in **Scheme 15**.

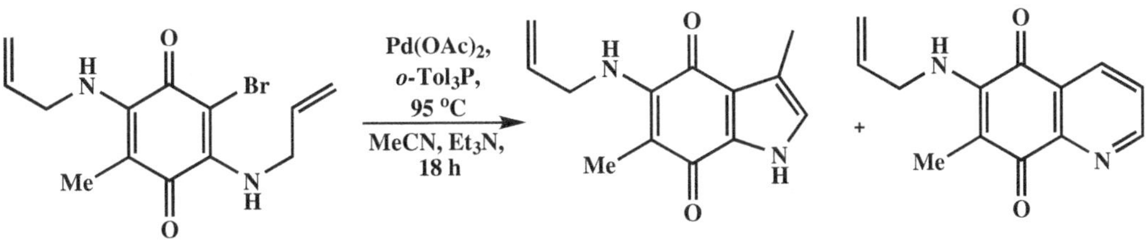

Scheme-15

Larock [41] has observed cross-coupling of *o*-iodoaniline and allylic alcohols for the formation of quinolines in moderate to good yields **(Scheme 16)**.

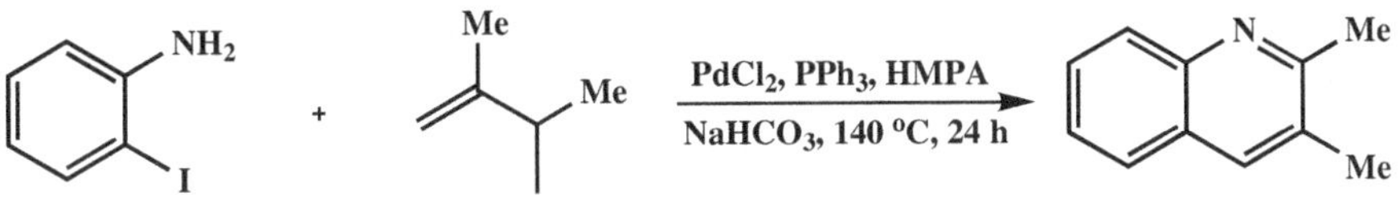

Scheme-16

Buckwald [42] and Hartwig [43] firstly observed direct Pd-catalyzed carbon-nitrogen bond formation for the synthesis of arylamines. The amine possessing aryl halides were reacted for the synthesis of tetrahydroquinoline in the presence of $Pd(PPh_3)_4$ and potassium carbonate **(Scheme 17)**.

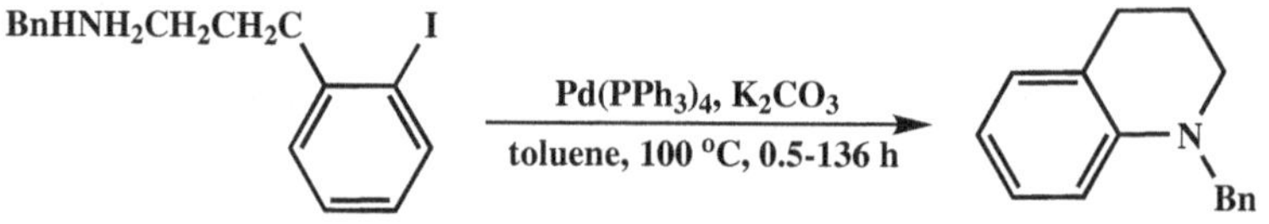
BnHNH2CH2CH2C
I
Pd(PPh3)4, K2CO3
toluene, 100 °C, 0.5-136 h
N
Bn

Scheme-17

Hatano and Mikami [44] described an ene-type cyclization of 1,7-enynes for highly enantioselective synthesis of quinoline through a cationic 2,2-bis(diphenyl-phosphanyl)-1,1-binaphthyl-Pd complex-catalyzed reaction **(Scheme 18)**.

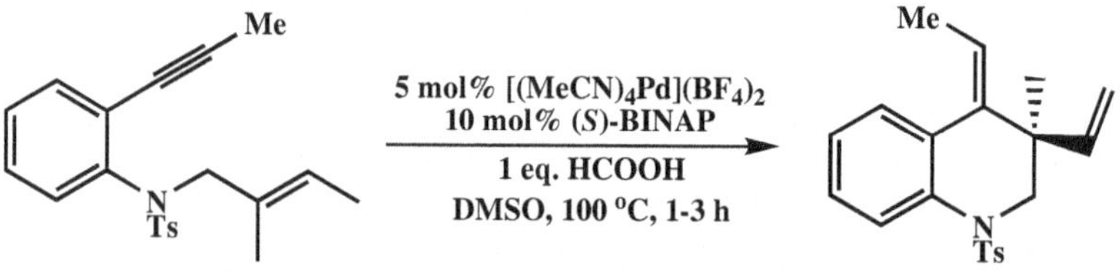
Me
N
Ts
5 mol% [(MeCN)4Pd](BF4)2
10 mol% (S)-BINAP
1 eq. HCOOH
DMSO, 100 °C, 1-3 h
Me
N
Ts

Scheme-18

2-Aryl-4-aminoquinolines were synthesized by Pd-mediated multi-component domino reaction of CO, 2-ethynylarylamine, PhI and primary amines [45a-b] as shown in **Scheme 19**. A triple domino sequence was proposed in this palladium-mediated reaction which involved carbonylative coupling of 2-ethynylaryamines and PhI followed by inter- and intramolecular nucleophilic addition to a C-C triple bond and C-O double bond, respectively.

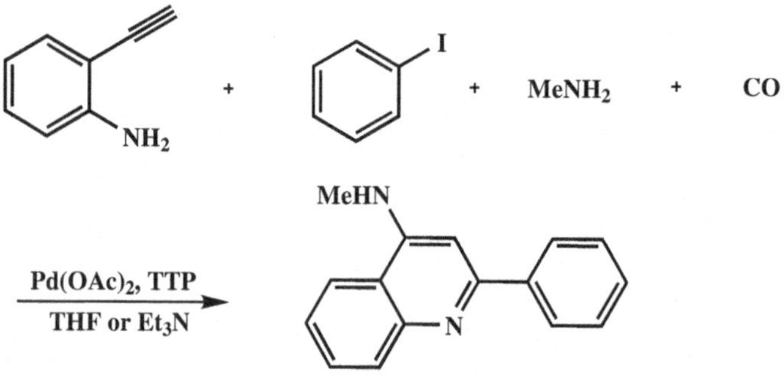
NH2
+
I
+
MeNH2
+
CO
Pd(OAc)2, TTP
THF or Et3N
MeHN
N

Scheme-19

Cho and Kim [46] reported a Heck coupling reaction of 2-iodoaniline with an α,β-unsaturated carbonyl. Substituted quinolines were obtained by palladium acetate catalysis as shown in **Scheme 20**.

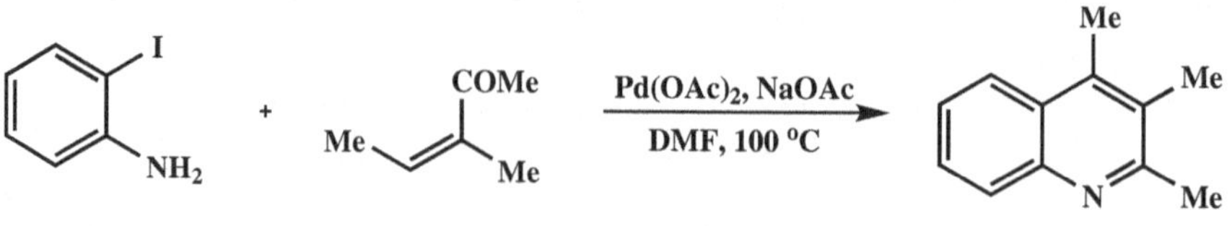
I
NH2
+
COMe
Me
Me
Pd(OAc)2, NaOAc
DMF, 100 °C
Me
Me
N
Me

Scheme-20

Gabriele [47-48] has reported the synthesis of quinolines by alkynylation of 2-ketoaniline derivatives followed by Pd-catalyzed cyclization **(Scheme 21)**. This cyclization occurred by a spontaneous dehydration upon ring closure. Hartwig *et al.* [49] described a sequential intermolecular and transannular, intermolecular Pd-catalyzed hydroamination of cycloheptatriene to synthesize biologically active azabicyclic tropene derivatives. Quinolines were also obtained as by-products in addition to tropenes. Pd(II) bromide was found to be an effective catalyst for the formation of quinolines from anilines *via ortho*-carbon-hydrogen activation of anilines [50]. The presence of 1-hexene favored the conversion of *N*-alkylanilines and the role of 1-hexene was highlighted although the actual role was not clear. A convenient synthesis of substituted quinolines was reported by regioselective Pd (or Cu)-catalyzed 6-*endo-dig* heteroannulation and dehydration of 1-(2-aminoaryl)-2-yn-1-ols in good to excellent yields. The crude substrates were easily prepared by Grignard reactions of 2-aminoaryl ketones with appropriate alkynylmagnesium bromide and were used for cyclization without further purification. By using same substrates in the presence of palladium iodide catalyst under oxidative conditions, quinoline-3-carboxylic esters were obtained *via* 6-*endo-dig* cyclization. Interestingly, under non-oxidative conditions, indol-2-acetic esters were obtained *via* 5-*exo-dig* cyclization.

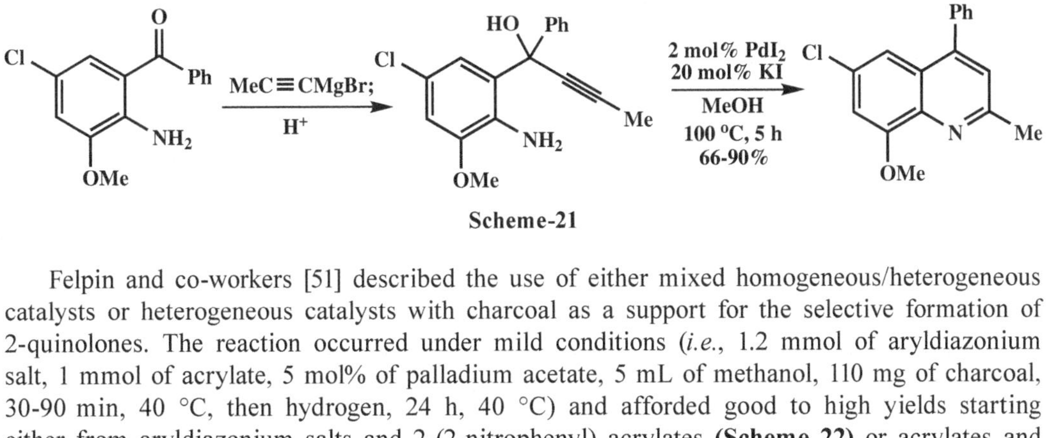

Scheme-21

Felpin and co-workers [51] described the use of either mixed homogeneous/heterogeneous catalysts or heterogeneous catalysts with charcoal as a support for the selective formation of 2-quinolones. The reaction occurred under mild conditions (*i.e.*, 1.2 mmol of aryldiazonium salt, 1 mmol of acrylate, 5 mol% of palladium acetate, 5 mL of methanol, 110 mg of charcoal, 30-90 min, 40 °C, then hydrogen, 24 h, 40 °C) and afforded good to high yields starting either from aryldiazonium salts and 2-(2-nitrophenyl) acrylates **(Scheme 22)** or acrylates and 2-nitrobenzenediazonium salts **(Scheme 23)** [52].

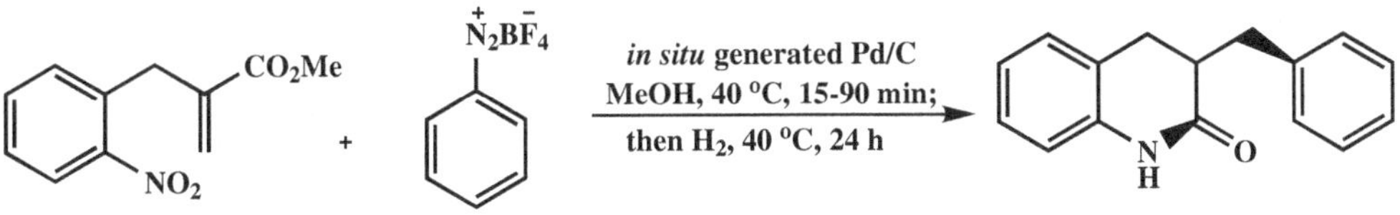

Scheme-22

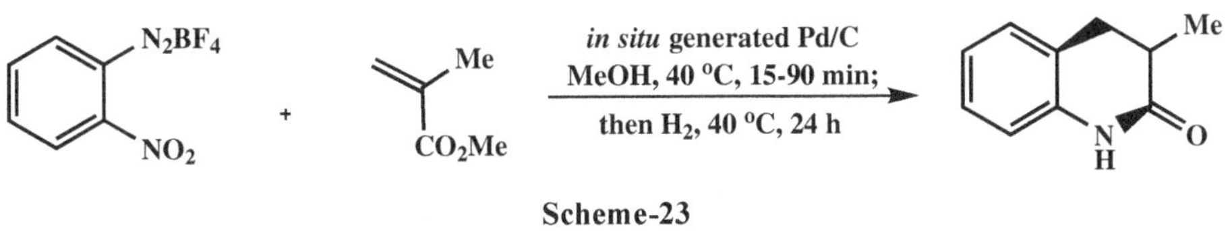

Scheme-23

The 2(1*H*)-quinolinones were formed *via* direct, simple, selective, and Pd-catalyzed oxidative cyclocarbonylation of *N*-monosubstituted-2-vinylanilines. The reaction was environmentally benign and has operational simplicity. The 2(1*H*)-quinolinones containing a number of substituents were formed in up to 97% yield **(Scheme 24)** [53].

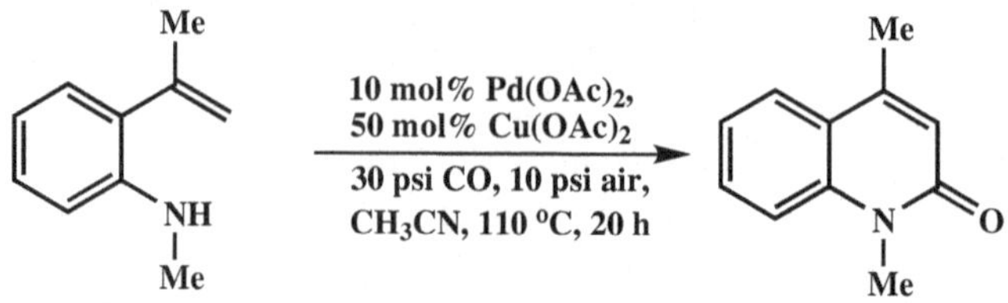

Scheme-24

The Pd(II) catalyst was regenerated by addition of amines to alkenes in the presence of external oxidant, due to rapid elimination of HX upon β-hydride elimination from Pd. However, in an alternative reaction aromatization occurred through β-X elimination without reductive elimination, and allowed the Pd to stay in palladium(II) state. This was exemplified in the work of Venturello [54], where quinolines were produced by Pd-catalyzed intramolecular addition of N-tosyl aniline derivatives to dienes **(Scheme 25)**. The reaction occurred by coordination of Pd catalyst to diene which initiated the nucleophilic attack. However, re-insertion and β-tosyl elimination followed by β-hydride elimination constructed the Pd(II) catalyst for further reaction. This method eliminated the requirement of external oxidants, and formed six-membered quinoline ring.

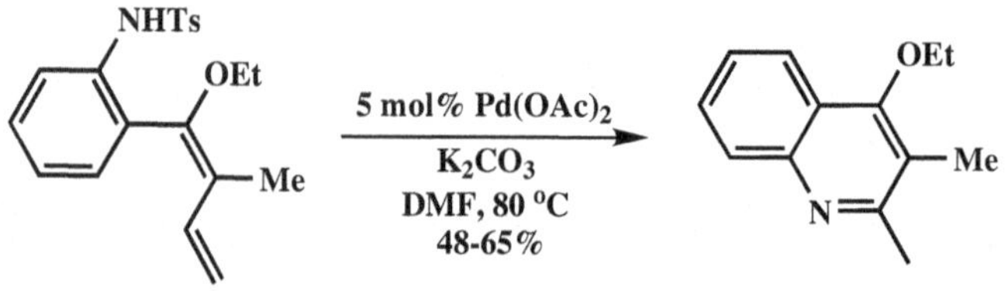

Scheme-25

Frederickson and co-workers [55] used Pd(II) salts in a oxime-nitrone-isoxazolidine cascade. They reported the formation of cyclic nitrone from α,β-unsaturated oxime **(Scheme 26)**. Here, oxime directly attacked the olefinic moiety which was activated by coordination to Pd(II) complexes.

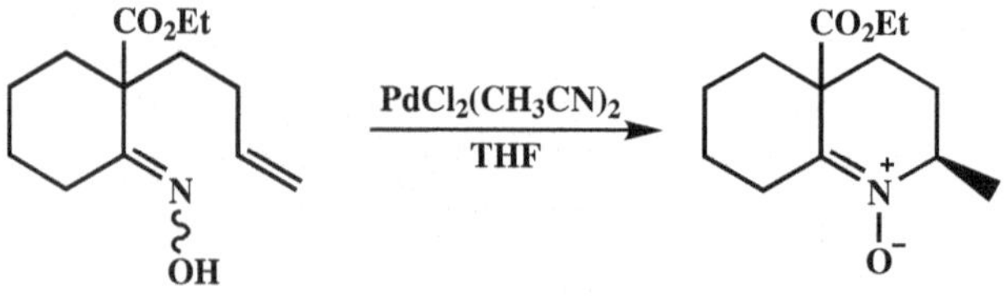

Scheme-26

A continuous flow process was developed for tandem nucleophilic aromatic substitution reaction of 1-methyl-homopiperazine with 2-fluoronitrobenzene and hydrogenation to afford aniline, an intermediate in flow processing of potent 5HT1B antagonist. In-line purification was achieved by flowing product solutions through glass columns consisting of quadrapure-benzylamine (QP-BZA) to scavenge hydrofluoric acid from nucleophilic aromatic substitution reaction and quadrapure thiourea (QP-TU) to scavenge leached Pd from hydrogenation reaction **(Scheme 27)** [56].

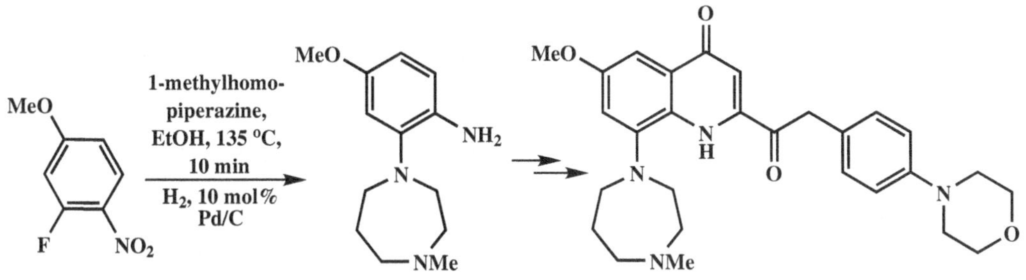

Scheme-27

The α,β-unsaturated ketone O-pentafluorobenzoyloximes underwent 5-*exo*-cyclization through alkylideneaminopalladium species. The Heck-type reaction of α,β-unsaturated ketone oximes containing α-OMe group proceeded *via* 6-*endo*-cyclization. Reasonable yield of pyridine derivatives was observed with TBAC **(Scheme 28-29)**. The reaction strategy of 6-*endo*-cyclization was not clear, but reaction must have started by oxidative addition of oximes. Many isoquinoline derivatives were formed from cyclization of o-allylphenyl ketone O-pentafluorobenzoyloxime in the presence of TBAC [57].

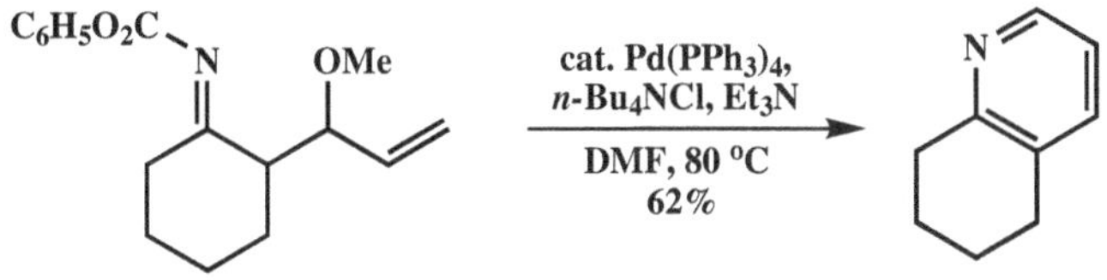

Scheme-28

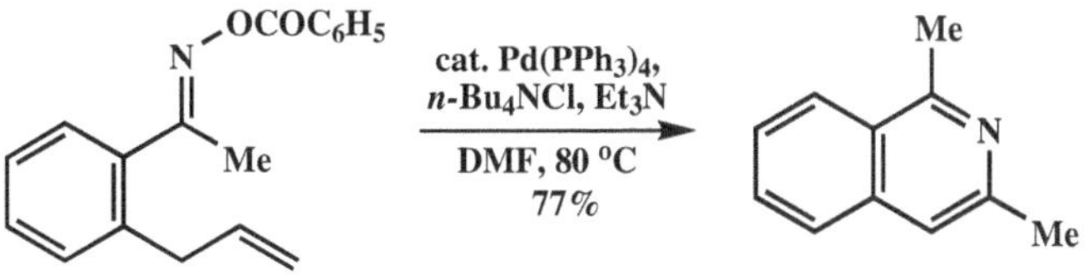

Scheme-29

An intramolecular MW assisted Mizoroki-Heck cyclization was carried out for the preparation of benzazepinones [58]. However, instead 61-78% yield was observed from 6-*exo-trig* derivative **(Scheme 30)**. The intramolecular Mizoroki-Heck reaction was performed with 98% yield in the presence of palladium acetate, triethylamine, and triphenylphosphine in CH_3CN. The reaction was carried out on solid-phase, binding the substrate to a resin and in solution. Both Mizoroki-Heck and Ugi reaction were performed on support. Six-membered rings were produced in solution in the same fashion starting from bromo-aryls [59].

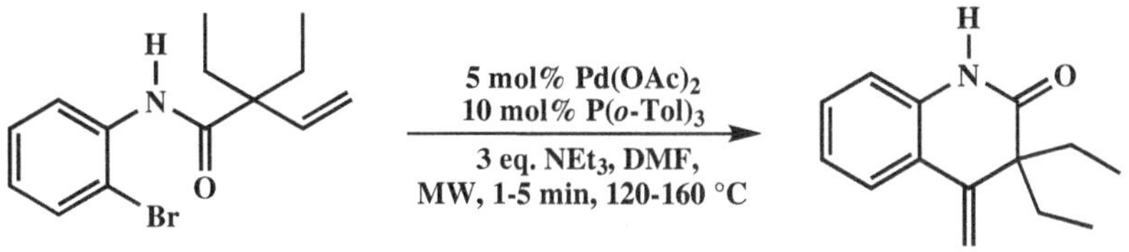

Scheme-30

Kaye et al. [60] used a Baylis-Hillman method for the synthesis of quinoline. The Baylis-Hillman products were provided when o-nitrobenzaldehyde was reacted with methyl (ethyl) vinyl ketones in 1,4-diazabicyclo[2.2.2]octane. The Baylis-Hillman products were reduced catalytically for direct cyclization to quinoline derivatives in low yields **(Scheme 31)**.

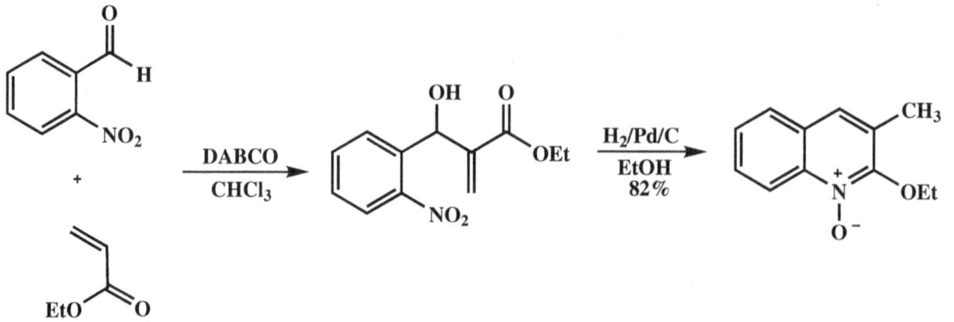

Scheme-31

Quinoline derivatives were obtained by Familoni and Klaas [60] following the reduction of Baylis Hillman products, prepared by treating 2-nitrobenzaldehyde with activated alkenes in the presence of catalyst, 1,4-diazabicyclo[2.2.2]octane. Use of methyl acrylate as activated alkene afforded quinolones **(Scheme 32)**, while the use of methyl vinyl ketone afforded 2,3-methyl quinoline *N*-oxide. In all cases, cyclization of reduced intermediate appeared to involve nucleophilic attack at carbonyl carbon rather than the vinylic carbon.

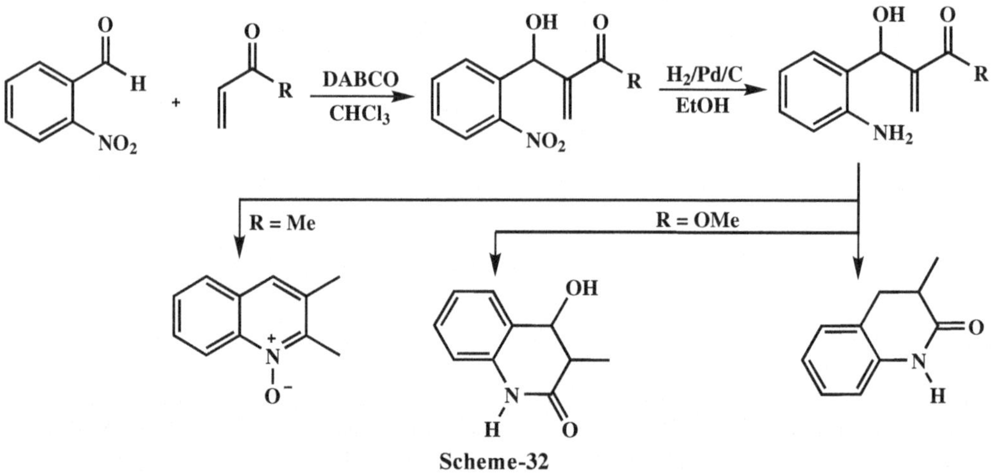

Scheme-32

Various biological molecules contain amidine moiety [61]. Sodium hydride was used for the protection of amine group by deprotonation followed by treatment with SEM ([2-(trimethylsilyl) ethoxy]methyl acetal) chloride. The protected species was reacted with boronic acid by extension of Liebeskind-Srogl thioether cross-coupling process **(Scheme 33)** [62-64].

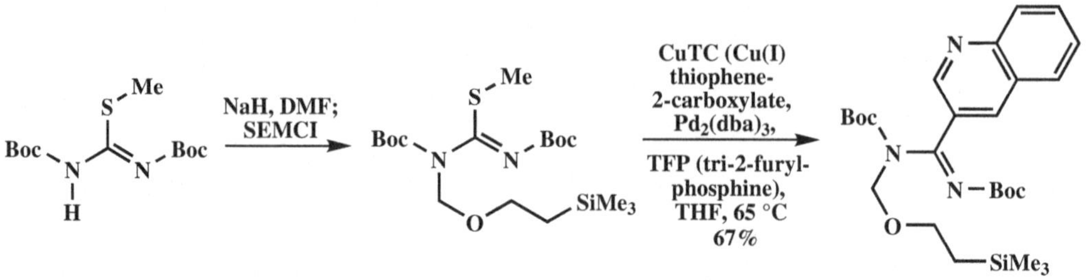

Scheme-33

Many of syntheses of 3-aminotetrahydroquinolines reported in the literature utilized a reduction of α-aminoamides to form the desired 1,2-diamine. The α-aminoamides were often readily available in enantiopure form from corresponding amino acid derivatives. These reductions have been carried out both before and after cyclization to form the tetrahydroquinoline ring. Bethuel and Gademann [65] used nitro-dopamine derivative in a lactamization reaction to form lactam, which was subsequently reduced with borane to yield the desired 3-aminotetrahydroquinoline **(Scheme 34)** [66].

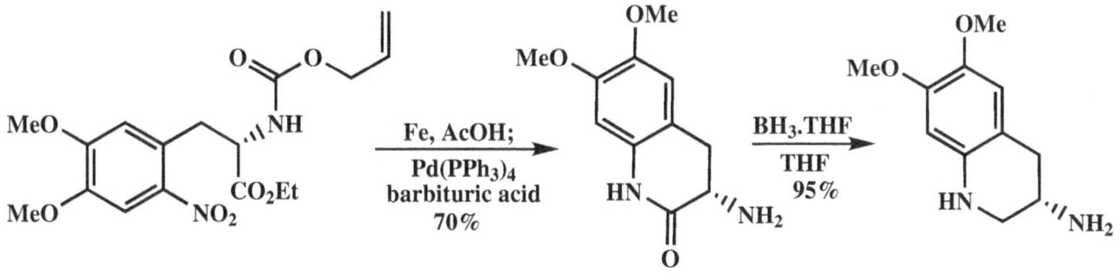

Scheme-34

Hamada and co-workers [67] synthesized 3-substituted 2,3-dihydroquinolin-4-ones through a Stetter reaction of *N*-allyl aniline in the presence of thiazolium salt, which in turn was synthesized from allylic amination of acetoxy α,β-unsaturated carbonyl compounds with 2-amino benzaldehyde derivatives in the presence of palladium(0) catalyst **(Scheme 35)** [29].

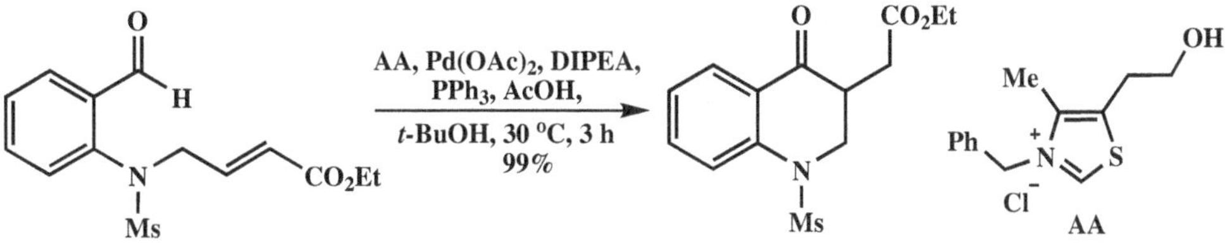

Scheme-35

A high yielding and highly diastereoselective synthesis of 3-aminotetrahydroquinolines was reported **(Scheme 36)**. This was achieved by utilizing a reductive nitro-Mannich reaction of nitroalkenes bearing a pendant *o*-bromo-substituted aromatic ring. Reduction of β-nitroamine products to 1,2-diamines provided substrates for selective intramolecular *N*-arylations to yield both five- and six-membered ring heterocycles. This synthesis was used to produce an array of 1,2-diamine containing fused heterocycles [68].

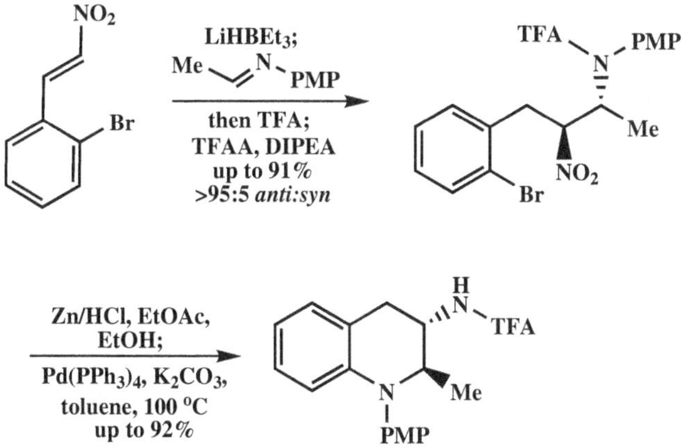

Scheme-36

The reductive cyclization of *N*-allyl aniline bearing ethenyl substituents on nitrogen gave azabicycle **(Scheme 37)** [29, 69].

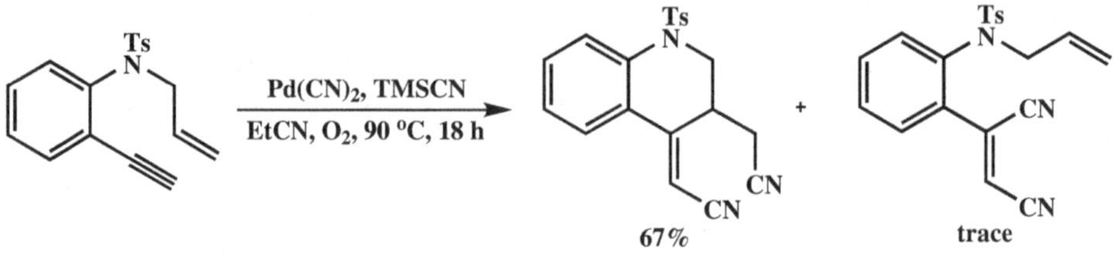

Scheme-37

The annealing of a cyclic amine ring onto an existing carbocyclic six-membered ring for the synthesis of hydroindole and hydroquinoline skeletons has already been carried out utilizing a wide range of chemistry [70]. A second example involved a catalytic hydrogenation under acidic conditions, which causes the reduction of both olefinic-bond and de-protection of benzyl carbamate of cyclohexene. The resulting intermediate spontaneously cyclized onto pendant keto group to generate hydroquinoline **(Scheme 38)** [71].

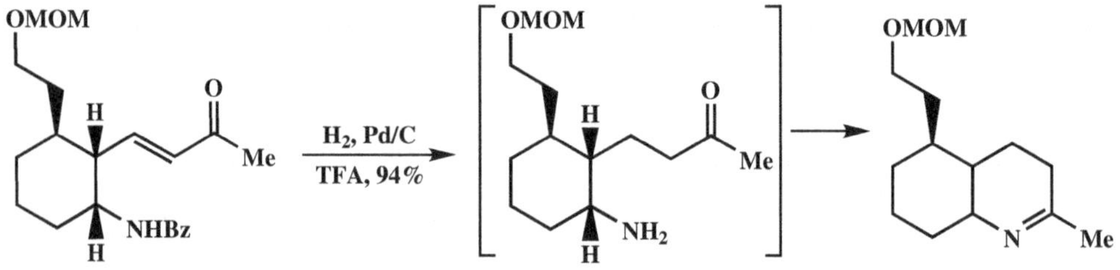

Scheme-38

On the basis of reaction conditions, *N*-tosylated *o*-allylanilines provided different cyclization products **(Scheme 39)** [72]. Product yields and catalyst stability were improved in the presence of compounds in which palladium(II) was coordinated to *N*-heterocyclic carbene ligands like IPr, IMes, or seven-membered heterocycle. The reactions also occurred with air rather than oxygen and carboxylic acid co-catalysts like benzoic acid or acetic acid [73].

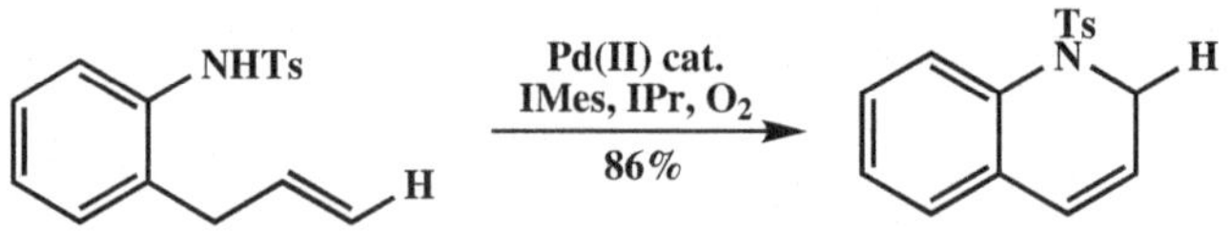

Scheme-39

Two species of European *Basidomycetes* (*Tricholoma sciodes* and *Tricholoma virgatum*) contain mushroom metabolites, indole derivatives. These mushroom metabolites were produced by this protocol [74]. For β,β-disubstituted styrenes an alkyl shift, similar to triethyl phosphite mediated reactions, can be reported [75]. Poor yields were obtained when the reaction was mediated by triethyl phosphate while the transition metal-mediated reactions afforded higher yields of indoles from β,β-disubstituted styrenes, without the formation of dimerization products or indoline-3-ones. Only quinoline was obtained in 23% yield from 2-nitrocinnamaldehyde and indole was not formed [76]. Similarly, quinolines were produced by reductive cyclization of 2-nitrochalcones in the presence of indium **(Scheme 40)** [77].

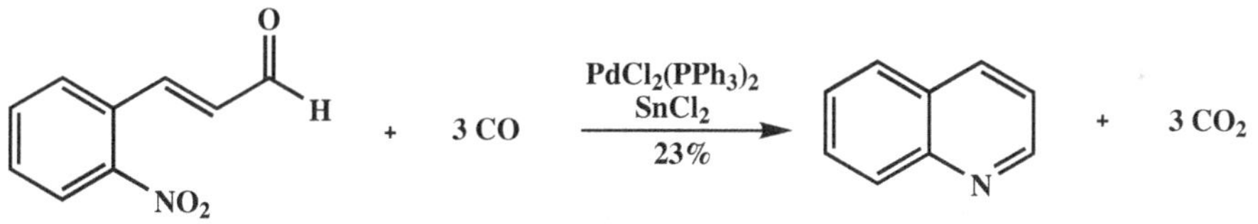

Scheme-40

Vieira and Alper [78] found a phosphine-free ionic domino rhodium-catalyzed route to tetrahydroquinolines *via* intramolecular hydroaminomethylation of 2-isopropenylanilines. The reaction was found to be highly chemo- and regioselective. Another regiospecific quinoline synthesis from α,β-unsaturated ketones and 2-aminophenylboronic acid derivatives was reported by Marsden et al. [79] **(Scheme 41)**.

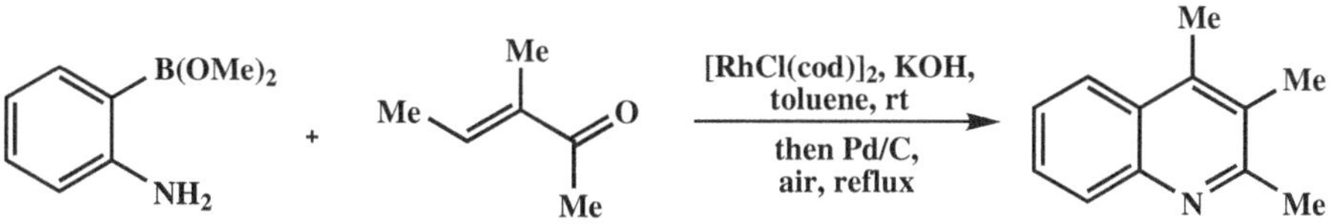

Scheme-41

For the control of selectivity in 2-substituted-4-quinolones, the nature of palladium catalysts, bases, ligands, solvents and additives was varied. The 2-substituted-4-quinolones were synthesized selectively *via* a one-pot two-step multi-catalysis in the presence of [PdCl$_2$(dppp)] catalysts and diethylamine **(Scheme 42)** [52, 80].

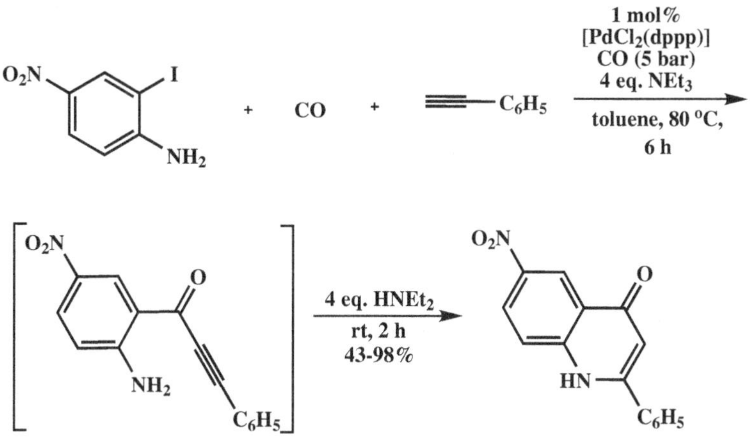

Scheme-42

Fujiwara [81] explained the effective metalation of aromatic carbon-hydrogen bonds at rt employing *in situ* generated highly-electrophilic platinum(II) and palladium(II) cationic moieties in TFA and led to regioselective inter- and intramolecular addition of simple arenes to carbon-carbon multiple bonds **(Scheme 43)**.

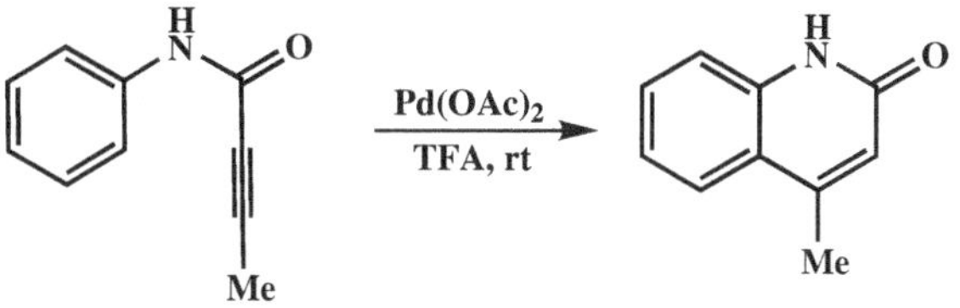

Scheme-43

8.3 Synthesis of isoquinolines

No product was observed from reaction mixture as TMS acetylene failed in current isoquinoline synthesis. Very limited success was noted in this method from 2-bromoarylaldehydes to 2'-bromoarylketones. The 1-substituted isoquinolines were not formed from 2'-bromoarylketones under optimized conditions for 2-bromoarylaldehydes. When 2'-iodoarylketones were used instead of 2'-bromoarylketones only very moderate yields were reported. The best case was where 18% yield was obtained. This one-pot reaction occurred by a coupling reaction of terminal acetylene and 2-bromoarylaldehyde in the presence of palladium catalyst, followed by imination and intramolecular annulation reactions **(Scheme 44)** [82].

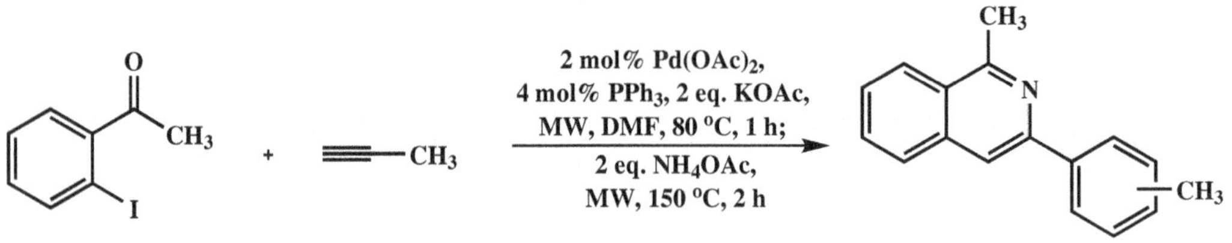

Scheme-44

The isoquinolines were synthesized under MW conditions by a one-pot reaction with Pd catalyst. The reaction of *o*-bromoarylaldehydes and terminal alkynes was performed by sequential coupling-imination-annulation reactions with NH$_4$OAc, and moderate to excellent yields (up to 86%) of a number of substituted furopyridines, isoquinolines, and thienopyridines were obtained **(Scheme 45)** [82].

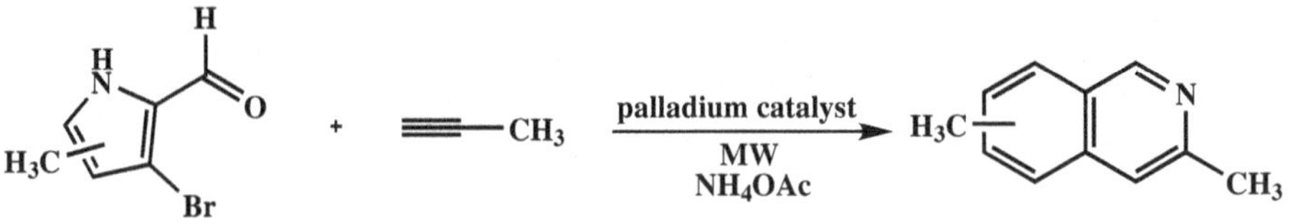

Scheme-45

The standard Sonogashira coupling conditions were applied in reaction of 4-methoxyphenyl acetylene, 2-bromobenzaldehyde, and NH$_4$OAc. The reaction occurred in one-step to form the isoquinolines in moderate yield (37%) by adding ammonium acetate initially to reaction mixture. The yield of product was enhanced to 62% when the reaction was performed in two sequential steps in one-pot reaction. Therefore, after the completion of Pd-catalyzed coupling ammonium acetate was added to reaction mixture. The desired isoquinolines were formed in 83% yield with superior effect of potassium acetate, among the other organic and inorganic bases investigated. Similar chemical yield was observed on reducing the loading of ammonium acetate and potassium acetate from 5 to 2 eq. Slightly lower yield (79%) was obtained at lower temperature (120 °C). The yield reduced when catalyst loading was decreased to 2 mol% of triphenylphosphine and 1 mol% of palladium acetate. Other ammonium salts such as ammonium bicarbonate, ammonium carbonate, and ammonium format provided inferior results as compared to ammonium acetate. In same reaction time, 60% yield was obtained when the reaction was conducted with oil bath heating. A number of 2-bromobenzaldehydes were utilized in this reaction, in which both electron-withdrawing and electron-donating substituents were compatible. Additionally, in this reaction both alkyl and aryl acetylenes were found to be compatible as well. Good to excellent yields were obtained with linear alkyl acetylenes. When sterically demanding 2-methoxyphenyl acetylene was employed yield was 75%. However, when more sterically demanding 3,3-dimethylbut-1-yne was used moderate yield (38%) was reported **(Scheme 46)** [82].

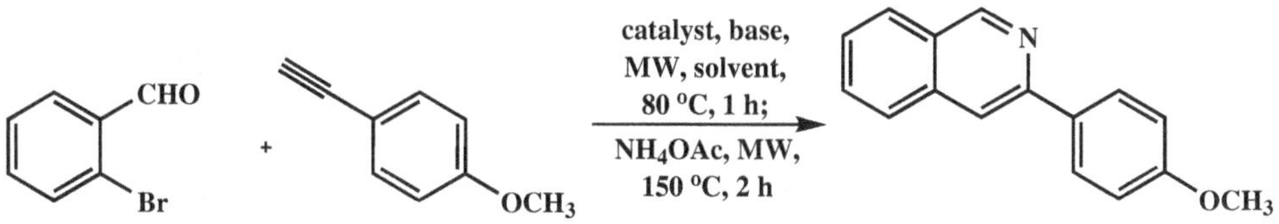

Scheme-46

Pictet-Spengler reaction of imino derivatives afforded highly functionalized chiral tetrahydro-isoquinolines. A catalytic enantioselective nitro-aldol reaction of nitromethane on arylaldehydes formed a stereo-defined chiral center in the presence of Cu-C2-symmetrical oligo-thiophene catalyst **(Scheme 47)** [83]. The amino alcohol was formed from nitro-alcohol and the amino alcohol was protected as fluorenylmethoxycarbamate. The silylation of hydroxy group was performed in this reaction, since amine protection was subsequently removed to form the primary amine. Transformation of amine into benzylidene imine was followed by a metallo-free ring closure which synthesized final product in satisfactory enantio- and diastereoselectivities [84-87].

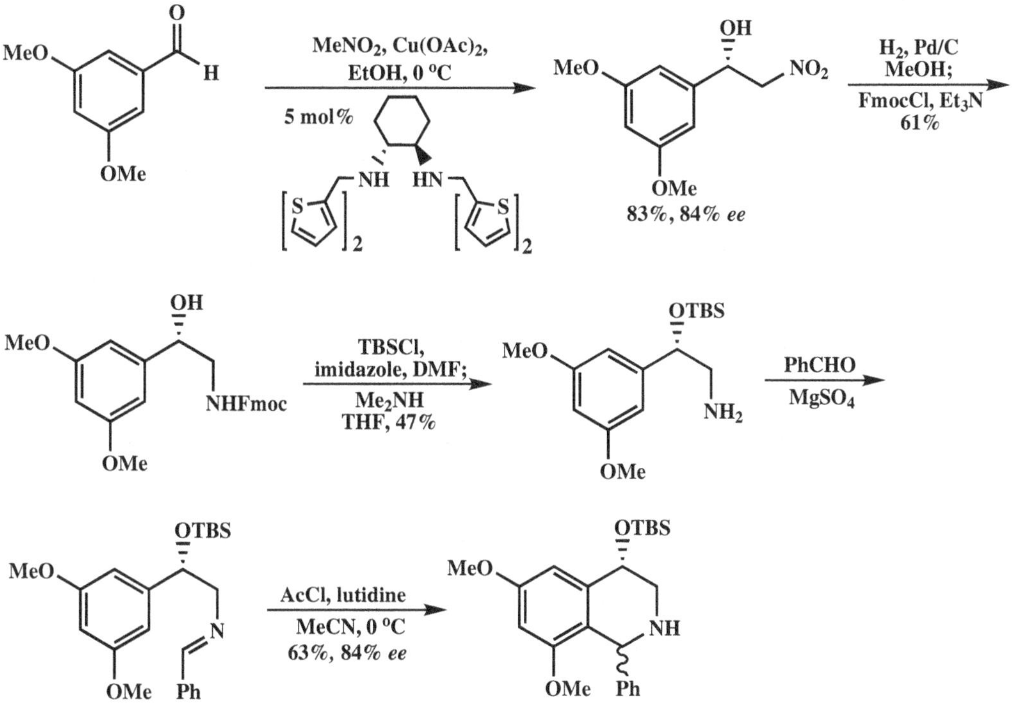

Scheme-47

Wu et al. [88] synthesized 1,2-dihydroisoquinolin-1-ylphosphonates by a tandem four-component reaction. The Sonogashira coupling proceeded between an alkyne and a 2-bromobenzaldehyde in catalytic amounts of $PdCl_2(PPh_3)_2$ and cuprous iodide. When aldehyde was completely transformed into coupling product (thin layer chromatography control), then a diethylphosphite and primary amine were added to reaction medium with concomitant addition of 10 mol% $Cu(OTf)_2$ which was required to complete the cyclization step. An imine intermediate was formed which attacked the triple bond activated by Cu(II) complex. The addition of diethylphosphite resulted in final trapping of iminium. Depending on the nature of substituents moderate to good yields were obtained **(Scheme 48)** [89].

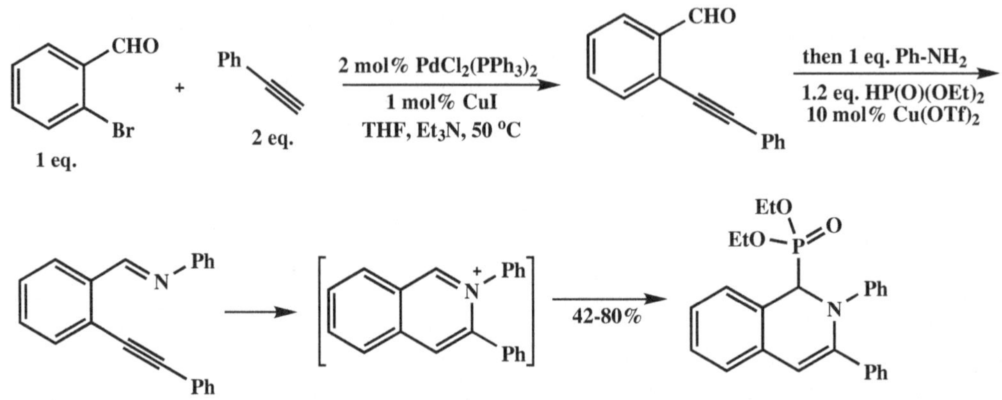

Scheme-48

Felpin et al. [90] developed a HRC protocol and reacted 2-(2-cyanoaryl)acrylates with aryldiazonium salt for the preparation of 4-benzyl-1,2-dihydroisoquinolin-3-ones. The reaction occurred under mild conditions (*i.e.* 1.2 mmol of aryldiazonium salt, 1 mmol of acrylate, 5 mL of methanol, 5 mol% of palladium acetate, 12 h, 40 °C; then 110 mg charcoal, hydrogen, 24 h, 50 °C) and afforded good to high yields of desired products **(Scheme 49)** [52].

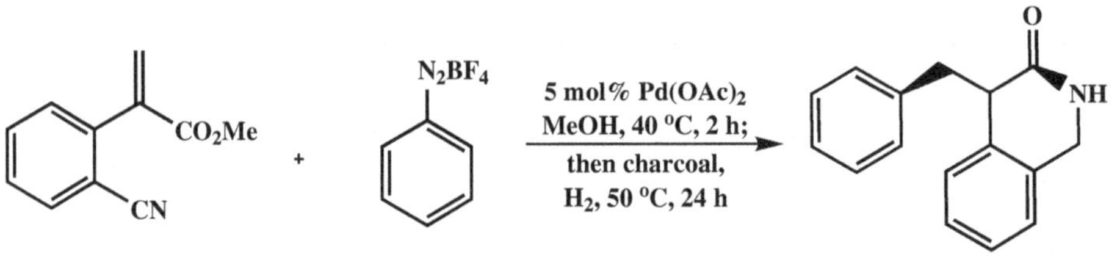

Scheme-49

The complex mixture possessing bis-arylated product as one of the major by-products was obtained by cyclization of starting substrate with PhI **(Scheme 50)**. For the synthesis of thiophenes similar carbon-hydrogen arylation chemistry was observed previously [91-92]. The desired mono-arylated product was observed in 18% yield and good purity (92%) only in one case of PhI [93].

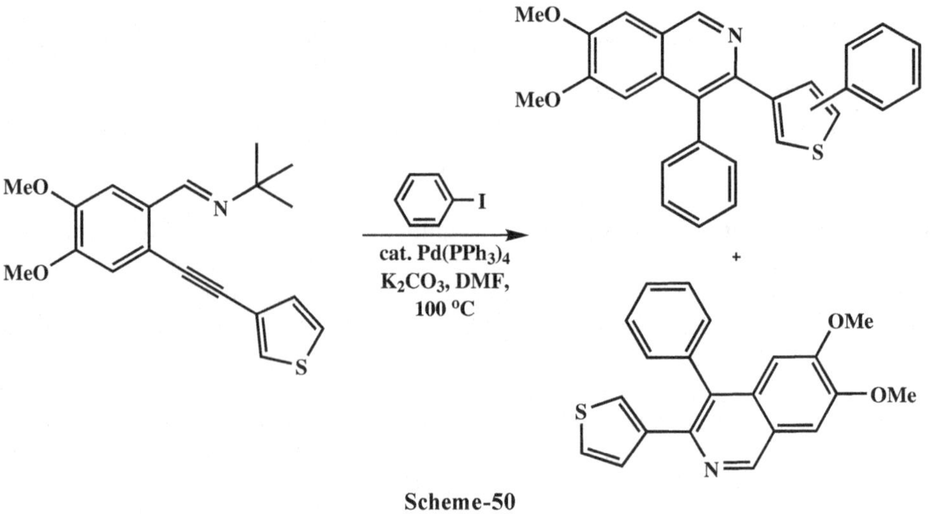

Scheme-50

The domino approach to isoquinolines has been successfully transformed into a valuable MW-assisted multi-component process starting from simple building blocks *o*-bromoarylaldehydes, terminal alkynes and aqueous NH$_3$, as depicted in **Scheme 51** [94].

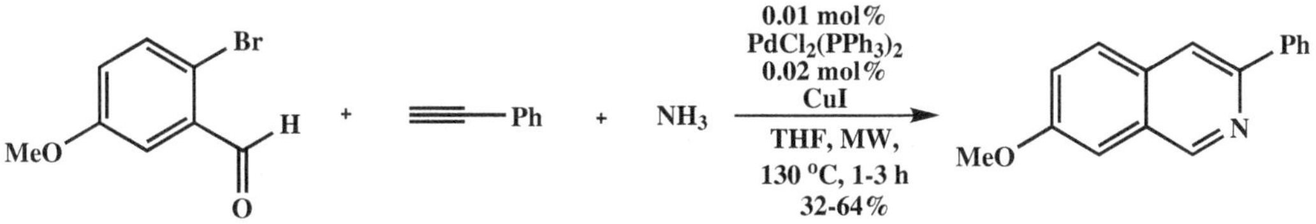

Scheme-51

Researchers have envisaged the synthesis of 5-hydroxy- or 1-hydroxy(acyloxy) methylisoquinoline as efficient substrates for a new regioselective oxidation of isoquinoline-5,8-dione anti-biotics based on a retrosynthetic analysis. For the preparation of a ketoxime, that is, a 1-azahexatriene system, began with 2,4-dimethoxy-3-methylbenzaldehyde. The 2-hydroxybenzaldehyde was synthesized from 2,4-dimethoxy-3-methylbenzaldehyde and boron tribromide, the formed 2-hydroxybenzaldehyde was transformed into benzyl ether. The phenol was obtained when benzaldehyde underwent Baeyer-Villiger reaction with *m*-CPBA. The triflate was formed when phenol was reacted with hexamethylenetetramine by Duff reaction in CH$_3$COOH, followed by treatment with trifluoromethanesulfonic anhydride. The ethenylbenzaldehyde was formed by cross-coupling reaction with vinyl tributyltin in Pd dichlorobistriphenylphosphine, then the formed ethenylbenzaldehyde underwent Grignard reaction with dimethylisopropyloxysilylmethylmagnesium chloride, followed by treatment with KF and 30% H$_2$O$_2$, to provide 1,2-diol. The 1,2-diol was selectively protected with *tert*-butyldimethylsilyl chloride (*tert*-butyldimethylsilyl chloride) to synthesize *tert*-butyldimethylsilyl ether, which was oxidized with PCC (pyridinium chlorochromate) to afford ketone. Then, the

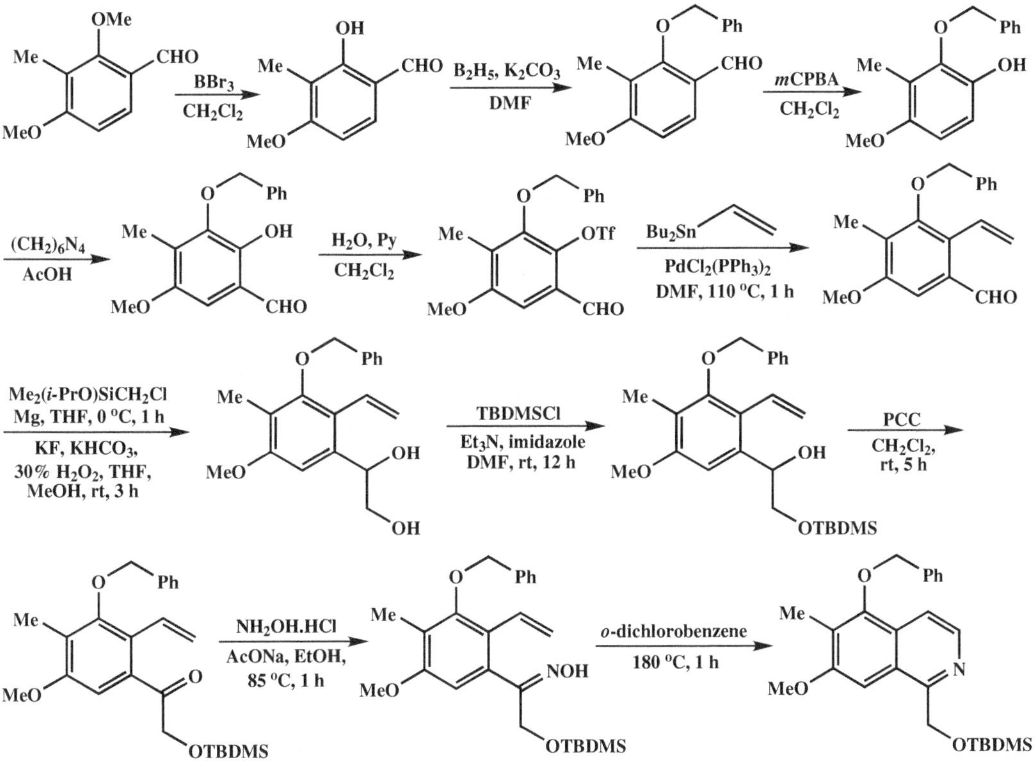

Scheme-52

ketone was reacted with hydroxylamine to provide ketoxime as 1-azahexatriene system. The ketoxime underwent thermal electrocyclic reaction at 180 °C in *o*-dichlorobenzene to deliver desired 5-benzyloxyisoquinoline **(Scheme 52)** [95a-b].

Zuckermann and Goff [96] explained a protocol for SPS of isoquinoline derivatives. The *trans*-4-bromo-2-butenoic acid was coupled to support through Rink linker with *N,N'*-diisopropylcarbodiimide. The support-bound amide was afforded on bromide displacement with a primary amine followed by acylation of resulting secondary amine with a 2-iodobenzoyl chloride. The (2*H*)-isoquinoline was formed by an intramolecular Heck reaction in the presence of Pd(PPh$_3$)$_4$ followed by cleavage with trifluoroacetic acid **(Scheme 53)**.

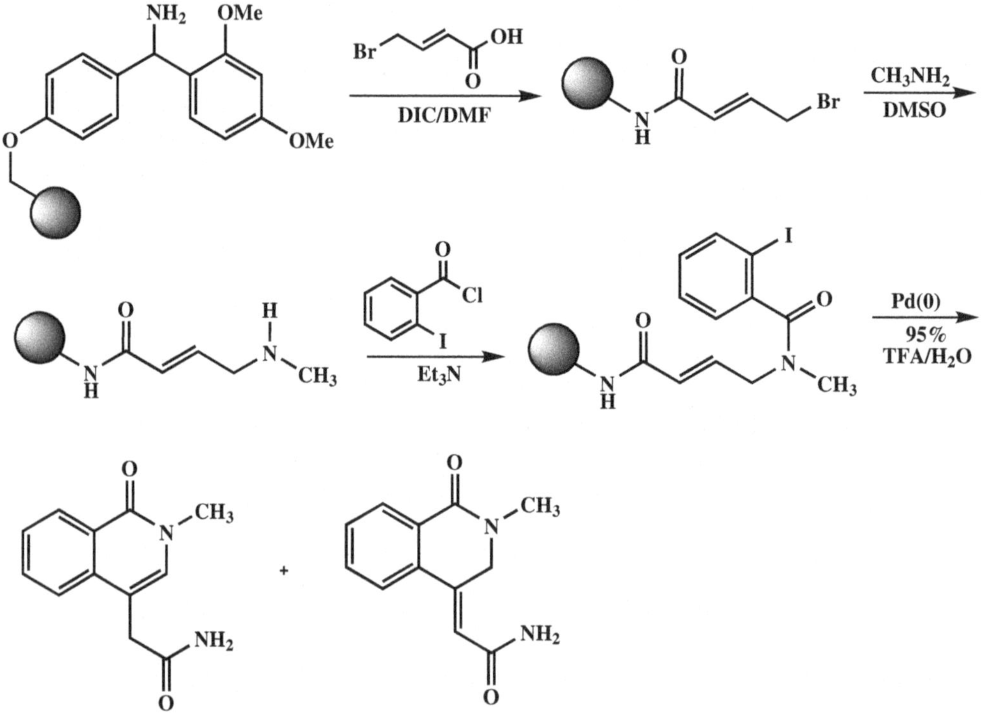

Scheme-53

The isoquinoline was produced *via* a catalytic 6-*exo*-cyclization. When TBAC was used in this reaction, improved yield was observed [97]. The isoquinoline derivatives were afforded by a Pd-catalyzed amino-Heck reaction of *o*-allylphenyl ketone oximes **(Scheme 54)**.

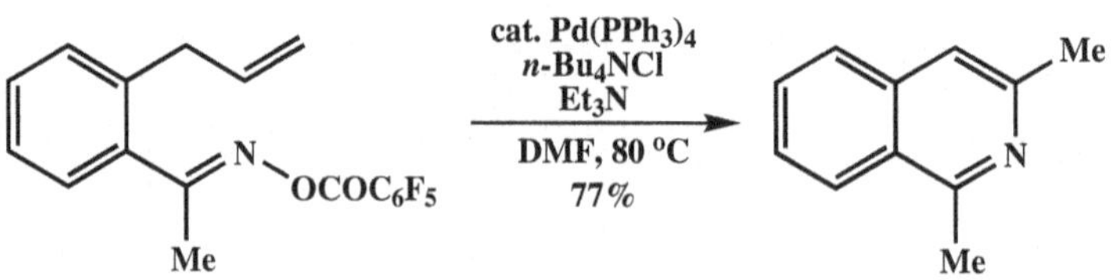

Scheme-54

Larock and co-workers [98-102] synthesized isoquinolines in good to high yields by the reaction of *t*-Bu imine of *o*-iodobenzaldehyde with alkynes in palladium acetate catalyst **(Scheme 55)**. In the area of isoquinoline synthesis Larock [103] has two approaches, the first being a Sonogashira cross-coupling strategy between halo-benzene and a terminal alkyne. This was followed by a 6-*endo-dig* cyclization to isoquinoline under thermal conditions [104-105]. The isoquinolines were synthesized by *N-t*-Bu imine cyclization pathway through non-oxidative addition/reductive elimination protocols. For instance, *o*-alkynyl substituted imine underwent Pd-catalyzed cyclization. The 2-substituted isoquinolines were formed with extra carbon unit in this reaction. Pfeffer et al. [106] explained a ring enlargement by alkyne insertions into palladium-carbon bond of cyclopalladated amines followed by subsequent ring closure for the controlled synthesis of isoquinoline [107]. When asymmetrical alkynes were employed, the reactions were found to be very regiospecific, and only one regioisomer was obtained with bulkier group closer to nitrogen. Among terminal alkynes, alkyl-substituted acetylenes did not succeed in this annulation reaction. However, the iminoalkyne intermediate possessing alkenyl, aryl, and alkyl substituents synthesized from these Pd-catalyzed reactions underwent Cu-catalyzed cyclization in short reaction times and excellent yields. This annulation approach was effective for alkenyl- or aryl-substituted alkynes. The reaction was extended to alkyl substituted alkynes when electron-rich imines were utilized [108]. The monosubstituted heterocyclic products were also formed from trimethylsilyl-substituted alkynes by this annulation strategy [23b, 109-110].

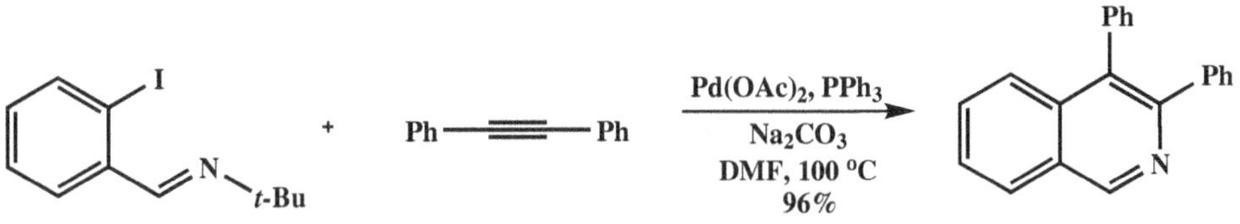

Scheme-55

Zhang and Larock [111] reported a cyclization of iminoalkynes for the synthesis of pyridine and isoquinoline derivatives. Iminoalkynes were produced in two-step method which involved a Sonogashira coupling of aryl and vinyl iodides or bromides and the conversion of aldehydes into *tert*-butylimines. The cyclization of iminoalkynes occurred by Pd or Cu catalysis or with electrophiles (iodine, ICl, PhSeCl, silver nitrate) (**Scheme 56**) [112-113].

The C1-substituted tetrahydroisoquinoline scaffolds were produced by a number of synthetic protocols [114-127]. A series of C1-substituted tetrahydroisoquinolines was synthesized *via* a Pd-catalyzed domino Heck-aza-Michael reaction (**Scheme 57**) [128a-b]. A catalytic system was needed for domino Heck-aza-Michael reaction which facilitated the fast Heck reaction between an electron-deficient terminal alkene and domino precursor. Followed by this reaction, aza-Michael cyclization occurred to prepare the *N*-heteroycle. The 2-bromophenethylamine was reacted with acrylates for the synthesis of tetrahydroisoquinolines using either palladium acetate/DavePhos or palladium acetate/triphenylphosphine in potassium carbonate and PhMe.

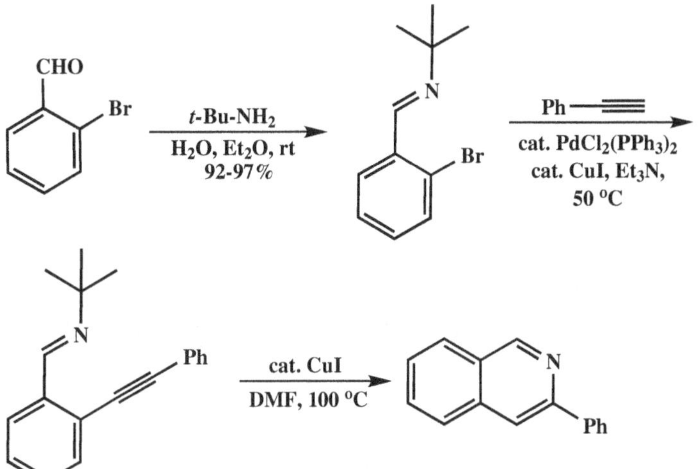

Scheme-56

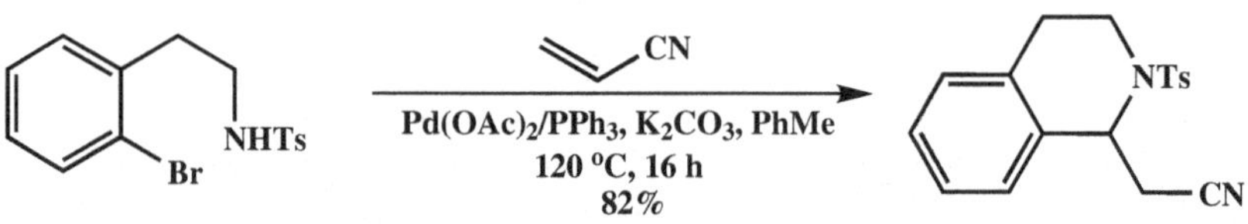

Scheme-57

The isolation of palladacycles was explained by Broggini and co-workers [129]. The β-hydride elimination was inhibited from s-alkylpalladium Heck intermediates during palladium-catalyzed intramolecular Heck reactions of N-allyl-2-halobenzylamines, which provided a number of stable bridged five-membered palladacycles with metal centre containing a Br atom and a triphenylphosphine ligand **(Scheme 58)** [29].

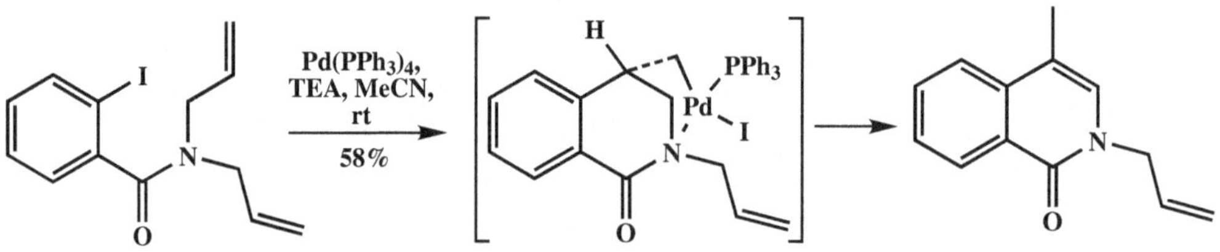

Scheme-58

Lin and Kazmaier [130] reported an intramolecular Stille coupling which transformed substituted vinylstannanes into isoquinoline derivatives **(Scheme 59)** [29].

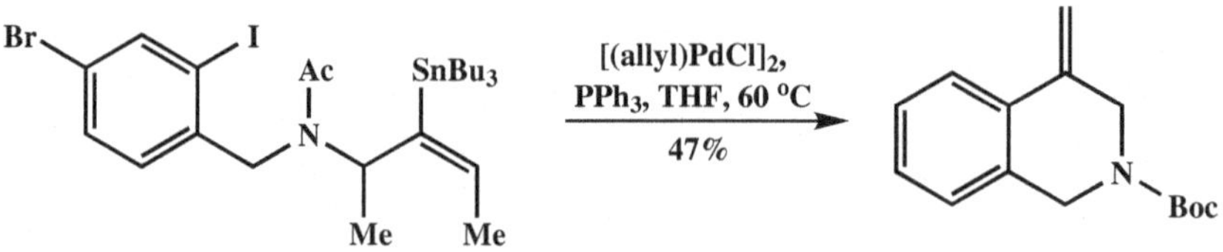

Scheme-59

Shi [131] applied phosphoramidite ligands in an intramolecular allylic amination for the synthesis of tetrahydroisoquinoline core **(Scheme 60)**. It was noted from this endeavor that both nucleophile substituents and allylic leaving groups played a critical role in stereoselectivity of this reaction. In case of allylic leaving groups, bulkier substituents afforded higher enantioselectivity (*t*-buty affording 77% *ee*). Higher enantioselectivity was achieved when trifluoroacetic acid amide was employed in place of tosylamide. The highest enantiomeric excess, 95% *ee*, was obtained with trifluoroacetic acid amide and phenyl carbonate substituents.

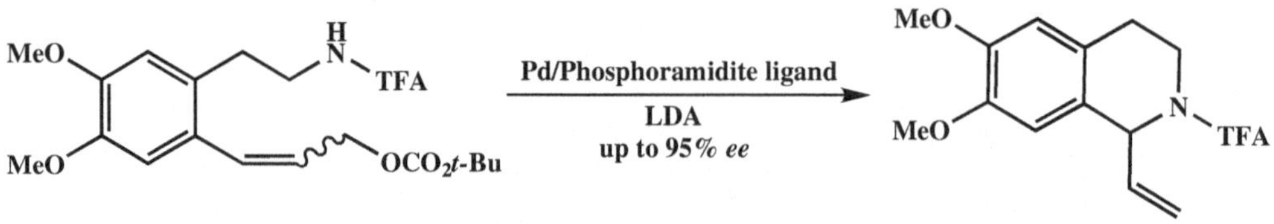

Scheme-60

Nagao and co-workers [132] synthesized isoquinolones in high yields by a ring-expansion of hydroxy methoxyallenylisoindolinones in palladium(0) catalyst **(Scheme 61)**. The hydridopalladium species were formed by oxidative addition of O-H bond of hydroxy methoxyallenylisoindolinones to Pd(0). Subsequently, allylpalladium intermediate was produced by intramolecular hydropalladation of hydridopalladium species. The isoquinolones were formed in one-atom ring-expansion which resulted in rearrangement of methylamino group of allylpalladium intermediate into allylpalladium functionality.

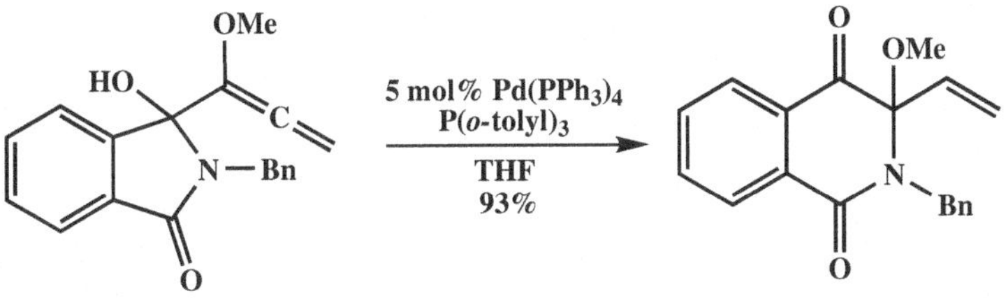

Scheme-61

Huang and Larock [133-134] synthesized isoquinolines in good to high yields when *o*-alkynylbenzaldimines were reacted *via* Pd-catalyzed cyclization/olefination reaction **(Scheme 62)**. An *ortho*-OMe group was introduced on benzene ring of alkynyl substituent to increase the yields of cyclized products. The reaction occurred *via* nucleophilic attack of nitrogen atom on electron-deficient alkyne, synthesis of alkenylpalladium intermediate, insertion of alkenes into carbon-palladium bond, and α-hydride elimination.

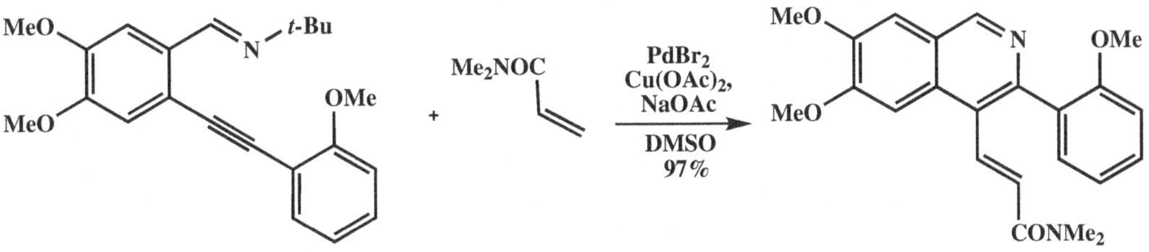

Scheme-62

The iminoalkynes were cyclized with PhI in the presence of Pd catalyst **(Scheme 63)** [135]. The 2-(phenylethynyl)benzaldehydes were produced from three 2-bromobenzaldehydes *via* Sonogashira reaction of phenyl acetylene. The 2-(phenylethynyl)benzaldehydes were transformed into *o*-(1-alkynyl)benzaldimine intermediates. A library of isoquinoline was prepared by Pd-catalyzed cyclization of iminoalkynes in many commercially available PhI [136]. The isoquinoline derivatives were formed by carbonylative version of this reaction with selected iodides. However, compound purities were lower in this carbonylative process [93].

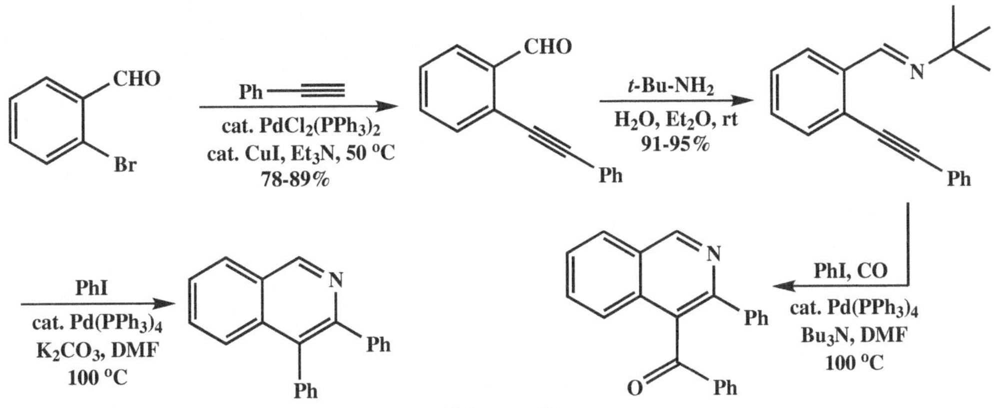

Scheme-63

The cross-coupling of *N-tert*-butyl-*o*-(1-alkynyl)-benzaldimines with allylic, aryl, and alkynyl halides produced 3,4-disubstituted isoquinolines in good yields in the presence of Pd$_2$(dba)$_3$ [137]. The acylpalladation of C-C triple bond and cyclization afforded 3-substituted 4-aroylisoquinolines with carbon monoxide and Pd(PPh$_3$)$_4$ **(Scheme 64)** [138].

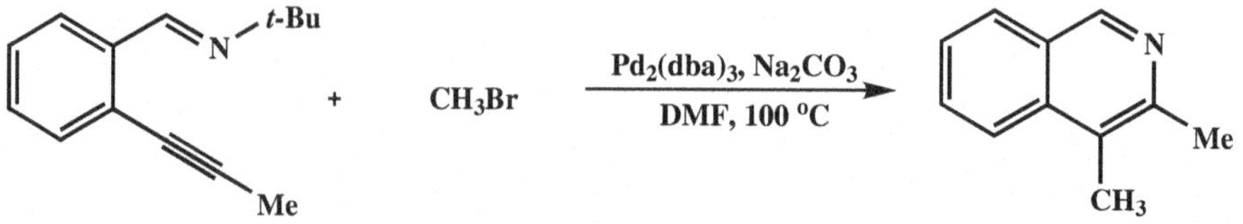

Scheme-64

Sole and co-workers [139-143], Gaertzen and Buchwald [144] and Hartwig and co-workers [145-146] reported this important synthetic protocol for the synthesis of heterocycles *via* Pd-catalyzed intramolecular arylation of esters, ketones, and amides. Honda and co-workers [147] synthesized isoquinoline alkaloids latifine and cherylline through intramolecular arylation of amides **(Scheme 65)**.

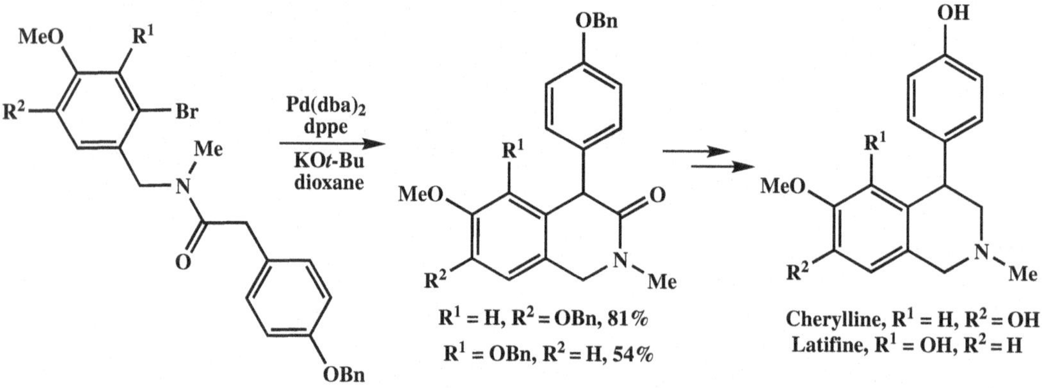

R^1 = H, R^2 = OBn, 81%
R^1 = OBn, R^2 = H, 54%

Cherylline, R^1 = H, R^2 = OH
Latifine, R^1 = OH, R^2 = H

Scheme-65

Grigg [148a] described a *de novo* intramolecular carbopalladation/cyclization-anion capture cascade process in the presence of palladium catalyst using allenamides **(Scheme 66)**. The palladium-π-allyl complex was produced by a selective carbopalladation/cyclization onto central allenic carbon after oxidative addition of palladium(0) to PhI. The allylic amines were obtained when π-allyl species were captured regioselectively by amines in potassium carbonate at sterically less hindered γ-allenic position (γ-attack). Although NMR studies have confirmed the γ-attack, to favor the more stable allylic amines an equilibration was established under reaction conditions. Intriguingly, utilization of silver carbonate altered the regioselectivity to favor α-attack as shown in vinyl aminal. The reaction occurred *via* cationic π-ally complex in the presence of silver carbonate, which favored α-attack and impede any ensuing equilibration [148b].

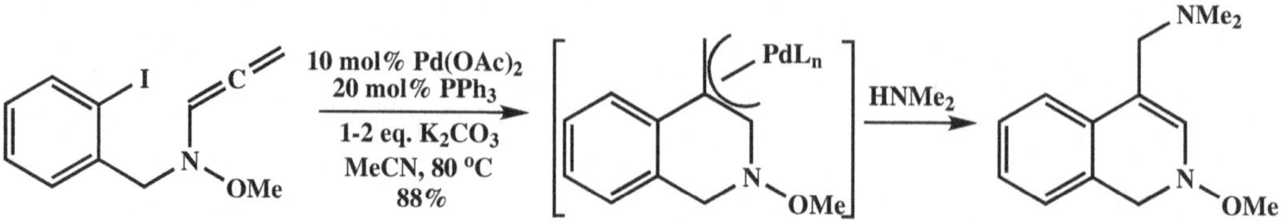

Scheme-66

The isoquinolones were produced when organostannanes were used as anion capture reagents in a Stille-type cross-coupling, although the regiochemistry was not as good. Again intriguing, silver carbonate has no significant effect on regioselectivity. Azides were obtained when NaN$_3$ was used as a capture reagent **(Scheme 67)**. Grigg [149-151] also observed a palladium-catalyzed cyclization-anion capturing cascade with organoboron reagents as anion transfer reagents **(Scheme 68)**. The Pd π-allyl complexes were obtained after carbopalladation/ cyclization. The Pd π-allyl complexes underwent transmetalation with boronic acids to afford isoquinolones after reductive elimination. Although minor isomer was also found, Suzuki-Miyaura type cross-coupling was favored predominantly at less hindered γ-allenic carbon and was overall highly regioselective regardless of the base used [148b].

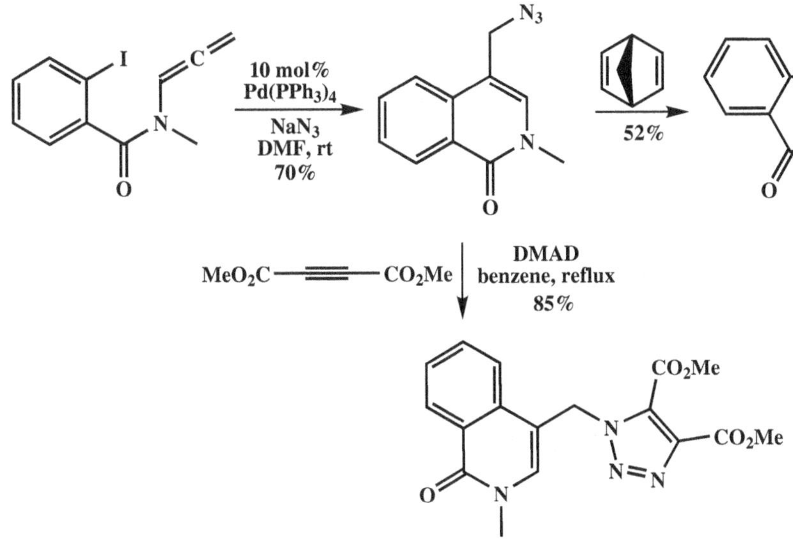

Scheme-67

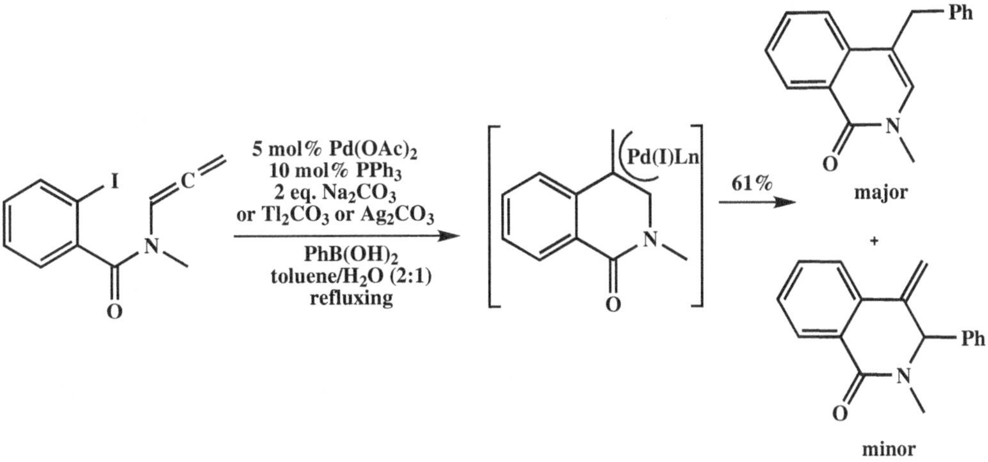

Scheme-68

Cheng [152] reported palladium-catalyzed cyclization-capture cascade in which bicyclic alkene was used for terminating process **(Scheme 69)**. The allenamide formed Pd π-allyl complex which underwent carbopalladation/cyclization cross-coupled with oxanorbornadiene to form the 1,2-dihydroisoquinoline in 78% yield. The *exo* face was favored by coordination of oxanorbornadiene to Pd π-allyl complex, and Pd-oxo complex was formed by an ensuing migratory insertion and β-oxy *syn*-elimination before zinc-reduction [148b].

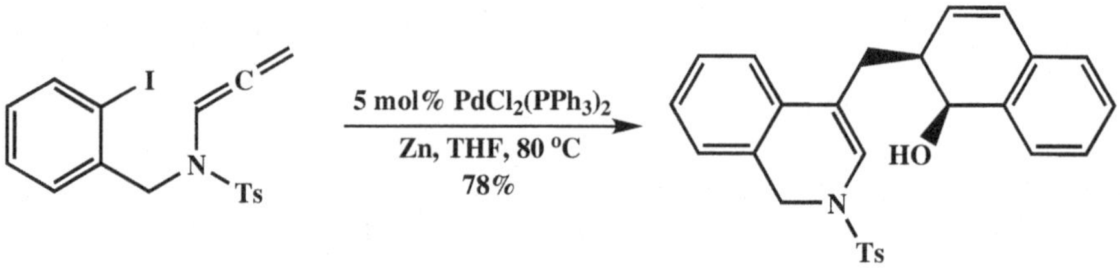

Scheme-69

Jia and co-workers [153] explained an efficient palladium-catalyzed domino reaction which involved a carbon-hydrogen activation procedure in substrates. The palladacycle intermediate was trapped with aryl or alkene functionality *via* a Heck reaction for the synthesis of tetracycle or tetrahydroisoquinoline, respectively **(Scheme 70)** [29].

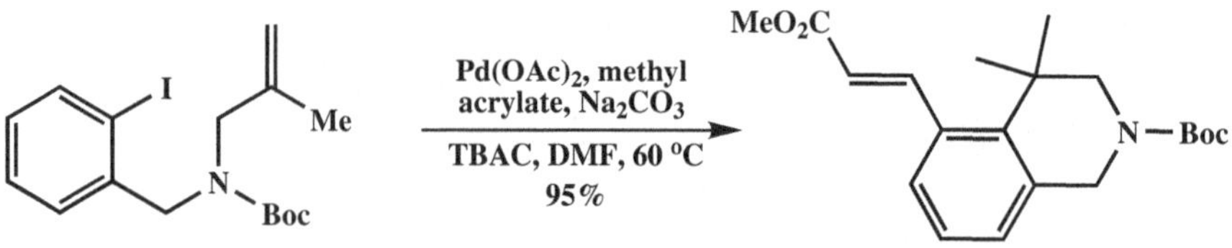

Scheme-70

Electron-rich allylbenzene derivatives such as methyleugenol, through Ritter reaction, were transformed into isoquinoline derivatives in the presence of $Pd(CH_3CN)_4(BF_4)_2$ [154]. Both dihydroisoquinoline ester (through CO insertion) and isoquinoline derivative (through spontaneous β-hydride elimination and olefin migration) were afforded **(Scheme 71)**.

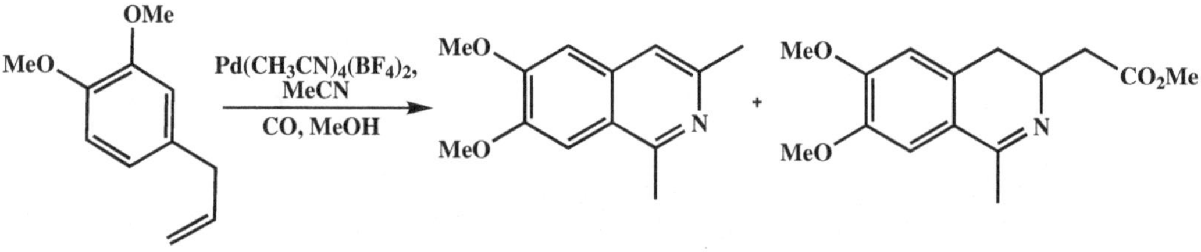

Scheme-71

A Pd(II) mediated domino carbon-hydrogen olefination/aza-Michael addition was developed for the synthesis of tetrahydroisoquinoline ketone derivatives **(Scheme 72)**. This process tolerated the presence of electron-withdrawing substituents on aromatic ring, however when methyl acrylate was employed, only Heck adduct was isolated [155].

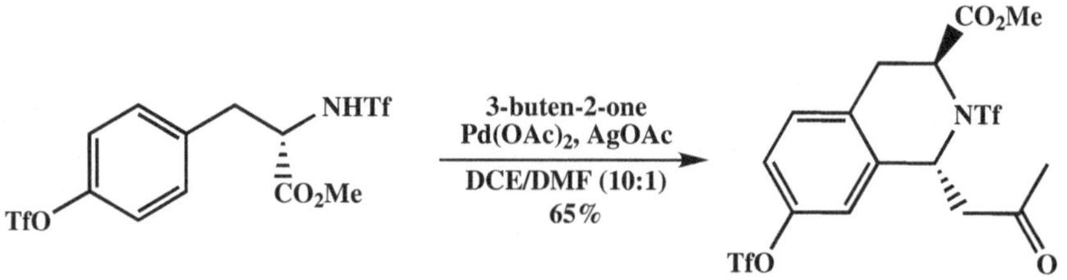

Scheme-72

Benzylamine acted as an amine substrate. The acryloyl chloride was added to a solution possessing benzylamine, and K_2CO_3 in PhMe. The mixture was stirred for one hr at rt, then palladium acetate/triphenylphosphine and 2-bromophenethylsulfonamide were added, and formed mixture was heated for 16 h at 120 °C **(Scheme 73)**. The desired tetrahydroisoquinoline was provided in an excellent yield (97%) [128a-b, 156].

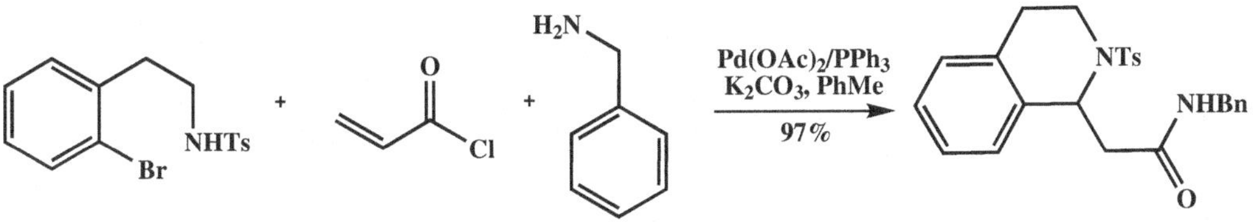

Scheme-73

The isoquinoline derivatives were formed from allylamines containing *o*-halobenzyl functionality on nitrogen. Liu and co-workers [157] used *N*-allyl benzylamines for the synthesis of 1,2,3,4-tetrahydroisoquinolines under ligand-free conditions through palladium-catalyzed reductive Heck cyclization **(Scheme 74)** [29].

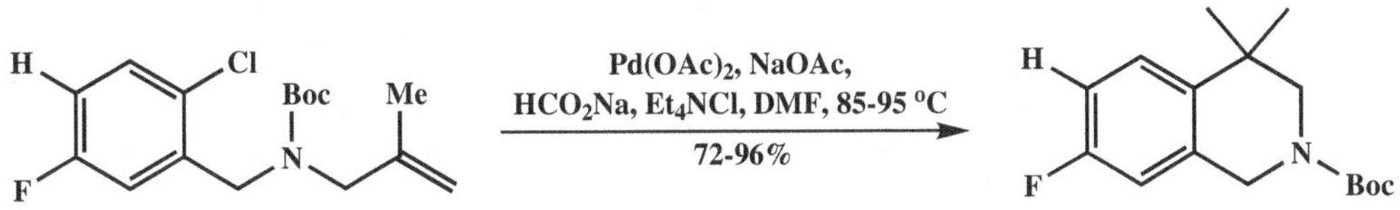

Scheme-74

In drug discovery programs many small molecules are in great demand. The fast synthesis of natural product-like compounds is of utmost importance and urgency for efficient and practical protocols [158-160]. Recently, through cascade reactions a small library of *H*-pyrazolo[5,1-*a*] isoquinolines was successfully synthesized [161]. The preliminary biological assays have shown that some of these compounds showed biological activities such as TC-PTP inhibitor, CDC25B inhibitor, and PTP1B inhibitor **(Scheme 75)**.

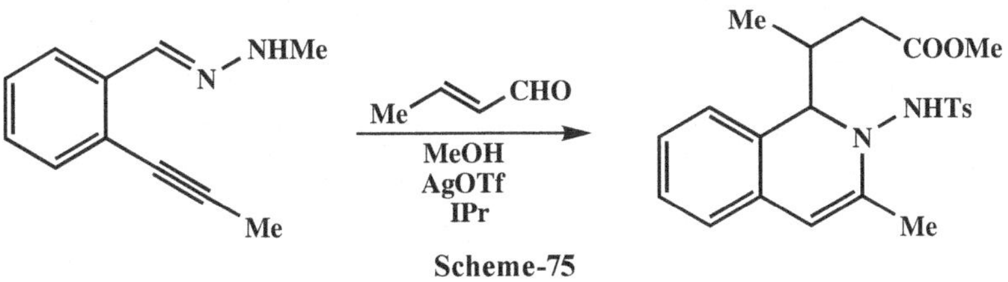

Scheme-75

During multi-component synthesis of functionalized tetrahydroisoquinolines it was observed that valine acrylamide led to a 3:7 mixture of diastereomers (40% *de*) following domino Heck-aza-Michael process **(Scheme 76)** [162].

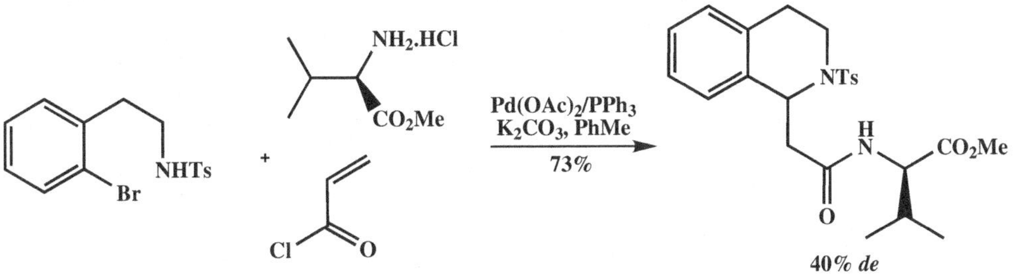

Scheme-76

Nandi and Ray [163] explained the palladium(0)-catalyzed 6-*exo-trig* cyclization of *N*-aryl allylamines for the synthesis of fused cyclopropa[*d*]-fused isoquinoline derivatives. The cyclopropa[*d*]-fused isoquinoline derivatives were provided *via* a domino reaction from *N*-methallylated derivatives under Heck reaction conditions (**Scheme 77**) [29].

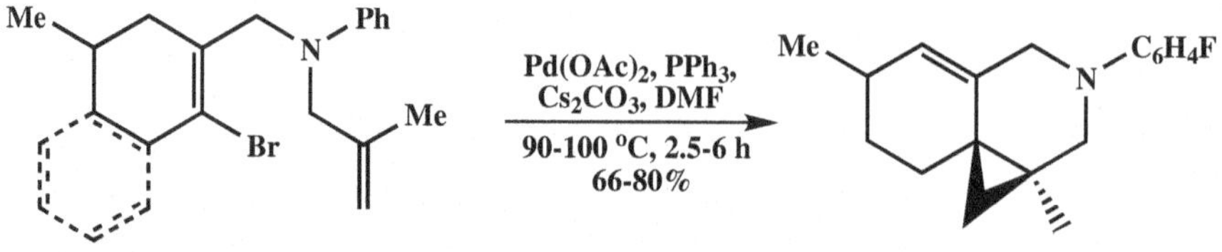

Scheme-77

The indolines were produced *via* a tandem carbon-hydrogen bond iodination/amination pathway in the presence of copper(I)/palladium(II) catalysts. The tetrahydroisoquinolines were synthesized by modifying this reaction under different reaction conditions and with different substrates (**Scheme 78**) [155, 164].

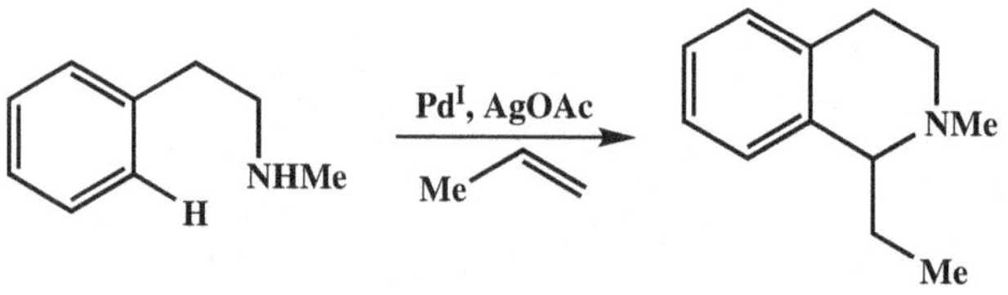

Scheme-78

Majumdar and co-workers [165] used different *N*-allylbenzamide derivatives for the synthesis of *N*-substituted 4-methyl- and 4-ethylisoquinolone derivatives *via* a ligand-free Heck cyclization in a single step (**Scheme 79**) [29].

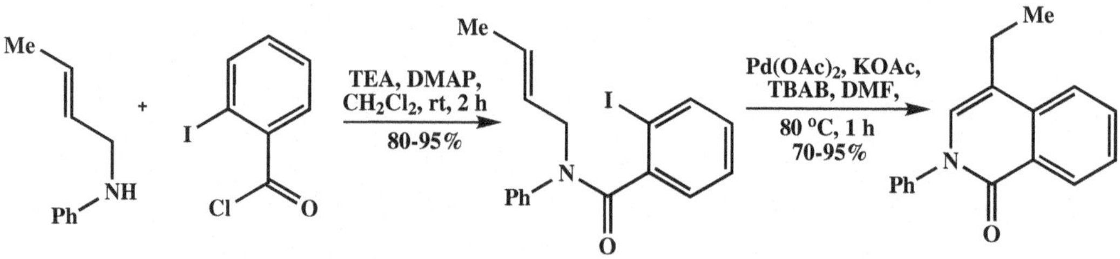

Scheme-79

The most widely used methods for the formation of isoquinoline rings are Bischler-Napieralski cyclization and Pictet-Spengler condensation [166]. However, the presence of two electron-releasing groups on aryl rings was needed in both of these protocols. The vinyl ketones were reacted through a tandem carbon-hydrogen alkenylation and aza-Michael addition for the synthesis of tetrahydroisoquinolines in high diastereoselectivity. However, the cyclization reaction described in **Scheme 80** does not need electron-releasing groups on aryl rings. The reaction was not retarded when trifluoromethylsulfonate group was present at *para* position. The electron-withdrawing chloro group was also tolerated as shown in tandem iodination and amination reaction. For the introduction of diversity at C1, inexpensive reagents olefins were utilized. This protocol was used for the synthesis of many heterocyclic compounds from natural amino acids such as tyrosine, phenylalanine, and tryptophan [155, 164, 167].

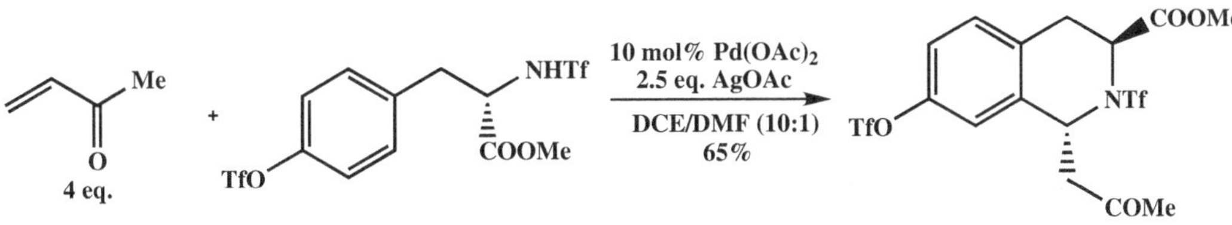

Scheme-80

With requisite chiral precursor in hand, the domino reaction was attempted using same conditions previously identified for the formation of tetrahydroisoquinolines **(Scheme 81)** [168].

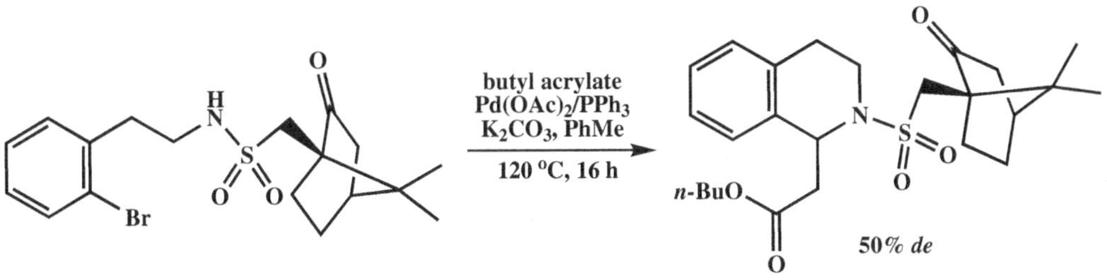

Scheme-81

Bonnaventure and Charette [169] explored an intramolecular Heck cyclization of iodobenzene with olefin of allylamine for the synthesis of tetrahydroisoquinoline with an exocyclic double bond **(Scheme 82)**. The hexahydroisoquinoline was formed by reduction of tetrahydroisoquinoline with PtO_2 [29].

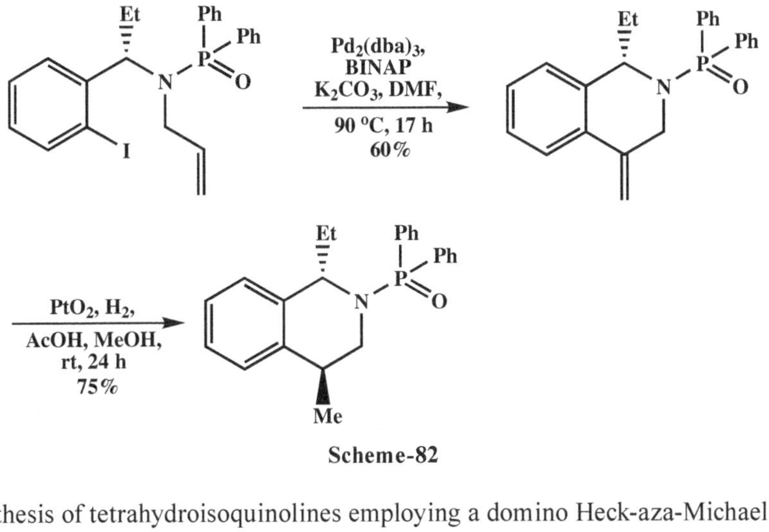

Scheme-82

The synthesis of tetrahydroisoquinolines employing a domino Heck-aza-Michael process was published in 2004 by Ferraccioli and co-workers [170]. The first step in this multi-component reaction was *o*-alkylation of PhI with bromoethylcarbamate to form the corresponding phenethylamine **(Scheme 83)** through a carbon-hydrogen activation process involving norbornene. The Heck reaction of aryl-iodide and *tert*-butylacrylate afforded conjugated Michael acceptor. Finally, formation of *N*-heterocycle through 1,4-addition of carbamate furnished a new ring system in an excellent yield of 68% for three-step process. Using bromopropylcarbamate substrate, this reaction sequence was also successfully applied to the synthesis of C1-substituted tetrahydro-2-benzazepines.

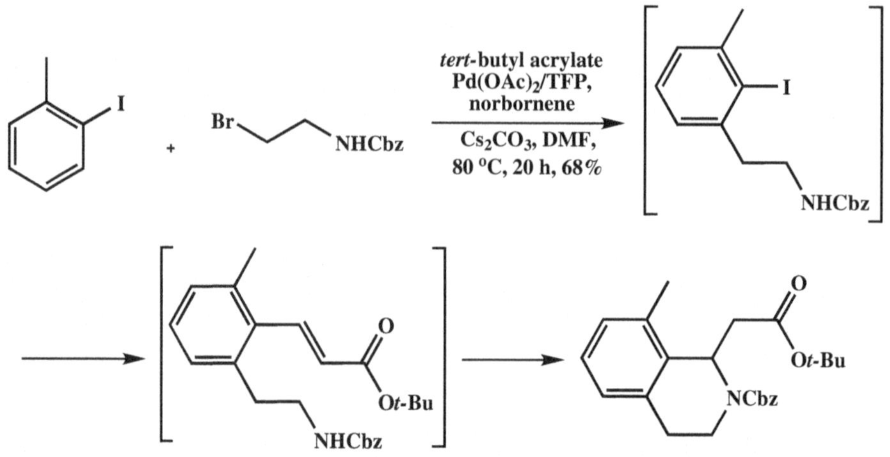

Scheme-83

Broggini and co-workers [171] utilized *N*-allylamides of 2-iodobenzoic acids for the direct preparation of 4-[(methoxycarbonyl)methyl]-3,4-dihydroisoquinolin-1-ones *via* palladium-catalyzed carbonylative Heck cyclization (**Scheme 84**) [29].

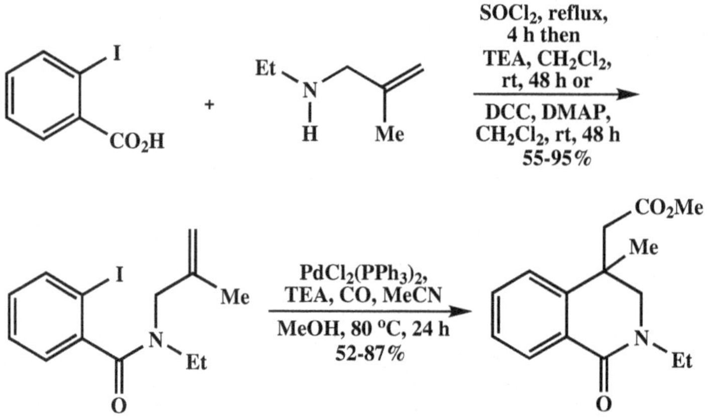

Scheme-84

Threadgill and co-workers [172] synthesized two isomeric isoquinolinones, 4-alkyl-5-nitro-3,4-dihydroisoquinolin-1-ones and 4-alkyl-5-nitroisoquinolin-1-ones *via* palladium-catalyzed Heck cyclizations of secondary and tertiary *N*-cinnamyl and *N*-allyl 2-iodo-3-nitrobenzamides (**Scheme 85**). The 4-alkyl-5-nitroisoquinolin-1-ones were formed in optimum yields with tetrabutylammonium chloride and rapid heating at 150 °C. The 4-benzyl- and 4-methyl-5-aminoisoquinolin-1-ones (potent inhibitors of PARP-1) were formed by hydrogenation of NO_2 groups. Significant increased potency for inhibition of human PARP-1 was observed for 4-substituted 5-aminoisoquinolin-1-ones (5-AIQ) [29].

The propargyl type 1,3-dipoles were produced by nucleophilic displacement of azides as trapping nucleophiles. The annelated triazoles were synthesized easily. The triazole derivatives were formed in one-pot manner by sequence of reactions *i.e.* insertion of allenes, allylic substitution and intramolecular 1,3-dipolar cycloaddition (**Scheme 86**) [173]. Good yields of isoquinolines were obtained by extrusion of nitrogen followed by an isomerization-aromatization with release of excessive allene and extended heating [174].

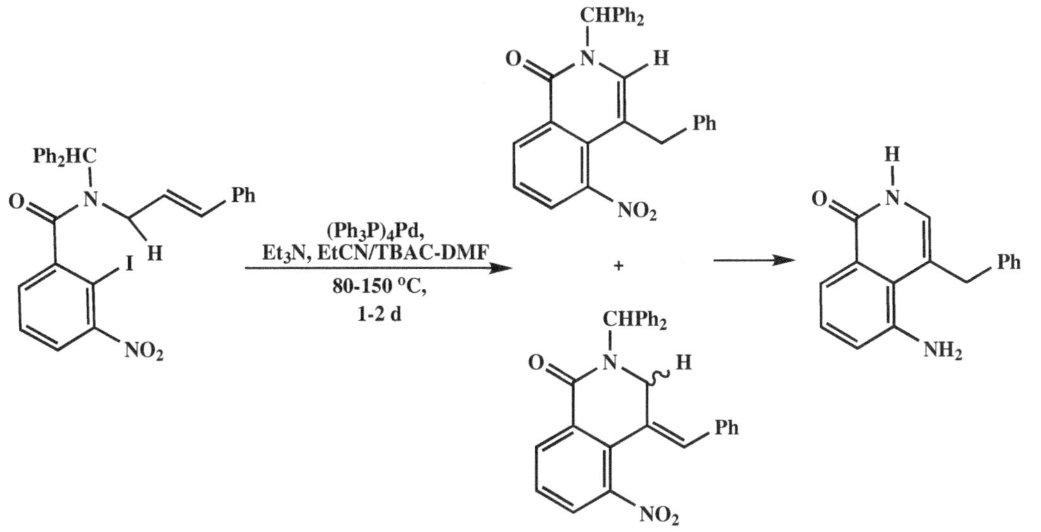

Scheme-85

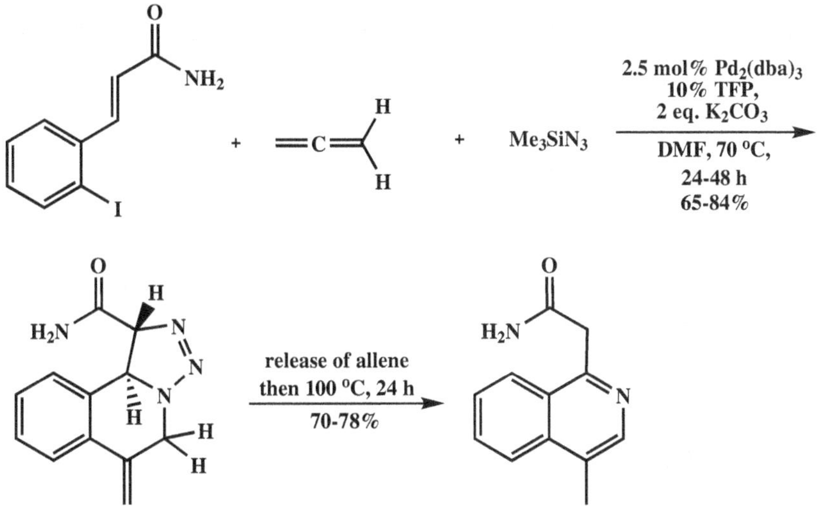

Scheme-86

Gowrisankar and co-workers [28] used allylamide in palladium-catalyzed Heck-type cyclization for the preparation of isoquinoline **(Scheme 87)** [29].

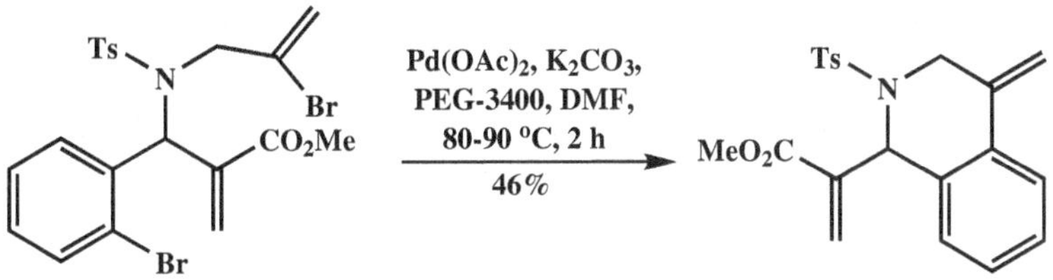

Scheme-87

Medicinal agents and natural products contain β-arylethylamine. Gaunt et al. [175] synthesized a variety of β-arylethylamine motifs *via* an amine directed palladium(II)-catalyzed carbon-hydrogen bond functionalization pathway. The reaction proceeded through carbon-hydrogen carbonylation, carbon-hydrogen arylation and carbon-hydrogen amination. This palladium(II)-catalyzed carbon-hydrogen bond carbonylation and carbon-hydrogen arylation occurred at rt and tolerated complex stereocentres and functionality **(Scheme 88)** [33, 176].

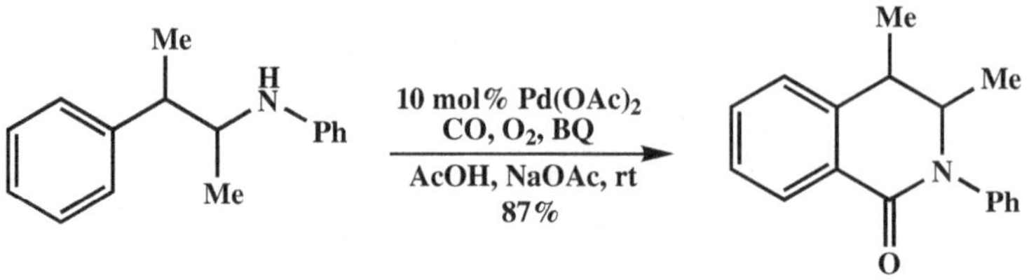

Scheme-88

The *o*-vinylbenzamides and *o*-vinylacetanilides were used for the synthesis of isoquinolinones and indoles, respectively **(Scheme 89)** [177]. The cyclizations in these cases were formally amidation reactions. An alkaloid skeleton like bukittinggine, a *daphniphyllum* alkaloid was synthesized by this same protocol [73, 178].

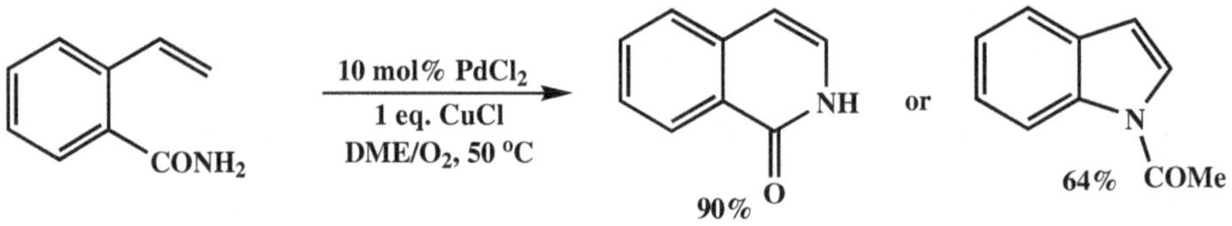

Scheme-89

Savic [179] reported a palladium-catalyzed carbopalladation/cyclization-anion capture cascade in the presence of acetate anion as a capturing nucleophile **(Scheme 90)**. The desired cyclized products were obtained from allenamides by intramolecular version of this reaction. However, a mixture of regioisomeric acetates was formed from allenamide when intermolecular version was performed [148b].

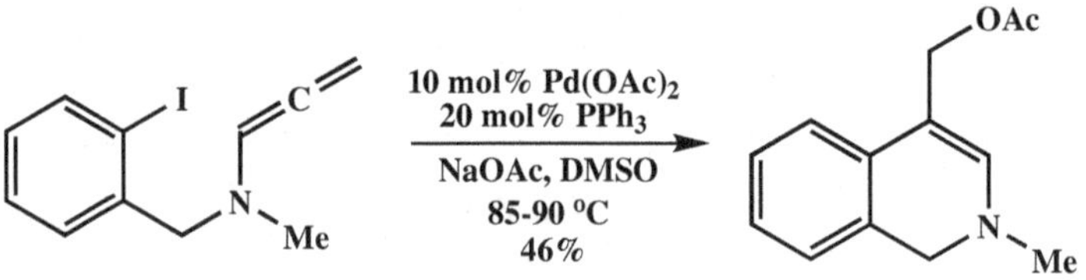

Scheme-90

REFERENCES

[1]   M.A.P. Martins, W. Cunico, C.M.P. Pereira, A.F.C. Flores, H.G. Bonacorso and N. Zanatta. 2004. 4-Alkoxy-1,1,1-trichloro-3-alken-2-ones: preparation and applications in heterocyclic synthesis. Curr. Org. Synth. 1: 391-403.

[2]   A. Domling. 2006. Recent developments in isocyanide based multi-component reactions in applied chemistry. Chem. Rev. 106: 17-89.

[3]   R.V.A. Orru and M. de Greef. 2003. Recent advances in solution-phase multi-component methodology for the synthesis of heterocyclic compounds. Synthesis 10: 1471-1499.

[4]   (a) N. Kaur. 2015. Metal catalysts: applications in higher-membered *N*-heterocycles synthesis. J. Iran. Chem. Soc. 12: 9-45.

(b) N. Kaur. 2015. Insight into microwave-assisted synthesis of benzo derivatives of five-membered *N,N*-heterocycles. Synth. Commun. 45: 1269-1300.

(c) N. Kaur. 2015. Synthesis of fused five-membered *N,N*-heterocycles using microwave irradiation. Synth. Commun. 45: 1379-1410.

(d) N. Kaur. 2014. Microwave-assisted synthesis of seven-membered *S*-heterocycles. Synth. Commun. 44: 3201-3228.

(e) N. Kaur. 2015. Six-membered *N*-heterocycles: microwave-assisted synthesis. Synth. Commun. 45: 1-34.

(f) N. Kaur. 2015. Polycyclic six-membered *N*-heterocycles: microwave-assisted synthesis. Synth. Commun. 45: 35-69.

[5]   K.C. Majumdar, A. Taher and P. Debnath. 2009. Palladium-catalyzed intramolecular biaryl coupling: a highly efficient avenue for benzannulated pyranoquinolines and julolidine derivatives. Synthesis 5: 793-800.

[6]   S. Obika, H. Kono, Y. Yasui, R. Yanada and Y. Takemoto. 2007. Concise synthesis of 1,2-dihydroisoquinolines and 1*H*-isochromenes by carbophilic Lewis acid-catalyzed tandem nucleophilic addition and cyclization of 2-(1-alkynyl)arylaldimines and 2-(1-alkynyl)arylaldehydes. J. Org. Chem. 72: 4462-4468.

[7]   P. Supsana, P.G. Tsoungas, A. Aubry, S. Skoulika and G. Varvounis. 2001. Oxidation of 1-acyl-2-naphthol oximes: peri- and *o*-cyclization and spiro cyclodimerization of naphthoquinone nitrosomethide intermediates. Tetrahedron 57: 3445-3453.

[8]   J.F. Sanz-Cervera, R. Blasco, J. Piera, M. Cynamon, I. Ibáñez, M. Murguia and S. Fustero. 2009. Solution versus fluorous versus solid-phase synthesis of 2,5-disubstituted 1,3-azoles. Preliminary anti-bacterial activity studies. J. Org. Chem. 74: 8988-8996.

[9]   D. Castagnolo, M. Pagano, M. Bernardini and M. Botta. 2009. Domino alkylation-cyclization reaction of propargyl bromides with thioureas/thiopyrimidinones: a new facile synthesis of 2-aminothiazoles and 5*H*-thiazolo[3,2-*a*]pyrimidin-5-ones. Synlett 13: 2093-2096.

[10]   L.F. Silva and S.A. Quintiliano. 2009. An expeditious synthesis of hexahydrobenzo[*f*]isochromenes and of hexahydrobenzo[*f*]isoquinoline *via* iodine-catalyzed Prins and aza-Prins cyclization. Tetrahedron Lett. 50: 2256-2260.

[11]   K.C. Majumdar, A.K. Pal, A. Taher and P. Debnath. 2007. Highly effective regioselective method for the synthesis of substituted coumarin and quinolone annulated heterocycles using Pd(0)-catalyzed reaction. Synthesis 11: 1707-1711.

[12]   X.-Y. Sun, C.-X. Wei, K.-Y. Chai, H.-R. Piao and Z.-S. Quan. 2008. Synthesis and anti-inflammatory activity evaluation of novel 7-alkoxy-1-amino-4,5-dihydro[1,2,4]triazole[4,3-*a*] quinolines. Arch. Pharm. Chem. Life Sci. 341: 288-293.

[13]   C.H. Lee and H.-S. Lee. 2011. Relaxant effect of quinoline derivatives on histamine-induced contraction of the isolated guinea pig trachea. J. Korean Soc. Appl. Biol. Chem. 54: 118-123.

[14]   M. Sankaran, C. Kumarasamy, U. Chokkalingam and P.S. Mohan. 2010. Synthesis, anti-oxidant and toxicological study of novel pyrimido quinoline derivatives from 4-hydroxy-3-acyl quinolin-2-one. Bioorg. Med. Chem. Lett. 20: 7147-7151.

[15]   V.R. Solomon and H. Lee. 2011. Quinoline as a privileged scaffold in cancer drug discovery. Curr. Med. Chem. 18: 1488-1508.

[16]   N. Ahmed, K.G. Brahmbhatt, S. Sabde, D. Mitra, I.P. Singh and K.K. Bhutani. 2010. Synthesis and anti-HIV activity of alkylated quinoline 2,4-diols. Bioorg. Med. Chem. Lett. 18: 2872-2879.

[17]   J.P. Wolfe, R.A. Rennels and S.L. Buchwald. 1996. Intramolecular palladium-catalyzed aryl amination and aryl amidation. Tetrahedron 52: 7525-7546.

[18]   Y. Wang and T.N. Huang. 1998. Solid-phase synthesis of heterocycles *via* palladium-catalyzed annulations. Tetrahedron Lett. 39: 9605-9608.

[19]   A.C. Tadd, A. Matsuno, M.R. Fielding and M.C. Willis. 2009. Cascade palladium-catalyzed alkenyl aminocarbonylation/intramolecular aryl amidation: an annulative synthesis of 2-quinolones. Org. Lett. 11: 583-586.

[20]   A. Dieudonne-Vatran, M. Azoulay and J.C. Florent. 2012. A new access to 3-substituted-1(2*H*)-isoquinolone by tandem palladium-catalyzed intramolecular aminocarbonylation annulation. Org. Biomol. Chem. 10: 2683-2691.

[21]   C.J. Ball and M.C. Willis. 2013. Cascade palladium- and copper-catalyzed aromatic heterocycle synthesis: the emergence of general precursors. Eur. J. Org. Chem. 3: 425-441.

[22]   X. Luo, E. Chenard, P. Martens, Y.-X. Cheng and M.J. Tomaszewshi. 2010. Practical synthesis of quinoxalinones *via* palladium-catalyzed intramolecular *N*-arylations. Org. Lett. 12: 3574-3577.

[23]   (a) G.S. Lemen and J.P. Wolfe. 2011. Cascade intramolecular *N*-arylation/intermolecular carboamination reactions for the construction of tricyclic heterocycles. Org. Lett. 13: 3218-3221.
       (b) J.C. Anderson, A. Noble and D.A. Tocher. 2012. Reductive nitro-Mannich route for the synthesis of 1,2-diamine containing indolines and tetrahydroquinolines. J. Org. Chem. 77: 6703-6727.

[24]   A.J. Peat and S.L. Buchwald. 1996. Novel syntheses of tetrahydropyrroloquinolines: applications to alkaloid synthesis. J. Am. Chem. Soc. 118: 1028-1030.

[25]   H.J.C. Deboves, C. Hunter and R.F.W. Jackson. 2002. Synthesis of 2-substituted indolines using sequential Pd-catalyzed processes. J. Chem. Soc. Perkin Trans. 1. 6: 733-736.

[26]   S. Wagaw, R.A. Rennels and S.L. Buchwald. 1997. Palladium-catalyzed coupling of optically active amines with aryl bromides. J. Am. Chem. Soc. 119: 8451-8458.

[27]   R.S. Colemen and W. Chen. 2001. A convergent approach to the mitomycin ring system. Org. Lett. 3: 1141-1144.

[28]   S. Gowrisankar, H.S. Lee, J.M. Kim and J.N. Kim. 2008. Pd-mediated synthesis of 2-arylquinolines and tetrahydropyridines from modified Baylis-Hillman adducts. Tetrahedron Lett. 49: 1670-1673.

[29]   S. Nag and S. Batra. 2011. Applications of allylamines for the syntheses of aza-heterocycles. Tetrahedron 67: 8959-9061.

[30]   Y.S. Park, M.Y. Cho, Y.B. Kwon, B.W. Yoo and C.M. Yoon. 2007. Amination of the Baylis-Hillman acetates in ethanol. Synth. Commun. 37: 2677-2685.

[31]   B.-L. Chen, B. Wang and G.-Q. Lin. 2010. Highly diastereoselective addition of alkynylmagnesium chlorides to *N-tert*-butanesulfinyl aldimines: a practical and general access to chiral α-branched amines. J. Org. Chem. 75: 941-944.

[32]   Z. Zhang, J. Tan and Z. Wang. 2008. A facile synthesis of 2-methylquinolines *via* Pd-catalyzed aza-Wacker oxidative cyclization. Org. Lett. 10: 173-175.

[33]   Z. Shi, C. Zhang, C. Tanga and N. Jiao. 2012. Recent advances in transition-metal catalyzed reactions using molecular oxygen as the oxidant. Chem. Soc. Rev. 41: 3381-3430.

[34]   R.C. Larock, H. Yang, P. Pace, S. Cacchi and G. Fabrizi. 1998. Synthesis of 2-vinylic dihydroindoles and tetrahydroquinolines *via* Pd-catalyzed cross-coupling of *o*-alkenyl anilides with vinylic halides and triflates. Tetrahedron Lett. 39: 1885-1888.

[35]   R.C. Larock, P. Pace and H. Yang. 1998. Synthesis of unexpected nitrogen heterocycles *via* Pd-catalyzed cross-coupling of *o*-isopropenyl and methallyl anilides with vinylic halides. Tetrahedron Lett. 39: 2515-2518.

[36]   R.C. Larock, P. Pace, H. Yang, C. Russell, S. Cacchi and G. Fabrizi. 1998. Synthesis of nitrogen heterocycles *via* Pd-catalyzed cross-coupling of *o*-alkenyl anilides with vinylic halides and triflates. Tetrahedron 54: 9961-9980.

[37]   R. Annunziata, S. Cenini, G. Palmisano and S. Tollari. 1996. 4(1*H*)-Quinolinone alkaloids. An efficient synthesis of graveoline by palladium-catalyzed reductive *N*-heterocyclization. Synth. Commun. 26: 495-501.

[38]   F. Ragaini, P. Sportiello and S. Cenini. 1999. Investigation of the possible role of arylamine formation in the *ortho*-substituted nitroarenes reductive cyclization reactions to afford heterocycles. J. Organomet. Chem. 577: 283-291.

[39]   J.-R. Wang and K. Manabe. 2010. Hydroxyterphenylphoshine- palladium catalyst for benzo[*b*]furan synthesis from 2-chlorophenols. Bifunctional ligand strategy for cross-coupling of chloroarenes. J. Org. Chem. 75: 5340-5342.

[40]   L.S. Hegedus, T.A. Mulhern and A. Mori. 1985. Palladium(0)-catalyzed syntheses of indoloquinones. J. Org. Chem. 50: 4282-4288.

[41] R.C. Larock and M.Y. Kuo. 1991. Palladium-catalyzed synthesis of quinolines from allylic alcohols and *o*-iodoaniline. Tetrahedron Lett. 32: 569-572.

[42] A.S. Guram and S.L. Buchwald. 1994. Palladium-catalyzed aromatic aminations with *in situ* generated aminostannanes. J. Am. Soc. Chem. 116: 7901-7902.

[43] F. Paul, J. Patt and J.F. Hartwig. 1994. Palladium-catalyzed formation of carbon-nitrogen bonds. Reaction intermediates and catalyst improvements in the hetero cross-coupling of aryl halides and tin amides. J. Am. Soc. Chem. 116: 5969-5970.

[44] M. Hatano and K. Mikami. 2003. Highly enantioselective quinoline synthesis *via* ene-type cyclization of 1,7-enynes catalyzed by a cationic BINAP-palladium(II) complex. J. Am. Soc. Chem. 125: 4704-4705.

[45] (a) G. Abbiati, A. Arcadi, V. Canevari, L. Capezzuto and E. Rossi. 2005. Palladium-assisted multi-component synthesis of 2-aryl-4-aminoquinolines and 2-aryl-4-amino(1,8)naphthyridines. J. Org. Chem. 70: 6454-6460.
(b) S. Madapa, Z. Tusi and S. Batra. 2008. Advances in the syntheses of quinoline and quinoline-annulated ring systems. Curr. Org. Chem. 12: 1116-1183.

[46] C.K. Cho and J.K. Kim. 2007. An approach for quinolines *via* palladium-catalyzed Heck coupling followed by cyclization. Tetrahedron Lett. 48: 3775-3778.

[47] B. Gabriele, R. Mancuso, G. Salerno, G. Ruffolo and P. Plastina. 2007. Novel and convenient synthesis of substituted quinolines by copper- or palladium-catalyzed cyclodehydration of 1-(2-aminoaryl)-2-yn-1-ols. J. Org. Chem. 72: 6873-6877.

[48] B. Gabriele, R. Mancuso, G. Salerno, E. Elvira Lupinacci, G. Ruffolo and M. Costa. 2008. Versatile synthesis of quinoline-3-carboxylic esters and indol-2-acetic esters by palladium-catalyzed carbonylation of 1-(2-aminoaryl)-2-yn-1-ols. J. Org. Chem. 73: 4971-4977.

[49] N. Sakai, A. Ridder and J.F. Hartwig. 2006. Tropene derivatives by sequential intermolecular and transannular, intramolecular palladium-catalyzed hydroamination of cycloheptatriene. J. Am. Soc. Chem. 128: 8134-8135.

[50] S. Anguille, J. Brunet, N.C. Chu, O. Diallo, C. Pages and S. Vincendeau. 2006. Platinum-catalyzed formation of quinolines from anilines. Aliphatic α-C-H activation of alkylamines and aromatic *ortho*-C-H activation of anilines. Organometallics 25: 2943-2948.

[51] F.-X. Felpin, J. Coste, C. Zakri and E. Fouquet. 2009. Preparation of 2-quinolones by sequential Heck reduction-cyclization (HRC) reactions by using a multi task palladium catalyst. Chem. Eur. J. 15: 7238-7245.

[52] L. Djakovitch, N. Batail and M. Genelot. 2011. Recent advances in the synthesis of *N*-containing heteroaromatics *via* heterogeneously transition metal catalyzed cross-coupling reactions. Molecules 16: 5241-5267.

[53] I.G. Fomina, Z.V. Dobrokhotova, M.A. Kiskin, G.G. Aleksandrov, O. Proshenkina, A.L. Emelina, V.N. Ikorskii, V.M. Novotortsev and I.L. Eremenko. 2007. Thermal decomposition of dinuclear complexes LM(μ-OOCR)$_4$ML (L is α-substituted pyridine). Russ. Chem. Bull. Int. Ed. 56: 1712-1721.

[54] A. Deagostino, V. Farina, C. Prandi, C. Zavattaro and P. Venturello. 2006. New metal-catalyzed synthesis of quinoline and chromene skeletons. Eur. J. Org. Chem. 15: 3451-3456.

[55] M. Fredelickson, R. Grigg, J. Markandu, M. Thornton-Pett and I. Redpath. 1997. X = Y-ZH systems as potential 1,3-dipoles. Catalytic palladium(II) mediated oxime-nitrone-isoxazolidine cascades. Tetrahedron 53: 15051-15060.

[56] Z. Qian, I.R. Baxendale and S.V. Ley. 2010. A flow process using microreactors for the preparation of a quinolone derivative as a potent 5HT1B antagonist preparation of a potent $5HT_{1B}$. Synlett 4: 505-508.

[57] K. Narasaka. 2002. Metal-assisted amination with oxime derivatives. Pure Appl. Chem. 74: 143-149.

[58] D.M. Garrido, D.F. Corbett, K.A. Dwornik, A.S. Goetz, T.R. Littleton, S.C. McKeown, W.Y. Mills, T.L. Smalley, C.P. Briscoe and A.J. Peat. 2006. Synthesis and activity of small molecule GPR40 agonists. Bioorg. Med. Chem. Lett. 16: 1840-1845.

[59] W. Bonrath and T. Netscher. 2005. Catalytic processes in vitamins synthesis and production. Appl. Catal. A: Gen. 280: 55-73.

[60] O.B. Familoni, P.T. Kaye and P.J. Klas. 1998. Application of Baylis-Hillman methodology in a novel synthesis of quinoline derivatives. Chem. Commun. 23: 2563-2564.

[61] C.L. Kusturin, L.S. Liebeskind and W.L. Neumann. 2002. A new catalytic cross-coupling approach for the synthesis of protected aryl and heteroaryl amidines. Org. Lett. 4: 983-985.

[62] L.S. Liebeskind and J. Srogl. 2002. Heteroaromatic thioether-boronic acid cross-coupling under neutral reaction conditions. Org. Lett. 4: 979-981.

[63] C. Savarin, J. Srogl and L.S. Liebeskind. 2001. Substituted alkyne synthesis under nonbasic conditions: copper carboxylate-mediated, palladium-catalyzed thioalkyne-boronic acid cross-coupling. Org. Lett. 3: 91-93.

[64] L.S. Liebeskind and J. Srogl. 2000. Thiol ester-boronic acid coupling. A mechanistically unprecedented and general ketone synthesis. J. Am. Chem. Soc. 122: 11260-11261.

[65] Y. Bethuel and K. Gademann. 2005. Synthesis and evaluation of the *bis-nor*-anachelin chromophore as potential cyanobacterial ligand. J. Org. Chem. 70: 6258-6264.

[66] A. Sahin, O. Cakmak, I. Demirtas, S. Okten and A. Tutar. 2008. Efficient and selective synthesis of quinoline derivatives. Tetrahedron 64: 10068-10074.

[67] T. Nemoto, T. Fukuda and Y. Hamada. 2006. Efficient synthesis of 3-substituted 2,3-dihydroquinolin-4-ones using a one-pot sequential multi-catalytic process: Pd-catalyzed allylic amination-thiazolium salt-catalyzed Stetter reaction cascade. Tetrahedron Lett. 47: 4365-4368.

[68] M.A. Khalilzadeh, A. Hosseini, M. Shokrollahzadeh, M.R. Halvagar, D. Ahmadi, F. Mohannazadeh and M. Tajbakhsh. 2006. HIO_4/Al_2O_3 as a new system for iodination of activated aromatics and 1,3-dicarbonyl compounds. Tetrahedron Lett. 47: 3525-3528.

[69] N. Charrier, E. Demont, R. Dunsdon, G. Maile, A. Naylor, A. O'Brien, S. Redshaw, P. Theobald, D. Vesey and D. Walter. 2006. Synthesis of indoles: efficient functionalization of the 7-position. Synthesis 38: 3467-3477.

[70] A.G. Schultz, M.A. Holoboski and M.S. Smyth. 1993. The first asymmetric synthesis of a lycorine alkaloid. Total synthesis of (+)-1-deoxylycorine. J. Am. Chem. Soc. 115: 7904-7905.

[71] L.E. Overman, D. Lesuisse and M. Hashimoto. 1983. Synthetic applications of *N*-acylamino-1,3-dienes. Importance of allylic interactions and stereoelectronic effects in dictating the steric course of the reaction of iminium ions with nucleophiles. An efficient total synthesis of (+)-gephyrotoxin. J. Am. Chem. Soc. 105: 5373-5379.

[72] M.M. Rogers, J.E. Wendlandt, I.A. Guzei and S.S. Stahl. 2006. Aerobic intramolecular oxidative amination of alkenes catalyzed by NHC-coordinated palladium complexes. Org. Lett. 8: 2257-2260.

[73] E.M. Beccalli, G. Broggini, M. Martinelli and S. Sottocornola. 2007. C-C, C-O, C-N Bond formation on sp^2 carbon by Pd(II)-catalyzed reactions involving oxidant agents. Chem. Rev. 107: 5318-5365.

[74] B.C. Soderberg, A.C. Chisnell, S.N. O'Neil and J.A. Shriver. 1999. Synthesis of indoles isolated from *Tricholoma* species. J. Org. Chem. 64: 9731-9734.

[75] C. Crotti, S. Cenini, A. Bossoli, B. Rindone and F. Demartin. 1991. Synthesis of carbazole by $Ru_3(CO)_{12}$-catalyzed reductive carbonylation of 2-nitrobiphenyl: the crystal and molecular structure of $Ru_3(\mu_3-NC_6H_4-o-C_6H_5)_2(CO)_9$. J. Mol. Catal. 70: 175-187.

[76] R. Han, S. Chen, S.J. Lee, F. Qi, X. Wu and B.H. Kim. 2006. Indium-mediated reductive cyclization of 2-nitrochalcones to quinolines. Heterocycles 68: 1675-1684.

[77] M. Akazome, T. Kondo and Y. Watanabe. 1992. Novel synthesis of indoles *via* palladium-catalyzed reductive *N*-heterocyclization of *o*-nitrostyrene derivatives. Chem. Lett. 5: 769-772.

[78] T.O. Vieira and H. Alper. 2007. Rhodium(I)-catalyzed hydroaminomethylation of 2-isopropenylanilines as a novel route to 1,2,3,4-tetrahydroquinolines. Chem. Commun. 26: 2710-2711.

[79] J. Horn, S.P. Marsden, A. Nelson, D. House and G.G. Weingarten. 2008. Convergent, regiospecific synthesis of quinolines from *o*-aminophenylboronates. Org. Lett. 10: 4117-4120.

[80] M. Genelot, A. Bendjeriou, V. Dufaud and L. Djakovitch. 2009. Optimized procedures for the one-pot selective syntheses of indoxyls and 4-quinolones by a carbonylative Sonogashira/cyclization sequence. Appl. Catal. A: Gen. 369: 125-132.

[81] C. Jia, D. Piao, J. Oyamada, W. Lu, T. Kitamura and Y. Fujiwara. 2000. Efficient activation of aromatic C-H bonds for addition to C-C multiple bonds. Science 287: 1992-1995.

[82] D. Yang, S. Burugupalli, D. Daniel and Y. Chen. 2012. Microwave-assisted one-pot synthesis of isoquinolines, furopyridines, and thienopyridines by palladium-catalyzed sequential coupling-imination-annulation of 2-bromoarylaldehydes with terminal acetylenes and ammonium acetate. J. Org. Chem. 77: 4466-4472.

[83] M. Bandini, F. Piccinelli, S. Tommasi, A. Umani-Ronchi and C. Ventrici. 2007. Highly enantioselective nitroaldol reaction catalyzed by new chiral copper complexes. Chem. Commun. 6: 616-618.

[84] R. Ballini and M. Petrini. 2009. Nitroalkanes as key building blocks for the synthesis of heterocyclic derivatives. ARKIVOC (ix): 195-223.

[85] D. Mujahidin and S. Doye. 2005. Enantioselective synthesis of (+)-(S)-laudanosine and (-)-(S)-xylopinine. Eur. J. Org. Chem. 13: 2689-2693.

[86] N. Uematsu, A. Fujii, S. Hashiguchi, Ikariya and R. Noyori. 1996. Asymmetric transfer hydrogenation of imines. J. Am. Chem. Soc. 118: 4916-4917.

[87] T.E. Muller, K.C. Hultzsch, M. Yus, F. Foubelo and M. Tada. 2008. Hydroamination: direct addition of amines to alkenes and alkynes. Chem. Rev. 108: 3795-3892.

[88] H. Zhou, H. Jin, S. Ye, X. He and J. Wu. 2009. Multicatalytic synthesis of 1,2-dihydroisoquinolin-1-ylphosphonates *via* a tandem four-component reaction. Tetrahedron Lett. 50: 4616-4618.

[89] D. Bouyssi, N. Monteiro and G. Balme. 2011. Amines as key building blocks in Pd-assisted multicomponent processes. Beilstein J. Org. Chem. 7: 1387-1406.

[90] J. Laudien, E. Fouquet, C. Zakri and F.-X. Felpin. 2010. A multi-task palladium catalyst involved in Heck-reduction-cyclization (HRC) sequences for the preparation of 4-benzyl-1,2-dihydroisoquinolin-3-ones: an unusual homogeneous-heterogeneous sustainable approach. Synlett 10: 1539-1543.

[91] A. Yokooji, T. Satoh, M. Miura and M. Nomura. 2004. Synthesis of 5,5'-diarylated 2,2'-bithiophenes *via* palladium-catalyzed arylation reactions. Tetrahedron 60: 6757-6763.

[92] L.-C. Campeau, M. Parisien, A. Jean and K. Fagnou. 2006. Catalytic direct arylation with aryl chlorides, bromides, and iodides: intramolecular studies leading to new intermolecular reactions. J. Am. Chem. Soc. 128: 581-590.

[93] S. Roy, S. Roy, B. Neuenswander, D. Hill and R.C. Larock. 2009. Palladium- and copper-catalyzed solution phase synthesis of a diverse library of isoquinolines. J. Comb. Chem. 11: 1061-1065.

[94] G. Abbiati, E. Beccalli, A. Marchesini and E. Rossi. 2001. Synthesis of β-carbolines from 2-acyl-1-benzenesulfonyl-3-iodo-1H-indoles. Synthesis 16: 2477-2483.

[95] (a) N. Kuwabara, H. Hayashi, N. Hiramatsu, T. Choshi, E. Sugino and S. Hibino. 1999. New regioselective total syntheses of anti-biotic renierol, renierol acetate, and renierol propionate from the 5-oxygenated isoquinoline. Chem. Pharm. Bull. 47: 1805-1807.

(b) N. Kuwabara, H. Hayashi, N. Hiramatsu, T. Choshi, T. Kumemura, J. Nobuhiro and S. Hibino 2004. Syntheses of the anti-biotic alkaloids renierone, mimocin, renierol, renierol acetate, renierol propionate, and 7-methoxy-1,6-dimethylisoquinoline-5,8-dione. Tetrahedron 60: 2943-2952.

[96] D.A. Goff and R.N. Zuckermann. 1995. Solid-phase synthesis of highly substituted peptoid 1(2H)-isoquinolinones. J. Org. Chem. 60: 5748-5749.

[97] H. Tsutsui and K. Narasaka. 2001. Synthesis of pyridine and isoquinoline derivatives by the palladium-catalyzed cyclization of olefinic ketone O-pentafluorobenzoyloximes. Chem. Lett. 30: 526-527.

[98] H. Zhang and R.C. Larock. 2001. Synthesis of β- and γ-carbolines by the palladium-catalyzed iminoannulation of internal alkynes. Org. Lett. 3: 3083-3086.

[99] H. Zhang and R.C. Larock. 2002. Synthesis of β- and γ-carbolines by the palladium-catalyzed iminoannulation of alkynes. J. Org. Chem. 67: 9318-9330.

[100] H. Zhang and R.C. Larock. 2003. Synthesis of annulated γ-carbolines and heteropolycycles by the palladium-catalyzed intramolecular annulation of alkynes. J. Org. Chem. 68: 5132-5138.

[101] R.V. Rozhkov and R.C. Larock. 2003. Synthesis of dihydrofurocoumarins *via* palladium-catalyzed annulation of 1,3-dienes by o-iodoacetoxycoumarins. Org. Lett. 5: 797-800.

[102] R.V. Rozhkov and R.C. Larock. 2003. An efficient approach to dihydrofurocoumarins *via* palladium-catalyzed annulation of 1,3-dienes by o-iodoacetoxycoumarins. J. Org. Chem. 68: 6314-6320.

[103] K.R. Roesch and R.C. Larock. 1999. Synthesis of isoquinolines and pyridines by the palladium- and copper-catalyzed coupling and cyclization of terminal acetylenes. Org. Lett. 1: 553-556.

[104] T. Sakamoto, A. Numata and Y. Kondo. 2000. The cyclization reaction of *o*-ethynylbenzalddehyde derivatives into isoquinoline derivatives. Chem. Pharm. Bull. 48: 669-672.

[105] A. Numata, Y. Kondo and T. Sakamoto. 1999. General synthetic method for naphthyridines and their *N*-oxides containing isoquinolinic nitrogen. Synthesis 2: 306-311.

[106] F. Maassarani, M. Pfeffer and G.L. Borgne. 1987. Reaction of cyclopalladated compounds. Controlled synthesis of heterocyclic compounds through ring enlargement by alkyne insertions into the palladium-carbon bonds of cyclopalladated amines followed by ring closure. Organometallics 6: 2029-2043.

[107] K.R. Roesch and R.C. Larock. 1998. Synthesis of isoquinolines and pyridines *via* palladium-catalyzed iminoannulation of internal acetylenes. J. Org. Chem. 63: 5306-5307.

[108] K.R. Roesch, H. Zhang and R.C. Larock. 2001. Synthesis of isoquinolines and pyridines by the palladium-catalyzed iminoannulation of internal alkynes. J. Org. Chem. 66: 8042-8051.

[109] T. Konno, J. Chae, T. Miyabe and T. Ishihara. 2005. Regioselective one-step synthesis of 4-fluoroalkylated isoquinolines *via* carbopalladation reaction of fluorine-containing alkynes. J. Org. Chem. 70: 10172-10174.

[110] H. Zhang and R.C. Larock. 2002. Synthesis of annulated γ-carbolines by palladium-catalyzed intramolecular iminoannulation. Org. Lett. 4: 3035-3038.

[111] H. Zhang and R.C. Larock. 2002. Synthesis of β- and γ-carbolines by the palladium/copper-catalyzed coupling and copper-catalyzed or thermal cyclization of terminal acetylenes. Tetrahedron Lett. 43: 1359-1362.

[112] H. Zhang and R.C. Larock. 2002. Synthesis of β- and γ-carbolines by the palladium/copper-catalyzed coupling and cyclization of terminal acetylenes. J. Org. Chem. 67: 7048-7056.

[113] G. Kirsch, S. Hesse and A. Comel. 2004. Synthesis of five- and six-membered heterocycles through palladium-catalyzed reactions. Curr. Org. Synth. 1: 47-63.

[114] E.D. Cox and J.M. Cook. 1995. The Pictet-Spengler condensation: a new direction for an old reaction. Chem. Rev. 95: 1797-1842.

[115] S.W. Youn. 2006. The Pictet-Spengler reaction: efficient carbon-carbon bond forming reaction in heterocyclic synthesis. Org. Prep. Proced. Int. 38: 505-591.

[116] A.B.J. Bracca and T.S. Kaufman. 2004. Synthetic approaches to carnegine, a simple tetrahydroisoquinoline alkaloid. Tetrahedron 60: 10575-10610.

[117] W.J. Huang, O.V. Singh, C.H. Chen and S.S. Lee. 2004. Synthesis of (+)-neospirodienone *via* an one-pot Bischler-Napieralski reaction and oxidative coupling by a hypervalent iodine reagent. Helv. Chim. Acta 87: 167-174.

[118] M. Krishna, D. Nirupam and C. Santanu. 2011. Palladium-mediated bis-arylation of inactivated and activated arenes. Synth. Commun. 41: 121-130.

[119] A.S. Capilla, M. Romero, M.D. Pujol, D.H. Caignard and P. Renard. 2001. Synthesis of isoquinolines and tetrahydroisoquinolines as potential anti-tumour agents. Tetrahedron 57: 8297-8303.

[120] D.S. Kashdan, J.A. Schwartz and H. Rapoport. 1982. Synthesis of 1,2,3,4-tetrahydroisoquinolines. J. Org. Chem. 47: 2638-2643.

[121] M. Nicoletti, D. O'Hagan and A.M.Z. Slawin. 2002. The asymmetric Bischler-Napieralski reaction: preparation of 1,3,4-trisubstituted 1,2,3,4-tetrahydroisoquinolines. J. Chem. Soc. Perkin Trans. 1. 1: 116-121.

[122] J. Selvakumar, A. Makriyannis and C.R. Ramanathan. 2010. An unusual reactivity of BBr$_3$: accessing tetrahydroisoquinoline units from *N*-phenethylimides. Org. Biomol. Chem. 8: 4056-4058.

[123] D. Enders, J.X. Liebich and G. Raabe. 2010. Organocatalytic asymmetric synthesis of *trans*-1,3-disubstituted tetrahydroisoquinolines *via* a reductive amination/aza-Michael sequence. Chem. Eur. J. 16: 9763-9766.

[124] M. Amat, V. Elias, N. Llor, F. Subrizi, E. Molins and J. Bosch. 2010. A general methodology for the enantioselective synthesis of 1-substituted tetrahydroisoquinoline alkaloids. Eur. J. Org. Chem. 21: 4017-4026.

[125] I. Schuster, L. Lazar and F. Fulop. 2010. Convenient synthesis of 1,2,3,4-tetrahydroisoquinoline-1-carboxylic acid derivatives *via* isocyanide-based, three-component reactions. Synth. Commun. 40: 2488-2498.

[126] L.F. Tietze, Y.F. Zhou and E. Topken. 2000. Synthesis of simple enantiopure tetrahydro-β-carbolines and tetrahydroisoquinolines. Eur. J. Org. Chem. 12: 2247-2252.

[127] L.F. Tietze, N. Rackelmann and I. Muller. 2004. Enantioselective total syntheses of the *Ipecacuanha* alkaloid emetine, the *Alangium* alkaloid tubulosine and a novel benzoquinolizidine alkaloid by using a domino process. Chem. Eur. J. 10: 2722-2731.

[128] (a) D.L. Priebbenow, S.G. Stewart and F.M. Pfeffer. 2011. A general approach to *N*-heterocyclic scaffolds using domino Heck-aza-Michael reactions. Org. Biomol. Chem. 9: 1508-1515.
(b) D.L. Priebbenow, F.M. Pfeffer and S.G. Stewart. 2011. A one-pot, three-component approach to functionalized tetrahydroisoquinolines using domino Heck-aza-Michael reactions. Eur. J. Org. Chem. 9: 1632-1635.

[129] E.M. Beccalli, E. Borsini, S. Brenna, S. Galli, M. Rigamonti and G. Broggini. 2010. σ-Alkylpalladium intermediates in intramolecular Heck reactions: isolation and catalytic activity. Chem. Eur. J. 16: 1670-1678.

[130] H. Lin and U. Kazmaier. 2009. Molybdenum-catalyzed α-hydrostannations of propargylamines as the key step in the synthesis of *N*-heterocycles. Eur. J. Org. Chem. 8: 1221-1227.

[131] C. Shi and I. Ojima. 2007. Asymmetric synthesis of 1-vinyltetrahydroisoquinoline through Pd-catalyzed intramolecular allylic amination. Tetrahedron 63: 8563-8570.

[132] Y. Nagao, A. Ueki, K. Asano, S. Tanaka, S. Sano and M. Shiro. 2002. Facile palladium(0)-catalyzed ring expansion reactions of hydroxy methoxyallenyl cyclic compounds *via* hydropalladation. Org. Lett. 4: 455-457.

[133] Q. Huang and R.C. Larock. 2002. Synthesis of isoquinolines by palladium-catalyzed cyclization, followed by a Heck reaction. Tetrahedron Lett. 43: 3557-3560.

[134] Q. Huang and R.C. Larock. 2003. Synthesis of 4-(1-alkenyl)isoquinolines by palladium(II)-catalyzed cyclization/olefination. J. Org. Chem. 68: 980-988.

[135] G. Dai and R.C. Larock. 2003. Synthesis of 3,4-disubstituted isoquinolines *via* palladium-catalyzed cross-coupling of 2-(1-alkynyl)benzaldimines and organic halides. J. Org. Chem. 68: 920-928.

[136] G. Dai and R.C. Larock. 2002. Synthesis of 3-substituted 4-aroylisoquinolines *via* Pd-catalyzed carbonylative cyclization of 2-(1-alkynyl)benzaldimines. J. Org. Chem. 67: 7042-7047.

[137] G. Dai and R.C. Larock. 2001. Synthesis of 3,4-disubstituted isoquinolines *via* palladium-catalyzed cross-coupling of *o*-(1-alkynyl)benzaldimines and organic halides. Org. Lett. 3: 4035-4038.

[138] G. Dai and R.C. Larock. 2002. Synthesis of 3-substituted 4-aroylisoquinolines *via* Pd-catalyzed carbonylative cyclization of *o*-(1-alkynyl)benzaldimines. Org. Lett. 4: 193-196.

[139] D. Sole, E. Peidro and J. Bonjoch. 2000. Palladium-catalyzed intramolecular coupling of vinyl halides and ketone enolates. Synthesis of bridged azabicyclic compounds. Org. Lett. 2: 2225-2228.

[140] D. Sole, L. Vallverdu, E. Peidro and J. Bonjoch. 2001. Palladium-catalyzed intramolecular annulation of 2-haloanilines and ketones: enolate arylation vs. nucleophilic addition to the carbonyl group. Chem. Commun. 18: 1888-1889.

[141] D. Sole, L. Vallverdu and J. Bonjoch. 2001. Palladium-catalyzed intramolecular coupling of aryl halides and ketone enolates: synthesis of hexahydro-2,6-methano-1-benzazocines. Adv. Synth. Catal. 343: 439-442.

[142] D. Sole, L. Vallverdu, X. Solans, M. Font-Bardia and J. Bonjoch. 2003. Intramolecular Pd-mediated processes of amino-tethered aryl halides and ketones: insight into the ketone α-arylation and carbonyl-addition dichotomy. A new class of four-membered azapalladacycles. J. Am. Chem. Soc. 125: 1587-1594.

[143] D. Sole, F. Diaba and J. Bonjoch. 2003. Nitrogen heterocycles by palladium-catalyzed cyclization of amino-tethered vinyl halides and ketone enolates. J. Org. Chem. 68: 5746-5749.

[144] O. Gaertzen and S.L. Buchwald. 2002. Palladium-catalyzed intramolecular α-arylation of α-amino acid esters. J. Org. Chem. 67: 465-475.

[145] K.H. Shaughnessy, B.C. Hamann and J.F. Hartwig. 1998. Palladium-catalyzed inter- and intramolecular α-arylation of amides. Application of intramolecular amide arylation to the synthesis of oxindoles. J. Org. Chem. 63: 6546-6553.

[146] S. Lee and J.F. Hartwig. 2001. Improved catalysts for the palladium-catalyzed synthesis of oxindoles by amide α-arylation. Rate acceleration, use of aryl chloride substrates, and a new carbene ligand for asymmetric transformations. J. Org. Chem. 66: 3402-3415.

[147] T. Honda, H. Namiki and F. Satoh. 2001. Palladium-catalyzed intramolecular δ-lactam formation of aryl halides and amide-enolates: syntheses of cherylline and latifine. Org. Lett. 3: 631-633.

[148] (a) R. Grigg, V. Sridharan and L-.H. Xu. 1995. Palladium-catalyzed cyclization-amination of allenes -effect of base on regioselectivity of formation of allylic amines. J. Chem. Soc. Chem. Commun. 18: 1903-1904.
(b) T. Lu, Z. Lu, Z.-X. Ma, Y. Zhang and R.P. Hsung. 2013. Allenamides: a powerful and versatile building block in organic synthesis. Chem. Rev. 113: 4862-4904.

[149] M. Gardiner, R. Grigg, V. Sridharan and N. Vicker. 1998. Cascade and sequential palladium catalyzed cyclization-azide capture-1,3-dipolar cycloaddition route to complex triazoles. Tetrahedron Lett. 39: 435-438.

[150] M. Gardiner, R. Grigg, M. Kordes, V. Sridharan and N. Vicker. 2001. One-pot sequential and cascade formation of triazoles *via* palladium catalyzed azide capture-1,3-dipolar cycloaddition. Tetrahedron 57: 7729-7735.

[151] R. Grigg, J.M. Sansano, V. Santhakumar, V. Sridharan, R. Thangavelanthum, M. Thornton-Pett and D. Wilson. 1997. Palladium catalyzed tandem cyclization-anion capture processes. Organoboron anion transfer agents. Tetrahedron 53: 11803-11826.

[152] K. Parthasarathy, M. Jeganmohan and C.-H. Cheng. 2006. Palladium-catalyzed multistep reactions involving ring closure of 2-iodophenoxyallenes and ring opening of bicyclic alkenes. Org. Lett. 8: 621-623.

[153] Z. Lu, C. Hu, J. Guo, J. Li, Y. Cui and Y. Jia. 2010. Water-controlled regioselectivity of Pd-catalyzed domino reaction involving a C-H activation process: rapid synthesis of diverse carbo- and heterocyclic skeletons. Org. Lett. 12: 480-483.

[154] M. Ashiq, M. Danish, M.A. Mohsin, S. Bari and F. Mukhtar. 2013. Chemistry of platinum and palladium metal complexes in homogeneous and heterogeneous catalysis: a mini review. Int. J. Sci: Basic Appl. Res. 7: 50-61.

[155] J.J. Li, T.S. Mei and J.Q. Yu. 2008. Synthesis of indolines and tetrahydroisoquinolines from arylethylamines by Pd-II-catalyzed C-H activation reactions. Angew. Chem. Int. Ed. 47: 6452-6455.

[156] L.F. Tietze, S.G. Stewart and M.E. Polomska. 2005. Intramolecular Heck reactions for the synthesis of the novel anti-biotic mesacarcin: investigation of catalytic, electronic and conjugative effects in the preparation of the hexahydroanthracene core. Eur. J. Org. Chem. 9: 1752-1759.

[157] P. Liu, L. Huang, Y. Lu, M. Dilmeghani, J. Baum, T. Xiang, J. Adams, A. Tasker, R. Larsen and M.M. Faul. 2007. Synthesis of heterocycles *via* ligand-free palladium catalyzed reductive Heck cyclization. Tetrahedron Lett. 48: 2307-2310.

[158] D.P. Walsh and Y.-T. Chang. 2006. Chemical genetics. Chem. Rev. 106: 2476-2530.

[159] P. Arya, D.T.H. Chou and M.-G. Baek. 2001. Diversity-based organic synthesis in the era of genomics and proteomics. Angew. Chem. Int. Ed. 40: 339-346.

[160] S.L. Schreiber. 2000. Target-oriented and diversity-oriented organic synthesis in drug discovery. Science 287: 1964-1969.

[161] S. Li, Y. Luo and J. Wu. 2011. Three-component reaction of N'-(2-alkynylbenzylidene)hydrazide, alkyne, with sulfonyl azide *via* a multicatalytic process: a novel and concise approach to 2-amino-H-pyrazolo[5,1-a]isoquinolines. Org. Lett. 13: 4312-4315.

[162] V. De Matteis, O. Dufay, D.C.J. Waalboer, F.L. van Delft, J. Tiebes and F.P.J.T. Rutjes. 2007. An improved ring-closing metathesis approach to fluorinated and trifluoromethylated nitrogen heterocycles. Eur. J. Org. Chem. 16: 2667-2675.

[163] S. Nandi and J.K. Ray. 2009. Palladium-catalyzed cyclization/cyclopropanation reaction for the synthesis of fused N-containing heterocycles. Tetrahedron Lett. 50: 6993-6997.

[164] J.-J. Li, T.-S. Mei and J.-Q. Yu. 2008. Synthesis of indolines and tetrahydroisoquinolines from arylethylamines by PdII-catalyzed C-H activation reactions. Angew. Chem. 120: 6552-6555.

[165] K.C. Majumdar, S. Chakravorty and K. Ray. 2008. Palladium-mediated direct synthesis of *N*-substituted 4-methyl- and 4-ethylisoquinolone derivatives. Synthesis 18: 2991-2995.

[166] M. Chrzanowska and M. Rozwadowska. 2004. Asymmetric synthesis of isoquinoline alkaloids. Chem. Rev. 104: 3341-3370.

[167] G. EspuLa, G. Arsequell, G. Valencia, J. Barluenga, J.M. Alvarez-Gutierrez, A. Ballesteros and J.M. Gonzalez. 2004. Regioselective postsynthetic modification of phenylalanine side chains of peptides leading to uncommon *o*-iodinated analogues. Angew. Chem. Int. Ed. 43: 325-329.

[168] A. Shirai, O. Miyata, N. Tohnai, M. Miyata, D.J. Procter, D. Sucunza and T. Naito. 2008. Total synthesis of (-)-martinellic acid *via* radical addition-cyclization-elimination reaction. J. Org. Chem. 73: 4464-4475.

[169] I. Bonnaventure and A.B. Charette. 2009. Stereoselective synthesis of *N*-heterocycles: application of the asymmetric Cu-catalyzed addition of Et_2Zn to functionalized alkyl and aryl imines. Tetrahedron 65: 4968-4976.

[170] R. Ferraccioli, D. Carenzi and M. Catellani. 2004. Synthesis of 1,2,3,4-tetrahydroisoquinolines and 2,3,4,5-tetrahydro-1*H*-2-benzazepines combining sequential palladium-catalyzed *ortho* alkylation/ vinylation with aza-Michael addition reactions. Tetrahedron Lett. 45: 6903-6907.

[171] G.A. Ardizzoia, E.M. Beccalli, E. Borsini, S. Brenna, G. Broggini and M. Rigamonti. 2008. Palladium-catalyzed cyclization/carbonylation as a direct route to 4-[(methoxycarbonyl)methyl]-3,4-dihydroisoquinolinones. Eur. J. Org. Chem. 33: 5590-5596.

[172] A. Dhami, M.F. Mahon, M.D. Lloyd and M.D. Threadgill. 2009. 4-Substituted 5-nitroisoquinolin-1-ones from intramolecular Pd-catalyzed reaction of *N*-(2-alkenyl)-2-halo-3-nitrobenzamides. Tetrahedron 65: 4751-4765.

[173] X. Gai, R. Grigg, S. Rajviroongit, S. Songarsa and V. Sridharan. 2005. Synthesis of triazolo- and tetrazolo-tetrahydroisoquinolines and isoquinolines *via* temperature controlled palladium catalyzed allene/azide incorporation/intramolecular 1,3-dipolar cycloaddition cascades. Tetrahedron Lett. 46: 5899-5902.

[174] D.M. D'Souza and T.J.J. Muller. 2007. Multi-component syntheses of heterocycles by transition-metal catalysis. Chem. Soc. Rev. 36: 1095-1108.

[175] B. Haffemayer, M. Gulias and M. Gaunt. 2011. Amine directed Pd(II)-catalyzed C-H bond functionalization under ambient conditions. J. Chem. Sci. 2: 312-315.

[176] E.M. Beccalli, G. Broggini, M. Martinelli, N. Masciocchi and S. Sottocornola. 2006. New 4-spiroannulated tetrahydroisoquinolines by a one-pot sequential procedure. Isolation and characterization of σ-alkylpalladium Heck intermediates. Org. Lett. 8: 4521-4524.

[177] T. Izumi, Y. Nishimoto, K. Kohei and A. Kasahara. 1990. Palladium-catalyzed synthesis of isocoumarin and 1-isoquinolinone derivatives. J. Heterocycl. Chem. 27: 1419-1424.

[178] C.H. Heathcock, J.A. Stafford and D.L. Clark. 1992. *Daphniphyllum* alkaloids. Total synthesis of (+)-bukittinggine. J. Org. Chem. 57: 2575-2585.

[179] S. Husinec, M. Petkovic, V. Savic and M. Simic. 2012. Synthesis of allyl acetates *via* palladium-catalyzed functionalization of allenes and 1,3-dienes. Synthesis 44: 399-408.

CHAPTER 9

Six-Membered Fused N-Heterocycles

9.1 Introduction

N-Heterocycles are a special group of organic compounds found in various pharmacologically active synthetic and natural products. The nature has provided us countless chemical substances which are biologically and structurally relevant. Among these heterocyclic compounds tetrahydroquinolines exhibit significant biological activity with different therapeutic targets. They show many uses in diverse fields like agro-chemistry, pharmaceuticals, and industry. They are also found in natural sources displaying plant growth regulation, insecticidal, anti-bacterial and pigment functions [1-6].

Fused six-membered nitrogen-containing heterocycles like benzimidazoisoquinolines and benzimidazoquinazolines are potent anti-tumor agents. Benzimidazo[2,1-*b*]benzo[*f*]isoquinoline ring system is present in pharmacologically active compounds and benzimidazo[2,1-*b*] quinazolines are potent immuno-suppressors [7-9]. Due to the importance of this motif in the field of medicinal chemistry and alkaloid synthesis, the control of enantioselective synthesis of substituted six-membered nitrogen heterocycles has been the subject of much attention [10]. The importance of these compounds lies in their uses in drug industries and it has been established that they are biologically active in many aspects [11-15]. These results have encouraged many researchers to pay attention on the modification of these compounds for the treatment of different diseases [16a-g].

9.2 Palladium assisted synthesis of six-membered *N*-heterocycles fused with other heterocycles

9.3 Synthesis of six-membered heterocycles fused with aromatics

The biologically active azabicyclic tropene ring system was obtained by double addition of aniline to a cyclic triene **(Scheme 1)** [17-18].

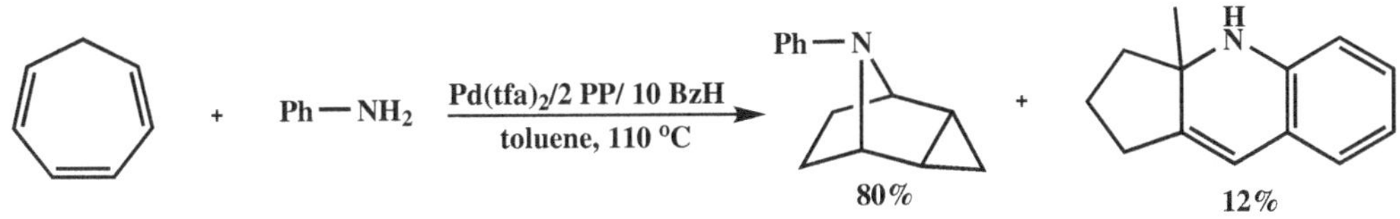

Scheme-1

Some of products formed in this reaction may be applied to a green emitter for electro-luminescence (EL) devices and displayed an intense luminescence in solid-state. Shi [19-20] synthesized tetrahydroquinoline derivatives with highly substituted cyclopentadienyl cores *via* Pd-catalyzed ring-expansion of indoles with alkynes through dual carbon-hydrogen bond activations in the presence of oxygen as oxidant. The NO_2 or nitrile groups were incorporated in benzene ring of indole units and halogen-bearing motifs work well in this reaction. This conversion involved one carbon-carbon bond cleavage, dual carbon-hydrogen bond activations, five new carbon-carbon bond formations, and ring-expansion of indole through rearrangement under mild reaction conditions (**Scheme 2**).

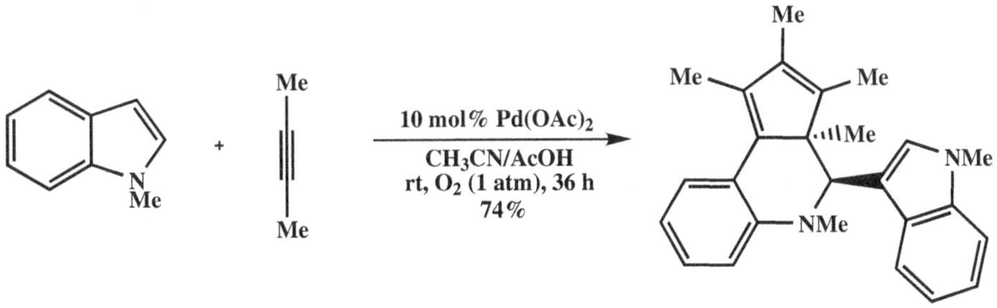

Scheme-2

Beydoun and Pfeffer [21] explained Pd-catalyzed annulation of internal alkynes with 1-iodo-8-(dimethyl)-naphthalene for the preparation of *N*-methylbenzo[*d,e*]quinolines (**Scheme 3**).

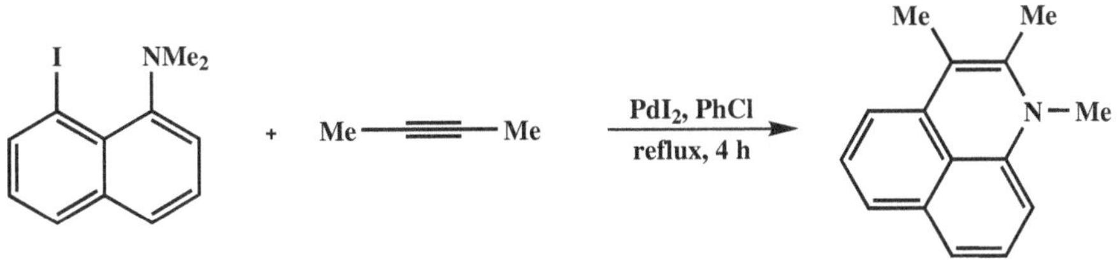

Scheme-3

Varying linkages containing substrates between two aryl groups (NRCO, CH_2O, SO_2NR) were synthesized. Other cyclic compounds were prepared by subjecting substrates to Pd-catalyzed direct arylation conditions (**Scheme 4-5**) [22]. However, the desired fused six-membered ring products were obtained in low yields.

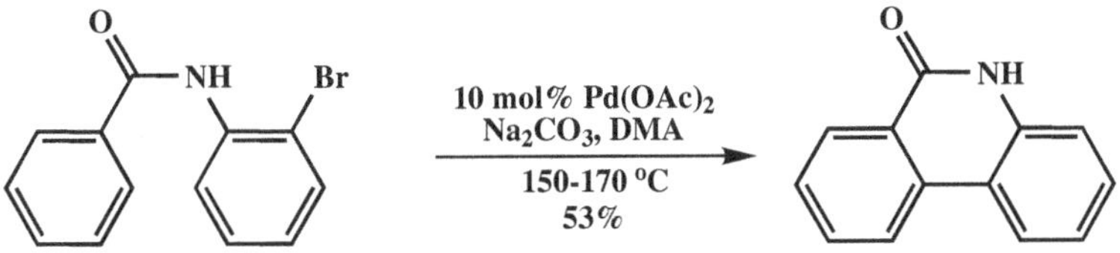

Scheme-4

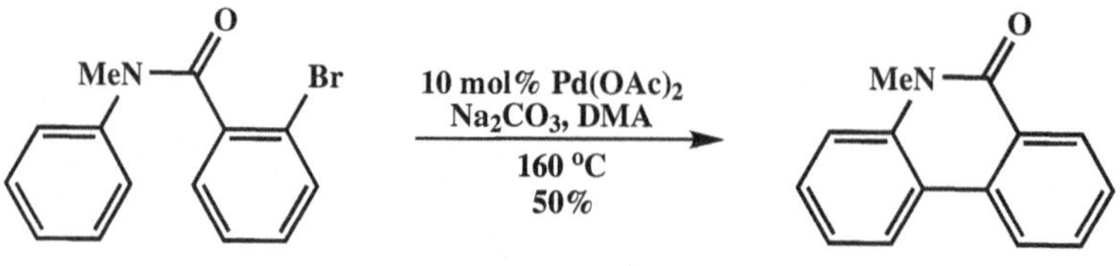

Scheme-5

Rawal [23] reported the use of Herrmann's catalyst and cesium carbonate for intramolecular arylation of phenolates in dimethylaniline **(Scheme 6)**. Good to excellent yields of a number of biaryl compounds bearing many linkages between two aryl groups were reported under these conditions.

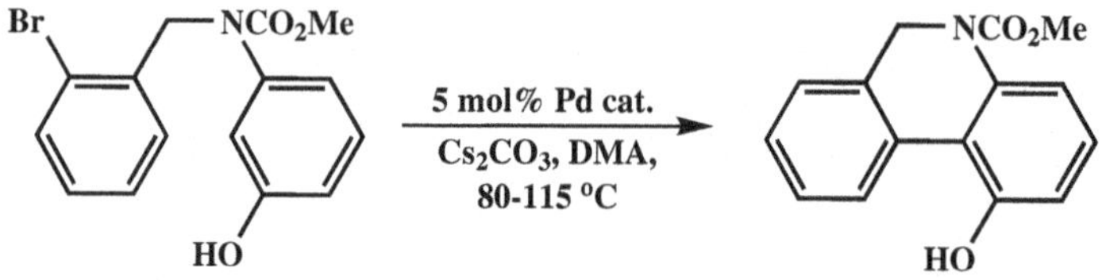

Scheme-6

Excellent yields of both electron-withdrawing and electron-donating substituents containing six-membered ring biaryl compounds were obtained **(Scheme 7)**. Nitrogen and alkyl bearing tethers were tolerated, but to ensure complete transformation higher catalyst loadings were needed [24].

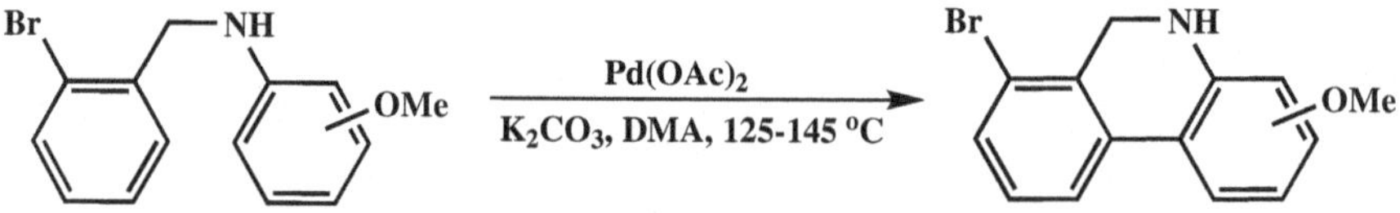

Scheme-7

Fagnou [25] reported intramolecular direct aryation of aryl bromides, chlorides, and iodides with this general and efficient catalyst system to synthesize a number of five- and six-membered carbo- and heterocyclic biaryl products **(Scheme 8)**.

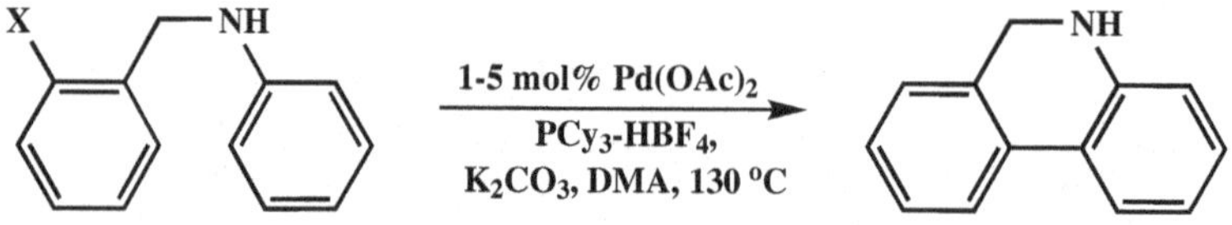

Scheme-8

Fagnou [25] reported Pd-catalyzed direct arylation reactions. The experiments described in **Schemes 9-10** were performed to see whether the catalyst would react preferentially with a more electron-rich or electron-poor arene. A small selectivity was reported in both cases, with preference for the more electron-rich arene, although this argument assumed that the reaction proceeded under Curtin-Hammett conditions.

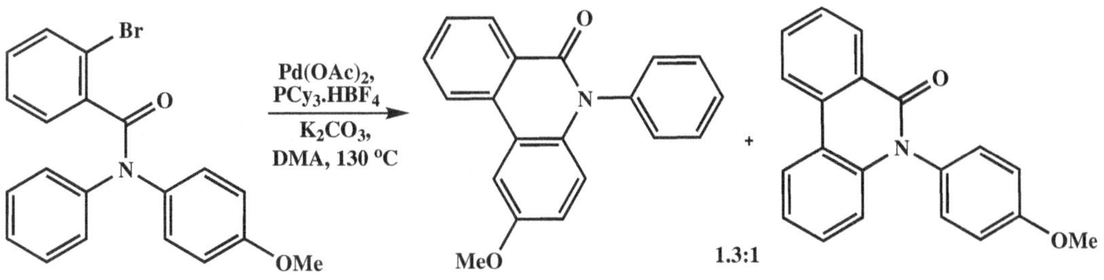

Scheme-9

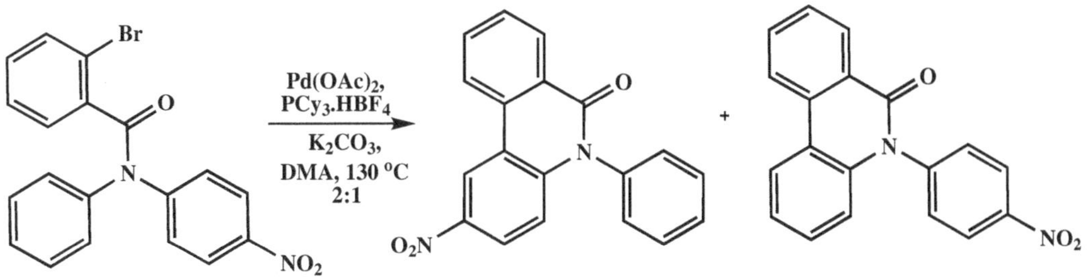

Scheme-10

This methodology, however, was limited to aryl bromides, with aryl chlorides no reaction occurred. However, upon implementation of an electron-rich *N*-heterocyclic carbene ligand, excellent yields of a number of functionalized five- and six-membered rings were obtained with varying tethers such as amine, ether, alkyl and amide moieties **(Scheme 11)** [26].

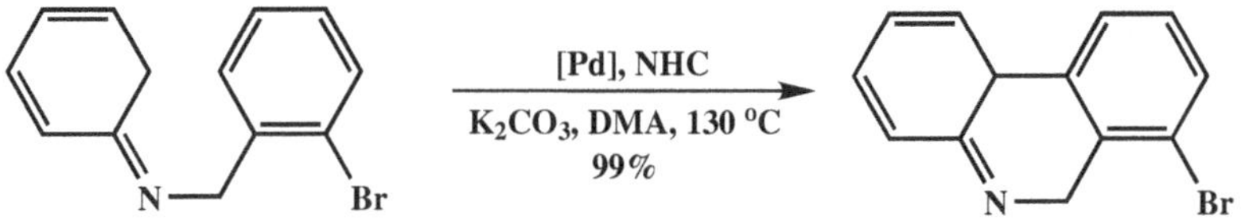

Scheme-11

The phenanthridine derivatives were produced by coupling reaction of *N*-sulfonyl-2-aminodiphenyls with electron-deficient alkenes under air in the presence of palladium acetate and copper acetate **(Scheme 12)** [27-28].

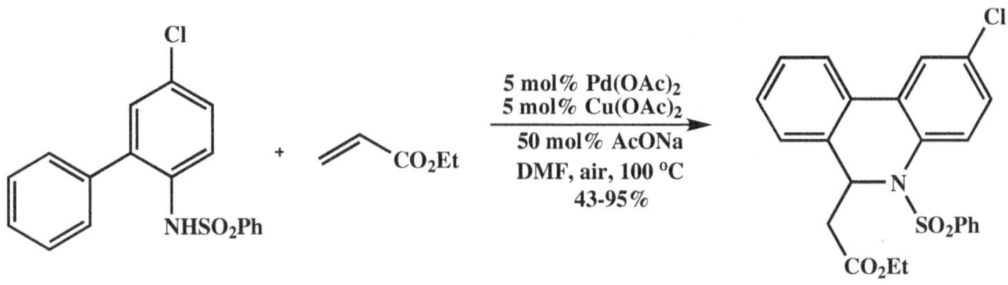

Scheme-12

A number of amine-, ether-, alkyl-, amide-, and alkenyl-based tethers were tolerated in this reaction. Many electron-donating and electron-withdrawing substituents were also compatible on both aryl moieties and produced the desired products in high regioselectivity and excellent yields. Furthermore, direct arylation of more sterically demanding substrates also occurred with this catalyst system **(Scheme 13)** [29].

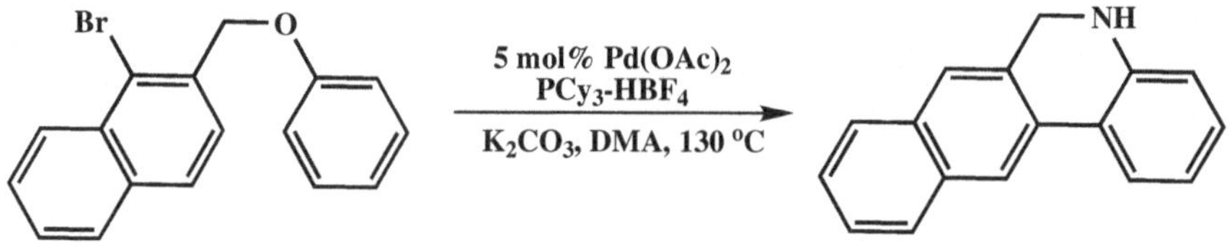

5 mol% Pd(OAc)$_2$
PCy$_3$-HBF$_4$

K$_2$CO$_3$, DMA, 130 °C

Scheme-13

Structural complexity was obtained by Ugi four-component transformation (Ugi-4CR) [30]. The Ugi four-component reaction adducts were converted into many cyclic scaffolds through post-Ugi reactions which provided a variety of medicinally important heterocyclic compounds. Among these heterocycles, benzofuran is present in many biologically active natural products. The benzofurans were prepared *via* Rap-Stoermer reaction of linear dipeptide-like Ugi-4CR adducts under MWI [31]. The benzofurans were formed in 43-90% yields when produced intermediate was reacted with salicylaldehydes in the presence of cesium carbonate in acetonitrile under controlled MW heating for 15-30 min at 80-140 °C. With benzofurans in hand, two different heterocyclic compounds such as 2-oxindoles and 5,6-dihydrophenanthridines were produced readily by intramolecular direct arylation and intramolecular *N*-arylation processes in the presence of Pd catalyst **(Scheme 14)** [32-35].

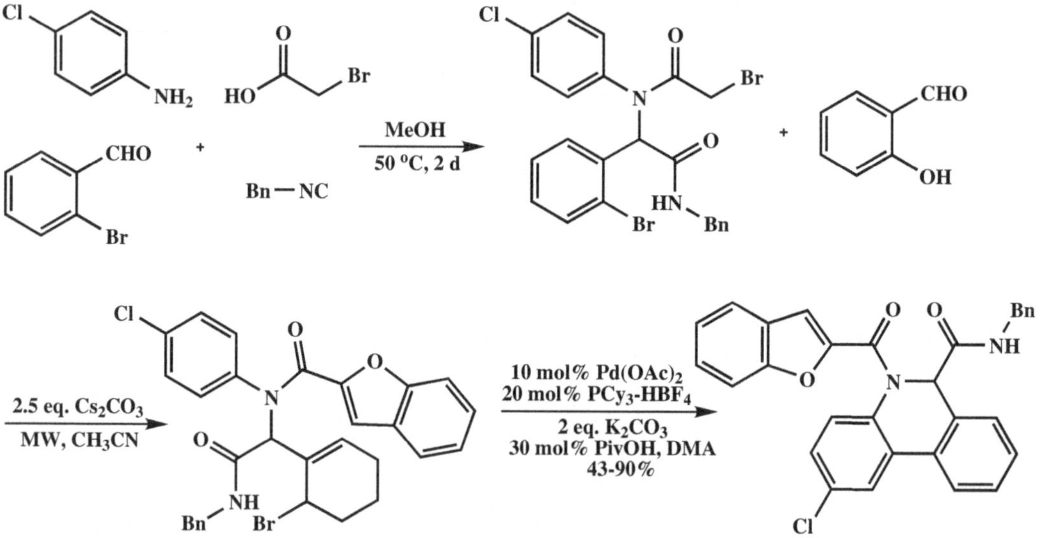

MeOH
50 °C, 2 d

2.5 eq. Cs$_2$CO$_3$
MW, CH$_3$CN

10 mol% Pd(OAc)$_2$
20 mol% PCy$_3$-HBF$_4$
2 eq. K$_2$CO$_3$
30 mol% PivOH, DMA
43-90%

Scheme-14

The coupling of electron rich aryl bromides with a boronic acid, which was prone to proto-deboronation, was difficult to conduct under conventional heating conditions [36]. Therefore this cross-coupling was carried out under MWI. According to optimized method [37-41], styrene and boronic acid were treated with [Pd(PPh$_3$)$_4$] as catalyst and sodium bicarbonate as base in a 1:1 mixture of H$_2$O and dimethylformamide at 150 °C and irradiation power of 150 W. This reaction afforded biaryl compound in an excellent yield of 84% in 15 min with a negligible degree of proto-deboronation, and homo-coupling products were not reported. The trimethoxy analogue was formed in 82% yield starting from styrene and boronic acid following the same method. However, reduction of NO$_2$ group of trimethoxy and biaryl intermediates was problematic, [42] using either granular tin or SnCl$_2$, failed, even after long heating **(Scheme 15)**. Invariably, the trimethoxy and biaryl were recovered. When NO$_2$ group was reduced with iron in refluxing ethanol with either ammonium hydroxide or with 6 N hydrogen chloride, a complex mixture was obtained, containing, phenanthridines. No substantial amount of anilines was obtained when reaction was performed by catalytic hydrogenation in the presence of palladium/carbon (10%) in methanol [43].

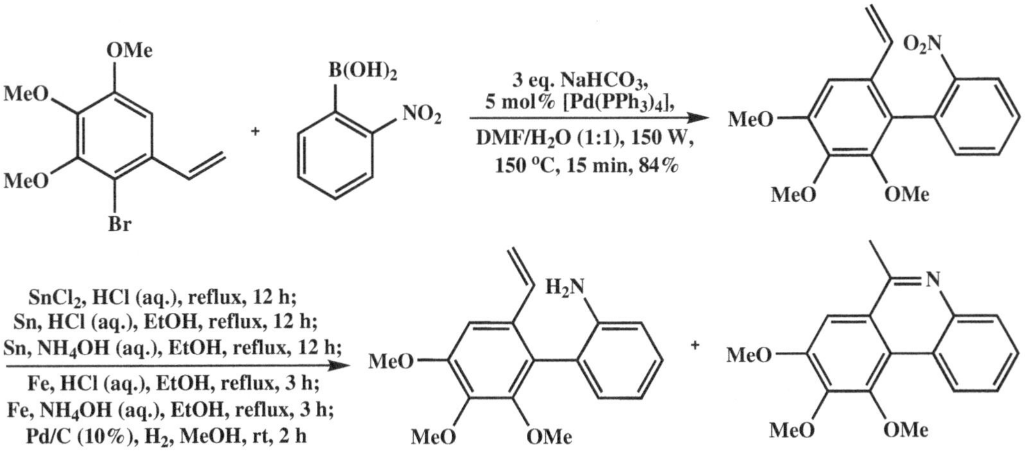

Scheme-15

The aryl bromides, iodides, and triflates were coupled using catalytic amounts of Pd **(Scheme 16)** [44-46]. For oxy-substituted haloarenes, these conditions worked well **(Scheme 17)**. The desired product was provided in poor yields with oxy-substituted aryl triflates. Similar conditions with 1,8-diazabicyclo[5.4.0]undec-7-ene base was also found to be effective for oxy-substituted aryl triflates [47]. These known reaction conditions were limited to either intramolecular or intermolecular variants of oxidative cross-couplings, and not applicable to both. Based on known cyclopalladations [48-49], it was found that *N*-methyl-*N*-phenylbenzamide underwent ring-closing oxidative cross-coupling to produce a six-membered lactam. The 5-methylphenanthridin-6(5*H*)-one was obtained in 60% yield when *N*-methyl-*N*-phenylbenzamide was subjected to same reaction conditions. Modest to good yields of phenanthridin-6(5*H*)-ones were afforded in this pathway. According to oxidative *o*-arylation of benzamides, more efficient transformations (60-77%) were reported when electron-donating groups were present on benzamide portion of substrates. For reaction efficiency a critical role was played by the position of electron rich substituent. 3-Methoxy-*N*-methyl-*N*-phenylbenzamide underwent lactam formation in 77% yield, while 4-methoxy-*N*-methyl-*N*-phenylbenzamide cyclized in a modest 33% yield. The *N*-methylcrinasiadine (natural product isolated from *Lapiedramartinezii* and *Hippeastrum equestre*) was generated from less electron rich *N*-methyl-*N*-phenylbenzo[*d*][1,3] dioxole-5-carboxamide [50-60].

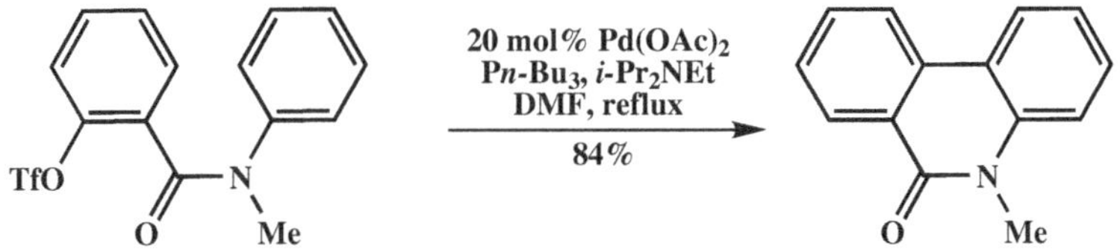

Scheme-16

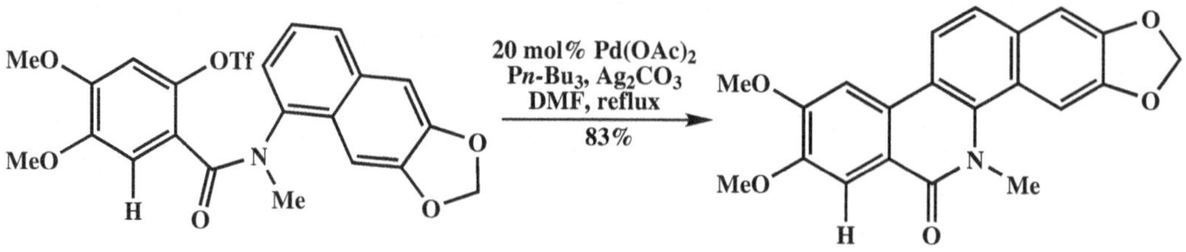

Scheme-17

Nandi and Ray [61] explained the cyclization of *N*-aryl allylamines *via* palladium(0)-mediated 6-*exo-trig* for the preparation of fused tetrahydropyridine derivatives. However, cyclopropa[*d*]-fused isoquinoline derivatives were provided *via* a domino sequence when *N*-methallylated derivatives were subjected to Heck reaction under same reaction conditions **(Scheme 18)** [62].

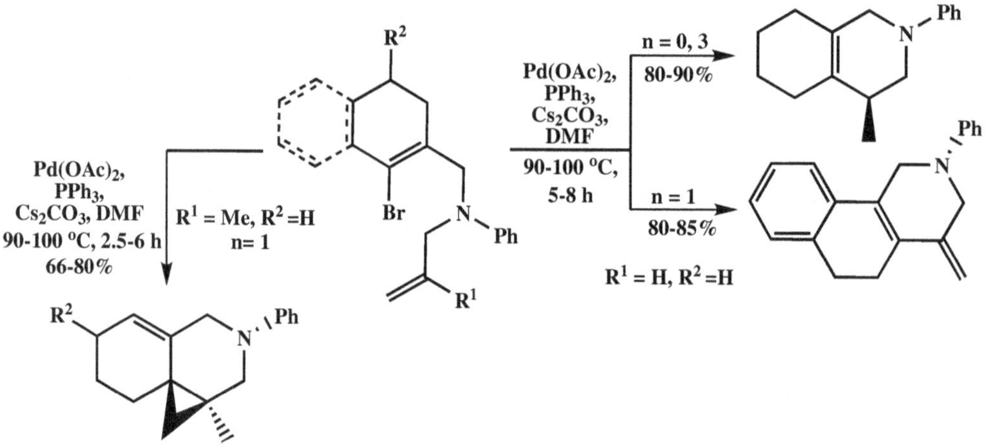

Scheme-18

Karthikeyan and Cheng [63] developed a catalytic system for the synthesis of phenanthridinones from methoxyamides and nonfunctionalized benzenes. The reaction furnished corresponding phenanthridinones in good to excellent yields under very mild conditions at rt. Similar to Wang's protocol the reaction proceeded *via* formation of arylated amide, followed by oxidative cyclization into phenanthridinone. The reaction represented an example of triple carbon-hydrogen bond activation processes, affording heterocyclic compounds from very simple starting materials. This method, however, has a regioselectivity issue when asymmetrically substituted arene was utilized. It also required a large excess of arene **(Scheme 19)** [64].

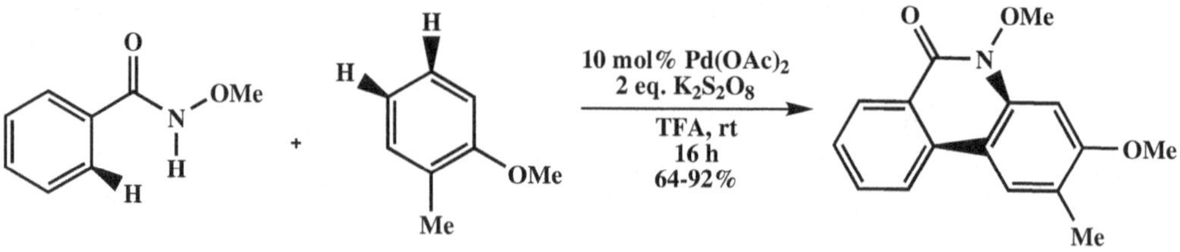

Scheme-19

Yang et al. [65] developed a two-step synthetic sequence to functionalized quinolines in high yields *via* an Ugi four-component reaction and Pd-catalyzed intramolecular arylation reaction as shown in **Scheme 20**. This highly efficient approach can be used to develop structurally diverse quinoline-based polycyclic compounds.

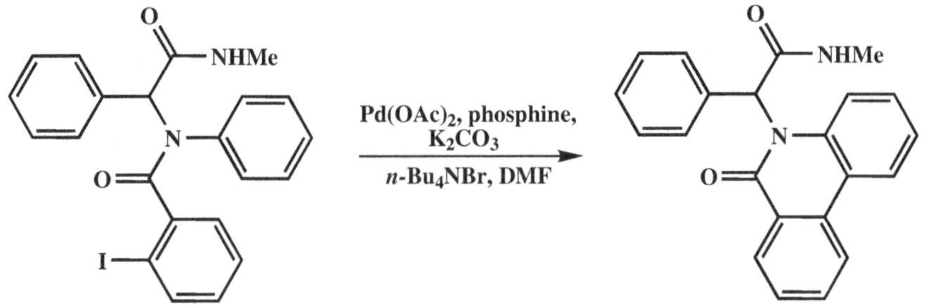

Scheme-20

The desired product was obtained in 100% transformation when solid support substrate was treated in the presence of palladium hydroxide/carbon, followed by cleavage with trifluoroacetic acid **(Scheme 21)**. It was not possible for two solid phases to interact, as the soluble catalyst species had leached into solution. The homogeneous ArI was reacted with palladium hydroxide/carbon in solid-phase thiol scavenger resin in second test. No reaction occurred in this case, which suggested that a homogeneous active catalyst was operative since this scavenger resin only removed homogeneous catalyst present in reaction [66].

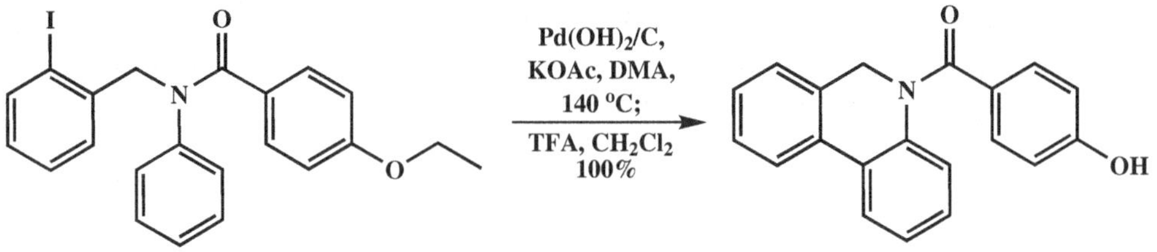

Scheme-21

Yang et al. [67] used easily accessible starting materials for the synthesis of isoquinoline in two steps through Ugi four-component reaction and palladium-catalyzed intramolecular Heck reaction. The procedure was similar to the preparation of quinolines as they reported later. By taking advantage of methodology developed by Konno et al. [68] a regioselective one-step synthesis of 4-fluoroalkylated isoquinolines was carried out using fluorine-containing alkynes. No 3-fluoroalkylated regioisomer was observed. A one-pot Pd-catalyzed alkylation/direct arylation synthesized 5,6-dihydro-pyrrolo[2,1-*a*]isoquinoline derivatives which involved an aromatic sp^2 carbon-hydrogen functionalization. The [*c*]annulated isoquinolines [69] were produced **(Scheme 22)** in two steps *via* Suzuki cross-coupling of boronic acids with α-iodoenones followed by hydrogenation. The highly oxygenated isoquinolines were formed by this efficient and mild method.

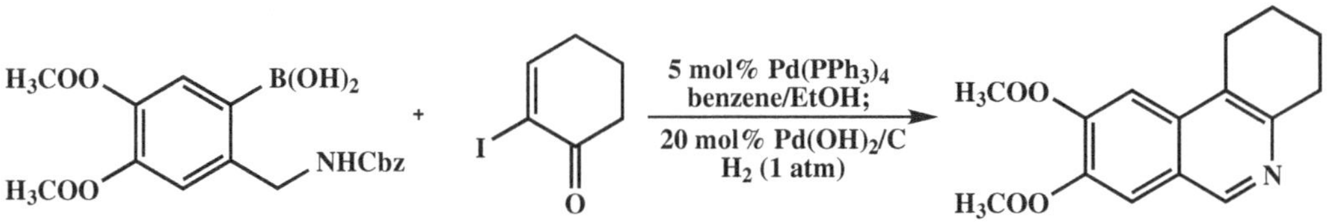

Scheme-22

Wang and co-workers [70] in 2010 reported a palladium-catalyzed reaction of methoxyamides and PhI in 2 eq. of Ag(I) oxide as an oxidant for the preparation of phenanthridinones. The reaction occurred *via* arylation in the presence of palladium catalyst followed by intramolecular CH-NH oxidative coupling **(Scheme 23)** [64].

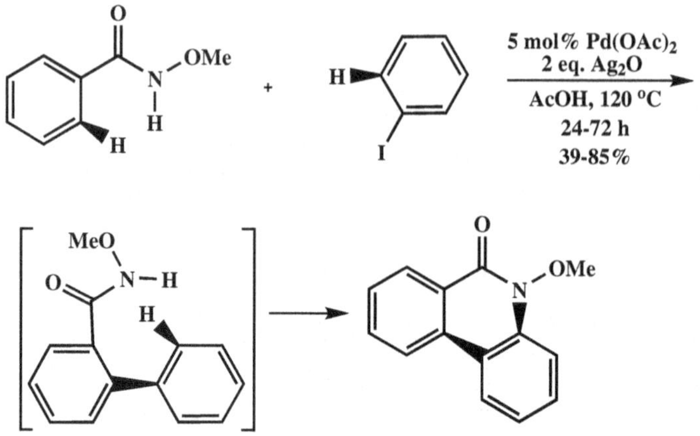

Scheme-23

This protocol was extended to tandem Heck/direct arylation reactions [71]. Both a chloride and a bromide containing substrates were treated with a Heck acceptor in the presence of 10 mol% of palladium acetate and P*t*-Bu$_3$-HBF$_4$. A number of substituted biaryl products were produced in good yields under these conditions *i.e.* 10 mol% palladium acetate and potassium carbonate at 130 °C in dimethylaniline **(Scheme 24)**.

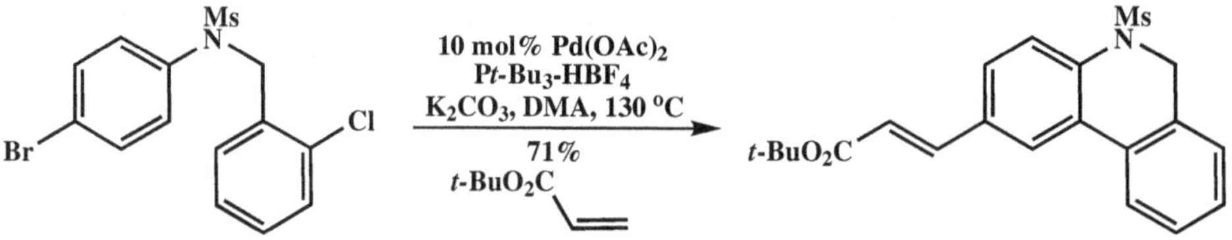

Scheme-24

The benzonaphthazepines were yielded regioselectively **(Scheme 25)** [72-73]. An unsubstituted naphthyl moiety bearing substrate was cyclized selectively at 8-, rather than the 2-position. The reaction proceeded *via* oxidative addition of Pd(0) to aryl bromide, followed by amine coordination to Pd(II) and regioselective electrophilic substitution of Pd(II) at 8-position. The product was obtained by subsequent reductive elimination. The same regioselectivity was reported with other substituted naphthyl rings with the exception when bulky substituents like 7-isopropoxynaphthalene was present. Subsequently, cyclization occurred to provide 2-cyclized product exclusively.

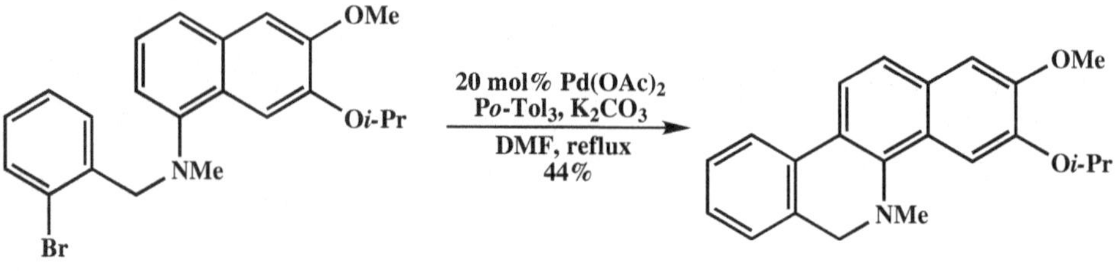

Scheme-25

Grigg [74] synthesized phenanthrene-type heterocyclic compounds through a [2+2+2]-cycloaddition in the presence of rhodium(I) catalyst followed by a direct arylation of newly produced aromatic functionality with Pd catalyst (**Scheme 26**).

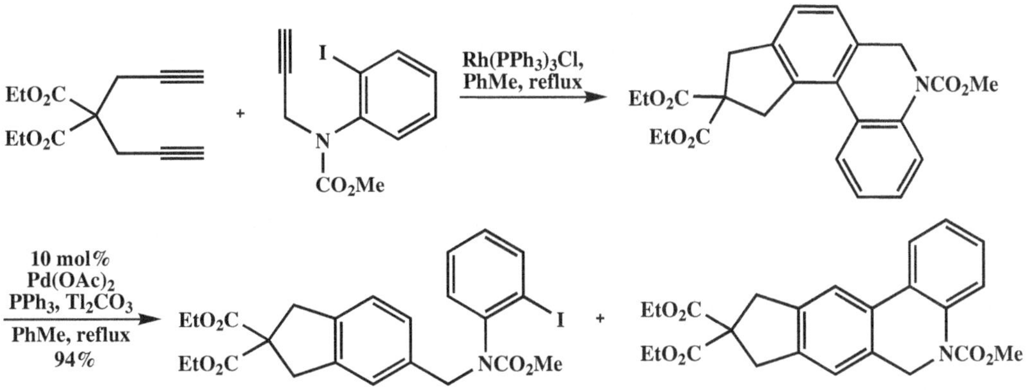

Scheme-26

While considerable research has been conducted on metal-nitrene amination of sp^3 carbon-hydrogen bonds, significant advancements were made only in oxidative amination of sp^2 carbon-hydrogen bonds. To this end, Sanford et al. [75] have reported stoichiometric studies with palladium(II) palladacycles where they can be oxidized with PhI=NTs (and derivatives of), a common aminating agent for intermolecular reactions with sp^3 carbon-hydrogen bonds [76-79]. Subsequent reductive elimination afforded aminated product (**Scheme 27**). The postulated intermediacy of a palladium(IV) imido species was supported by known reactions with analogous palladium(IV) oxo complexes [80-81] and supported by the formation of C-Cl and C-OAc by-products which were usually formed from reductive elimination of palladium(IV) centers [82-84].

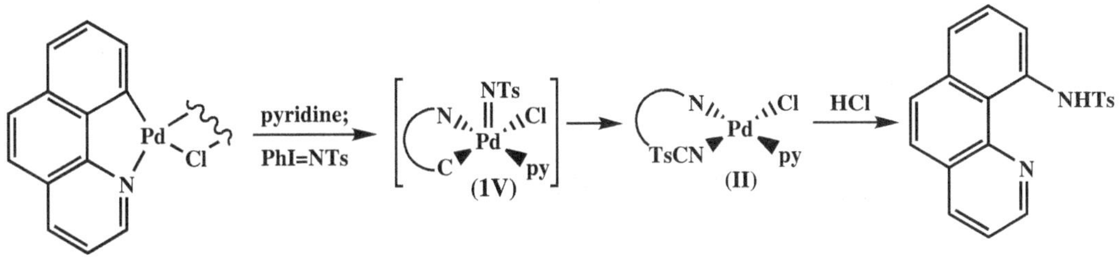

Scheme-27

De Kimpe et al. [85] synthesized dimethoxy derivative through an intramolecular Heck reaction of *N*-protected 2-(allylamino)methyl-3-bromo-1,4-dimethoxynaphthalene. The formed dimethoxy derivative was utilized for the synthesis of *N*-protected 1,2-dihydrobenz[*g*] isoquinoline-5,10-dione. This pathway was extended to *N*-protected 2-((allylamino) methyl)-3-bromo-1,4-naphthoquinone for the preparation of 4-methyl derivatives (**Scheme 28-29**) [62].

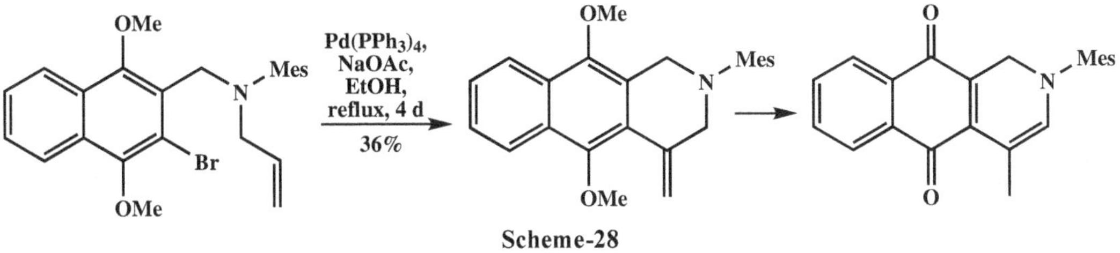

Scheme-28

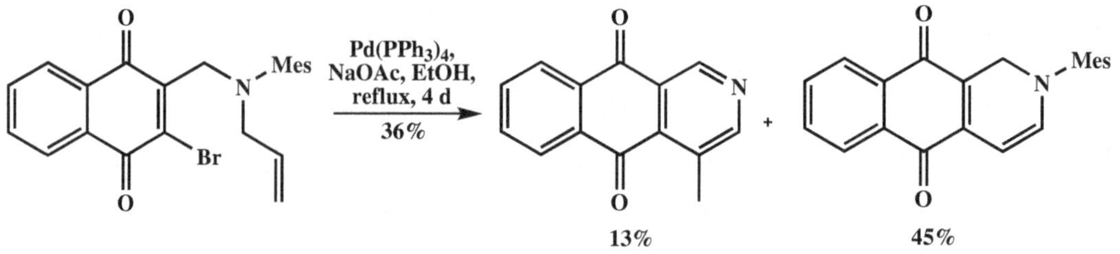

Scheme-29

Vazquez and Dominguez [86] utilized allenamide for the preparation of a tetracyclic unit of protoberberine **(Scheme 30)**. The acid-catalyzed intramolecular electrophilic aromatic substitution of allenamide occurred through *N*-acyliminium ion. Good yield of desired cyclization product was obtained, and subsequently 6-*exo* Heck reaction afforded methylene protoberberine.

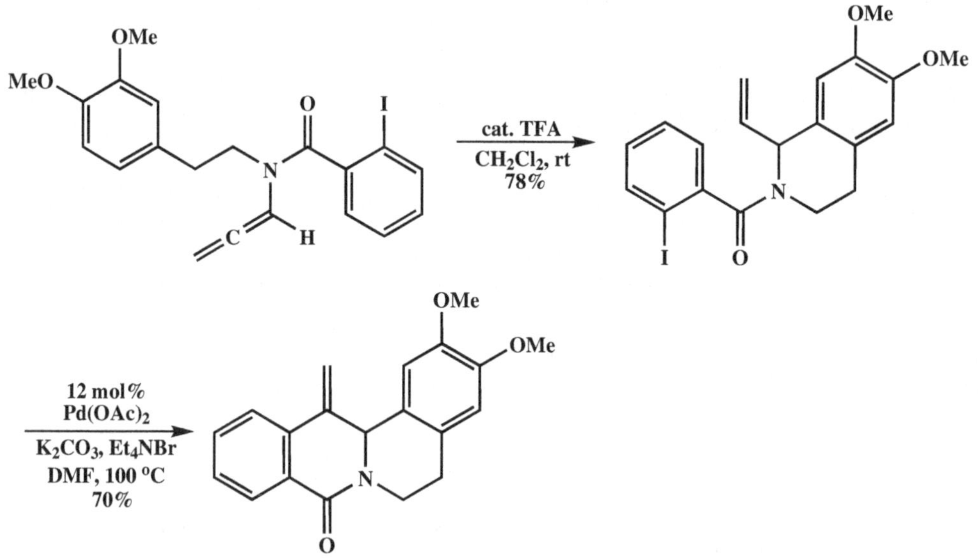

Scheme-30

Electron-donating groups containing arenes were more reactive than with electron-withdrawing counterparts. The reaction occurred *via* a free-amine-directed carbon-hydrogen cleavage. The cycloamination product was formed when alkenylated products were reacted under alkenylation reaction conditions **(Scheme 31)**. In the absence of Pd catalyst the cycloamination did not occur and in the absence of Cu salts reaction rate was very slow [87-92].

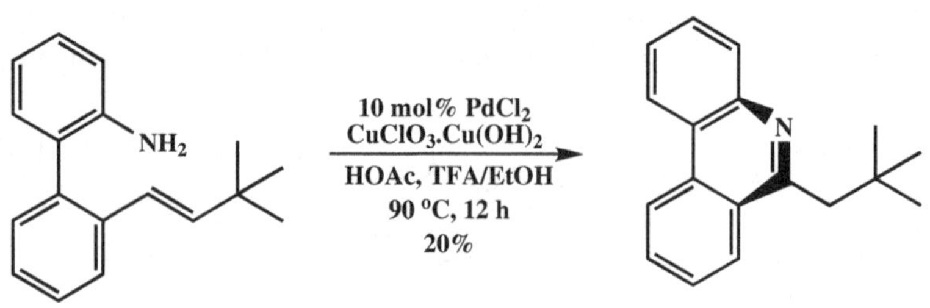

Scheme-31

The Stille reaction tolerated many functional groups and made it effective for the synthesis of complex pyridine derivatives [93]. The organostannane was generated *in situ* through Pd-mediated reaction of a pyridyl triflate or halide with hexamethylditin **(Scheme 32)** [94-95].

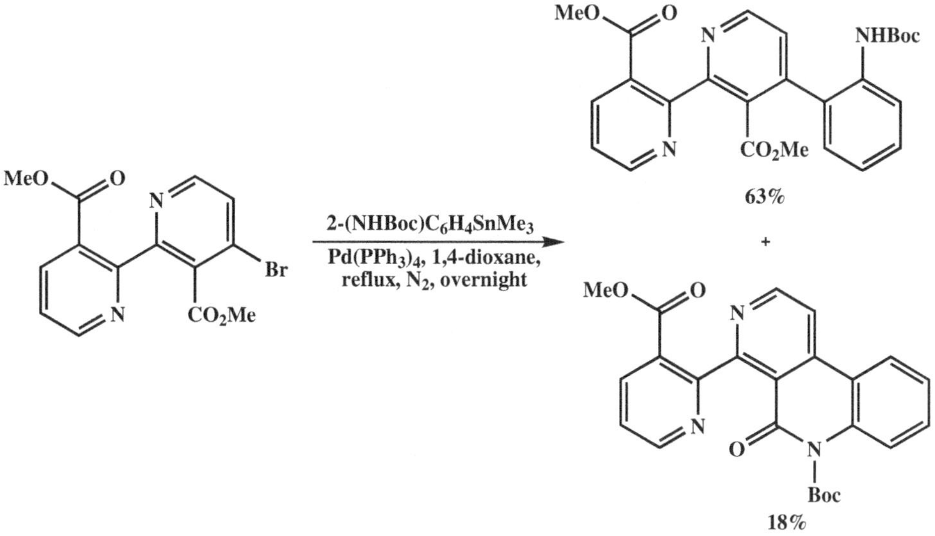

Scheme-32

The benzo[*h*][1,6]naphthyridines were synthesized using pyridine as basal support for iminyl radical and aromatic acceptor. The 2-aryl-3-formyl-pyridine derivatives were prepared when 2-bromonicotinaldehyde underwent coupling with phenylboronic acids in the presence of palladium catalyst. The 2-aryl-3-formyl-pyridine derivatives were transformed smoothly into oxime ethers. Oxime ethers were irradiated under microwaves to afford very satisfactory yield of benzo[*h*][1,6]naphthyridine. The benzo[*h*][1,6]naphthyridines bearing useful moiety at 8-position were easily produced from precursors with Br and CN substituents. Some of benzo[*h*] [1,6]naphthiridine derivatives were reported in the literature [96-98], but none of them was commercially available **(Scheme 33)** [99].

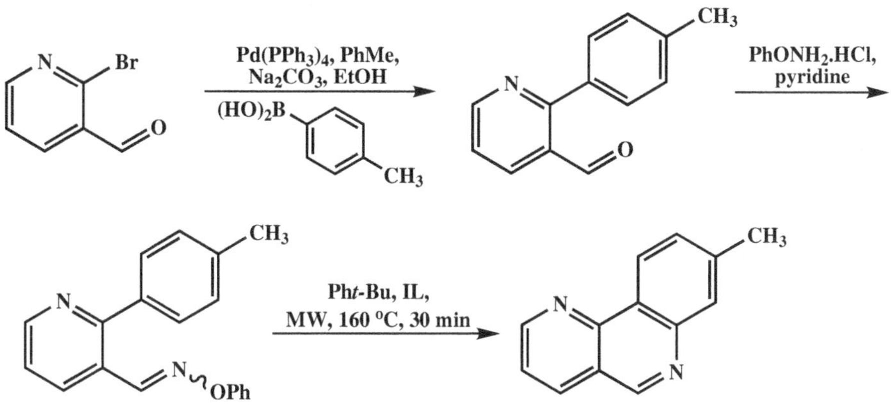

Scheme-33

The azaaromatics possess many biological activities [100]. 2-Formylbiphenyls were synthesized in yields ranging from 62% to 71% by coupling of 2-bromobenzaldehyde with many aromatic boronic acids in the presence of palladium catalyst [101]. The formed 2-formylbiphenyls were transformed into *O*-phenyl oximes upon treatment with PhONH$_2$·HCl. Individual precursors were then irradiated under microwaves in *t*-BuPh with emimPF$_6$ for 30 min. This protocol provided parent phenanthridine in 76% yield along with phenol. The reaction was equally successful for a precursor containing an electron-releasing substituent (OMe), and for precursors bearing electron-withdrawing substituents (CN, Br). For further functional group transformations the 3-cyano- and 3-bromophenanthridines were convenient. The benzo[*k*]phenanthridine was accessible through an analogous route. Previously, it had been made by cyclization of aryl formamides [102], photocyclization of 4-phenyl-3-vinylquinolines [103], and an anionic/aryne cyclization and *in situ* oxidation sequence starting from 2-bromonaphthyl-2-fluorophenylamine. Under standard reaction conditions, MWI of naphthalene containing precursor in *t*-BuPh afforded benzo[*k*]phenanthridine in 64% yield **(Scheme 34)**.

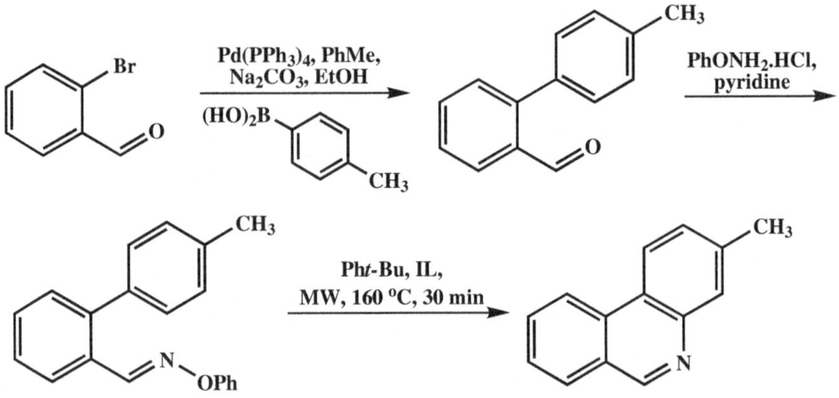

Scheme-34

Zhu [104] was able to use an aryne annulation to complete the same molecules while maintaining an alternative approach from functionalized oximes. The role of Pd in reaction was not clear, but it might assist in N-O bond cleavage after hetero-Diels-Alder reaction to form the core of product **(Scheme 35)**.

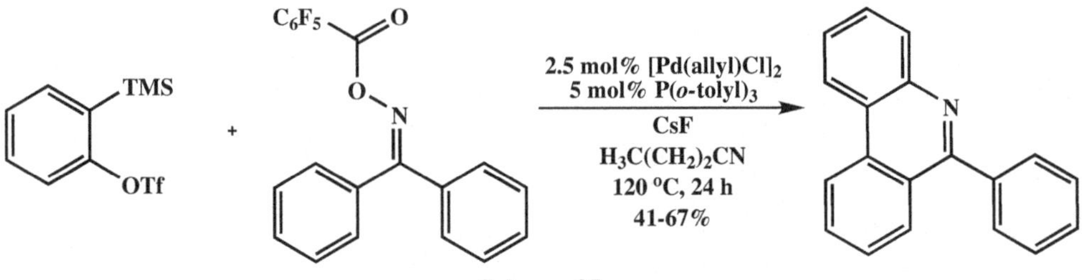

Scheme-35

9.4 Synthesis of six-membered heterocycles fused with five-membered heterocycles

Malinakova et al. [105] developed a powerful novel methodology for copper(I)-catalyzed three-component coupling of imines, vinylstannanes, or alkynes and *o*-bromoaroyl chlorides followed by an intramolecular palladium(0)-catalyzed 1,2-bisarylation of an olefin or an alkyne in amides to deliver substituted indenoisoquinolines. The advantage of this methodology was that various functional groups can be introduced from each component. The reaction proceeded by initial

Ag-catalyzed cycloisomerization of alkynyl imines to form isoquinolinium species followed by dipolar cycloaddition of alkynes, leading to formation of dihydropyrroles, which were finally isomerized and oxidized to afford the desired pyrrolo-isoquinolines **(Scheme 36)** [106].

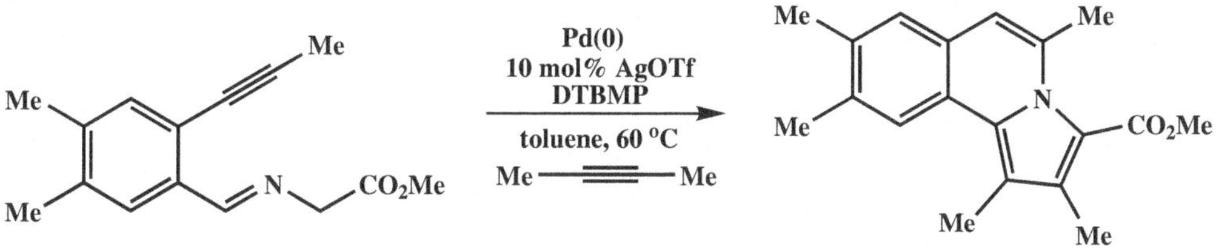

Scheme-36

The unsubstituted bromoalkyl pyrroles were reacted with a variety of aryl iodides using palladium chloride catalyst. Lautens et al. [107] extended their norbornene-mediated sequential coupling in the presence of Pd catalyst for annulation of pyrroles. Good to excellent yields of annulated pyrroles were reported when electron-poor aromatics, which contained one blocking group *ortho* to iodide functionality, were utilized. The desired annulated pyrroles were also formed when electron-rich aromatics were employed although in somewhat lower yields **(Scheme 37)**.

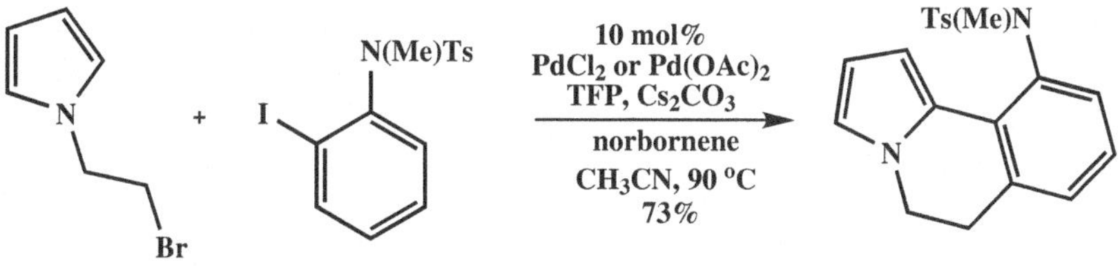

Scheme-37

Pyrrole ring is present in biologically active compounds such as lamellarin and lettowianthine. Under reaction conditions the silyl protected aryl iodides were also compatible and were de-protected *in situ* to afford alcohol product **(Scheme 38)**. Excellent yield of annulated pyrrole was provided with PhI **(Scheme 39)** [108-111].

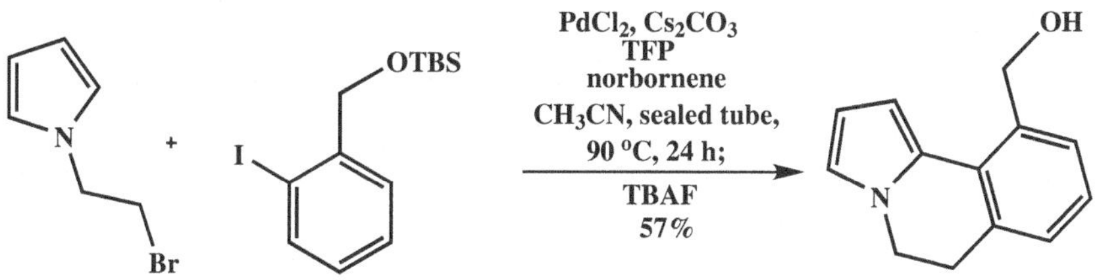

Scheme-38

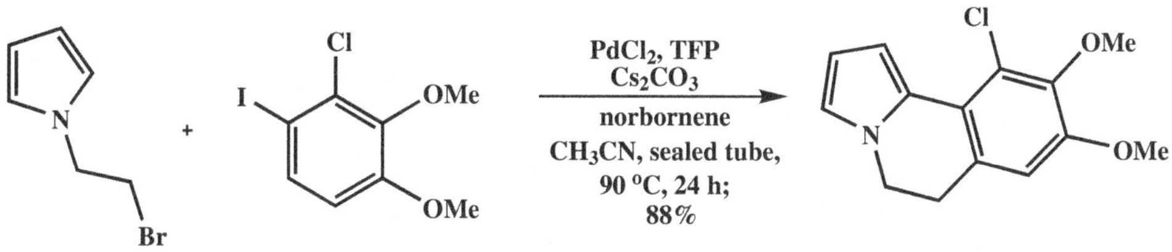

Scheme-39

The aromatic Finkelstein reaction was utilized only once for the synthesis of natural product by Furstner and Kennedy [112] for the generation of cytotoxic *Tylophora* alkaloids antofine and cryptopleurine. Suzuki coupling of 1-bromo-2-iodo-4-methoxybenzene afforded an intermediate. The formed intermediate underwent a bromide-iodide exchange using either a standard lithiation-iodination sequence or Buchwald's procedure using excess of sodium iodide together with CuI and diamine to give more reactive iodide. Then, the formed iodide synthesized antofine and cryptopleurine **(Scheme 40)**. Although for both procedures the yields were comparable, the standard lithiation was, however, preferred because long reaction times were needed in second case. A vinylic Finkelstein reaction was also used for the synthesis of 1-iodo-2-methylpropene from bromide during synthetic studies toward total synthesis of kaitocephalin [113-114].

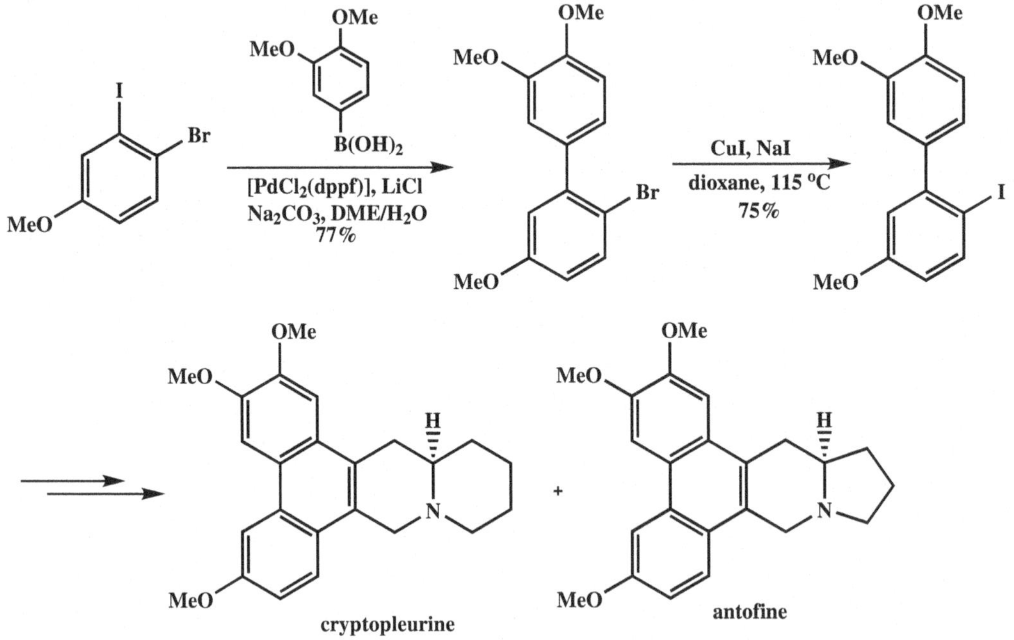

Scheme-40

Ozaki [115] have focused their attention on the formation of 6-membered ring. Interestingly, when compound was heated under standard conditions, the ring closure product was formed smoothly in 75% yield **(Scheme 41)**.

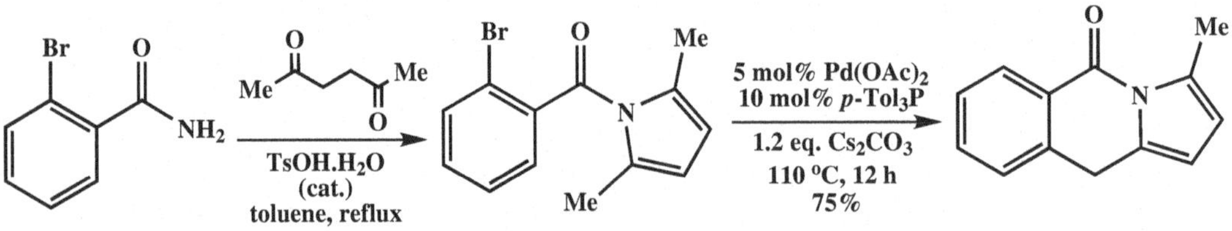

Scheme-41

The tricyclic compounds were synthesized in 74-85% yield from *N*-acylpyrrolamides under usual reaction conditions **(Scheme 42)** [116].

The carboamination reactions were extended to *N*-protected γ-aminoalkenes for the preparation of interesting compounds which could not be obtained using transformations of γ-*N*-(arylamino) alkenes. A palladium-catalyzed carboamination of substrate was conducted with methyl-2-bromobenzoate, which afforded intermediate in 73% yield. The tetrahydropyrroloisoquinolin-5-one was obtained in 95% yield when intermediate was treated with acid or base **(Scheme 43)** [117-122].

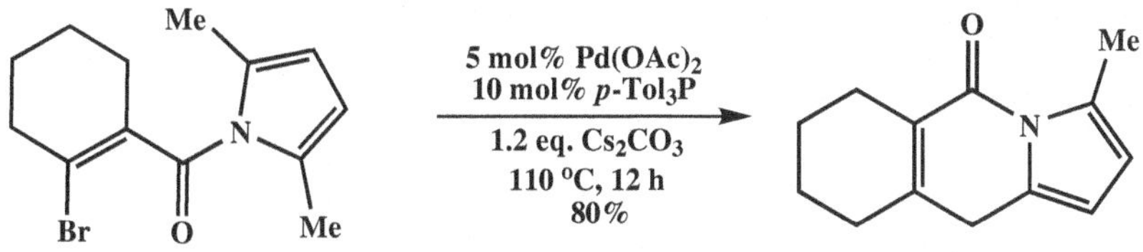

Scheme-42

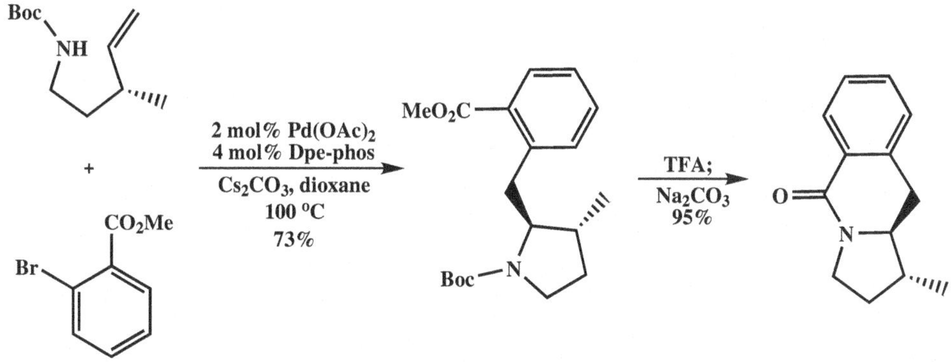

Scheme-43

The pyrrolo[1,2-*b*]isoquinolines were formed in 75-81% yield under standard conditions from readily available amides **(Scheme 44)** [123]. The amide reacted under milder conditions. The heterocyclic compound was generated in 79% yield when amide was heated with 5 mmol% of palladium acetate for 5 h at 80 °C [124a-b]. The oxidized naphthyl derivative was also present in crude reaction mixture **(Scheme 45)** [125-129].

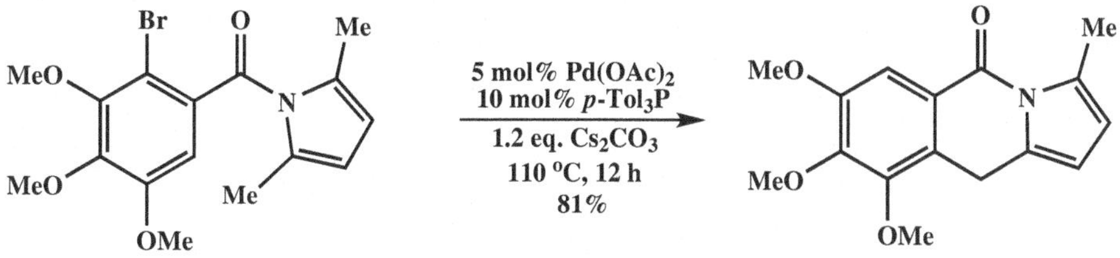

Scheme-44

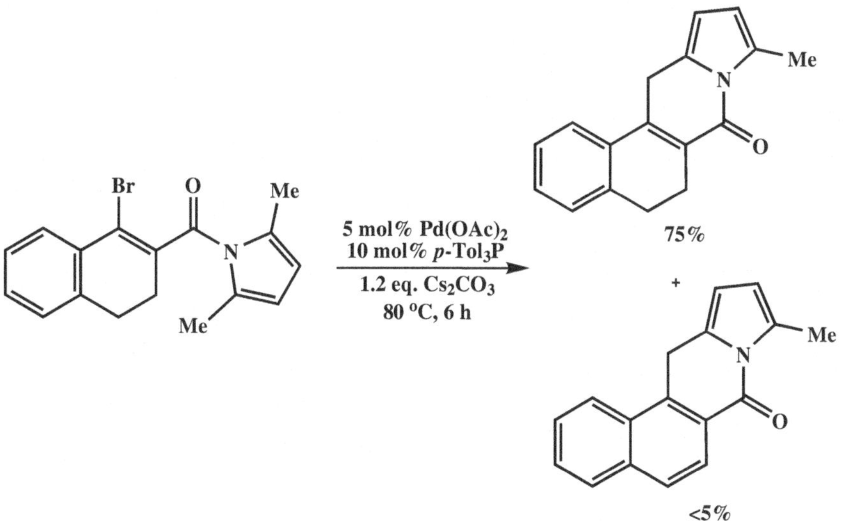

Scheme-45

The domino Suzuki cross-coupling and carbon-hydrogen activation product was formed in 65% yield when dibromoarylpyrrole was reacted with phenylboronic acid in the presence of 10 mol% of palladium acetate and 20 mol% of *p*-Tol₃P. The amount of phenylboronic acid utilized in this reaction was important. In the presence of an excess of phenylboronic acid, the double Suzuki cross-coupling product was produced. The starting substrate dibromoaryl pyrrole and mono-Suzuki cross-coupling product was obtained without any trace of carbon-hydrogen activation product if 0.9 eq. of phenylboronic acid was used **(Scheme 46)** [130-131].

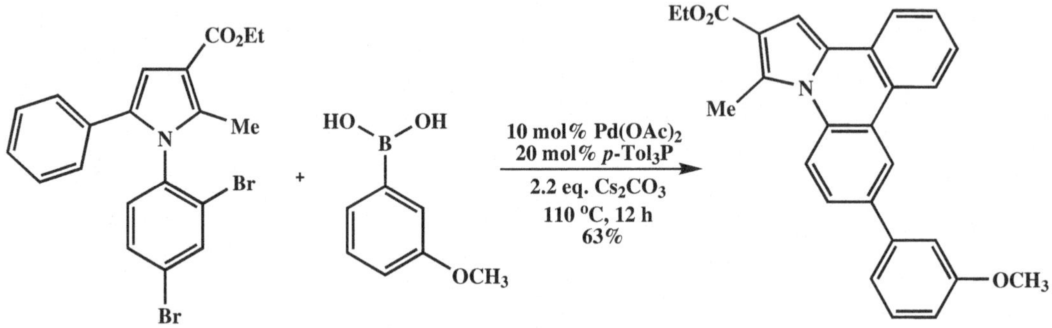

Scheme-46

The carbon-hydrogen activation and cross-coupling product was reported in 89% yield when 3-methyloxyl benzeneboronic acid was utilized. The desired product was also provided in 59% yield when dibromo substrate was reacted with 3-methyloxyl benzeneboronic acid under these conditions **(Scheme 47)** [132].

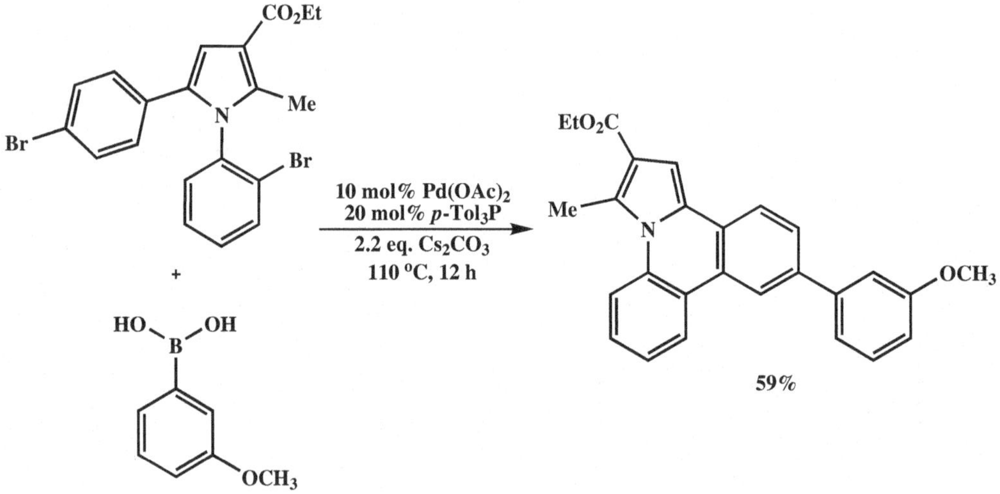

Scheme-47

Substrates bearing nitrogen in a ring were also cyclized [133-135]. The desired tetracyclic product was obtained in excellent yield from six-membered tetrahydroquinoline **(Scheme 48-49)**, while the desired product was formed in low yield under similar conditions when five-membered dihydroindole was utilized. The same product was formed in higher yield when substrate containing iodide on dihydroindole moiety was used.

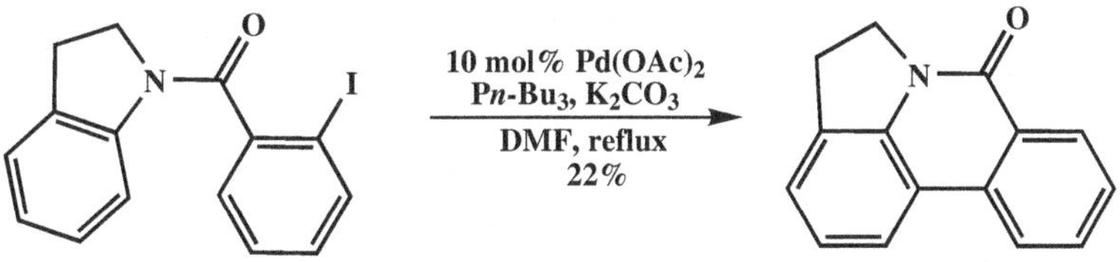

Scheme-48

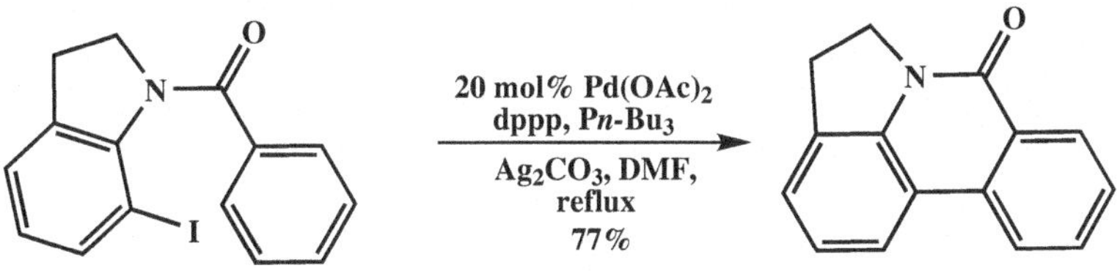

Scheme-49

A number of alkaloids, like indoles [136-139], indazoles [140-141], benzimidazoles [142-143], benazepines [144-145], phenazines [146], carbapenems [147] the mitomycin ring system [148], carbolines [149] and polyheterocycles [150] were synthesized by this protocol. The aminocyclization of vinyl and aryl iodides in the presence of Pd catalyst afforded pharmacologically active natural products, like dehydrobufotenine **(Scheme 50)** [151].

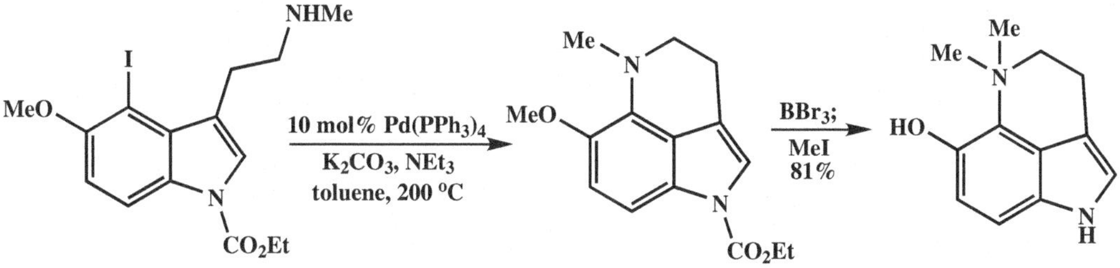

Scheme-50

The iodoindoles containing a tethered arene were cyclized **(Scheme 51)** [74]. A single dihydroazaphenanthrene derivative was provided in 62% yield by this method, despite the possibility of regioselectivity issues.

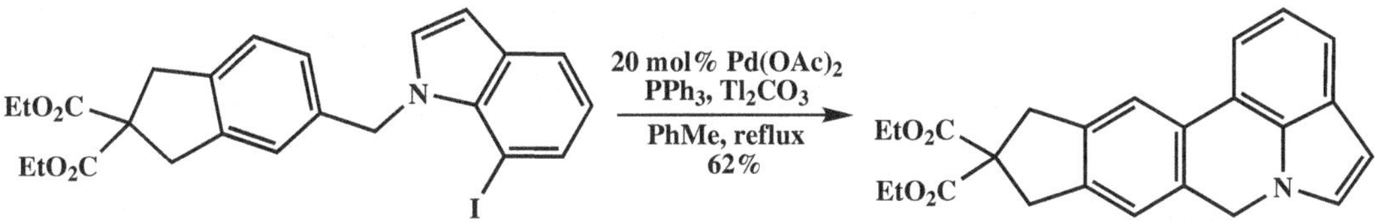

Scheme-51

For the anti-neophobic mitochondrial diazepam binding inhibitor receptor, Kozikowski [152] developed a new class of ligands. Following Kozikowski's report, Garratt [153] synthesized a large library of five-, six-, and seven-membered annulated indoles under same reaction conditions for probing the active site of receptor for melatonin **(Scheme 52)**.

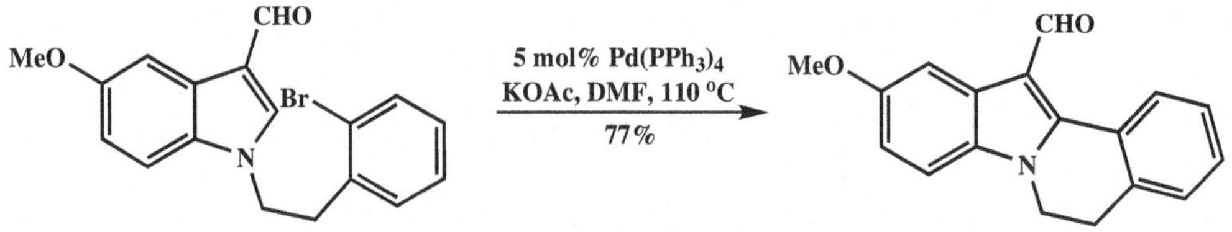

Scheme-52

A triaza analogue of a "crushed-fullerene" fragment was synthesized by a direct arylation [154]. Under reaction conditions the arylation of carbazole occurred in quantitative yields **(Scheme 53-54)**. Interestingly, a nearly equal mixture of products was obtained with a non-symmetrical carbazole which created a doubt on a proposed electrophilic aromatic substitution mechanism.

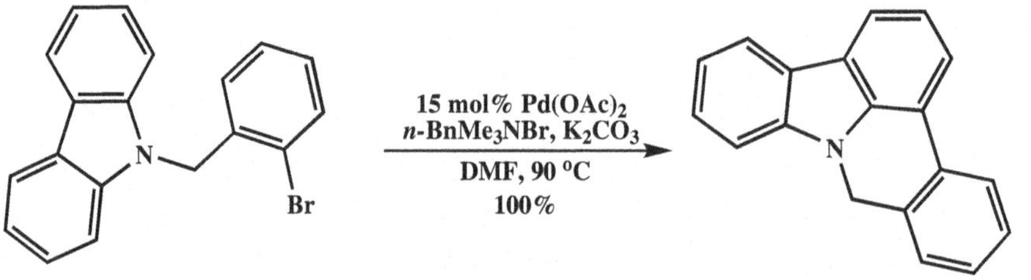

Scheme-53

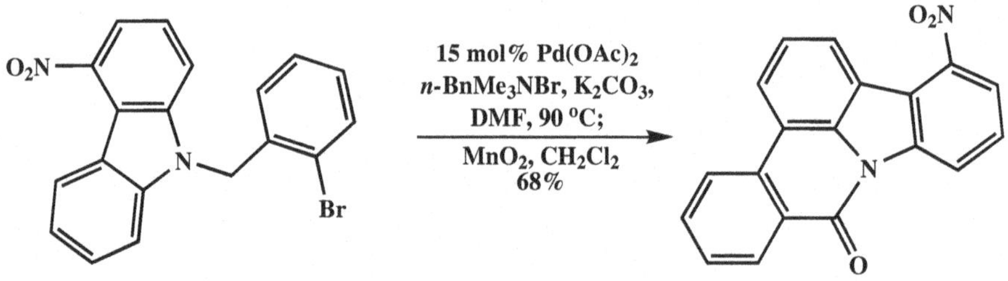

Scheme-54

The blockage of second position of an indole bearing an aryl bromide tethered at nitrogen was an example of direct arylation at arene portion of indole **(Scheme 55)**. The core structures of hippadine and pratosine were subsequently prepared by this protocol [155].

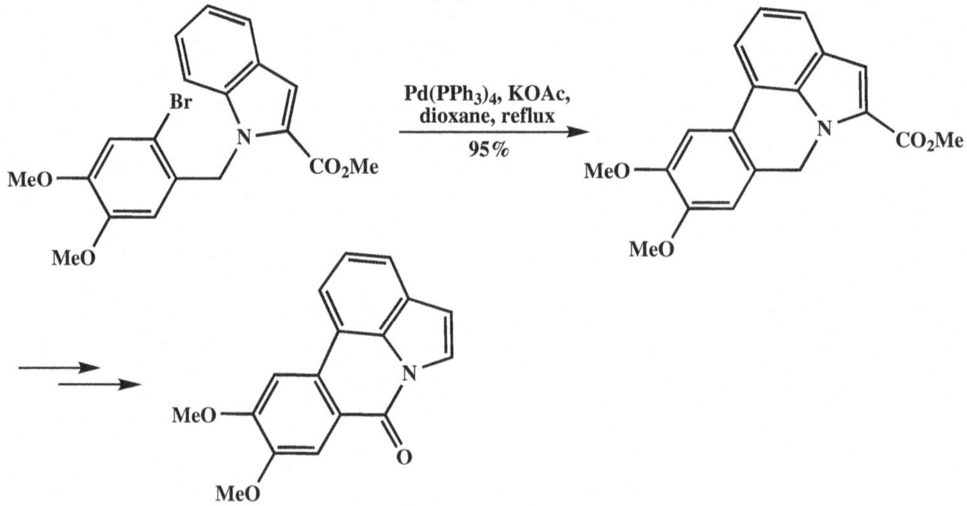

Scheme-55

Although anticipated products were obtained from most of the examined substrates, reactions of starting material with aryl bromides afforded surprising results **(Scheme 56)**. The desired products were not obtained, but instead moderate yield of intermediate was reported with excellent diastereoselectivity [156].

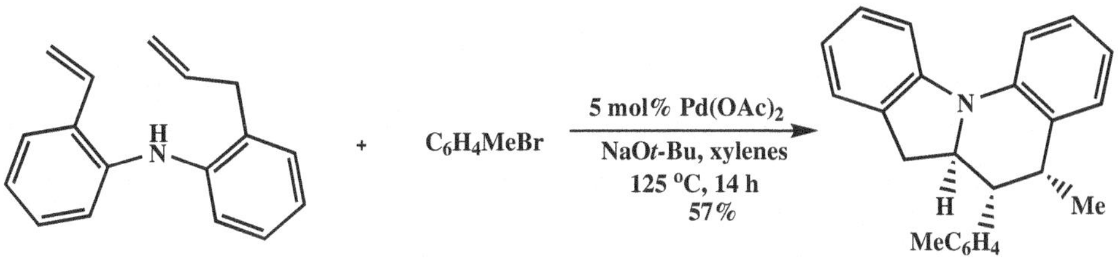

Scheme-56

The starting substrates were transformed into products without any migration of deuterium label **(Scheme 57)**. In contrast, products were obtained with migration of a deuterium atom to C5-methyl group when substrate contained deuterium atoms on terminal carbon of allyl group [157-159].

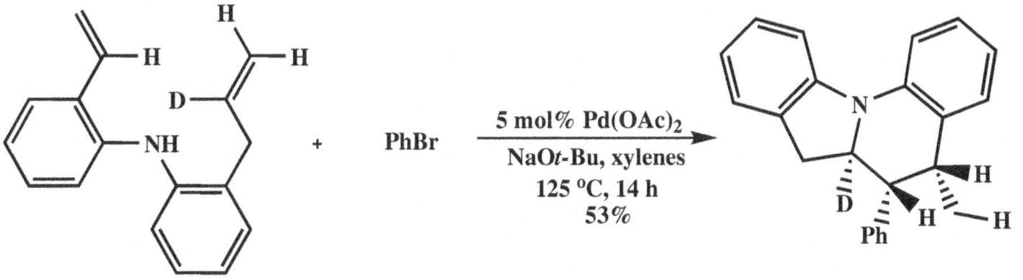

Scheme-57

The *Amaryllidaceae* alkaloids are biologically active natural product targets which attracted the attention of synthetic community [160]. Various synthetic protocols have been developed for the synthesis of these compounds due to their biological activity. Harayama [161] prepared this interesting scaffold by an intramolecular direct arylation of *N*-(2-halobenzyl)indulines with Pd catalyst. In most of the reactions, a low-yielding mixture of oxidized benzylindole and reduced benzylindoline as well as oxidized dihydropyrrolophenanthridone and cyclized dihydro-pyrrolophenanthridine was obtained. Many alkaloids such as assoanine, anhydrolycorine, oxoassoanine, and anhydrolycorin-7-one were produced using this method **(Scheme 58)**.

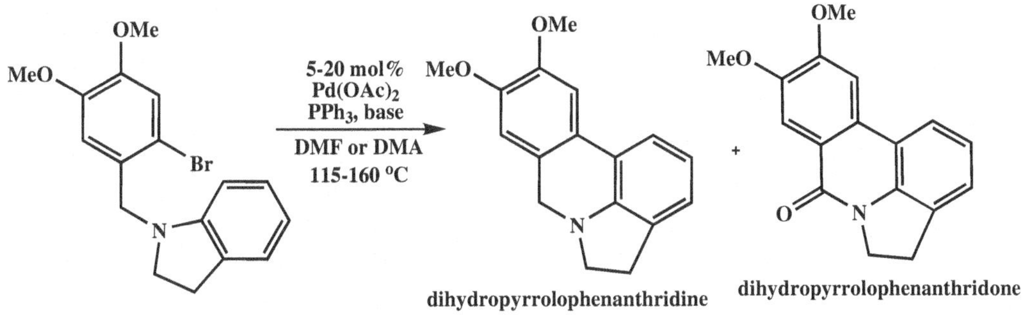

dihydropyrrolophenanthridine   **dihydropyrrolophenanthridone**

Scheme-58

Garden [162-163] used spirodioxolanes for the preparation of a class of related *Amaryllidaceae* alkaloids, in turn spirodioxolanes were produced from *N*-benzylisatin derivatives. The problem of regioselective cyclization at indole C-7 position was avoided using these substrates. These substrates underwent intramolecular direct arylation to provide excellent yields of desired cyclized compounds under Jeffery's conditions. A variety of alkaloid derivatives such as hippadine, dehydroanhydrolycorine, anhydrolycorin-7-one, and anhydrolycorine were obtained by subsequent manipulation of this core compound **(Scheme 59)**.

10 mol% Pd(OAc)$_2$
n-Bu$_4$NBr, KOAc,
DMF, 100 °C
95%

Y= H$_2$, dehydroanhydrolycorine
Y= O, hippadine

+

Y= H$_2$, anhydrolycorine
Y= O, anhydrolycorin-7-one

Scheme-59

Following various reports of BINOL-based (1,1′-bi-2-naphthol) ligands in asymmetric allylic alkylation, the Ojima [164-165] laboratory successfully applied their novel phosphoramidite biphenol-based ligands to two asymmetric allylic substitution reactions. The lycorane, involved in key step in the total synthesis of alkaloid following key allylic alkylation step, was obtained in >99% enantiomeric excess **(Scheme 60)**.

Pd/Ligand
LDA

5 steps

>99% *ee*

Scheme-60

Mori et al. [166] described the total synthesis of erythrocarine by using a number of important reaction sequences and ring-closing metathesis of dienyne as key step. The reaction of starting compound and trimethylsilylacetylene in the presence of Pd catalyst afforded alkyne which was then condensed with nitromethane to afford NO_2 derivative. Treatment of NO_2 derivative with lithium aluminium hydride followed by Boc-protection afforded corresponding alkyne. The ring-closing metathesis precursors were formed from alkyne by applying a number of reaction sequences. When a dichloromethane solution of dienyne hydrochloride was treated with 10 mol% of Grubbs' 1st generation catalyst at room temperature for 18 h, the corresponding cyclized product was reported in almost quantitative yield. Treatment of cyclized product with potassium carbonate in methanol gave corresponding alcohol, erythrocarine (**Scheme 61**) [167].

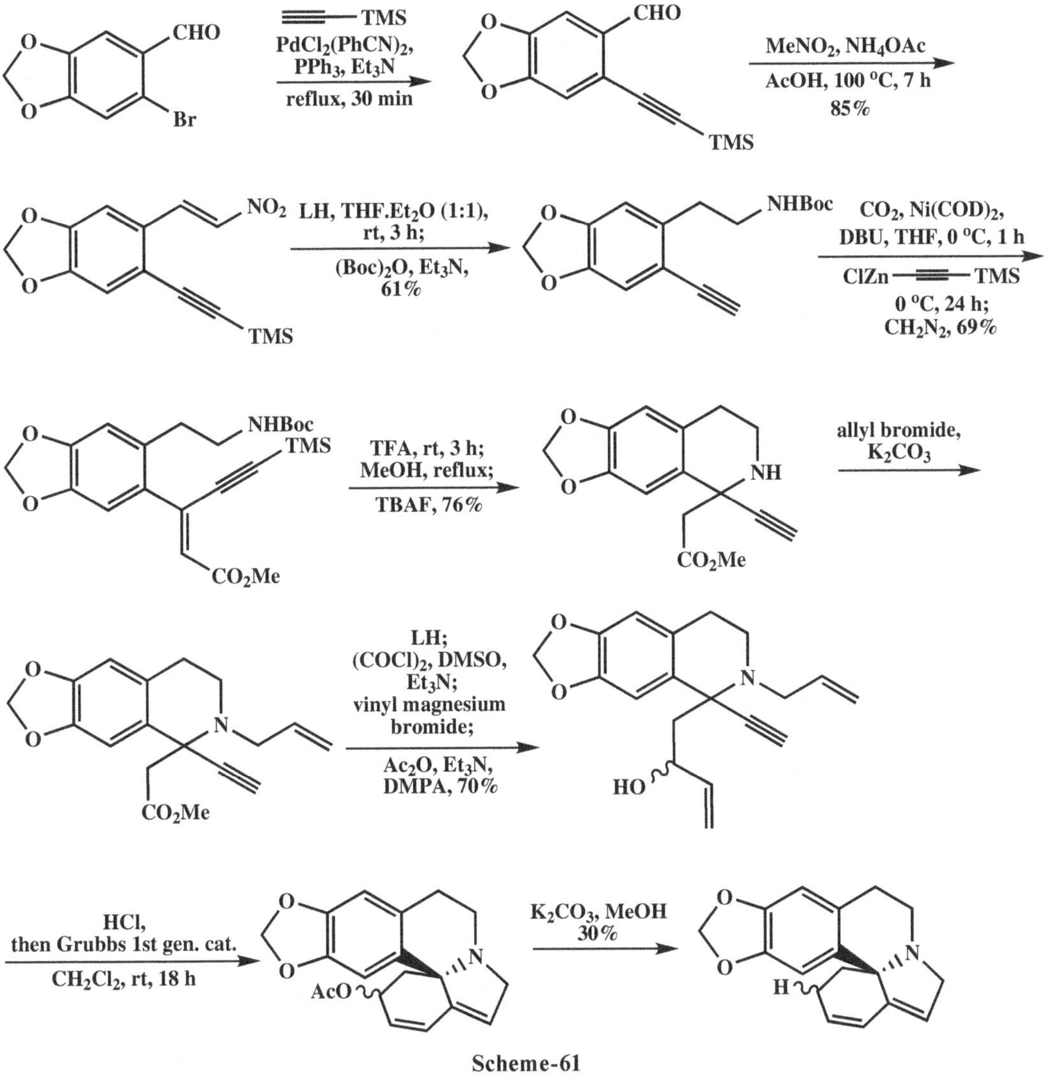

Scheme-61

Mejia-Oneto and Padwa [168-169] reported an intramolecular cyclization of allylamine derivative to synthesize the indole core of aspidophytine in the presence of palladium salt (**Scheme 62**) [62].

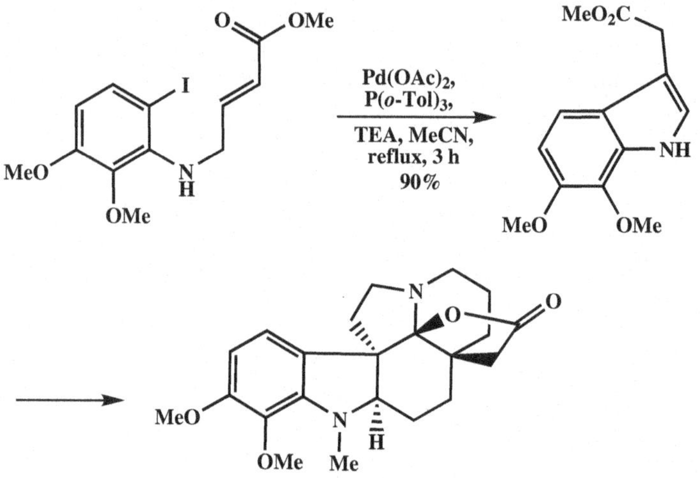

Scheme-62

Alberico et al. [170-171] produced annulated *N*-containing heterocyclic compounds by direct arylation reactions. An intermolecular *o*-alkylation of an aromatic carbon-hydrogen bond with *N*-bromoalkyl heterocycle, in the presence of norbornene and Pd catalyst, formed a tethered intermediate **(Scheme 63)** [172]. Catellani [173-176] proposed a mechanism for the initial step which involved a palladium(II)/palladium(IV) catalytic cycle. The formed species then underwent an intramolecular direct arylation to synthesize aryl-*N*-heteroaryl bond at 2 position of *N*-heteroaryl compound. Herein, *N*-bromoalkyl heterocyclic compounds were reacted with *o*-substituted aryl iodides for the preparation of functionalized annulated pyrroles, indoles, azaindoles, and pyrazoles [111].

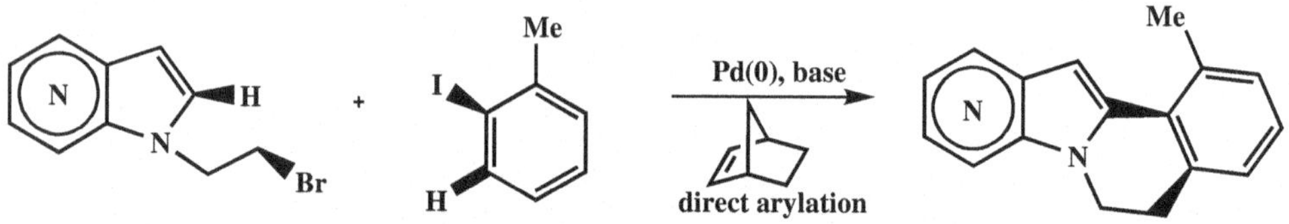

Scheme-63

An intramolecular coupling of ArI onto protected pyrrole occurred in 70% yield [177]. Beccalli et al. [178] at the same time independently reported a related intramolecular cyclization of many aryl halides onto a tethered *N*-methylpyrrole derivative **(Scheme 64)**. Good to excellent yields of pharmaceutically interesting tricyclic heterocyclic compounds were formed. However, the pyrrole, with aryl halide tethered by an amide group at C2 on pyrrole, does not underwent reaction at (now most reactive) C5 site, but instead reaction at kinetically accessible C3 position afforded product.

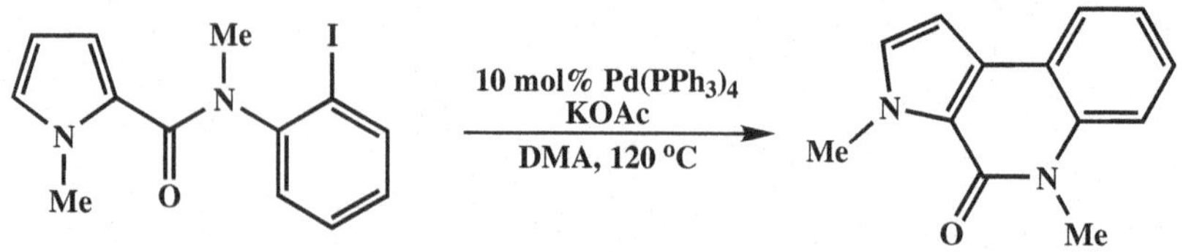

Scheme-64

The 2-iodoanilines were reacted with 2,3-dihydro-1*H*-pyrrole under MWI using 10 mol% of Pd(PPh₃)₄ and potassium carbonate at 170 °C in 1,4-dioxane for 1 h to afford 2,3-dihydro

-1*H*-pyrrolo[3,2-*c*]quinoline core in 60% yield **(Scheme 65)**. But, 2,3-dihydro-1*H*-pyrrolo[3,2-*c*] quinoline was formed in 44% yield from the reaction of 2-iodoanilines and 2,3-dihydro-1*H*-pyrrole in refluxing PhMe for 24 h [179].

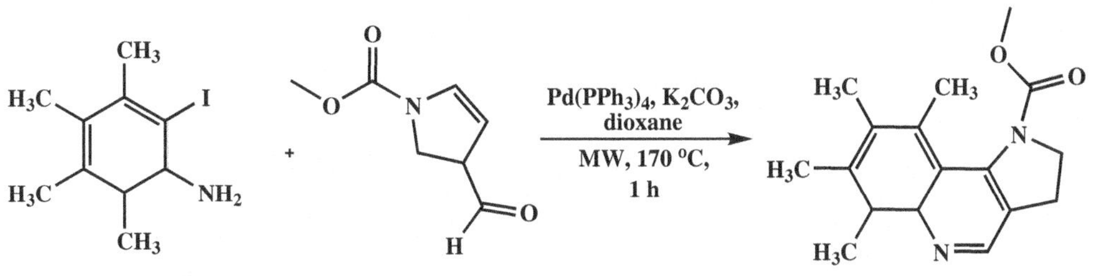

Scheme-65

While Pd participation aryne annulation reactions were relatively rare, Zhang [180] reported an intramolecular Pd-mediated method to form indolophenanthridines **(Scheme 66)**. The palladium-phosphine catalyst performed an oxidative addition into aryl bromide, and added across an aryne equivalent to generate aryl Pd intermediate. Ring closure resulted from carbopalladation of Pd to forge the carbon-carbon bond between arene and indole, yielding product.

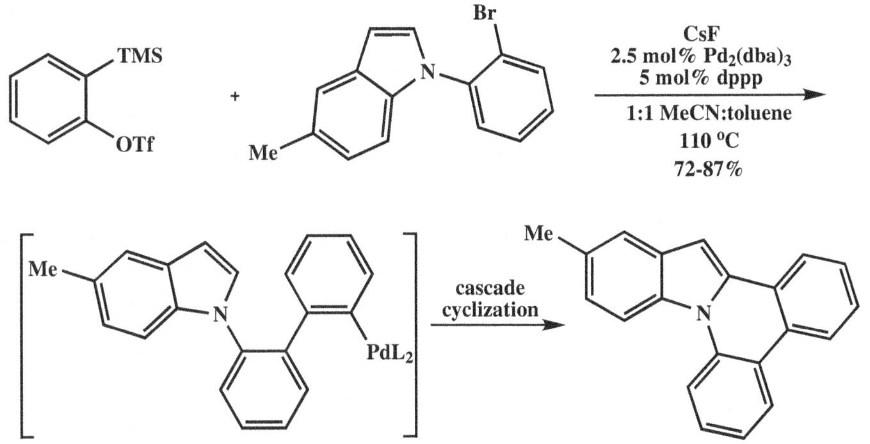

Scheme-66

In drug discovery programs large collections of small molecules are in great demand. For rapid construction of natural product-like compounds the pursuit of efficient and practical approaches is of utmost importance and urgency [181-183]. A small library of *H*-pyrazolo[5,1-*a*] isoquinolines was constructed successfully through cascade reactions **(Scheme 67)** [184].

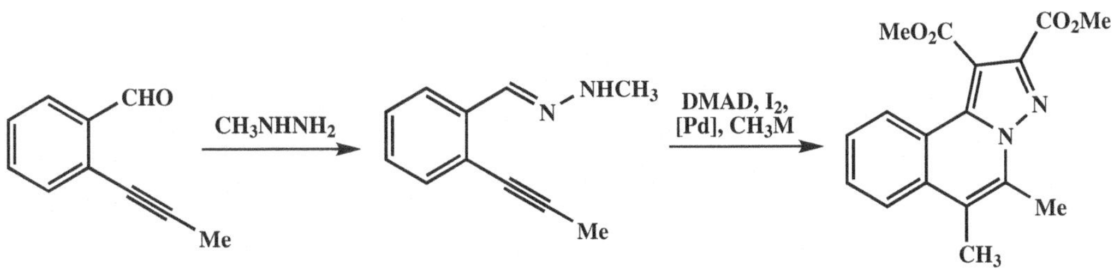

Scheme-67

The 5-butyl-l-methyl-1*H*-imidazo[4,5-*c*]quinolin-4(5*H*)-one (potent anti-asthmatic) was synthesized by an intramolecular heteroaryl Heck reaction [185]. Attempts to cyclize the free amide were unsuccessful. The desired target compound was afforded by alkylation of amide NH followed by treatment with palladium acetate under Jeffery's conditions (for smooth cyclization) **(Scheme 68)**.

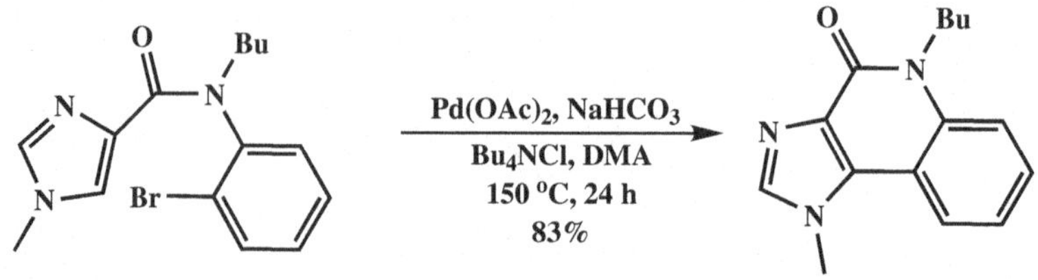

Scheme-68

The terminal alkynes, 2-bromoarylaldehydes, and 1,2-phenylenediamines were reacted under MWI by tandem process for direct and efficient preparation of benzimidazo[2,1-*a*]isoquinolines. This reaction occurred through Sonogashira coupling, 5-*endo*-cyclization, oxidative aromatization, and 6-*endo*-cyclization in a single synthetic operation **(Scheme 69)** [186-187].

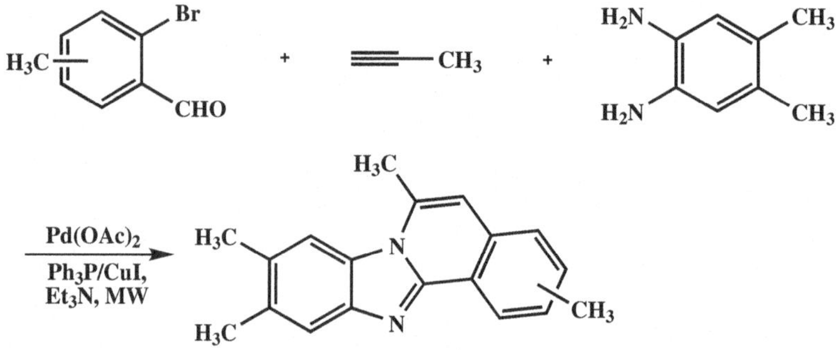

Scheme-69

Dominguez [188] reported the preparation of pyrazolophenanthridines *via* a Pd-catalyzed direct arylation of arylsubstituted pyrazoles **(Scheme 70)**. The resulting cyclization using palladium acetate, potassium carbonate, lithium chloride, and *n*-Bu$_4$Br in a sealed tube generated a number of pyrazolophenanthridines in dimethylformamide at 110 °C in 42-65% yields.

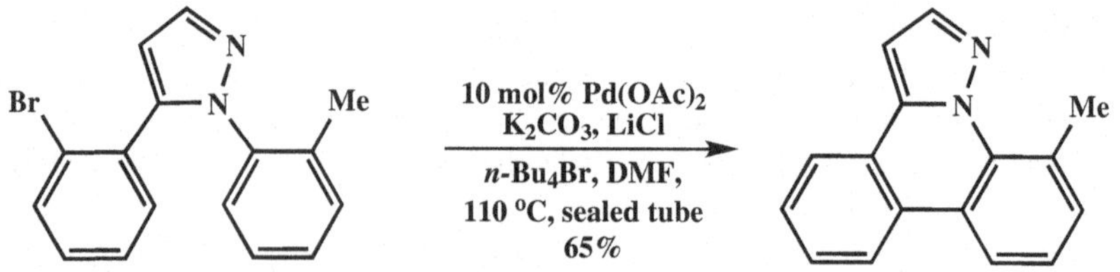

Scheme-70

The γ-aminobutyric acid receptor ligand 2-aryloxazolo-[4,5-*c*]quinolin-4(5*H*)-one was prepared by a intramolecular direct arylation. The fused tricyclic product was formed in 63% yield when ArI was coupled with isoxazole **(Scheme 71)**. If C5 was blocked, thermodynamic control generally directs arylation to carbon that gives lowest energy product, for example with

C5-substituted imidazole, which arylates at C4 forming a 6-membered ring product, rather than reaction at C2 to give a 7-membered ring product **(Scheme 72)**. Sometimes regioselectivity of arylation was controlled simply by having only one carbon-hydrogen available to react, as with substituted oxazole [189].

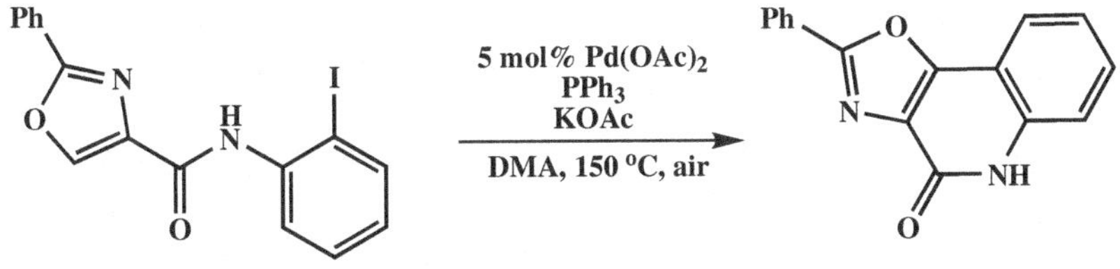

Scheme-71

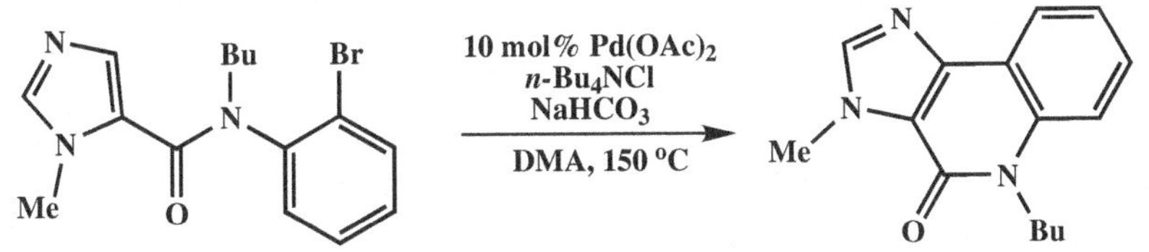

Scheme-72

The *N*-(2-azidophenyl)imines were synthesized by the reaction of 2-azidoaniline and aromatic aldehydes. The formed *N*-(2-azidophenyl)imines were treated with trimethylphosphine followed by with diphenylketene to afford 6,11-dihydrobenzimidazo[1,2-*b*]isoquinolines in excellent yields. The reaction occurred through a formal [4+2] intramolecular cycloaddition of ketenimine with imine function of intermediates. Good yields of benzimidazo[1,2-*b*]isoquinolines were obtained upon refluxing of 6,11-dihydrobenzimidazo[1,2-*b*]isoquinolines with palladium/carbon in PhMe **(Scheme 73)** [187, 190-191].

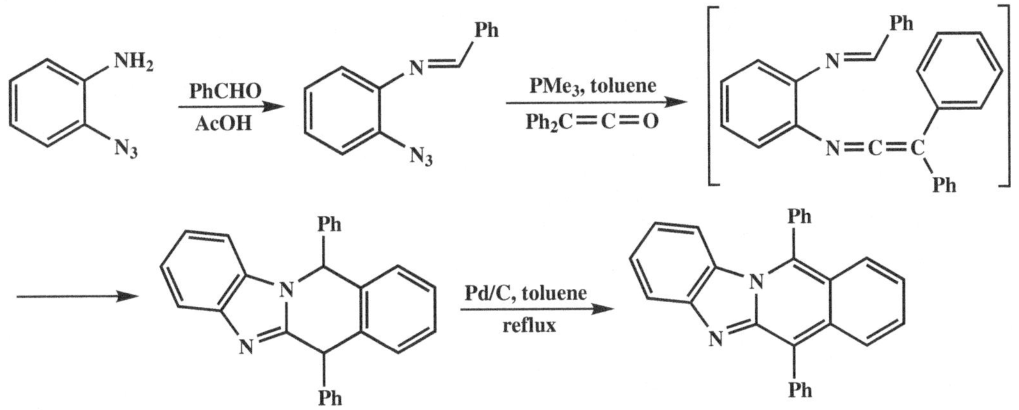

Scheme-73

The iodination of terminal alkynes with *N*-iodomorpholine afforded substrates for CuAAC (azide alkyne cycloaddition) reaction [192]. The substituted 5-iodo-1,2,3-triazoles were produced by copper azide alkyne cycloaddition reaction. The 5-iodo-1,2,3-triazoles underwent a Heck reaction or a carbon-hydrogen bond functionalization to generate the expected fused triazole **(Scheme 74)** [193-200].

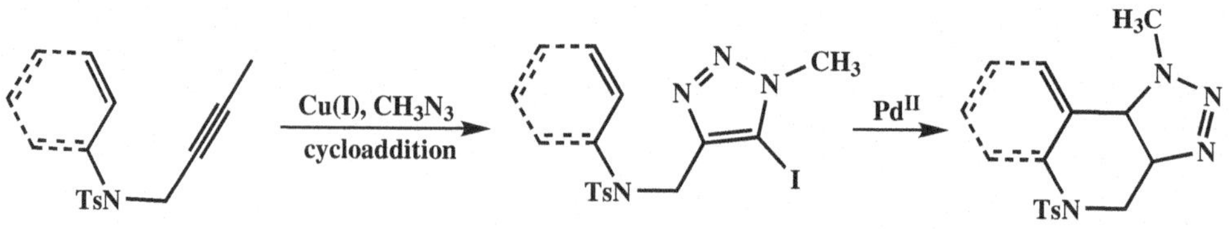

Scheme-74

The synthesis of lycorane by an intramolecular direct arylation of furan with ArI was unsuccessful [201]. Although cyclization occurred in 57% yield **(Scheme 75)**, all attempts for the transformation of cyclized product into required lycorane precursor were failed, forcing the exploration of an alternate route.

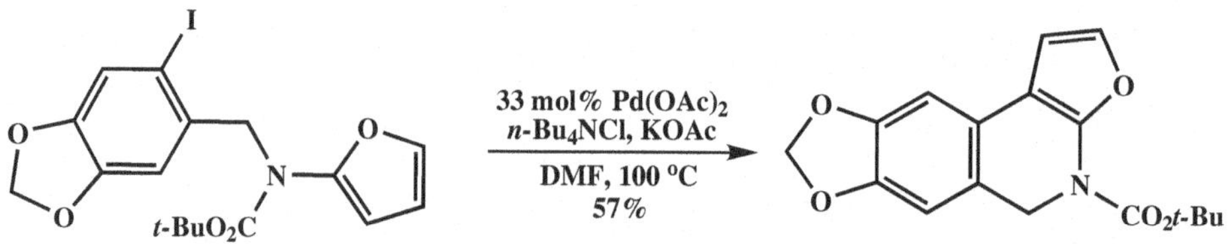

Scheme-75

Organotin reagents $RSnMe_3$ and $RSnBu_3$ were a valuable source of complexity and diversity. They were stable and readily available and were easily interfaced with relay switch reagents. The tris-cyclization-anion capture occurred as shown in **Scheme 76**. The reaction occurred through a Pd-catalyzed [2+2+2]-cycloaddition followed by oxidative addition of palladium(0) [202-209].

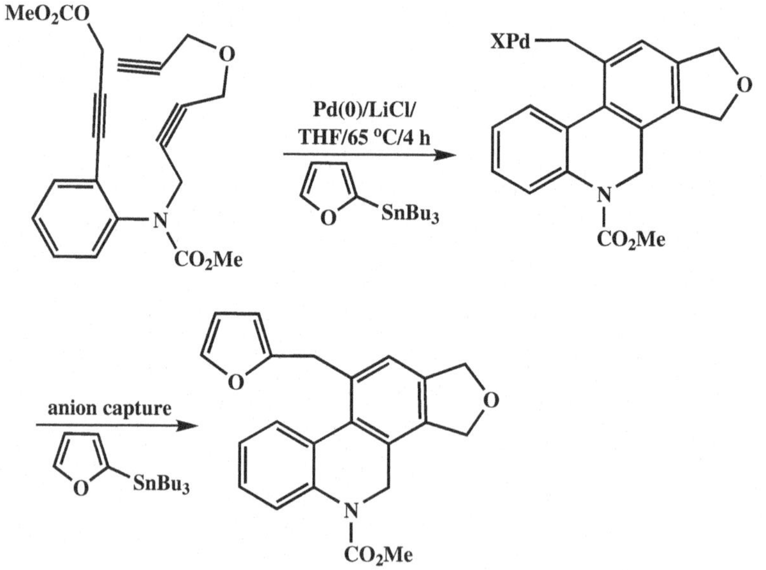

Scheme-76

A novel palladium reagent was prepared from palladium acetate, 1,3-bis(diphenylphosphino) propane, and tributylphosphine. The nitidine and chelerythrine were synthesized through aryl-aryl cyclization reaction in the presence of palladium reagent. This protocol was very versatile for coupling reaction of arene and aromatic triflate as well as for coupling of arene and aromatic halide **(Scheme 77)** [210].

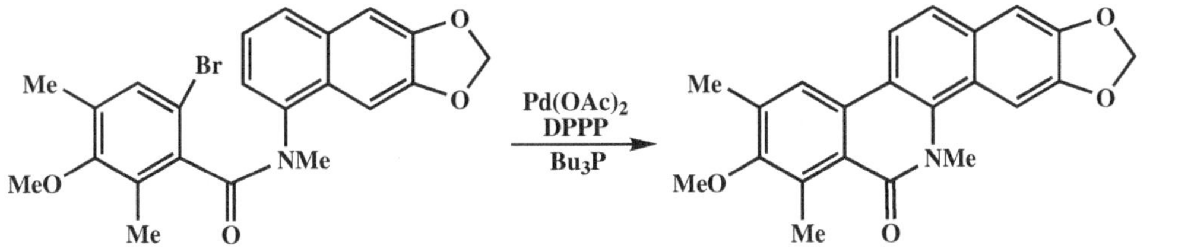

Scheme-77

It has been found that *N*-carbamates [211] and amides [212] can promote analogous processes under optimized conditions **(Scheme 78)**. With this route, *N*-methylcrinasiadine was formed in three steps.

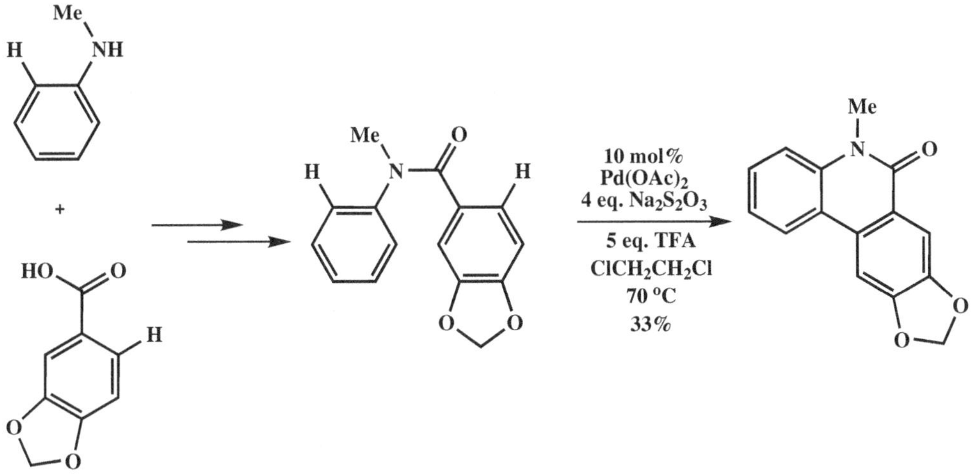

Scheme-78

The benzyl *N*-[2-(2,4-cyclohexadienyl)ethyl]carbamate underwent intramolecular 1,4-chloroamidation reaction for the total synthesis of lycorane alkaloid **(Scheme 79)** [28, 213].

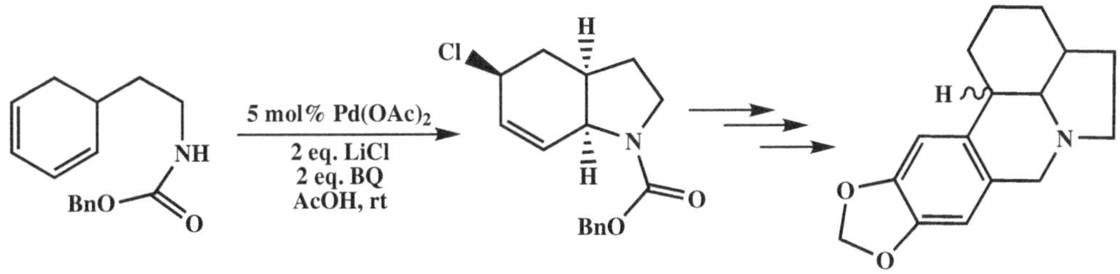

Scheme-79

Seven-membered benzazepinone ring systems were constructed upon cyclization onto C-3 position of benzothiophene [177]. A similar cyclization was also employed for the synthesis of a number of six-membered ring thiophene analogues **(Scheme 80)** [178].

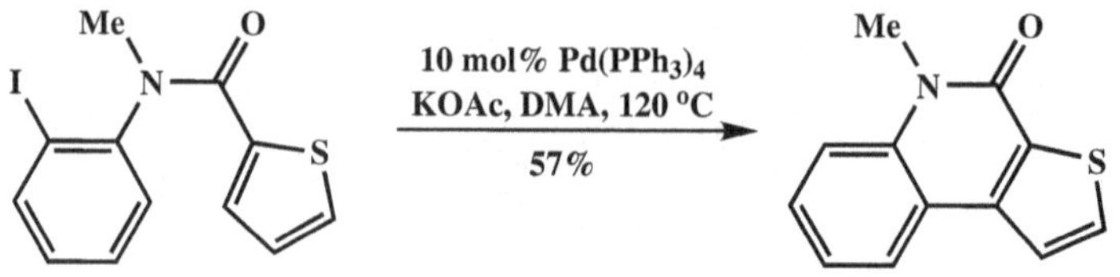

Scheme-80

The benzothiophene acted as a support for iminyl radical and acceptor. The 3-bromo-benzothiophene-2-carbaldehyde was utilized for the formation of precursor. This precursor was irradiated under MW for the synthesis of benzo[*b*]thieno[2,3-*c*]quinoline **(Scheme 81)** [214-217].

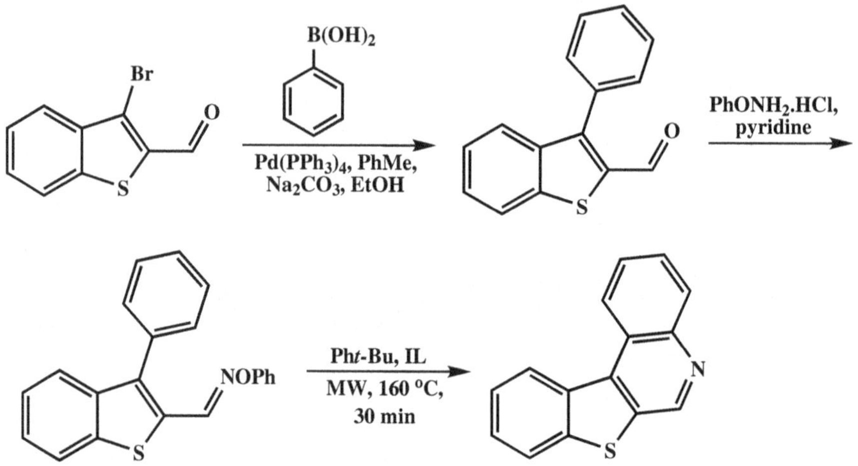

Scheme-81

The 2-acetamido-3-phenylheteroarenes underwent Bischler-Napieralski cyclization to form the 5-methylbenzo[*b*]heteroaryl[2,3-*c*]isoquinolines [218], in turn 2-acetamido-3-phenylheteroarenes were produced by cross-coupling reactions starting either from bromides or triflates in the presence of Pd catalyst **(Scheme 82)** [219].

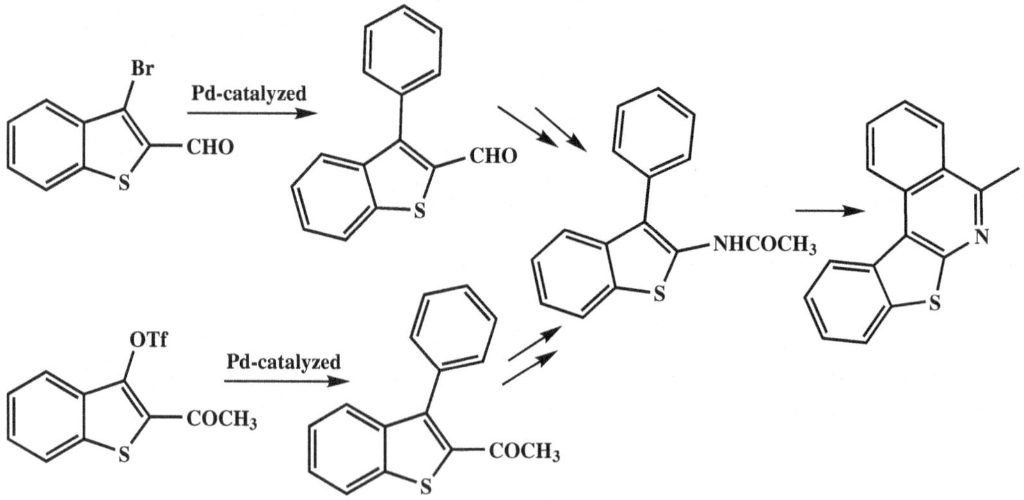

Scheme-82

9.5 Synthesis of six-membered heterocycles fused with six-membered heterocycles

These quinoline compounds were of special interest due to their structural similarity to ellipticine, a potent anti-tumor compound. A family of 6-substituted 4,5,3,2,2-pyrido[3c]quinolines and 6-substituted indolo[3,2-c]quinolines was produced in this method. To prevent the deiodination of starting substrate during Pd-catalyzed cyclization, the secondary amide was protected **(Scheme 83)** [220].

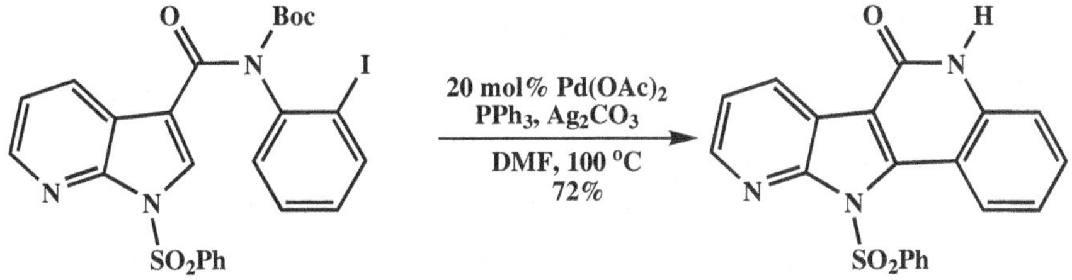

Scheme-83

Curran and Du [221] synthesized 11*H*-indolizino[1,2-*b*]quinolin-9-ones in high yields *via* a Pd-catalyzed cascade reaction of isonitriles with 6-iodo-*N*-propargylpyridone **(Scheme 84)**.

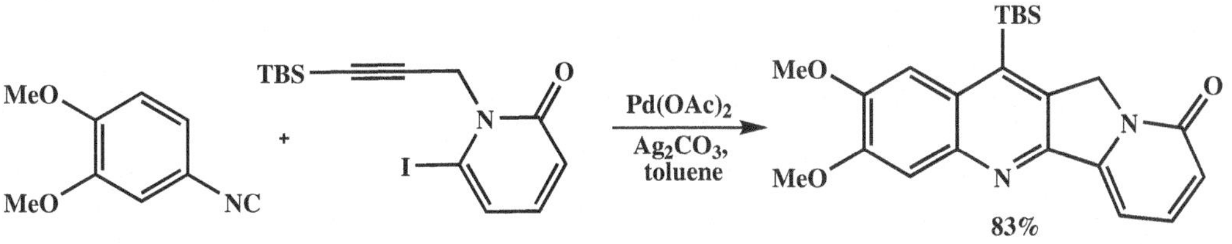

Scheme-84

This hydroamination/cyclization protocol was extended for the construction of opium alkaloids (*S*)-(-)-xylopinine and (*S*)-(+)-laudanosine **(Scheme 85)** [222]. The aminoalkyne was generated by Sonogashira coupling of ArI and phenyl acetylene followed by de-protection of amide. The 3,4-dihydroisoquinoline was formed in high regioselectivity *via* titanium-catalyzed hydroamination/cyclization of aminoalkyne. The 3,4-dihydroisoquinoline was reduced by asymmetric transfer hydrogenation using Noyori's [223] chiral ruthenium catalyst with high enantioselectivity. The 1,2,3,4-tetrahydroisoquinoline *via* reductive amination afforded (*S*)-(+)-laudanosine directly, while (*S*)-(-)-xylopinine was synthesized by Pictet-Spengler cyclization of 1,2,3,4-tetrahydroisoquinoline [18, 224].

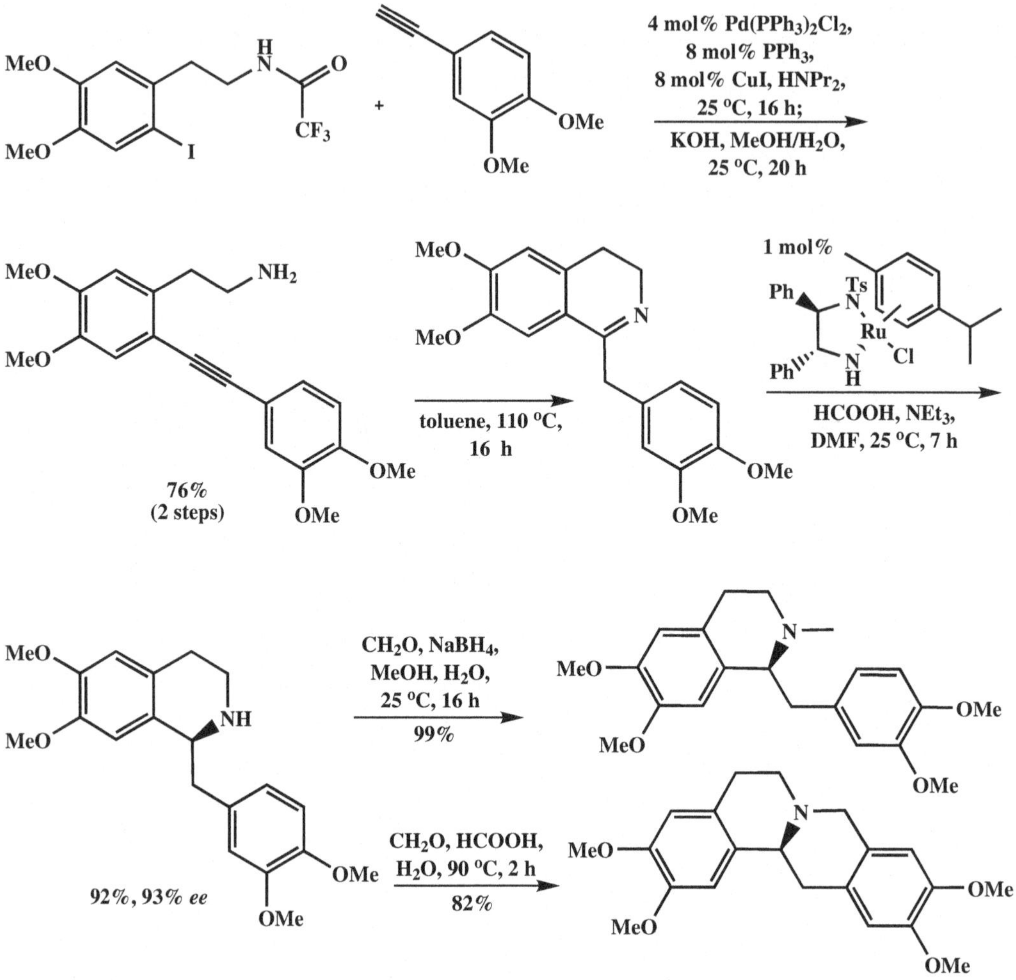

Scheme-85

9.6 Synthesis of six-membered heterocycles fused with seven-membered heterocycles

The 1,4-benzodiazepine-2,5-dione derivatives were prepared (**Scheme 86-87**). The reaction occurred efficiently with "ligandless" Pd acetate catalyst to afford the desired polyheterocycle from bisaryl diiodide [225].

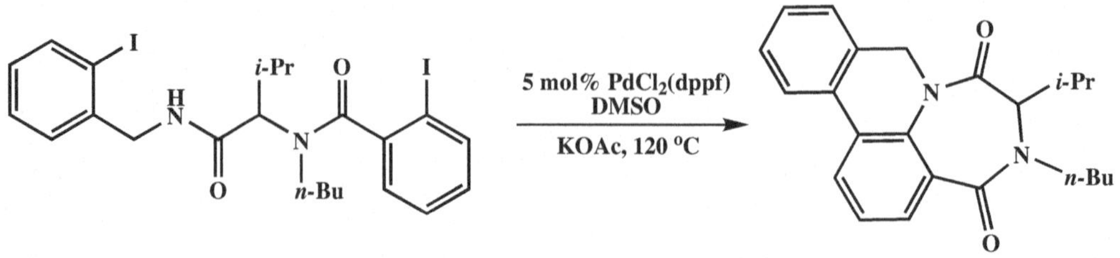

Scheme-86

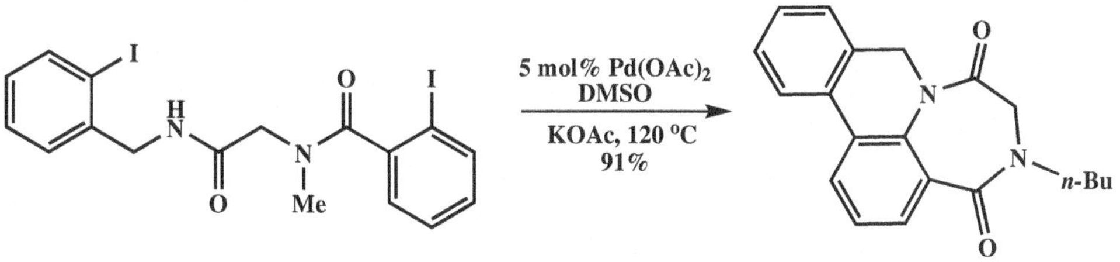

Scheme-87

The silatecans DB-67 and DB-91 were formed using Pd-catalyzed reaction of isonitrile and (*S*)-iodopyridones **(Scheme 88)** [226-230].

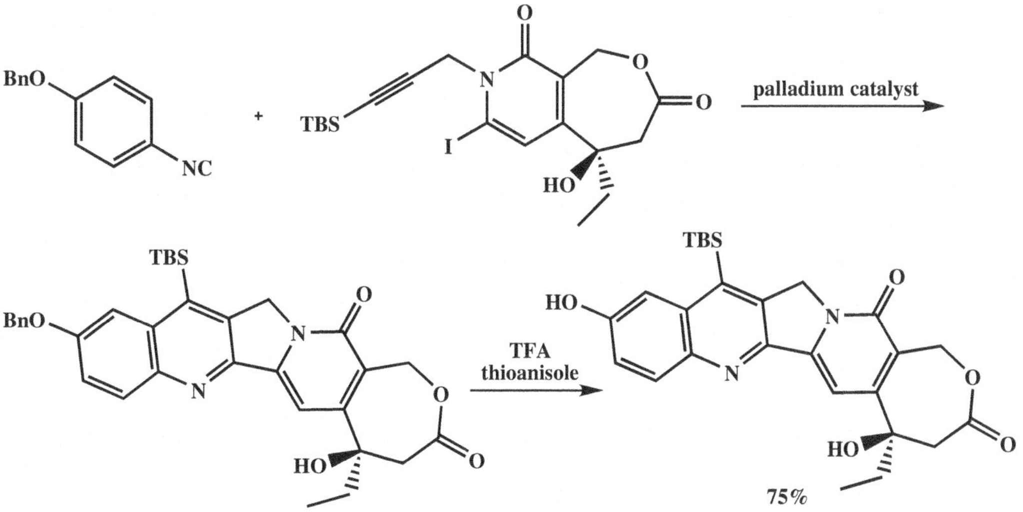

Scheme-88

Grigg [231] reported this protocol which involved anion capture as a part of intramolecular cascade **(Scheme 89)**. This protocol was also initiated *via* same carbopalladation/cyclization and the formation of Pd π-allyl complexes but followed by their interception, through an intramolecular nucleophilic addition, leading to polycyclic isoquinolones.

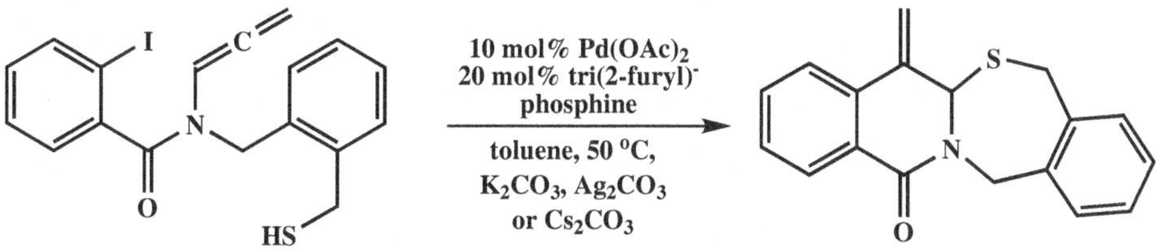

Scheme-89

REFERENCES

[1]   V. Kouznetsov. 2009. Recent synthetic developments in a powerful imino Diels-Alder reaction (Povarov reaction): application to the synthesis of *N*-polyheterocycles and related alkaloids. Tetrahedron. 65: 2721-2750.

[2]   A.D. Kinghorn, Y.W. Chin and S.M. Swanson. 2009. Discovery of natural product anti-cancer agents from biodiverse organisms. Curr. Opin. Drug Discov. Devel. 12: 189-196.

[3]   A. Marella, O.P. Tanwar, R. Saha, M.R. Ali, S. Srivastava, M. Akhter, M. Shaquiquzzaman and M.M. Alam. 2013. Quinoline: a versatile heterocyclic. Saudi Pharm. J. 21: 1-12.

[4]   C.M. Nunes, I. Reva, T.M.V.D. Pinho e Melo and R. Fausto. 2012. UV-Laser photochemistry of isoxazole isolated in a low-temperature matrix. J. Org. Chem. 77: 8723-8732.

[5]   X. Ma, W. Zhou and R. Brun. 2009. Synthesis, *in vitro* anti-trypanosomal and anti-bacterial activity of phenoxy, phenylthio or benzyloxy substituted quinolones. Bioorg. Med. Chem. Lett. 19: 986-989.

[6]   R.E. Khidre and B.F.A. Wahab. 2013. Synthesis of 5-membered heterocycles using benzoylacetonitriles as synthon. Turk. J. Chem. 37: 685-711.

[7]   L.W. Deady, T. Rodemann, G.J. Finalay, B.C. Baguley and W.A. Denny. 2001. Synthesis and cytotoxic activity of carboxamide derivatives of benzimidazo[2,1-*a*]isoquinoline and pyrido[3′,2′:4,5] imidazo[2,1-*a*]isoquinoline. Anticancer Drug Des. 15: 339-346.

[8]   R.D. Carpenter, K.S. Lam and M.J. Kurth. 2007. Microwave-mediated heterocyclization to benzimidazo[2,1-*b*]quinazolin-12(5*H*)-ones. J. Org. Chem. 72: 284-287.

[9]   D. Alberico, M.E. Scott and M. Lautens. 2007. Aryl bond formation by transition-metal-catalyzed direct arylation. Chem. Rev. 107: 174-238

[10]   H.-P. Husson and J. Royer. 1999. Chiral non-racemic *N*-cyanomethyloxazolidines: the pivotal system of the CN(R,S) method. Chem. Soc. Rev. 28: 383-394.

[11]   A.J. Walz and R.J. Sunberg. 2000. Synthesis of 8-methoxy-1-methyl-1*H*-benzo[*de*][1,6]naphthyridin-9-ol (isoaaptamine) and analogues. J. Org. Chem. 65: 8001-8010.

[12]   A.M. Thompson, C.J.C. Connolly, J.M. Hamby, S. Boushelle, B.G. Hartl, A.M. Amar, A.J. Kraker, D.L. Driscoll, R.W. Steinkampf, S.J. Patmore, P.W. Vincent, B.J. Roberts, W.L. Elliott, W. Klohs, W.R. Leopold, H.D.H. Showalter and W.A. Denny. 2000. 3-(3,5-Dimethoxyphenyl)-1,6-naphthyridine-2,7-diamines and related 2-urea derivatives are potent and selective inhibitors of the fGF receptor-1 tyrosine kinase. J. Med. Chem. 43: 4200-4211.

[13]   K. Mogilaiah and K. Vidya. 2006. Synthesis and anti-bacterial activity of 1,3,4-oxadiazolyl-l,8-naphthyridines. Indian J. Chem. 42B: 1905-1908.

[14]   M.S. Saeed, M.G. Elerafi, R. Mohamed. 2011. Synthesis of benzo-fused six-membered aromatic heterocycles. Der Chemica Sinica 2: 66-69.

[15]   P. Majumdar, A. Pati, M. Patra, R.K. Behera and A.K. Behera. 2014. Acid hydrazides, potent reagents for synthesis of oxygen-, nitrogen-, and/or sulfur-containing heterocyclic rings. Chem. Rev. 114: 2942-2977.

[16]   (a) N. Kaur. 2015. Environmentally benign synthesis of five-membered 1,3-*N,N*-heterocycles by microwave irradiation. Synth. Commun. 45: 909-943.
        (b) N. Kaur. 2015. Advances in microwave-assisted synthesis for five-membered *N*-heterocycles synthesis. Synth. Commun. 45: 432-457.
        (c) N. Kaur. 2014. Microwave-assisted synthesis of five-membered *S*-heterocycles. J. Iran. Chem. Soc. 11: 523-564.
        (d) N. Kaur. 2015. Review on the synthesis of six-membered *N,N*-heterocycles by microwave irradiation. Synth. Commun. 45: 1145-1182.
        (e) N. Kaur. 2015. Greener and expeditious synthesis of fused six-membered *N,N*-heterocycles using microwave irradiation. Synth. Commun. 45: 1493-1519.
        (f) N. Kaur. 2015. Applications of microwaves in the synthesis of polycyclic six-membered *N,N*-heterocycles. Synth. Commun. 45: 1599-1631.
        (g) N. Kaur. 2015. Synthesis of five-membered *N,N,N*- and *N,N,N,N*-heterocyclic compounds: applications of microwaves. Synth. Commun. 45: 1711-1742.

[17]   N. Sakai, A. Ridder and J.F. Hartwig. 2006. Tropene derivatives by sequential intermolecular and transannular, intramolecular palladium-catalyzed hydroamination of cycloheptatriene. J. Am. Soc. Chem. 128: 8134-8135.

[18]   T.E. Muller, K.C. Hultzsch, M. Yus, F. Foubelo and M. Tada. 2008. Hydroamination: direct addition of amines to alkenes and alkynes. Chem. Rev. 108: 3795-3892.

[19] Z. Shi, B. Zhang, Y. Cui and N. Jiao. 2010. Palladium-catalyzed ring-expansion reaction of indoles with alkynes: from indoles to tetrahydroquinoline derivatives under mild reaction conditions. Angew. Chem. Int. Ed. 49: 4036-4041.

[20] Z. Shi, C. Zhang, C. Tanga and N. Jiao. 2012. Recent advances in transition-metal catalyzed reactions using molecular oxygen as the oxidant. Chem. Soc. Rev. 41: 3381-3430.

[21] N. Beydoun and M. Pfeffer. 1990. Synthesis of *N*-methylbenzo[*d,e*]quinolines. Synthesis 8: 729-731.

[22] D.E. Ames and A. Opalko. 1984. Palladium-catalyzed cyclization of 2-substituted halogenoarenes by dehydrohalogenation. Tetrahedron 40: 1919-1925.

[23] D.D. Hennings, S. Iwasa and V.H. Rawal. 1997. Anion-accelerated palladium-catalyzed intramolecular coupling of phenols with aryl halides. J. Org. Chem. 62: 2-3.

[24] L.-C. Campeau, M. Parisien and K. Fagnou. 2004. Biaryl synthesis *via* direct arylation: establishment of an efficient catalyst for intramolecular processes. J. Am. Chem. Soc. 126: 9186-9187.

[25] L.-C. Campeau, M. Parisien, A. Jean and K. Fagnou. 2006. Catalytic direct arylation with aryl chlorides, bromides, and iodides: intramolecular studies leading to new intermolecular reactions. J. Am. Chem. Soc. 128: 581-590.

[26] L.-C. Campeau, P. Thanssandote and K. Fagnou. 2005. High-yielding intramolecular direct arylation reactions with aryl chlorides. Org. Lett. 7: 1857-1860.

[27] M. Miura, T. Tsuda, T. Satoh, S. Pivsa-Art and M. Nomura. 1998. Oxidative cross-coupling of *N*-(2'-phenylphenyl)benzene-sulfonamides or benzoic and naphthoic acids with alkenes using a palladium-copper catalyst system under air. J. Org. Chem. 63: 5211-5215.

[28] E.M. Beccalli, G. Broggini, M. Martinelli and S. Sottocornola. 2007. C-C, C-O, C-N Bond formation on sp^2 carbon by Pd(II)-catalyzed reactions involving oxidant agents. Chem. Rev. 107: 5318-5365.

[29] N. Kaur. 2018. Photochemical reactions as key steps in five-membered *N*-heterocycles synthesis. Synth. Commun. 48: 1259-1284.

[30] Y.J. Shang, C. Wang, X.W. He, K. Ju, M. Zhang, S.Y. Yu and J.P. Wu. 2010. DMAP-catalyzed cascade reaction: one-pot synthesis of benzofurans in water. Tetrahedron 66: 9629-9633.

[31] G. Kumaraswamy, G. Ramakrishna, R. Raju and M. Padmaja. 2010. An expedient synthesis of enantioenriched substituted (2-benzofuryl)arylcarbinols *via* tandem Rap-Stoermer and asymmetric transfer hydrogenation reactions. Tetrahedron 66: 9814-9818.

[32] B. Liegault, D. Lapointe, L. Caron, A. Vlassova and K. Fagnou. 2009. Establishment of broadly applicable reaction conditions for the palladium-catalyzed direct arylation of heteroatom-containing aromatic compounds. J. Org. Chem. 74: 1826-1834.

[33] S. Chaudhary and W.W. Harding. 2011. Synthesis of C-homoaporphines *via* microwave-assisted direct arylation. Tetrahedron 67: 569-575.

[34] S.I. Gorelsky, D. Lapointe and K. Fagnou. 2008. Analysis of the concerted metalation-deprotonation mechanism in palladium-catalyzed direct arylation across a broad range of aromatic substrates. J. Am. Chem. Soc. 130: 10848-10849.

[35] X.L. Xing, J.L. Wu, J.L. Luo and W.-M. Dai. 2006. C-N Bond-linked conjugates of dibenz[*b, f*][1,4]oxazepines with 2-oxindole. Synlett 13: 2099-2103.

[36] P. Appukkuttan, A.B. Orts, R.P. Chandran, J.L. Goeman, J. van der Eycken, W. Dehaen and E. van der Eycken. 2004. Generation of a small library of highly electron-rich 2-(hetero)aryl-substituted phenethylamines by the Suzuki-Miyaura reaction: a short synthesis of an apogalanthamine analogue. Eur. J. Org. Chem. 15: 3277-3285.

[37] A. Padwa, W.F. Rieker and R.J. Rosenthal. 1985. Studies dealing with the intramolecular ene reaction of cyclopropene derivatives. J. Am. Chem. Soc. 107: 1710-1717.

[38] M.E. Jung, P.Y.S. Lam, M.M. Mansuri and L.M. Speltz. 1985. Stereoselective synthesis of an analog of podophyllotoxin by an intramolecular Diels-Alder reaction. J. Org. Chem. 50: 1087-1105.

[39] R.D. Clark and Jahangir. 1989. Synthetic studies on the lithiated toluamide-imine cycloaddition route to (+)-corydalic acid methyl ester. J. Org. Chem. 54: 1174-1178.

[40] S.V. Gagnier and R.C. Larock. 2003. Palladium-catalyzed carbonylative cyclization of unsaturated aryl iodides and dienyl triflates, iodides, and bromides to indanones and 2-cyclopentenones. J. Am. Chem. Soc. 125: 4804-4807.

[41] M. Harmata and X. Hong. 2003. The intramolecular, stereoselective addition of sulfoximine carbanions to α,β-unsaturated esters. J. Am. Chem. Soc. 125: 5754-5756.

[42] P. Appukkuttan, E. van der Eycken and W. Dehaen. 2005. Microwave-enhanced cadogan cyclization: an easy access to the 2-substituted carbazoles and other fused heterocyclic systems. Synlett 1: 127-133.

[43] P. Appukkuttan, W. Dehaen and E.V. Eycken. 2007. Microwave-assisted transition-metal-catalyzed synthesis of N-shifted and ring-expanded buflavine analogues. Chem. Eur. J. 13: 6452-6460.

[44] T. Harayama, A. Hori, Y. Nakano, T. Akiyama, H. Abe and Y. Takeuchi. 2002. Aryl-aryl coupling reaction catalyzed by a palladium reagent prepared from Pd(OAc)$_2$ and n-Bu$_3$P. Heterocycles 58: 159-164.

[45] T. Harayama, H. Toko, K. Kubota, H. Nishioka, H. Abe and Y. Takeuchi. 2002. Studies on the selective intramolecular biaryl coupling reaction of 2-triflyloxy-6-halobenzanilides using a palladium reagent. Heterocycles 58: 175-181.

[46] T. Harayama, Y. Kawata, C. Nagura, T. Sato, T. Miyagoe, H. Abe and Y. Takeuchi. 2005. Effect of oxygen substituents on the regioselectivity of the Pd-assisted biaryl coupling reaction of benzanilides. Tetrahedron Lett. 46: 6091-6094.

[47] H. Nishioka, Y. Shoujiguchi, H. Abe, Y. Takeuchi and T. Harayama. 2004. Intramolecular Pd-catalyzed biaryl coupling reaction of N-aryl-2-triflyloxybenzamides using Pd(OAc)$_2$, 1,3-bis[diphenylphosphino] propane, Bu$_3$P and DBU. Heterocycles 64: 463-466.

[48] X. Zhao, C.S. Yeung and V.M. Dong. 2010. Palladium-catalyzed o-arylation of O-phenylcarbamates with simple arenes and sodium persulfate. J. Am. Chem. Soc. 132: 5837-5844.

[49] J. Dupont, C.S. Consorti and J. Spencer. 2005. The potential of palladacycles: more than just precatalysts. Chem. Rev. 105: 2527-2571.

[50] W. Doepke, H.P. Lam, E. Gruendemann, M. Bartoszek and S. Flatau. 1995. Alkaloids from *Hippeastrum equestre* herb. Pharmazie 50: 511-512.

[51] R. Suau, A.I. Gomez and R. Rico. 1990. Ismine and related alkaloids from *Lapiedra martinezii*. Phytochemistry 29: 1710-1712.

[52] G. Cahiez, A. Moyeux, J. Buendia and C. Duplais. 2007. Manganese- or iron-catalyzed homocoupling of Grignard reagents using atmospheric oxygen as an oxidant. J. Am. Chem. Soc. 129: 13788-13789.

[53] G. Cahiez, C. Chaboche, F. Mahuteau-Betzer and M. Ahr. 2005. Iron-catalyzed homo-coupling of simple and functionalized arylmagnesium reagents. Org. Lett. 7: 1943-1946.

[54] M.G. Banwell, B.D. Bissett, S. Busato, C.J. Cowden, D.C.R. Hockless, J.W. Holman, R.W. Read and A.W. Wu. 1995. Trifluoromethanesulfonic anhydride-4-(N,N-dimethylamino)pyridine as a reagent combination for effecting Bischler-Napieraiski cyclization under mild conditions: application to total syntheses of the *Amaryllidaceae* alkaloids N-methylcrinasiadine, anhydrolycorinone, hippadine and oxoassoanine. J. Chem. Soc. Chem. Commun. 24: 2551-2553.

[55] M.G. Banwell and C.J. Cowden. 1994. Convergent routes to the [1,3]dioxolo[4,5-j]phenanthridin-6(5H)-one and 2,3,4,4a-tetrahydro[1,3]dioxolo[4,5-j]phenanthridin-6(5H)-one nuclei. Application to syntheses of the *Amaryllidaceae* alkaloids crinasiadine, N-methylcrinasiadine and trisphaeridine. Aust. J. Chem. 47: 2235-2254.

[56] W.R. Bowman, H. Heaney and B.M. Jordan. 1991. Oxidation during reductive cyclizations using Bu$_3$SnH. Tetrahedron 47: 10119-10128.

[57] J. Grimshaw, R. Hamilton and J. Trocha-Grimshaw. 1982. Electrochemical reactions. Reductive cyclization of i-(2-halogenophenyl)-j-phenyl compounds: a general reaction. J. Chem. Soc. Perkin Trans. 1 229-234.

[58] R.K.-Y. Zee-Cheng, S.-J. Yan and C.C. Cheng. 1978. Anti-leukemic activity of ungeremine and related compounds. Preparation of analogs of ungeremine by a practical photochemical reaction. J. Med. Chem. 21: 199-203.

[59] A. Mondon and K. Krohn. 1972. Synthese des narciprimins und verwandter verbindungen. Chem. Ber. 105: 3726-3747.

[60] H.S. Forrest, R.D. Haworth, A.R. Pinder and T.S. Stevens. 1949. Experiments on the synthesis of the *Chelidonium* alkaloids. J. Chem. Soc. 1311-1313.

[61]   S. Nandi and J.K. Ray. 2009. Palladium-catalyzed cyclization/cyclopropanation reaction for the synthesis of fused *N*-containing heterocycles. Tetrahedron Lett. 50: 6993-6997.

[62]   S. Nag and S. Batra. 2011. Applications of allylamines for the syntheses of aza-heterocycles. Tetrahedron 67: 8959-9061.

[63]   J. Karthikeyan and C.-H. Cheng. 2011. Synthesis of phenanthridinones from *N*-methoxybenzamides and arenes by multiple palladium-catalyzed C-H activation steps at room temperature. Angew. Chem. Int. Ed. 50: 9880-9883.

[64]   A.V. Gulevich and V. Gevorgyan. 2012. Synthesis of fused heterocycles *via* Pd-catalyzed multiple aromatic C-H activation reactions. Chem. Heterocycl. Comp. 48: 17-20.

[65]   Z. Ma, Z. Xiang, T. Luo, K. Lu, Z. Xu, J. Chen and Z. Yang. 2006. Synthesis of functionalized quinolines *via* Ugi and Pd-catalyzed intramolecular arylation reactions. J. Comb. Chem. 8: 696-704.

[66]   M. Parisien, D. Valette and K. Fagnou. 2005. Direct arylation reactions catalyzed by Pd(OH)$_2$/C: evidence for a soluble palladium catalyst. J. Org. Chem. 70: 7578-7584.

[67]   Z. Xiang, T. Luo, K. Lu, J. Cui, X. Shi, R. Fathi, J. Chen and Z. Yang. 2004. Concise synthesis of isoquinoline *via* the Ugi and Heck reactions. Org. Lett. 6: 3155-3158.

[68]   T. Konno, J. Chae, T. Miyabe and T. Ishihara. 2005. Regioselective one-step synthesis of 4-fluoroalkylated isoquinolines *via* carbopalladation reaction of fluorine-containing alkynes. J. Org. Chem. 70: 10172-10174.

[69]   G. Pandey and M. Balakrishnan. 2008. Suzuki cross-coupling/reductive debenzyloxycarbonylation sequence for the syntheses of [*c*]annulated isoquinolines: application for the syntheses of pancratistatin-like isoquinolines. J. Org. Chem. 73: 8128-8131.

[70]   G.-W. Wang, T.-T. Yuan and D.-D. Li. 2011. One-pot formation of C-C and C-N bonds through palladium-catalyzed dual C-H activation: synthesis of phenanthridinones. Angew. Chem. Int. Ed. 50: 1380-1383.

[71]   J.-P. Leclerc, M. Andre and K. Fagnou. 2006. Tandem Heck, direct arylation, and hydrogenation: two or three sequential reactions from a single catalyst. J. Org. Chem. 71: 1711-1714.

[72]   T. Harayama, T. Sato, A. Hori, H. Abe and Y. Takeuchi. 2003. Novel synthesis of naphthobenzazepines from *N*-bromobenzylnaphthylamines by regioselective C-H activation utilizing the intramolecular coordination of an amine to Pd. Synlett 8: 1141-1144.

[73]   T. Harayama, T. Sato, A. Hori, H. Abe and Y. Takeuchi. 2004. Novel synthesis of a new skeletal compound benzonaphthazepine by regioselective C-H activation utilizing the intramolecular coordination of an amine to Pd. Synthesis 9: 1446-1456.

[74]   R. Grigg, V. Savic and V. Tambyrajah. 2000. Phenanthrene type heterocycles *via* Rh(I) catalyzed [2+2+2]-cycloaddition and Pd(0) catalyzed arylation. Tetrahedron Lett. 41: 3003-3006.

[75]   A.R. Dick, M.S. Remy, J.W. Kampf and M.S. Sanford. 2007. Carbon-nitrogen bond-forming reactions between palladacycles and hypervalent iodine reagents. Organometallics 26: 1365-1370.

[76]   Y. Kohmura and T. Katsuki. 2001. Mn(salen)-catalyzed enantioselective C-H amination. Tetrahedron 42: 3339-3342.

[77]   M. Yamawaki, H. Tsutsui, S. Kitagaki, M. Anada and S. Hashimoto. 2002. Dirhodium(II) tetrakis [*N*-tetrachlorophthaloyl-(*S*)-*tert*-leucinate]: a new chiral Rh(II) catalyst for enantioselective amidation of C-H bonds. Tetraheron Lett. 43: 9561-9564.

[78]   M.M. Diaz-Requejo, T.R. Belderrain, M.C. Nicasio, S. Trofimenko and P.J. Perez. 2003. Cyclohexane and benzene amination by catalytic nitrene insertion into C-H bonds with the copper-homoscorpionate catalyst TpBr$_3$CuNCMe. J. Am. Chem. Soc. 125: 12078-12079.

[79]   M.R. Fructos, S. Trofimenko, M.M. Diaz-Requejo and P.J. Perez. 2006. Facile amine formation by intermolecular catalytic amidation of carbon-hydrogen bonds. J. Am. Chem. Soc. 128: 11784-11791.

[80]   K. Kamaraj and D. Bandyopadhyay. 1999. Mechanism of palladium-carbon bond oxidation: dramatic solvent effect. Organometallics 18: 438-446.

[81]   K. Kamaraj and D. Bandyopadhyay. 1997. Oxene versus non-oxene reactive intermediates in iron(III) porphyrin catalyzed oxidation reactions: organometallic compounds as diagnostic probes. J. Am. Chem. Soc. 119: 8099-8100.

[82]   A.R. Dick, J.W. Kampf and M.S. Sanford. 2005. Unusually stable palladium(IV) complexes: detailed mechanistic investigation of C-O bond-forming reductive elimination. J. Am. Chem. Soc. 127: 12790-12791.

[83]   D. Kalyani, A.R. Dick, W.Q. Anani and M.S. Sanford. 2006. Scope and selectivity in palladium-catalyzed directed C-H bond halogenation reactions. Tetrahedron 62: 11483-11498.

[84]   D. Kalyani, A.R. Dick, W.Q. Anani and M.S. Sanford. 2006. A simple catalytic method for the regioselective halogenation of arenes. Org. Lett. 8: 2523-2526.

[85]   J. Jacobs, B.M. Mbala, B. Kesteleyn, G. Diels and N. De Kimpe. 2008. Straightforward palladium-mediated synthesis of *N*-substituted 1,2-dihydrobenz[*g*]isoquinoline-5,10-diones. Tetrahedron 64: 6364-6371.

[86]   A. Navarro-Vázquez, D. Rodriguez, M.F. Martinez-Esperon, A. Garcia, C. Saa and D. Dominguez. 2007. Acid-catalyzed cyclization of acyliminium ions derived from allenamides. A new entry to protoberberines. Tetrahedron Lett. 48: 2741-2743.

[87]   K. Muniz. 2007. Advancing palladium-catalyzed C-N bond formation: bisindoline construction from successive amide transfer to internal alkenes. J. Am. Chem. Soc. 129: 14542-14543.

[88]   S.L. Marquard, D.C. Rosenfeld and J.F. Hartwig. 2010. C(sp^3)-N bond-forming reductive elimination of amines: reactions of bisphosphine-ligated benzylpalladium(II) diarylamido complexes. Angew. Chem. 122: 805-808; Angew. Chem. Int. Ed. 49: 793-796.

[89]   L.D. Julian and J.F. Hartwig. 2010. Intramolecular hydroamination of unbiased and functionalized primary aminoalkenes catalyzed by a rhodium aminophosphine complex. J. Am. Chem. Soc. 132: 13813-13822.

[90]   S.V. Pronin, M.G. Tabor, D.J. Jansen and R.A. Shenvi. 2012. A stereoselective hydroamination transform to access polysubstituted indolizidines. J. Am. Chem. Soc. 134: 2012-2015.

[91]   A. Iglesias, R. Alvarez, A.R. de Lera and K. Muniz. 2012. Palladium-catalyzed intermolecular C(sp^3)-H amidation. Angew. Chem. 124: 2268-2271; Angew. Chem. Int. Ed. 51: 2225-2228.

[92]   Z. Liang, L. Ju, Y. Xie, L. Huang and Y. Zhang. 2012. Free-amine-directed alkenylation of (sp^2)-H and cycloamination by palladium catalysis. Chem. Eur. J. 18: 15816-15821.

[93]   L. Bijeire, L. Legentil, J. Bastide, F. Darro, C. Rochart and E. Delfourne. 2004. A total synthesis of subarine, a marine alkaloid related to the pyridoacridine family. Eur. J. Org. Chem. 9: 1891-1893.

[94]   S.A. Hitchcock, D.R. Mayhugh and G.S. Gregory. 1995. Selectivity in palladium(0)-catalyzed cross-coupling reactions: application to a tandem Stille reaction. Tetrahedron Lett. 36: 9085-9088.

[95]   N. Zhang, L. Thomas and B. Wu. 2001. Palladium-catalyzed selective cross-coupling between 2-bromopyridines and aryl bromides. J. Org. Chem. 66: 1500-1502.

[96]   B. Bachowska and T. Zujewska. 2001. Chemistry and applications of benzonaphthyridines. ARKIVOC (vi): 77-84.

[97]   A. Nadin, J.M.S. Lopez, A.P. Owens, D.M. Howells, A.C. Talbot and T. Harrison. 2003. New synthesis of 1,3-dihydro-1,4-benzodiazepin-2(2*H*)-ones and 3-amino-1,3-dihydro-1,4-benzodiazepin-2(2*H*)-ones: Pd-catalyzed cross-coupling of imidoyl chlorides with organoboronic acids. J. Org. Chem. 68: 2844-2852.

[98]   A. Godard and G. Queguiner. 1982. Synthesis of benzonaphthyridines. J. Heterocycl. Chem. 19: 1289-1296.

[99]   J.Y. Bass, J.A. Caravella, L. Chen, K.L. Creech, D.N. Deaton, K.P. Madauss, H.B. Marr, R.B. McFadyen, A.B. Miller, W.Y. Mills, F. Navas, D.J. Parks, T.L. Smalley, P.K. Spearing, D. Todd, S.P. Williams and G.B. Wisely. 2011. Conformationally constrained farnesoid X receptor (FXR) agonists: heteroaryl replacements of the naphthalene. Bioorg. Med. Chem. Lett. 21: 1206-1213.

[100] P.A. Keller. 2005. Hetarenes and related ring systems. Sci. Synth. 15: 1065-1088.

[101] S.P. Khanapure, D.S. Garvey, D.V. Young, M. Ezawa, R.A. Earl, R.D. Gaston, X. Fang, M. Murty, A. Martino, M. Shumway, M. Trocha, P. Marek, S.W. Tam, D.R. Janero and L.G. Letts. 2003. Synthesis and structure-activity relationship of novel, highly potent metharyl and methcycloalkyl cyclooxygenase-2 (COX-2) selective inhibitors. J. Med. Chem. 46: 5484-5504.

[102] J.H. Boyer and J.R. Patel. 1978. Cyclization from aryl formamides in phosphorus oxychloride and tin(IV) chloride. Synthesis 3: 205-205.

[103] M. Islami-Moghaddam, H. Mansouri-Torshizi, A. Divaslar and A. Saboury. 2009. Synthesis, characterization, cytotoxic and DNA binding studies of diimine platinum(II) and palladium(II) complexes of short hydrocarbon chain ethyldithiocarbamate ligand. J. Iran. Chem. Soc. 6: 552-569.

[104] T. Gerfaud, C. Xie, L. Neuville and J. Zhu. 2011. Protecting group free total synthesis of (*E*)- and (*Z*)-alstoscholarine. Angew. Chem. Int. Ed. 50: 3954-3957.

[105] T.T. Jayanth, L. Zhang, T.S. Johnson and H.C. Malinakova. 2009. Sequential Cu(I)/Pd(0)-catalyzed multicomponent coupling and annulation protocol for the synthesis of indenoisoquinolines. Org. Lett. 11: 815-818.

[106] S. Su and J.A. Porco. 2007. Synthesis of pyrrolo-isoquinolines related to the lamellarins using silver-catalyzed cycloisomerization/dipolar cycloaddition. J. Am. Chem. Soc. 129: 7744-7745.

[107] C. Blaszykowski, E. Aktoudianakis, C. Bressy, D. Alberico and M. Lautens. 2006. Preparation of annulated nitrogen-containing heterocycles *via* a one-pot palladium-catalyzed alkylation/direct arylation sequence. Org. Lett. 8: 2043-2045.

[108] N. Lettowianthine, D. Lamellarin, M.H.H. Kunya, S.A. Jonker, J.J. Makangara, R. Waibel and H. Achenbach. 2000. *Aporphinoid* alkaloids and other constituents from *Lettowianthus stellatus*. Phytochemistry 53: 1067-1073.

[109] M. Facompre, C. Tardy, C. Bal-Mahieu, P. Colson, C. Perez, I. Manzanares, C. Cuevas and C. Bailly. 2003. Lamellarin D: a novel potent inhibitor of topoisomerase I. Cancer Res. 63: 7392-7399.

[110] D. Pla, A. Marchal, C.A. Olsen, F. Albericio and M. Alvarez. 2005. Modular total synthesis of lamellarin D. J. Org. Chem. 70: 8231-8234.

[111] C. Blaszykowski, E. Aktoudianakis, D. Alberico, C. Bressy, D.G. Hulcoop, F. Jafarpour, A. Joushaghani, B. Laleu and M. Lautens. 2008. A palladium-catalyzed alkylation/direct arylation synthesis of nitrogen-containing heterocycles. J. Org. Chem. 73: 1888-1897.

[112] A. Furstner and J.W.J. Kennedy. 2006. Total syntheses of the *Tylophora* alkaloids cryptopleurine, (-)-antofine, (-)-tylophorine, and (-)-ficuseptine C. Chem. Eur. J. 12: 7398-7410.

[113] R.G. Vaswani and A.R. Chamberlin. 2008. Stereocontrolled total synthesis of (-)-kaitocephalin. J. Org. Chem. 73: 1661-1681.

[114] G. Evano, N. Blanchard and M. Toumi. 2008. Copper-mediated coupling reactions and their applications in natural products and designed biomolecules synthesis. Chem. Rev. 108: 3054-3131.

[115] S. Ozaki, M. Adachi, S. Sekiya and R. Kamikawa. 2003. Cyclization of aryl acyl radicals generated from *S*-(4-cyano)phenyl thiolesters by a nickel complex catalyzed electroreduction. J. Org. Chem. 68: 4586-4589.

[116] K. Ohe, K. Miki, T. Yokoi, F. Nishino and S. Uemura. 2000. Novel pyranylidene complexes from group 6 transition metals and β-ethynyl α,β-unsaturated carbonyl compounds. Organometallics 19: 5525-5528.

[117] J.P. Wolfe. 2008. Stereoselective synthesis of saturated heterocycles *via* Pd-catalyzed alkene carboetherification and carboamination reactions. Synlett 19: 2913-2937.

[118] J.P. Wolfe. 2007. Palladium-catalyzed carboetherification and carboamination reactions of γ-hydroxy- and γ-aminoalkenes for the synthesis of tetrahydrofurans and pyrrolidines. Eur. J. Org. Chem. 4: 571-582.

[119] J.E. Ney and J.P. Wolfe. 2004. Palladium-catalyzed synthesis of *N*-aryl pyrrolidines from γ-(*N*-arylamino) alkenes: evidence for chemoselective alkene insertion into Pd-N bonds. Angew. Chem. Int. Ed. 43: 3605-3608.

[120] J. Ney and J.P. Wolfe. 2005. Selective synthesis of 5- or 6-aryl octahydrocyclopenta[*b*]pyrroles from a common precursor through control of competing pathways in a Pd-catalyzed reaction. J. Am. Chem. Soc. 127: 8644-8651.

[121] M.B. Bertrand and J.P. Wolfe. 2005. Carbamoylimidazolium and thiocarbamoylimidazolium salts: novel reagents for the synthesis of ureas, thioureas, carbamates, thiocarbamates and amides. Tetrahedron 61: 6447-6459.

[122] M.B. Bertrand, J.D. Neukom and J.P. Wolfe. 2008. Mild conditions for Pd-catalyzed carboamination of *N*-protected hex-4-enylamines and 1-, 3-, and 4-substituted pent-4-enylamines. Scope, limitations, and mechanism of pyrrolidine formation. J. Org. Chem. 73: 8851-8860.

[123] M.B. Bertrand, M.L. Leathen and J.P. Wolfe. 2007. Mild conditions for the synthesis of functionalized pyrrolidines *via* Pd-catalyzed carboamination reactions. Org. Lett. 9: 457-460.

[124] (a) Z. Li, Z. Jin and R. Huang. 2001. Isolation, total synthesis and biological activity of phenan-throindolizidine and phenanthroquinolizidine alkaloids. Synthesis 16: 2365-2378.
        (b) D.N. Mai and J.P. Wolfe. 2010. Asymmetric palladium-catalyzed carboamination reactions for the synthesis of enantiomerically enriched 2-(arylmethyl)- and 2-(alkenylmethyl)pyrrolidines. J. Am. Chem. Soc. 132: 12157-12159.

[125] W. Zeng and S.R. Chemler. 2008. Total synthesis of (*S*)-(+)-tylophorine *via* enantioselective intramolecular alkene carboamination. J. Org. Chem. 73: 6045-6047.

[126] A. McIver, D.D. Young and A. Dieters. 2008. A general approach to triphenylenes and azatriphenylenes: total synthesis of dehydrotylophorine and tylophorine. Chem. Commun. 39: 4750-4752.

[127] Z. Wang, Z. Li, K. Wang and Q. Wang. 2010. Efficient and chirally specific synthesis of phenanthro-indolizidine alkaloids by Parham-type cycloacylation. Eur. J. Org. Chem. 2: 292-299.

[128] L.M. Rossiter, M.L. Slater, R.E. Gissert, S.A. Sakwa and R.J. Herr. 2009. A concise palladium-catalyzed carboamination route to (+/-)-tylophorine. J. Org. Chem. 74: 9554-9557.

[129] T.L. Gilchrist and M.A.M. Healy. 1993. Preparation of 1-substituted-3,4-dihydronaphthalene-2-carboxaldehyde *N,N*-dimethylhydrazones by palladium(0) coupling, and their electrocyclic ring closure. Tetrahedron 49: 2543-2556.

[130] S.A. Worlikar, B. Neuenswander, G.H. Lushington and R.C. Larock. 2009. Highly substituted indole library synthesis by palladium-catalyzed coupling reactions in solution and on a solid support. J. Comb. Chem. 11: 875-879.

[131] R. Samanta and A.P. Antonchick. 2011. Palladium-catalyzed double C-H activation directed by sulfoxides in the synthesis of dibenzothiophenes. Angew. Chem. Int. Ed. 50: 5217-5220.

[132] P. Knochel, W. Dohle, N. Gommermann, F.F. Kneisel, F. Kopp, T. Korn, I. Sapountzis and V.A. Vu. 2003. Highly functionalized magnesium organometallics prepared *via* a halogen-metal exchange. Angew. Chem. 115: 4438-4456.

[133] T. Harayama, H. Toko, A. Hori, T. Miyagoe, T. Sato, H. Nishioka, H. Abe and Y. Takeuchi. 2003. Synthetic studies on pyrrolophenanthridone skeleton from 1-benzoyl-7-iododihydroindole derivatives using palladium-assisted biaryl coupling reactions. Heterocycles 61: 513-520.

[134] T. Harayama, T. Sato, A. Hori, H. Abe and Y. Takeuchi. 2005. Palladium-assisted biaryl coupling reaction of 1-(2-iodobenzoyl)-1,2,3,4-tetrahydroquinoline. Heterocycles 66: 527-530.

[135] T. Harayama, A. Hori, H. Abe and Y. Takeuchi. 2006. Regioselectivity in the biaryl coupling reactions of 1-[(1,3-benzodioxol-5-yl)methyl]-7-iodo-2,3-dihydroindole using palladium reagent. Heterocycles 67: 385-390.

[136] J.A. Brown. 2000. Synthesis of *N*-aryl indole-2-carboxylates *via* an intramolecular palladium-catalyzed annulation of didehydrophenylalanine derivatives. Tetrahedron Lett. 41: 1623-1626.

[137] M. Watanabe, T. Yamamoto and M. Nishiyama. 2000. A new palladium-catalyzed intramolecular cyclization: synthesis of 1-aminoindole derivatives and functionalization of their carbocylic rings. Angew. Chem. Int. Ed. 39: 2501-2504.

[138] H. Siebeneicher, I. Bytschkov and S. Doye. 2003. A flexible and catalytic one-pot procedure for the synthesis of indoles. Angew. Chem. Int. Ed. 42: 3042-3044.

[139] R. Omar-Amrani, A. Thomas, E. Brenner, R. Schneider and Y. Fort. 2003. Efficient nickel-mediated intramolecular amination of aryl chlorides. Org. Lett. 5: 2311-2314.

[140] J.J. Song and N.K. Yee. 2000. A novel synthesis of 2-aryl-2*H*-indazoles *via* a palladium-catalyzed intramolecular amination reaction. Org. Lett. 2: 519-521.

[141] J.J. Song and N.K. Yee. 2001. Synthesis of 1-aryl-1*H*-indazoles *via* the palladium-catalyzed cyclization of *N*-aryl-*N'*-(*o*-bromobenzyl)hydrazines and [*N*-aryl-*N'*-(*o*-bromobenzyl)-hydrazinato-*N'*]-triphenylphosphonium bromides. Tetrahedron Lett. 42: 2937-2940.

[142] C.T. Brain and S.A. Brunton. 2002. An intramolecular palladium-catalyzed aryl amination reaction to produce benzimidazoles. Tetrahedron Lett. 43: 1893-1895.

[143] C.T. Brain and J.T. Steer. 2003. An improved procedure for the synthesis of benzimidazoles, using palladium-catalyzed aryl-amination chemistry. J. Org. Chem. 68: 6814-6816.

[144] M. Catellani, C. Catucci, G. Celentano and R. Ferraccioli. 2001. Palladium-catalyzed synthesis of enantiopure 1,2,4,5-tetrahydro-1,4-benzodiazepin-3-(3*H*)-one derivatives. Synlett 6: 803-805.

[145] B.J. Margolis, J.J. Swidorski and B.N. Rogers. 2003. An efficient assembly of heterobenzazepine ring systems utilizing an intramolecular palladium-catalyzed cycloamination. J. Org. Chem. 68: 644-647.

[146] T. Emoto, N. Kubosaki, Y. Yamagiwa and T. Kamikawa. 2000. A new route to phenazines. Tetrahedron Lett. 41: 355-358.

[147] Y. Kozawa and M. Mori. 2002. Synthesis of 3-alkoxycarbonyl-1β-methylcarbapenem using palladium-catalyzed amidation of vinyl halide. Tetrahedron Lett. 43: 111-114.

[148] R.S. Colemen and W. Chen. 2001. A convergent approach to the mitomycin ring system. Org. Lett. 3: 1141-1144.

[149] A. Abouabdellah and R.H. Dodd. 1998. A new approach to the synthesis of functionalized pyrido[2,3-*b*]indoles by way of a palladium-catalyzed ring closing reaction between the *N*-1 and C-9a positions. Tetrahedron Lett. 39: 2119-2122.

[150] G. Cuny, M. Bois-Choussy and J. Zhu. 2003. One-pot synthesis of polyheterocycles by a palladium-catalyzed intramolecular *N*-arylation/C-H activation/aryl-aryl bond-forming domino process. Angew. Chem. Int. Ed. 42: 4774-4777.

[151] A.J. Peat and S.L. Buchwald. 1996. Novel syntheses of tetrahydropyrroloquinolines: applications to alkaloid synthesis. J. Am. Chem. Soc. 118: 1028-1030.

[152] A.P. Kozikowski, D. Ma, J. Brewer, S. Sun, E. Costa, E. Romeo and A. Guidotti. 1993. Chemistry, binding affinities, and behavioral properties of a new class of "anti-neophobic" mitochondrial DBI receptor complex (mDRC) ligands. J. Med. Chem. 36: 2908-2920.

[153] R. Faust, P.J. Garratt, R. Jones, L.-K. Yeh, A. Tsotinis, M. Panoussopoulou, T. Calogeropoulou, M.-T. The and D. Sugden. 2000. Mapping the melatonin receptor. 6. Melatonin agonists and antagonists derived from 6*H*-isoindolo[2,1-*a*]indoles, 5,6-dihydroindolo[2,1-*a*]isoquinolines, and 6,7-dihydro-5*H*-benzo[*c*]azepino[2,1-*a*]indoles. J. Med. Chem. 43: 1050-1061.

[154] B. Gomez-Lor and A.M. Echavarren. 2004. Synthesis of a triaza analogue of crushed-fullerene by intramolecular palladium-catalyzed arylation. Org. Lett. 6: 2993-2996.

[155] Y. Miki, H. Shirokoshi and K. Matsushita. 1999. Intramolecular palladium-catalyzed cyclization of methyl 1-(2-bromobenzyl)indole-2-carboxylates: synthesis of pratosine and hippadine. Tetrahedron Lett. 40: 4347-4348.

[156] A.H. Roy and J.F. Hartwig. 2001. Reductive elimination of aryl halides from palladium(II). J. Am. Chem. Soc. 123: 1232-1233.

[157] Q.H. Huang, A. Fazio, G.X. Dai, M.A. Campo and R.C. Larock. 2004. Pd-catalyzed alkyl to aryl migration and cyclization: an efficient synthesis of fused polycycles *via* multiple C-H activation. J. Am. Chem. Soc. 126: 7460-7461.

[158] T. Kesharwani, A.K. Verma, D. Emrich, J.A. Ward and R.C. Larock. 2009. Studies in acyl C-H activation *via* aryl and alkyl to acyl "through space" migration of palladium. Org. Lett. 11: 2591-2593.

[159] S. Ma and Z. Gu. 2005. 1,4-Migration of rhodium and palladium in catalytic organometallic reactions. Angew. Chem. Int. Ed. Engl. 44: 7512-7517.

[160] Z. Jin. 2005. *Amaryllidaceae* and *Sceletium* alkaloids. Nat. Prod. Rep. 22: 111-126.

[161] T. Harayama, A. Hori, H. Abe and Y. Takeuchi. 2003. Concise synthesis of pyrrolophenanthridine alkaloids using a Pd-catalyzed biaryl coupling reaction with regioselective C-H activation. Heterocycles 60: 2429-2434.

[162] S.J. Garden, J.C. Torres and A.C. Pinto. 2000. An investigation of a palladium catalyzed biaryl synthesis of pyrrolophenanthridine derivatives. Extension of the Heck reaction. J. Braz. Chem. Soc. 11: 441-446.

[163] J.C. Torres, A.C. Pinto and S.J. Garden. 2004. Application of a catalytic palladium biaryl synthesis reaction, *via* C-H functionalization, to the total synthesis of *Amaryllidaceae* alkaloids. Tetrahedron 60: 9889-9900.

[164] B.D. Chapsal and I. Ojima. 2005. Total synthesis of enantiopure (+)-γ-lycorane using highly efficient Pd-catalyzed asymmetric allylic alkylation. Org. Lett. 8: 1395-1398.

[165] B.D. Chapsal and I. Ojima. 2006. Catalytic asymmetric transformations with fine-tunable biphenol-based monodentate ligands. Tetrahedron: Asymmetry 17: 642-657.

[166] K. Shimizu, M. Takimoto and M. Mori. 2003. Novel synthesis of heterocycles having a functionalized carbon center *via* nickel-mediated carboxylation: total synthesis of erythrocarine. Org. Lett. 5: 2323-2325.

[167] K.C. Majumdar, S. Muhuri, R.U. Islam and B. Chattopadhyay. 2009. Synthesis of five- and six-membered heterocyclic compounds by the application of the metathesis reactions. Heterocycles 78: 1109-1169.

[168] J.M. Mejia-Oneto and A. Padwa. 2006. Application of the Rh(II) cyclization/cycloaddition cascade for the total synthesis of (±)-aspidophytine. Org. Lett. 8: 3275-3278.

[169] J.M. Mejia-Oneto and A. Padwa. 2008. Total synthesis of the alkaloid (±)-aspidophytine based on carbonyl ylide cycloaddition chemistry. Helv. Chim. Acta 91: 285-302.

[170] C. Bressy, D. Alberico and M. Lautens. 2005. A route to annulated indoles *via* a palladium-catalyzed tandem alkylation/direct arylation reaction. J. Am. Chem. Soc. 127: 13148-13149.

[171] A. Martins, D. Alberico and M. Lautens. 2006. Synthesis of polycyclic heterocycles *via* a one-pot *o*-alkylation/direct heteroarylation sequence. Org. Lett. 8: 4827-4829.

[172] N.R. Deprez and M.S. Sanford. 2007. Reactions of hypervalent iodine reagents with palladium: mechanisms and applications in organic synthesis. Inorg. Chem. 46: 1924-1935.

[173] M. Catellani, F. Frignani and A. Rangoni. 1997. A complex catalytic cycle leading to a regioselective synthesis of *o,o'*-disubstituted vinylarenes. Angew. Chem. Int. Ed. Engl. 36: 119-122.

[174] M. Catellani, C. Mealli, E. Motti, P. Paoli, E. Perez-Carreno and P.S. Pregosin. 2002. Palladium-arene interactions in catalytic intermediates: an experimental and theoretical investigation of the soft rearrangement between η^1 and η^2 coordination modes. J. Am. Chem. Soc. 124: 4336-4346.

[175] M. Catellani. 2003. Catalytic multistep reactions *via* palladacycles. Synlett 3: 298-313.

[176] M. Catellani. 2005. Novel methods of aromatic functionalization using palladium and norbornene as a unique catalytic system. Top. Organomet. Chem. 14: 21-53.

[177] L. Joucla, A. Putey and B. Joseph. 2005. Synthesis of fused heterocycles with a benzazepinone moiety *via* intramolecular Heck coupling. Tetrahedron Lett. 46: 8177-8179.

[178] E.M. Beccalli, G. Broggini, M. Martinelli, G. Paladino and C. Zoni. 2005. Synthesis of tricyclic quinolones and naphthyridones by intramolecular Heck cyclization of functionalized electron-rich heterocycles. Eur. J. Org. Chem. 10: 2091-2096.

[179] M.J. Tomaszewski, A. Whalley and Y.-J. Hu. 2008. A one-pot synthesis of 2,3-dihydro-1*H*-pyrrolo[3,2-*c*]quinolines. Tetrahedron Lett. 49: 3172-3175.

[180] C. Xie, Y. Zhang, Z. Huang and P. Xu. 2007. Synthesis of indolo[1,2-*f*]phenanthridines from palladium-catalyzed reactions of arynes. J. Org. Chem. 72: 5431-5434.

[181] D.P. Walsh and Y.-T. Chang. 2006. Chemical genetics. Chem. Rev. 106: 2476-2530.

[182] P. Arya, D.T.H. Chou and M.-G. Baek. 2001. Diversity-based organic synthesis in the era of genomics and proteomics. Angew. Chem. Int. Ed. 40: 339-346.

[183] S.L. Schreiber. 2000. Target-oriented and diversity-oriented organic synthesis in drug discovery. Science 287: 1964-1969.

[184] S. Li, Y. Luo and J. Wu. 2011. Three-component reaction of *N'*-(2-alkynylbenzylidene)hydrazide, alkyne, with sulfonyl azide *via* a multicatalytic process: a novel and concise approach to 2-amino-*H*-pyrazolo[5,1-*a*]isoquinolines. Org. Lett. 13: 4312-4315.

[185] T. Kuroda and F. Suzuki. 1991. Synthesis of 1*H*-imidazo[4,5-*c*]quinolin-4(5*H*)-one *via* palladium-catalyzed cyclization of *N*-(2-bromophenyl)-1*H*-imidazole-4-carboxamide. Tetrahedron Lett. 32: 6915-6918.

[186] N. Okamoto, K. Sakurai, M. Ishikura, K. Takeda and R. Yanada. 2009. One-pot concise syntheses of benzimidazo[2,1-*a*]isoquinolines by a microwave-accelerated tandem process. Tetrahedron Lett. 50: 4167-4169.

[187] K.M. Dawood and B.F. Abdel-Wahab. 2010. Synthetic routes to benzimidazole-based fused polyheterocycles. ARKIVOC (i): 333-389.

[188] S. Hernandez, R. SanMartin, I. Tellitu and E. Dominguez. 2003. Toward safer methodologies for the synthesis of polyheterocyclic systems: intramolecular arylation of arenes under Mizoroki-Heck reaction conditions. Org. Lett. 5: 1095-1098.

[189] K.J. Hodgetts and M.T. Kershaw. 2003. Synthesis of 2-aryl-oxazolo[4,5-*c*]quinoline-4(5*H*)-ones and 2-aryl-thiazolo[4,5-*c*]quinoline-4(5*H*)-ones. Org. Lett. 5: 2911-2914.

[190] M. Alajarin, A. Vidal, F. Tovar and C. Conesa. 1999. Formal [4+2] intramolecular cycloaddition ketenimine-imine. Synthesis of benzimidazo[1,2-*b*]isoquinolines. Tetrahedron Lett. 40: 6127-6130.

[191] M. Alajarin, A. Vidal and F. Tovar. 2000. Periselective intramolecular [4+2] cycloadditions of ketenimines: synthesis of pyrido[1,2-*a*]benzimidazoles. Tetrahedron Lett. 41: 7029-7032.

[192] M. Koyama, N. Ohtani, F. Kai, I. Moriguchi and S. Inouye. 1987. Synthesis and quantitative structure-activity relationship analysis of *N*-triiodoallyl- and *N*-iodopropargylazoles. New anti-fungal agents. J. Med. Chem. 30: 552-562.

[193] P. Thansandote and M. Lautens. 2009. Construction of nitrogen-containing heterocycles by C-H bond functionalization. Chem. Eur. J. 15: 5874-5883.

[194] G.P. McGlacken and L.M. Bateman. 2009. Recent advances in aryl-aryl bond formation by direct arylation. Chem. Soc. Rev. 38: 2447-2464.

[195] L. Ackermann, R. Vicente and A.R. Kapdi. 2009. Transition-metal-catalyzed direct arylation of (hetero)arenes by C-H bond cleavage. Angew Chem. Int. Ed. 48: 9792-9826.

[196] R.F. Heck. 1979. Palladium-catalyzed reactions of organic halides with olefins. Acc. Chem. Res. 12: 146-151.

[197] A. Meijere and F.E. Meyer. 1995. Fine feathers make fine birds: the Heck reaction in modern garb. Angew Chem. Int. Ed. Engl. 33: 2379-2411.

[198] E. Negishi, C. Coperet, S.M. Ma, S.Y. Liou and F. Liu. 1996. Cyclic carbopalladation. A versatile synthetic methodology for the construction of cyclic organic compounds. Chem. Rev. 96: 365-394.

[199] I.P. Beletskaya and A.V. Cheprakov. 2000. The Heck reaction as a sharpening stone of palladium catalysis. Chem. Rev. 100: 3009-3066.

[200] J.M. Schulman, A.A. Friedman, J. Panteleev and M. Lautens. 2012. Synthesis of 1,2,3-triazole-fused heterocycles *via* Pd-catalyzed cyclization of 5-iodotriazoles. Chem. Commun. 48: 55-57.

[201] A. Padwa, M.A. Brodney and S.M. Lynch. 2001. Formal total synthesis of (±)-γ-lycorane and (±)-1-deoxylycorine using the [4+2]-cycloaddition/rearrangement cascade of furanyl carbamates. J. Org. Chem. 66: 1716-1724.

[202] R. Grigg, R. Rasul and V. Savic. 1997. Palladium catalyzed triscyclization-anion capture queuing cascades. Tetrahedron Lett. 38: 1825-1828.

[203] R. Grigg and V. Sridharan. 1998. Heterocycles *via* Pd catalyzed molecular queuing processes. Relay switches and the maximization of molecular complexity. Pure Appl. Chem. 70: 1047-1057.

[204] T. Harayama, H. Akamatsu, K. Okamura, T. Miyagoe, T. Akiyama, H. Abe and Y. Takeuchi. 2001. Synthesis of trisphaeridine and norchelerythrine through palladium-catalyzed aryl-aryl coupling reactions. J. Chem. Soc. Perkin Trans. 1 5: 523-528.

[205] M.G. Banwell, D.W. Lupton, X. Ma, J. Renner and M.O. Sydnes. 2004. Synthesis of quinolines, 2-quinolones, phenanthridines, and 6(5*H*)-phenanthridinones *via* palladium[0]-mediated Ullmann cross-coupling of 1-bromo-2-nitroarenes with β-halo-enals, -enones, or -esters. Org. Lett. 6: 2741-2744.

[206] E. Bacque, M.E. Qacemi and S.Z. Zard. 2004. Tin-free radical cyclizations for the synthesis of 7-azaoxindoles, 7-azaindolines, tetrahydro[1,8]naphthyridines, and tetrahydro-5*H*-pyrido[2,3-*b*]azepin-8-ones. Org. Lett. 6: 3671-3674.

[207] D.H.R. Barton, B. Garcia, H. Togo and S.Z. Zard. 1986. Radical decarboxylative addition onto protonated heteroaromatic (and related) compounds. Tetrahedron Lett. 27: 1327-1330.

[208] F. Minisci, E. Vismara and F. Fontana. 1989. Recent developments of free-radical substitutions of heteroaromatic bases. Heterocycles 28: 489-519.

[209] B. Gabriele, R. Mancuso, L. Veltri, V. Maltese and G. Salerno. 2012. Synthesis of substituted thiophenes by palladium-catalyzed heterocyclodehydration of 1-mercapto-3-yn-2-ols in conventional and nonconventional solvents. J. Org. Chem. 77: 9905-9909.

[210] T. Harayama, T. Akiyama, Y. Nakano and K. Shibaike. 1998. Synthesis of naphtho[2,3-*b*]indolizine-6,11-dione derivatives by iodine oxidation of 2-alkyl-1,4-naphthoquinones in the presence of substituted pyridines. Heterocycles 48: 1993-2002.

[211] C.S. Yeung, X. Zhao, N. Borduas and V.M. Dong. 2010. Pd-catalyzed *o*-arylation of phenylacetamides, benzamides, and anilides with simple arenes using sodium persulfate. Chem. Sci. 1: 331-336.

[212] C.S. Yeung and V.M. Dong. 2011. Pd-catalyzed *o*-arylation of *N*-aryloxazolidinones with simple arenes using sodium persulfate. Synlett 7: 974-978.

[213] J.-E. Backvall, P.G. Andersson, G.B. Stone and A. Gogoll. 1991. Synthesis of (+)-α- and (+)-γ-lycorane *via* a stereocontrolled organopalladium route. J. Org. Chem. 56: 2988-2993.

[214] S. Deprets and G. Kirsch. 2002. New synthesis of substituted 6-methylbenzo[*b*]furo-, -thieno-, and -seleno[2,3-*c*]quinolines, and heterocyclic analogues. ARKIVOC (i): 40-48.

[215] T. Itoh and T. Mase. 2007. A novel practical synthesis of benzothiazoles *via* Pd-catalyzed thiol cross-coupling. Org. Lett. 9: 3687-3689.

[216] J.K. Luo, H. Kudo, R.F. Federspiel and R.N. Castle. 1995. The synthesis of novel polycyclic heterocyclic ring systems *via* photocyclization. J. Heterocycl. Chem. 32: 317-322.

[217] J.D. McKenney and R.N. Castle. 1987. The synthesis of [1]benzothieno[2,3-*c*]quinolines, [1]benzothieno[2,3-*c*][1,2,4]triazolo[4,3-*a*]quinoline, and [1]benzothieno[2,3-*c*]tetrazolo[1,5-*a*]quinoline. J. Heterocycl. Chem. 24: 1525-1529.

[218] S. Deprets and G. Kirsch. 2000. Synthesis of 5-methylbenzo[*b*]thieno[2,3-*c*]isoquinolines and 5-methylbenzo[*b*]seleno[2,3-*c*]isoquinolines. Eur. J. Org. Chem. 7: 1353-1357.

[219] G. Kirsch, S. Hesse and A. Comel. 2004. Synthesis of five- and six-membered heterocycles through palladium-catalyzed reactions. Curr. Org. Synth. 1: 47-63.

[220] A. Mouaddib, B. Joseph, A. Hasnaoui and J.-Y. Merour. 2000. Synthesis of indolo[3,2-*c*]quinoline and pyrido[3′,2′ : 4,5] [3,2-*c*]quinoline derivatives. Synthesis 4: 549-556.

[221] D.P. Curran and W. Du. 2002. Palladium-promoted cascade reactions of isonitriles and 6-iodo-*N*-propargylpyridones: synthesis of mappicines, camptothecins, and homocamptothecins. Org. Lett. 4: 3215-3218.

[222] D. Mujahidin and S. Doye. 2005. Enantioselective synthesis of (+)-(*S*)-laudanosine and (-)-(*S*)-xylopinine. Eur. J. Org. Chem. 13: 2689-2693.

[223] N. Uematsu, A. Fujii, S. Hashiguchi, T. Ikariya and R. Noyori. 1996. Asymmetric transfer hydrogenation of imines. J. Am. Chem. Soc. 118: 4916-4917.

[224] S. Hesse and G. Kirsch. 2003. Synthesis of pyridine-fused ring systems from β-chloroacroleins: a comparison of three different pathways. Synthesis 5: 717-722.

[225] G. Cuny, M. Bois-Choussy and J. Zhu. 2004. Palladium- and copper-catalyzed synthesis of medium- and large-sized ring-fused dihydroazaphenanthrenes and 1,4-benzodiazepine-2,5-diones. Control of reaction pathway by metal-switching. J. Am. Chem. Soc. 126: 14475-14484.

[226] S. Cacchi. 1999. Heterocycles *via* cyclization of alkynes promoted by organopalladium complexes. J. Organomet. Chem. 576: 42-64.

[227] R. Grigg and V. Sridharan. 1999. Palladium catalyzed cascade cyclization-anion capture, relay switches and molecular queues. J. Organomet. Chem. 576: 65-87.

[228] R.C. Larock. 1999. Palladium-catalyzed annulations. J. Organomet. Chem. 576: 111-124.

[229] Y. Yu, J.M. Ostresh and R.A. Houghten. 2003. Solid-phase synthesis of indolines *via* palladium-catalyzed cyclization. Tetrahedron Lett. 44: 2569-2572.

[230] R.C. Larock and E.K. Yum. 1991. Synthesis of indoles *via* palladium-catalyzed heteroannulation of internal alkynes. J. Am. Chem. Soc. 113: 6689-6690.

[231] R. Grigg, I. Koppen, M. Rasparini and V. Sridharan. 2001. Synthesis of spiro- and fused heterocycles by palladium catalyzed carbo- and heteroannulation cascades of allenes. Chem. Commun. 11: 964-965.

CHAPTER 10

Six-Membered N,N-Heterocycles

10.1 Introduction

Heterocyclic chemistry is the most interesting branch of organic chemistry and of utmost theoretical and practical importance [1]. As a result of this a great deal of research conducted in chemistry is devoted to heterocyclic chemistry [2a-f]. Heterocycles are widely distributed in nature. It is expanding and vast field of chemistry due to obvious use of compounds derived from heterocycles in medicine, pharmacy, plastic, agriculture, polymer and other areas [3a-b]. Due to their biological activities heterocycles are employed in the treatment of infectious diseases. Various heterocycles prepared in laboratories are successfully used as clinical agents [4-5].

Six-membered aromatic rings possessing two nitrogen atoms including quinazolinones, phthalazinones, pyrimidinones, and pyrimidines, exhibit a wide spectrum of pharmacological properties and therefore they are interesting target compounds in medicinal and pharmaceutical chemistry. The pathways for transformation of hydrocarbon substrates into nitrogen-containing products with the assistance of metal catalysts are the focus of investigation in synthetic organic chemistry [6-10]. Over 90% of pharmaceutical have at least one nitrogen atom in their structure and out of seven about one reaction in the pharmaceutical industry involved the formation of a C-N bond. N-Heterocycles occur in a variety of biologically active and natural compounds. Efficient protocols for the preparation of N-containing heterocycles are of fundamental importance and represent a major challenge in synthetic chemistry [11-16].

10.2 Palladium assisted synthesis of six-membered heterocycles with two nitrogen heteroatoms

10.3 Synthesis of six-membered two nitrogen-containing heterocycles

Six-membered heterocyclic compounds were synthesized conveniently by catalytic hetero-Diels-Alder reaction **(Scheme 1)**. The hetero-Diels-Alder reaction was classified into two groups: (a) [4+2]-cycloaddition of 1,3-dienes with a heteroatom-heteroatom double bond or carbon-heteroatom (b) [4+2]-cycloaddition of α,β-unsaturated carbonyl compounds with olefins [17-20].

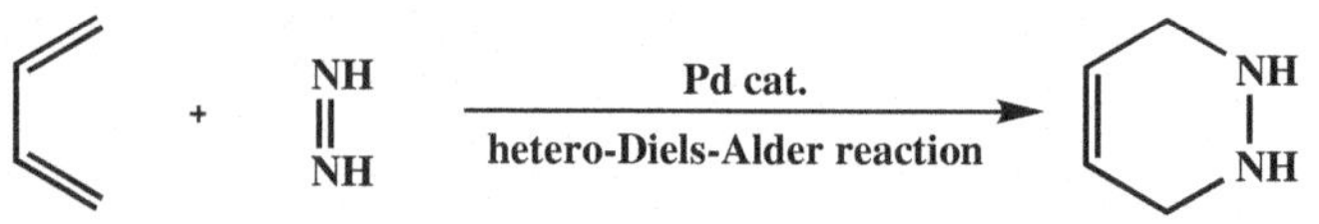

Scheme-1

The pyrimidine ring was prepared from tagged substrates through aldol condensation and cycloaddition reactions. The intermediates and boronic acids formed biaryl compounds *via* Suzuki reactions. The formed biaryl compounds were reacted with amine to form products or reacted with formic acid to afford traceless de-tagged products (**Scheme 2**) [21-22].

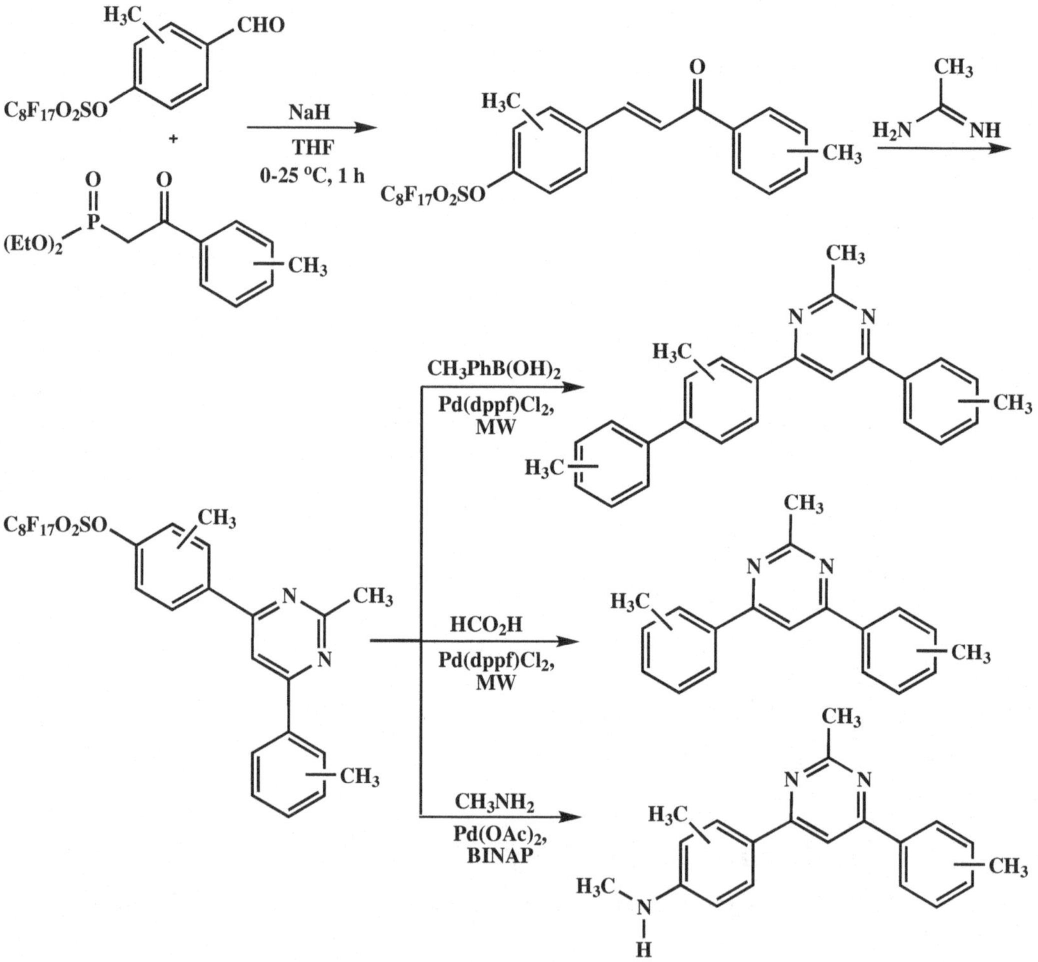

Scheme-2

Karpov and Muller [23-24] produced a class of alkynones by a catalytic Sonogashira method: terminal acetylenes were reacted with acid chlorides in the presence of only one eq. of amine base to form the highly electrophilic ynones concomitantly consigning an essentially neutral reaction medium. Subsequently, the unsaturated functionality underwent Michael additions with a variety of nucleophiles. Pharmacologically active class of pyrimidines was prepared by the reaction of amidinium salts as amidine precursors in an excess of Na_2CO_3. The disubstituted derivatives were formed upon cleavage of trimethylsilyl under mild conditions when "notorious" trimethylsilyl alkynones were reacted. The carbonylative alkynylation of aryl iodides, alkynes and CO was performed by an alternative catalytic three-component reaction for the synthesis of ynones. Polysubstituted pyrimidines were synthesized upon subsequent addition of an amidinium salt in the sense of a four-component reaction **(Scheme 3)** [25-26].

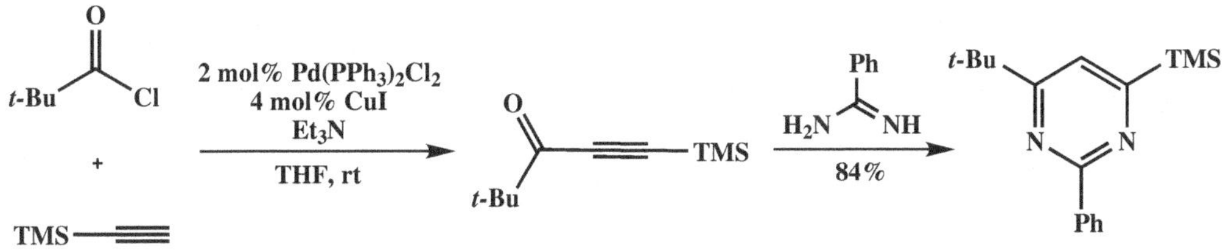

Scheme-3

Hogrefe [27] synthesized protected nucleoside by an alternative method as depicted in **Scheme 4**. Initially, allylamine was reacted with 3,5-di-*tert*-butyl-1,2-benzoquinone to form the 2-vinyl-4,6-di-*tert*-butylbenzoxazole. The desired nucleoside was generated when 2-vinyl-4,6-di-*tert*-butylbenzoxazole was coupled with 5-iodo-3,5-di-*O*-benzoyl-deoxyuridine under Heck conditions [28].

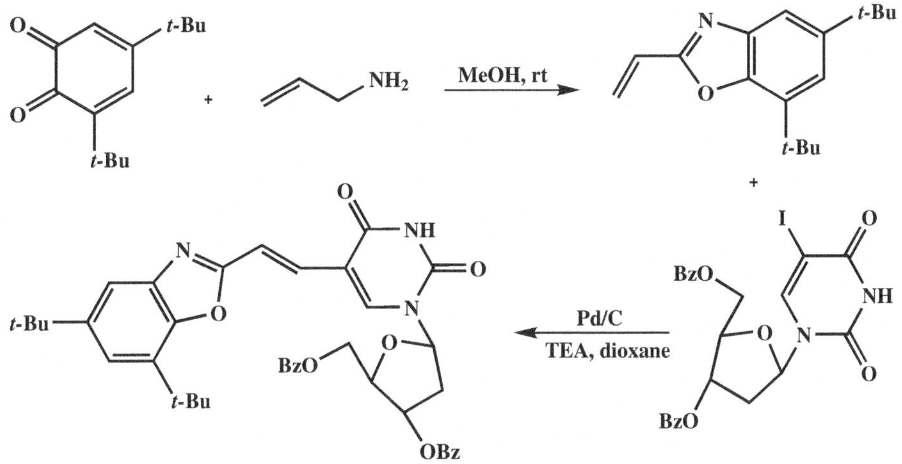

Scheme-4

The pyrimidine motifs were synthesized following the same strategy as for terpyridine. Firstly they synthesized diol **(Scheme 5)**, as main core motif as previously described [29] and further functionalized this structure with carboxyl groups and triple bonds.

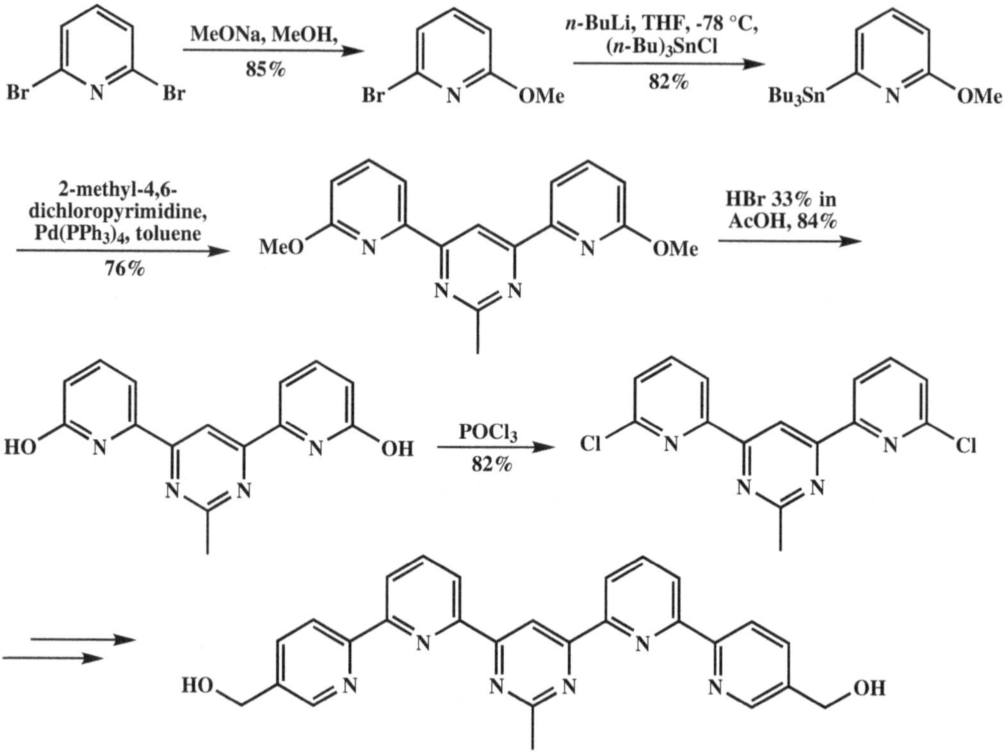

Scheme-5

Ferber and co-workers [30] synthesized 3,5-disubstituted piperazinones in quantitative yields through an intramolecular allylic amination of starting compound in the presence of palladium(II) catalyst and lithium chloride without a re-oxidizing system **(Scheme 6)**. Reversed stereoselectivity was observed when the reaction was carried out without lithium chloride [28].

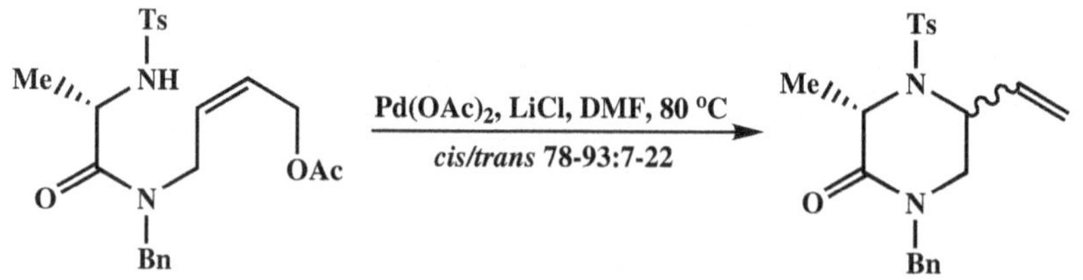

Scheme-6

Effective reaction conditions were optimized in piperidine-forming reactions. The use of a catalyst composed of $Pd_2(dba)_3$ and 1,4-bis(diphenylphosphino)butane or $P(2\text{-fur})_3$ provided satisfactory results with several aryl bromide coupling partners **(Scheme 7)** [30].

Wolfe and co-workers [31a-b] synthesized highly diastereo- and enantiomerically enriched *cis*-2,6-disubstituted piperazines. The carboamination reaction of alkenyl or aryl halides and substituted *N*-allyl ethylenediamine derivatives occurred in the presence of palladium catalyst **(Scheme 8)** [28].

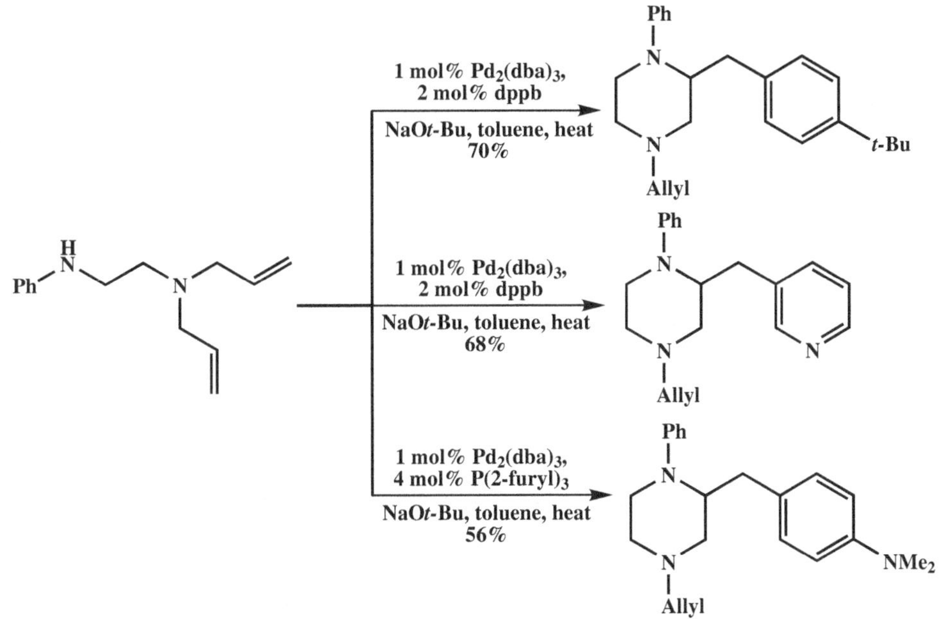

Scheme-7

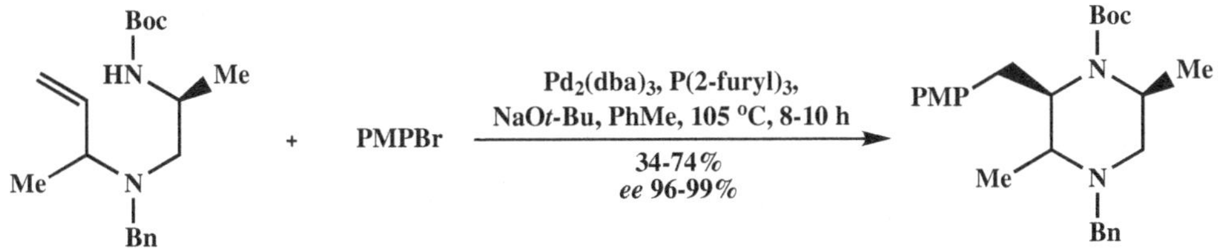

Scheme-8

Nakhla [32] reported a complementary method for the synthesis of *trans*-2,6-disubstituted piperazines *via* palladium-catalyzed hydroamination reactions **(Scheme 9)**. The palladium-activated olefin was attacked by nucleophilic amine which was followed by protonolysis to release the product. However, this transformation was limited to the preparation of compounds bearing a methyl group in 2-position. The authors proposed an allylic strain argument to explain the formation of 2,6-*trans*-substituent disubstituted piperazine whereby it oriented itself in pseudo-axial position in order to avoid A(1,3) the strain in transition state. The tridentate palladium catalyst was believed to inhibit the hydride elimination of intermediate palladium-alkyl species.

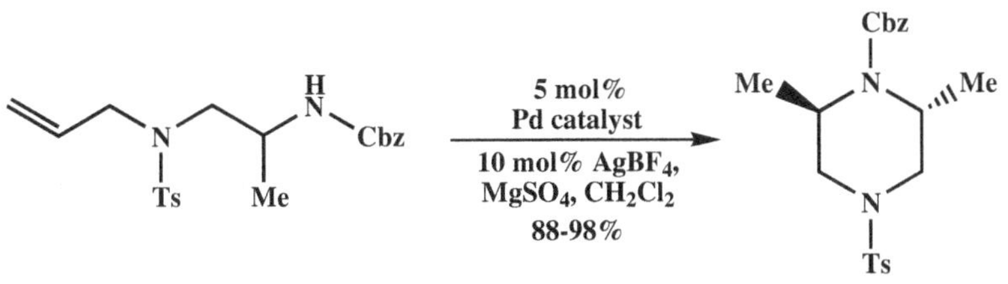

Scheme-9

Cochran and Michael [33] explained a stereoselective pathway for the conversion of unactivated alkenes into enantiopure *trans*-2,6-disubstituted piperazines by palladium-catalyzed intramolecular hydroamination with differently protected nitrogen atoms. The reaction occurred through inhibition of β-hydride elimination **(Scheme 10)** [28].

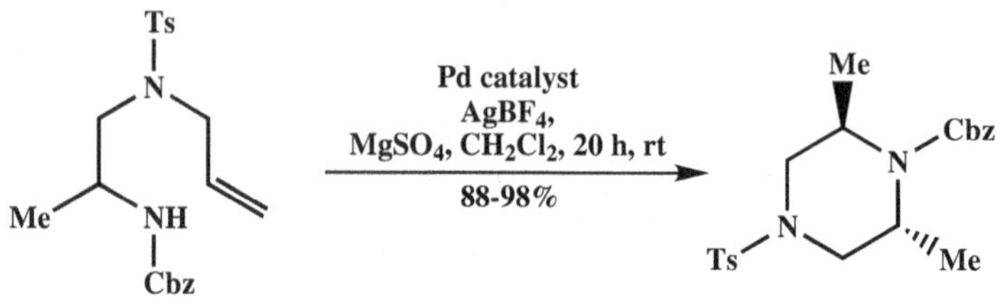

Scheme-10

The intramolecular *syn*-aminopalladation step in the catalytic cycle might be slow relative to analogous five-membered ring process due to entropy. They hypothesized that they could potentially circumvent the difficulties associated with an entropically slower transformation by installing an amine in tether, which would assist in bringing the two ends of molecule together, therefore facilitating the more challenging cyclization **(Scheme 11)** [34].

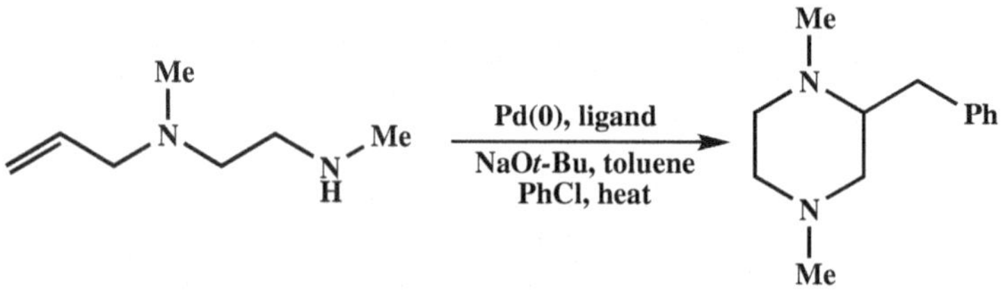

Scheme-11

To determine whether other protecting groups on N1 would undergo carboamination reaction, Boc-protected substrate was prepared from Boc-glycine in two steps. This substrate underwent carboamination reaction to provide piperazine in good yield, further demonstrating the greater ease of cyclization of 1,2-diamino olefins relative to carbon analog. These results demonstrated the viability of this strategy for piperazine synthesis, and set out to prepare more highly substituted derivatives **(Scheme 12)** [35].

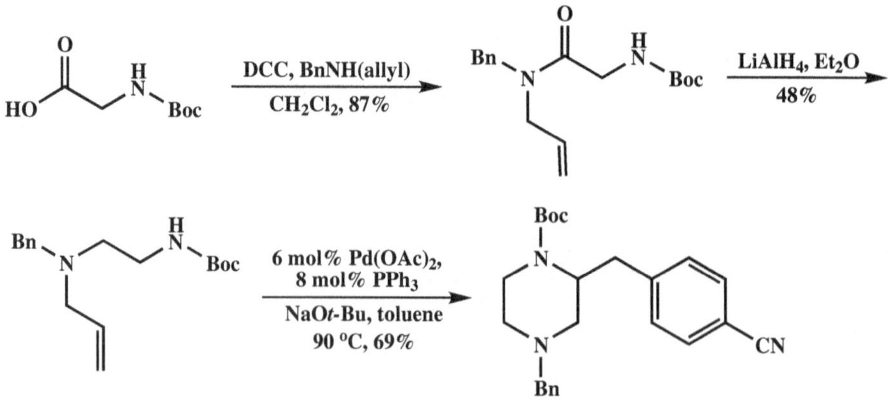

Scheme-12

The palladium-catalyzed carboamination reactions of starting compounds were examined using reaction conditions optimized for the synthesis of 2,6-disubstituted piperazines. These conditions required slight modification as it was necessary to employ higher temperatures (xylenes, 140 °C) in order to effect consumption of starting material. The reactions [36-37] proceeded in good to moderate yields and modest levels of diastereoselectivity **(Scheme 13-14)**.

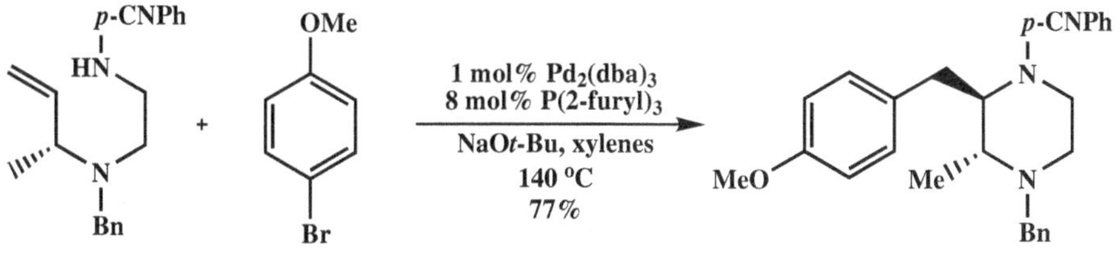

Scheme-13

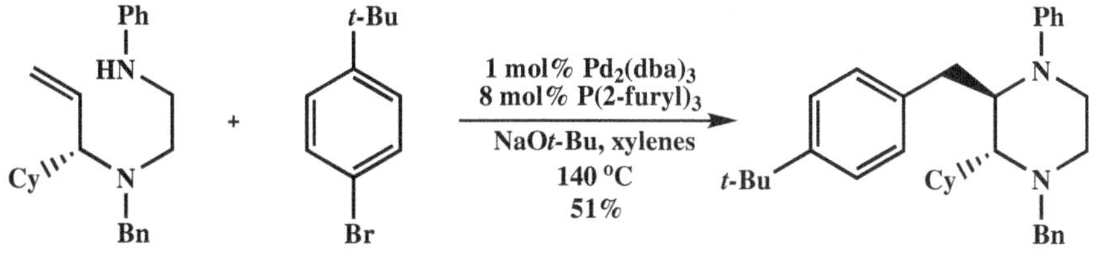

Scheme-14

The major diastereomer observed in 2,3-disubstituted piperazine cyclizations was *trans*-diastereomer. The modest stereocontrol resulted from equatorial or axial positioning of allylic substituent in transition state is shown in **Scheme 15-16**. The minor diastereomer was less favored due to unfavorable 1,3-diaxial interactions. These reactions required more forcing conditions in order that they may go to completion and were therefore conducted in xylenes at 140 °C [38-39].

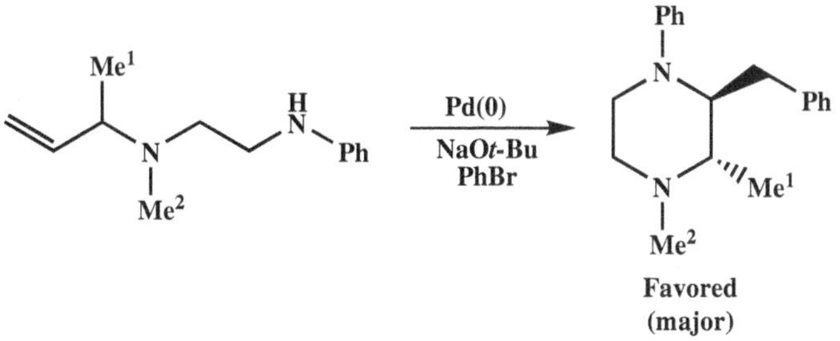

Scheme-15

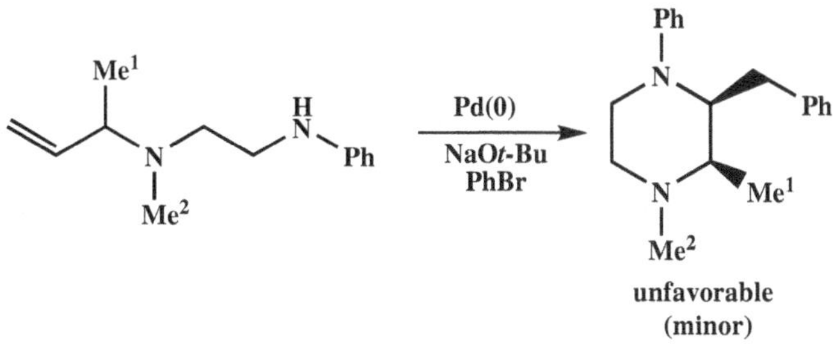

Scheme-16

10.4 Synthesis of six-membered two nitrogen-containing polyheterocycles

Savic [40a] reported the use of acetate anion as a capturing nucleophile in palladium-catalyzed carbopalladation/cyclization-anion capture cascade **(Scheme 17)**. The allenamides afforded desired cyclized products by intramolecular version of this reaction. However, a mixture of regioisomeric acetates was obtained from allenamide with intermolecular version [40b].

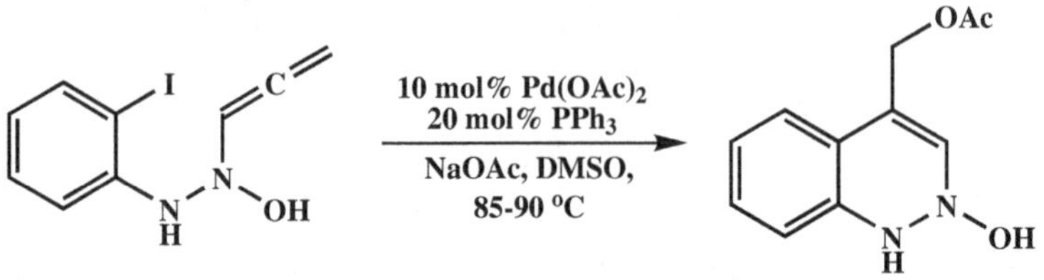

Scheme-17

Grigg et al. [41] used *o*-halogenated cinnamates and related compounds in a three-component reaction for the preparation of phthalazones with the help of CO and hydrazine derivatives. The reaction occurred by carbonylation of starting PhI to afford an acylpalladium species. The formed acylpalladium species was intercepted by hydrazine nucleophile to provide an acylhydrazide intermediate. This obtained intermediate underwent intramolecular Michael addition to afford di-*N,N'*- and mono-*N*-phthalazones on the basis of whether a 1,2-disubstituted or monosubstituted hydrazine derivative was employed. To improve the efficiency of each reaction a proper choice of reaction conditions and catalyst was required **(Scheme 18)** [42].

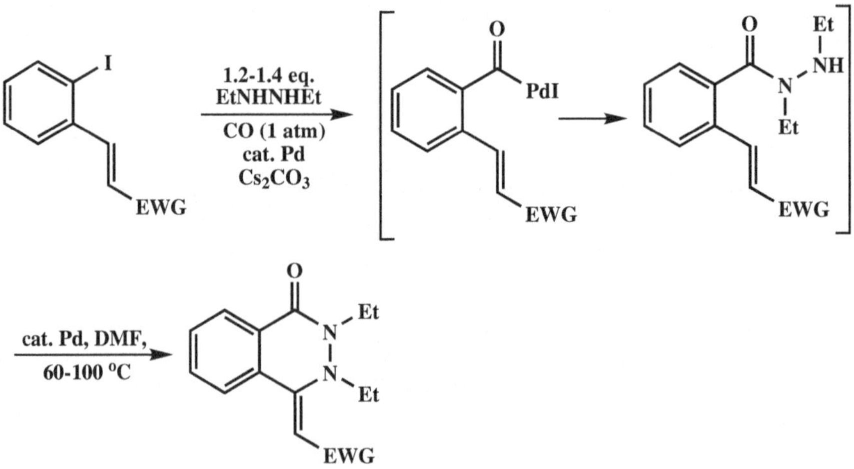

Scheme-18

Grigg [43] explained a *de novo* intramolecular carbopalladation/cyclization-anion capture reaction of allenamides using palladium catalyst **(Scheme 19)**. A selective carbopalladation/cyclization onto central allenic carbon was performed to produce the palladium-π-allyl complex after oxidative addition of palladium(0) to ArI. Allylic amines were prepared when π-allyl species was captured regioselectively by amines at sterically less hindered γ-allenic position (γ-attack) in the presence of potassium carbonate. This regioselectivity was altered with silver carbonate to favor the α-attack. The reaction occurred through cationic π-ally complex when silver carbonate was utilized which favored α-attack and impeded any ensuing equilibration [40b].

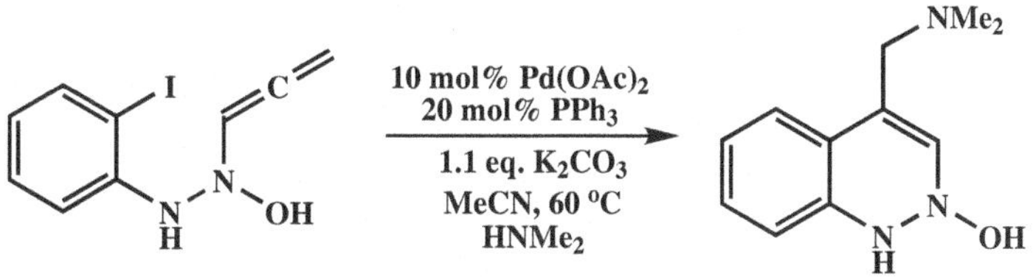

Scheme-19

The Suzuki cross-coupling of tosyl phthalazone and phenyl boronic acid was performed to obtain the second conformationally-restricted heterocycle, resulting in the synthesis of final product in good yield (77%) in only 20 min **(Scheme 20)** [44-45].

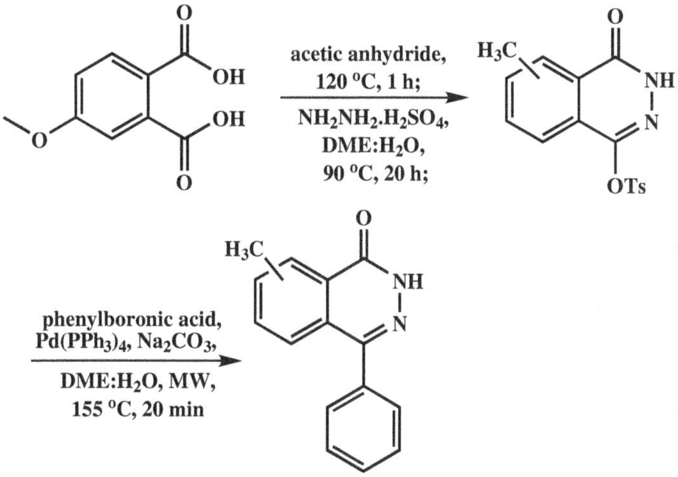

Scheme-20

Brase and co-workers [46] generated cinnolines by a Richter type solid-phase reaction. Starting from benzylaminomethyl polystyrene and substituted *o*-haloanilines, the *o*-haloaryl resins were synthesized. The Pd catalyst was utilized for cross-coupling reaction with alkynes. The cinnolines were formed by Richter cleavage reaction with hydrochloric or hydrobromic acid **(Scheme 21)**.

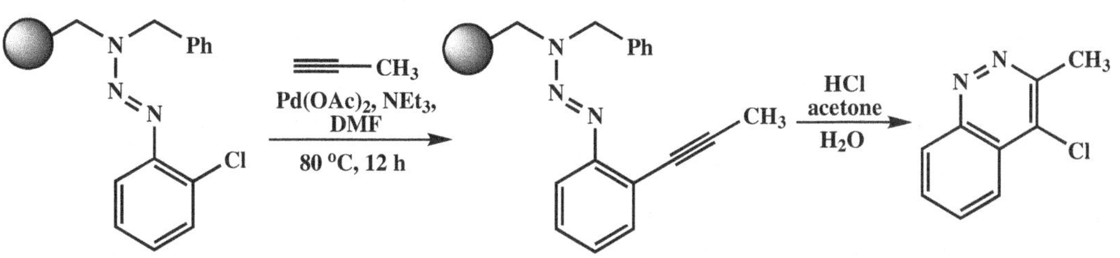

Scheme-21

The anthranilamide was used as a substrate due to its superior performance in Niementowski reaction, and was reacted with different ketones. Different 2,2-disubstituted 2,3-dihydroquinazolin-4(1*H*)-ones were formed in yields 66 to 95%. The reaction time was reduced dramatically as compared to conventional process. Excellent yields were obtained with an aliphatic ketone, and the reaction occurred equally well with cyclohexanone to afford 2-spiro substituted 2,3-dihydroquinazolin-4(1*H*)-one. However, with benzophenone a low yield was provided even though the irradiation time was prolonged to 20 min. In comparison to conventional methods this new protocol has benefits of a rapid and clean conversion and a good substrate tolerance. These were generally lower than that achieved in case of anthranilamide, especially when aromatic amide was used. The coupling of anthranilic acid or anthranilamide in the presence of acid catalyst was performed with amide under MWI **(Scheme 22)** [47-48].

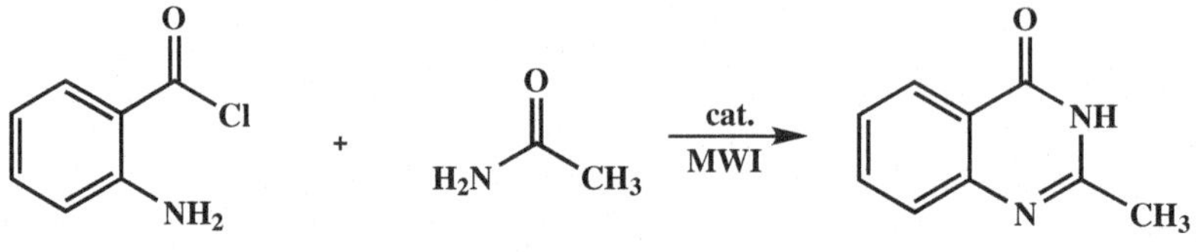

Scheme-22

In 2004, Beccalli and co-workers [49] described aerobic palladium(II)-catalyzed cyclization of tosylated *N*-allylanthranilamides. They found that, by using different base and solvent combinations, 2-vinylquinazolin-4-ones and 2-methylene-1,4-benzodiazepin-5-ones could be obtained regioselectively. The intramolecular amidation of tosylated *N*-allylanthranilamides in the presence of palladium(II) catalyst afforded 1,4-benzodiazepin-5-ones and quinazolin-4-ones **(Scheme 23)** [50].

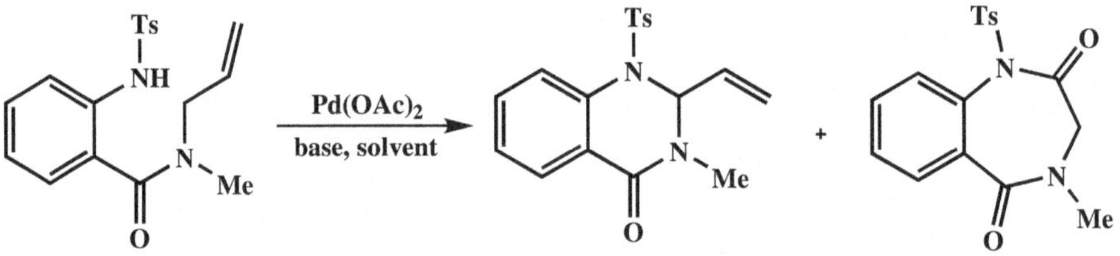

Scheme-23

Backvall [51] reported that good yields of carboamination products *i.e.* 2-(*α*-styryl) quinazolin-4-one derivatives were obtained when switched to palladium(0) catalyst along with aryl iodide **(Scheme 24)** [40b].

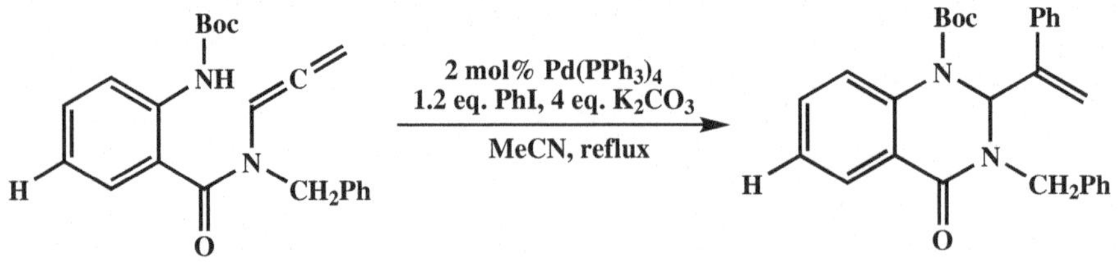

Scheme-24

Although application of reported cyclization conditions resulted in the formation of palladium black without conversion of starting material, the systematic use of a phase-transfer catalyst and an oxygen atmosphere on the basis of literature data [52-53] provided alkylated quinazoline in 69% yield as a single diastereomer **(Scheme 25)**. The *cis-N*-allyl-*N*-methyl analogue gave alkylated quinazolin as a single diastereomer, albeit in lower yield.

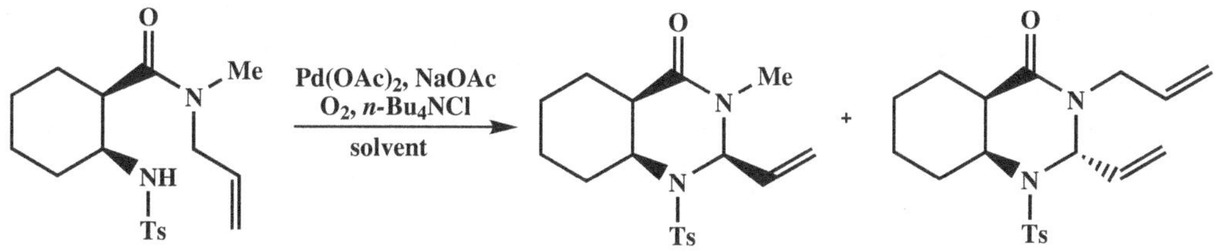

Scheme-25

The cyclization of *trans*-carboxamides was performed under optimized conditions in dimethylsulphoxide to afford a close to 1:1 mixture of two compounds (**Scheme 26**). On the basis of X-ray crystallography and two-dimensional NMR studies it was found that first-eluted compound was *trans* analogue of *trans*-carboxamides and the later-eluted one was *trans*-cyclohexane-fused 1,5-diazocin-6-one [54-55].

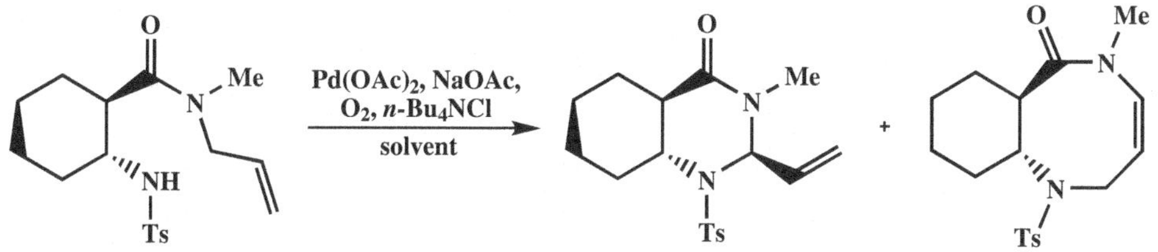

Scheme-26

Willis et al. [56] reported that under catalytic conditions *N*-(*o*-halophenyl)imidate substrates were utilized for the synthesis of benzimidazole precursors. These starting substrates were also used in the preparation of quinazolinones *via* carbonylation step. This catalytic method to obtain benzimidazoles was slightly modified which allowed the construction of a number of 2,3-disubstituted quinazolinones (**Scheme 27**) in good yields from aryl bromide substrates [57]. The mechanism proposed an initial Pd-catalyzed aminocarbonylation followed by a base-induced cyclization. The imidolyl chloride substrates were not used to prepare such quinazolinone [58].

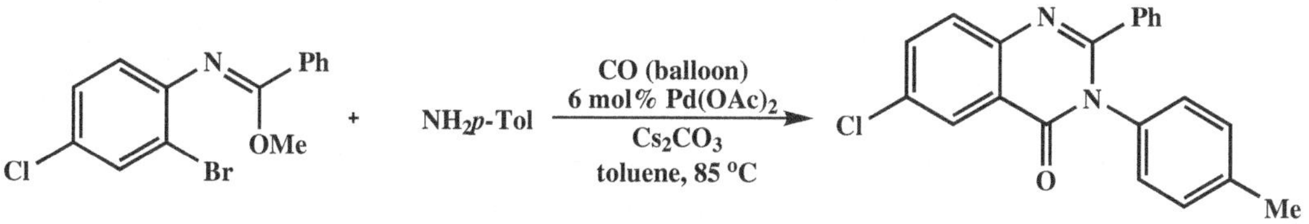

Scheme-27

The reaction of *o*-halobenzoates and monoalkyl ureas *via* tandem Pd-catalyzed arylation-ester amidation sequence produced many quinazolinediones. The 3-*N*-alkyl isomers were obtained regioselectively (**Scheme 28**) [59].

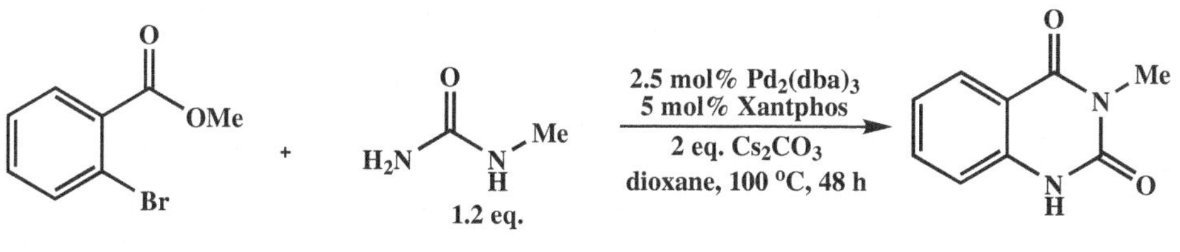

Scheme-28

Fueloep and co-workers [60] reported that *trans*- and *cis*-*N*-allyl-2-aminocyclohexane-carboxamides were transformed into cyclohexane-fused 1,5-diazocin-6-ones and pyrimidin-4-ones through *cis*-amino palladation *via* intramolecular oxidative cyclization in the presence of palladium(II) catalyst **(Scheme 29-30)**. Both diastereo- and regioselectivity of reaction was influenced depending on the solvent [28].

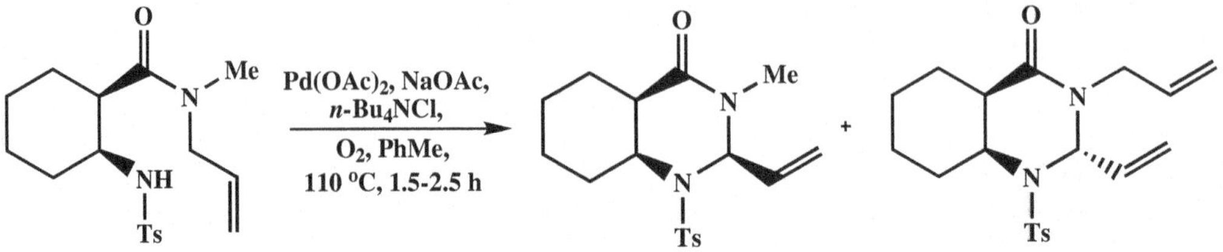

Scheme-29

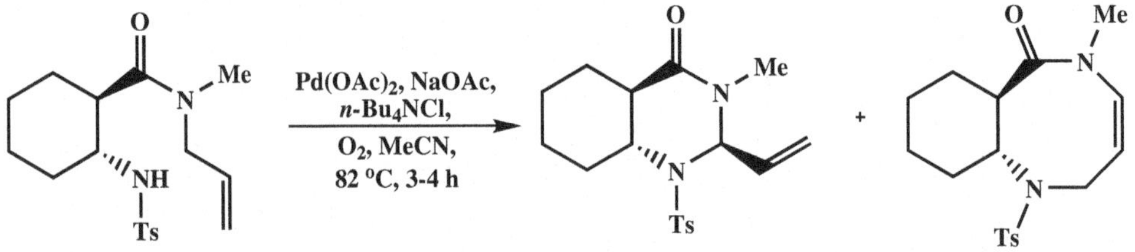

Scheme-30

Many isoindolinones were produced by this method **(Scheme 31)**. In some cases hydroxylated isoindolines were also synthesized along with isoindolinones. The hydroxylated isoindolines were produced from isoindolinones during the work-up. In each case isoindolinones and hydroxylated isoindolines were generated in high yields. This protocol was utilized for the synthesis of a natural product, glycosminine, from *N*-acetyl-2-bromoaniline derivative in a one-pot reaction. The *N*-acetyl-2-bromoaniline derivative, Pd(PPh$_3$)$_4$, and potassium carbonate were heated at 100 °C overnight under CO to afford glycosminine in 40% yield. The mechanism has proposed that acylpalladium complex was reacted with an enol part of acylpalladium complex to form benzoxazinone [61-62].

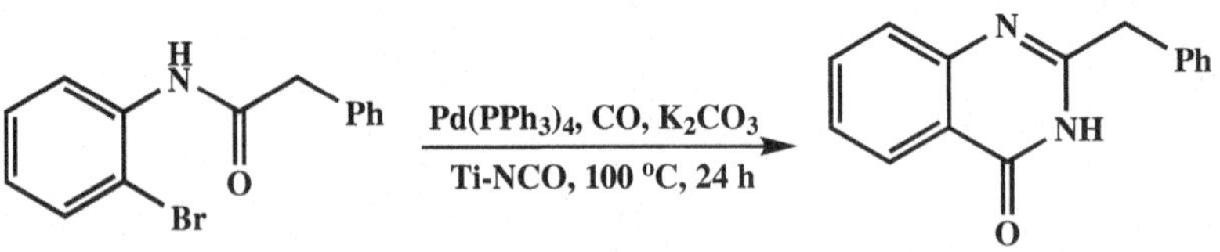

Scheme-31

The 6,7-disubstituted quinazolin-4(3*H*)-one was synthesized in 87% yield when 5-benzyloxy-4-methoxy-2-aminobenzamide was reacted with formamide in CH$_3$COOH (1 eq.) under MWI for 5 min at 300 W [63]. The reaction time reduced significantly by this protocol. In contrast to this, the thermal reaction of 6-benzyloxy-7-methoxyquinazolin-4(3*H*)-one and formamide occurred at 190 °C in 5 h [64]. The 4-chloro substituted quinazoline was formed in 68% yield upon reacting 6,7-disubstituted quinazolin-4(3*H*)-one in the presence of an excess amount of phosphoryl chloride. Then, the 4-anilino substituted derivative was formed in 93% yield from 4-chloro substituted quinazoline and 3-chloro-4-fluoroaniline. The debenzylation of 4-anilino substituted derivative was carried out smoothly upon hydrogenolysis over palladium/carbon in ethanol to afford the de-protected product in 85% yield. Finally, the etherification of 6-hydroxyl substituted quinazoline was attempted with 4-(3-chloropropyl)morpholine [65] in the presence of dimethylformamide upon heating at 90 °C for 3.5 h in a mild base **(Scheme 32)**.

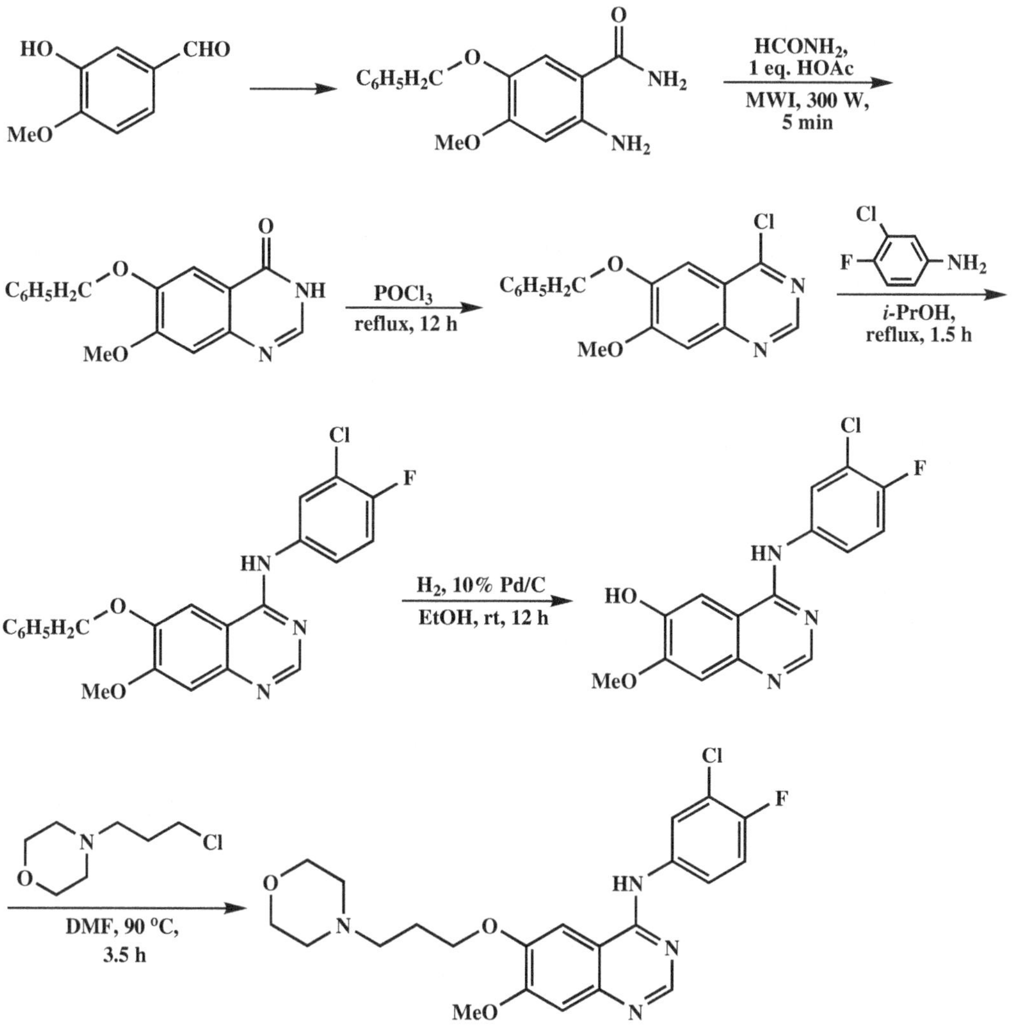

Scheme-32

The cyclization-oxidation with *o*-phenyldiamine analogs produced quinoxaline derivatives. Then, the quinoxaline-phenyl substituted compounds were produced by coupling with 4-fluoro phenyl boronic acid through Suzuki coupling in the presence of PdCl$_2$(dppf).DCM, *tert*-BuNH$_2$, sodium carbonate in isopropyl alcohol-water. The imidazo[1,2-*a*]pyridine was produced under MWI [66-68] using aluminium(III) chloride and propanoic anhydride at 100 °C for 20 min to provide an acylated product. The bromo compound was afforded by bromination [69-70] at α-carbon of acylated product in the presence of Br$_2$ in dichloromethane and diethyl ether at 0 °C-room temperature for 2 h. The bromo compound was alkylated with *N*-Boc-phenyl diamine using triethyl amine in CH$_3$CN for 12 h at 80 °C, and further cyclization-oxidation was performed *in situ* using CF$_3$COOH under refluxed condition for 4 h to provide bromo quinoxaline. The formed bromo quinoxaline *via* Suzuki coupling was further coupled with 4-fluorophenylboronic acid, [71-72] using PdCl$_2$(dppf).DCM, *tert.* BuNH$_2$, sodium carbonate in isopropyl alcohol-water under reflux conditions for 16 h, to afford quinoxaline derivative **(Scheme 33)** [73].

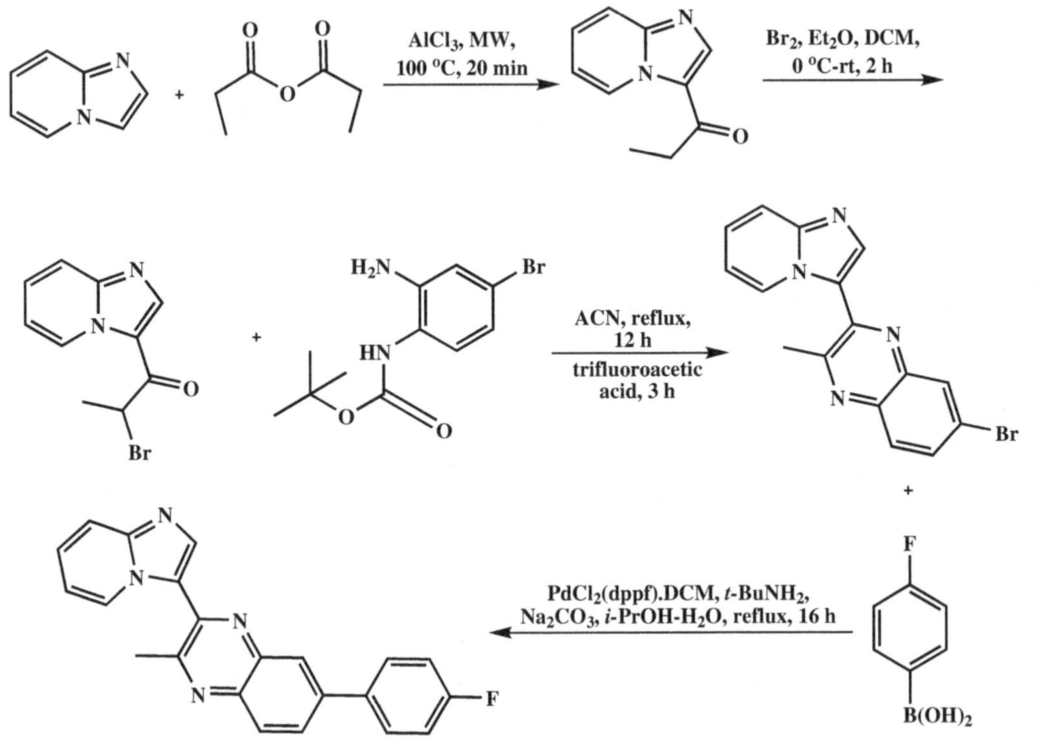

Scheme-33

The 4-acyl-1,2,3,4-tetrahydroquinoxalin-2-one library was synthesized by thermal and MW methods and it has been found that under MWI all the three steps afforded higher yields in less reaction times. Different types of reaction conditions were evaluated (for both protocols) for the optimization of experiments. Because of much faster reaction times in the MW runs a higher degree of optimization could be achieved. Whereas the thermal protocol needed 37 working days for optimization and validation to reach the final target structure, this could be achieved within 2 working days with microwaves **(Scheme 34)** [74].

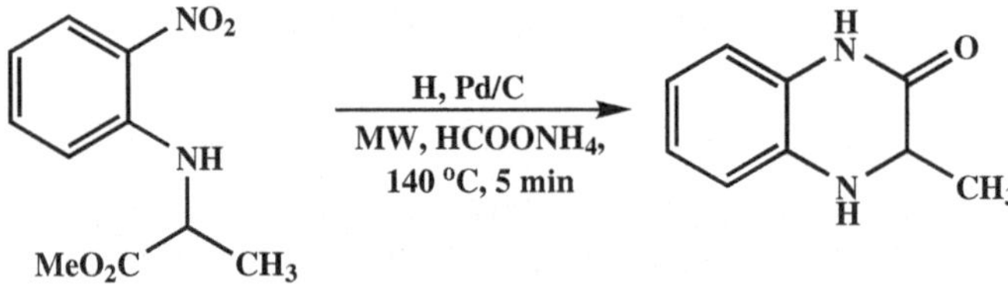

Scheme-34

Soderberg [75-76] reported the reductive deoxygenations of nitroaromatics in the presence of palladium(0) species with different ligands. Mixtures of 3,4-dihydroquinoxalines and 1,2-dihydro-quinoxalines were obtained when enamines were reacted with CO in the presence of 1,3-bis-(diphenylphosphino)propane and palladium(0). Soderberg also reported the preparation of 1,2-dihydro-4(3H)-carbazolones through a reductive N-heteroannulation step with palladium(0) catalyst. The enamine was used for the synthesis of 3,3-dimethyl-3,4-dihydro-1H-quinoxaline-2-one and 3,3-dimethyl-3,4-dihydro-quinoxaline. The yield of products was improved upon addition of a catalytic amount of 1,10-phenanthroline to reaction mixture **(Scheme 35)**.

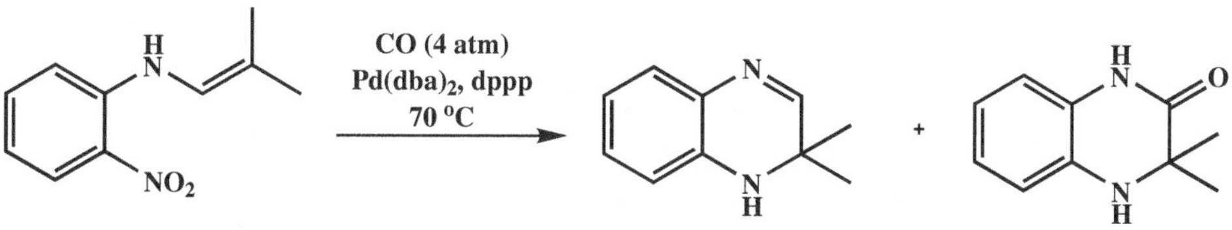

Scheme-35

The nucleophilic substitution of 6-fluoroquinoxaline with nitrogen-containing heterocyclic compounds and amines under computer-controlled MWI produced a small library of 6-aminoquinoxalines. The 4-fluoro-*o*-phenylenediamine was formed upon reduction of 4-fluoro-2-nitroaniline by catalytic hydrogenation in 10% palladium/carbon. The 6-fluoroquinoxalines were obtained by condensation of 4-fluoro-2-nitroaniline with 1,2-dioxo compounds. The 6-fluoroquinoxaline (1 eq.) was refluxed with pyrrolidine (2 eq.) in dimethyl sulfoxide in the presence of K_2CO_3 (2 eq.). After 30 min, 16% of expected 6-(1-pyrrolidinyl)-quinoxaline and 21% of unreacted starting material 6-fluoroquinoxaline were obtained. When reflux time was increased to 3 h, the starting material 6-fluoroquinoxaline disappeared, more side products were produced, and yield of substituted 6-(1-pyrrolidinyl)-quinoxaline was only slightly increased to 22%. MWI was employed to improve the nucleophilic substitution reaction. When a mixture of 6-fluoroquinoxaline (1 eq.), pyrrolidine (2 eq.) and K_2CO_3 (2 eq.) in DMF was exposed to MWI for 30 min at 120 °C, the starting material 6-fluoroquinoxaline was detected in considerable amounts and the yield of substituted product 6-(1-pyrrolidinyl)-quinoxaline was not improved. When solvent was changed from dimethylformamide to dimethylsulphoxide or *N*-methyl pyrrolidone and reaction temperature was raised to 200 °C, a moderate yield improvement was reported for the reaction in *N*-methyl-2-pyrrolidone, but in dimethylsulphoxide the reaction was completed within 30 min to afford the best yield (93%). The effect of base, 1,8-diazabicyclo[5,4,0] undec-7-ene or sodium hydroxide, was also evaluated, but more side products were detected and no yield improvements were reported in both cases. The yield also decreased when amount of pyrrolidine was reduced to one eq. Distinctly, in outcome of reactions, the concentration of nucleophile played an important role. Regardless of whether the reaction temperature was decreased or raised, the yield was not improved. It was reported that more by-products were produced at higher temperature and reaction was incomplete at temperatures lower than 200 °C. The yield decreased upon reducing the reaction time. These results indicated that optimized reaction conditions involved a mixture of 6-fluoroquinoxaline (one eq.), pyrrolidine (two eq.) and K_2CO_3 (two eq.) in dimethylsulphoxide under MWI for 30 min at 200 °C. The influence of substituents on quinoxaline ring was also reported. The product was obtained in excellent yields within 30 min when 2,3-difuryl substituted 6-fluoroquinoxaline was reacted with cyclic secondary amines, but to complete the reaction of 2,3-dimethyl- or 2,3-di-*p*-tolyl-substituted 6-fluoroquinoxaline with amines the reaction times needed to be prolonged **(Scheme 36)** [77].

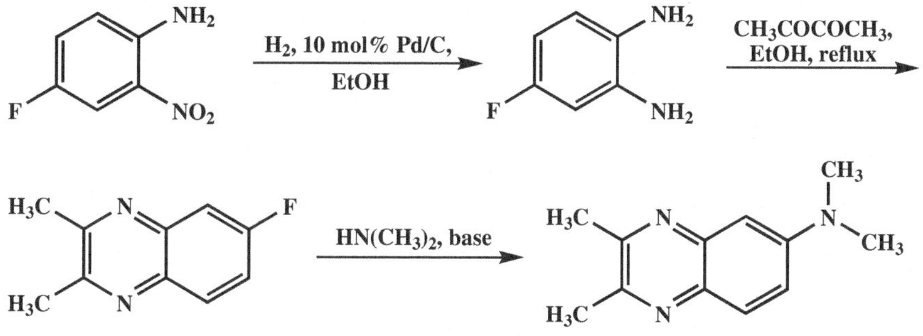

Scheme-36

The *o*-phenylenediamines provided tetrahydroquinoxalines as shown in **Scheme 37** [78]. The substituted *N*-allyl-1,2-phenylenediamine or *N*-allyl-ethylenediamine derivatives were utilized for the installation of different groups at C-2, C-6, N-1, and N-4 and synthesis of 2,3-disubstituted piperazines as well as tetrahydroquinoxalines [28].

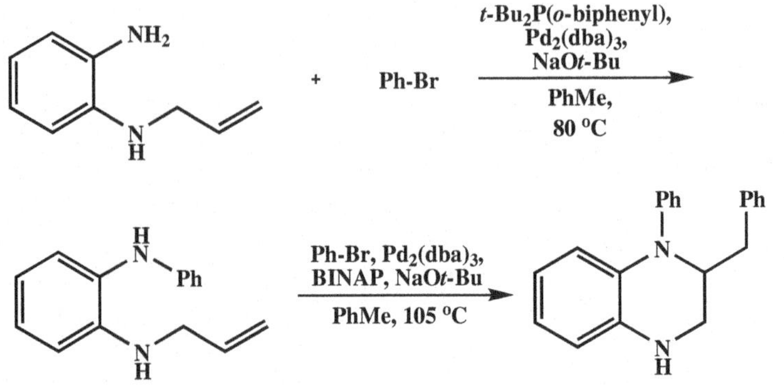

Scheme-37

Heterocyclic compounds were synthesized by a domino reaction which involved reduction of NO_2 group of *N*-allyl-*o*-nitroaniline coupled with Michael addition of formed amine onto allylic double bond. Beifuss et al. [79-80] reported a reductive domino cyclization of *N*-allyl-2-nitroanilines in the presence of $P(OEt)_3$ for the preparation of 1,2,3,4-tetrahydroquinoxalines in one-step under microwave irradiation **(Scheme 38)** [28].

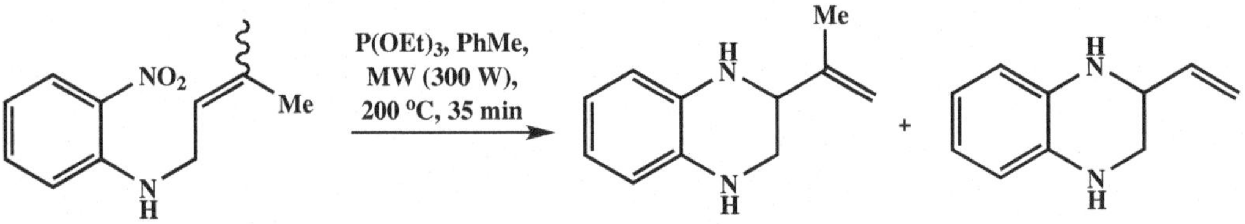

Scheme-38

This reaction afforded 2-methylenedihydroquinoxaline from starting substrate, not confirming the hypothesis that propargyl derivative reacted *via* allene intermediate **(Scheme 39)** [81-83].

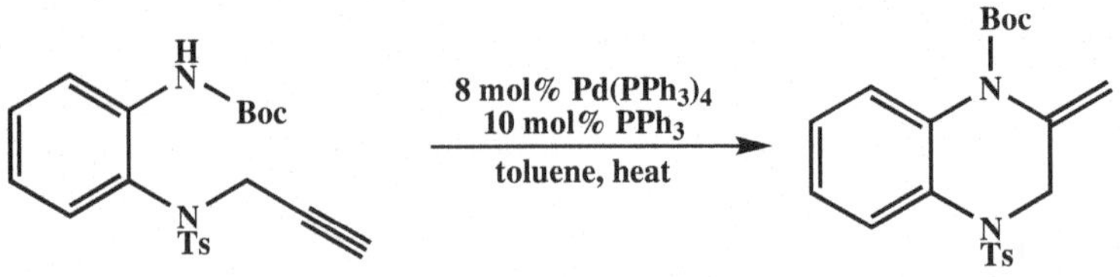

Scheme-39

The reductive cyclization of nitroalkene occurred with excess sodium borohydride-sodium ethoxide or with palladium acetate-carbon monoxide-mediated reductive heteroannulation, but poor yield of 1,2,3,4-tetrahydroquinoxaline was reported due to the formation of a mixture of products during the reaction **(Scheme 40)**. Nevertheless, the yield of product was improved upon increasing the catalytic load of palladium acetate [28, 84].

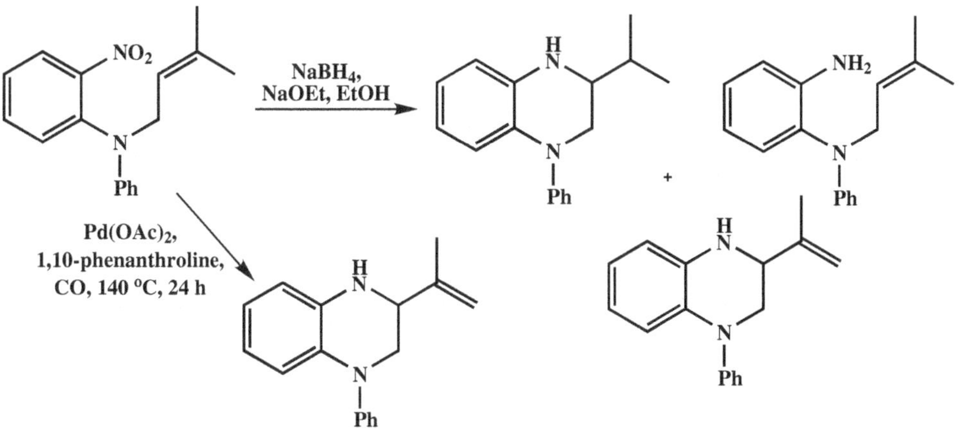

Scheme-40

10.5 Synthesis of six-membered two nitrogen-containing heterocycles fused with aromatics

The six-membered carbo- and heterocyclic rings were formed *via* intramolecular direct arylation of aryl bromides and aryl iodides in the presence of palladium hydroxide/carbon **(Scheme 41)** [85].

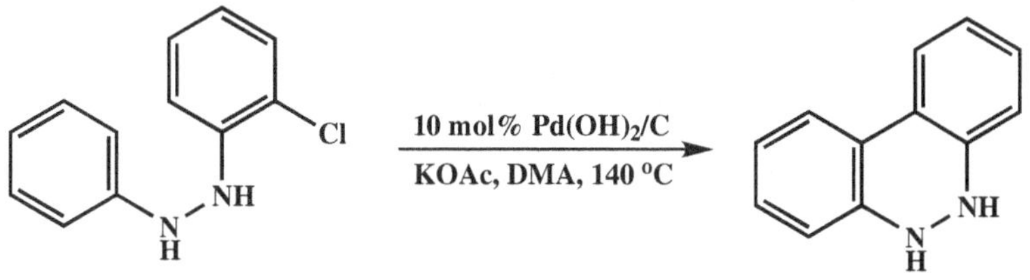

Scheme-41

Fagnou [86] reported the intramolecular direct aryation of aryl bromides, chlorides, and iodides with an efficient catalyst system **(Scheme 42)** for the synthesis of several five- and six-membered hetero- and carbocyclic biaryl compounds.

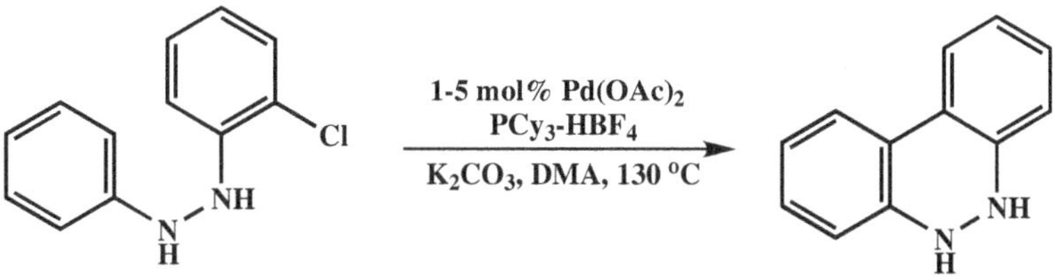

Scheme-42

While for direct arylation of aryl bromides the aforementioned catalytic system was found to be extremely effective, cyclized products were obtained in poor yields or no reaction occurred at all with aryl chlorides. Fagnou [87] reported new conditions using electron-rich *N*-heterocyclic carbene ligands [88]. A range of functionalized five- and six-membered rings were synthesized in excellent yields with varying tethers such as amine, ether, alkyl, and amide moieties in the presence of 1-3 mol% of catalyst, electron-rich *N*-heterocyclic carbene ligand, and potassium carbonate in dimethylaniline **(Scheme 43)**. This methodology, however, was limited to aryl bromides, no reaction occurred with aryl chlorides.

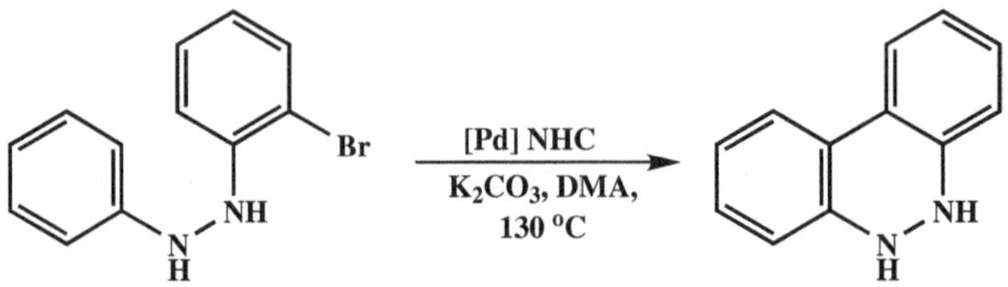

Scheme-43

Both electron-withdrawing and electron-donating substituents containing six-membered ring biaryl compounds were synthesized in excellent yields **(Scheme 44)**. Furthermore, nitrogen-and alkyl-possessing tethers were tolerated, but higher catalyst loadings were required for complete transformation [89].

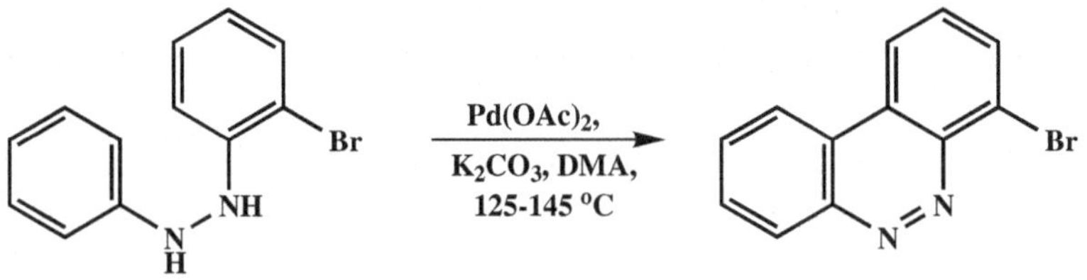

Scheme-44

Sharifi [90] utilized open containers and domestic oven for coupling of alkyl amines and aryl bromides. The most efficient catalyst was found to be Pd pre-catalyst Pd[P(*o*-tolyl)$_3$]$_2$Cl$_2$ in the presence of *t*-BuONa base and PhMe solvent. A similar method was reported by Hallberg [91] at about the same time for arylation of aryl and alkyl amines. The reaction was completed under mono-modal MWI of closed reaction vessels within 4 min in dimethylformamide, duplicating the standard method. Without compromising the high yield, high-temperature MW conditions afforded an improved reaction rate **(Scheme 45)** [92].

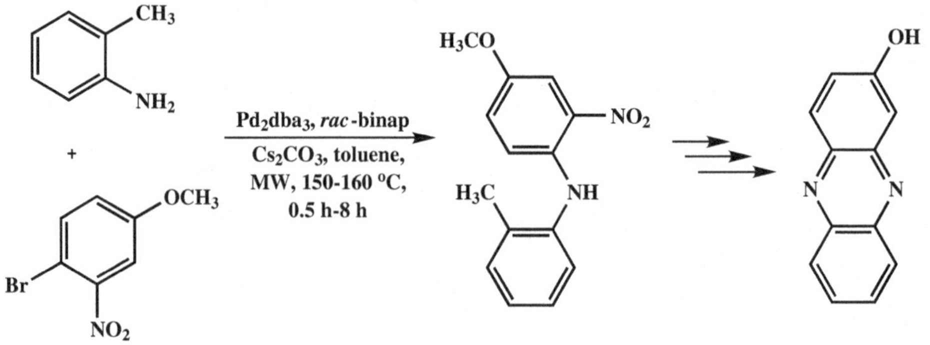

Scheme-45

The *N*-allylated phenazinones were synthesized through one-step or two steps reactions such as deoxygenation of NO$_2$ group and *N*-heterocyclization using a catalytic system such as carbon monoxide-palladium(II) or Buchwald-Hartwig [93-94] *N*-arylation of aryl halides. The Buchwald-Hartwig reaction was carried out with different substrates in the presence of palladium(0), *rac*-2,2-bis(diphenyl-phosphanyl)-1,1-binaphthyl, cesium carbonate as base and PhMe as solvent; [95] *N*-allyl 2-nitrodiphenylamine was a key precursor for direct ring closure through deoxygenation reaction to afford a compound; the tertiary amines were key precursors for a two-step cyclization reaction, through the reduction of NO$_2$ group to amino group followed by a possible intramolecular cyclization **(Scheme 46)**.

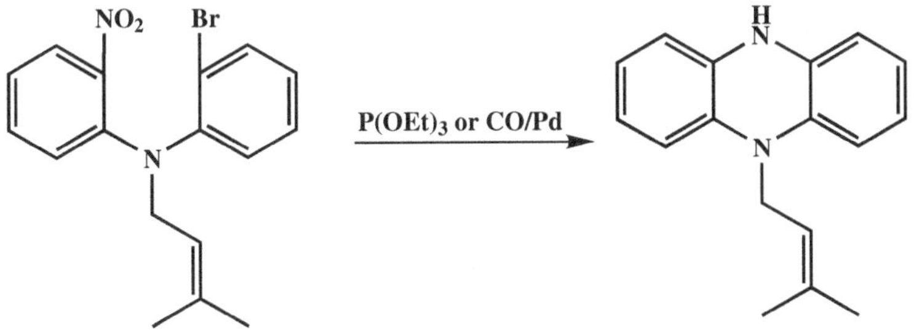

Scheme-46

Under optimized reaction conditions (2 mol% of Pd$_2$(dba)$_3$, 16 mol% of P(2-fur)$_3$), substrates were converted to products in good yield and with excellent diastereocontrol. A NOESY-2D experiment revealed the stereochemical outcome of transformation to be *syn*-addition across the olefin, which provided additional evidence for *syn*-amino-palladation mechanism proposed in **Scheme 47-48**. Side-allyl formation and consequently products in these reactions originated with the loss of diamine component of starting material [96].

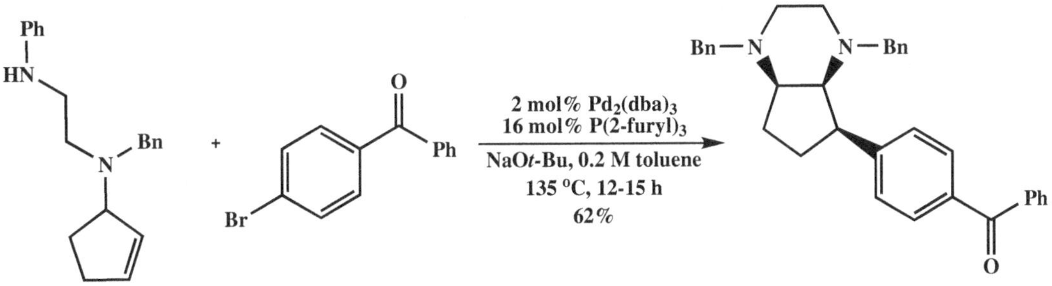

Scheme-47

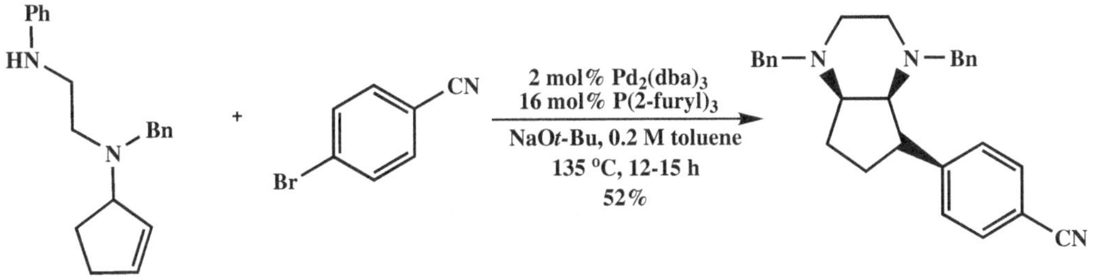

Scheme-48

10.6   Synthesis of six-membered two nitrogen-containing heterocycles fused with other heterocycles

The HWE reagent diethylphosphonoacetic acid was attached to *N*-terminus of amino acids on Rink amide resin. Horner-Wadsworth-Emmons reaction with a number of α,β-unsaturated aldehydes resulted in high transformation to diene amides. The triazolopyridazines were formed by subsequent [4+2]-cycloaddition with 4-substituted urazines, followed by cleavage of product from resin **(Scheme 49)** [97].

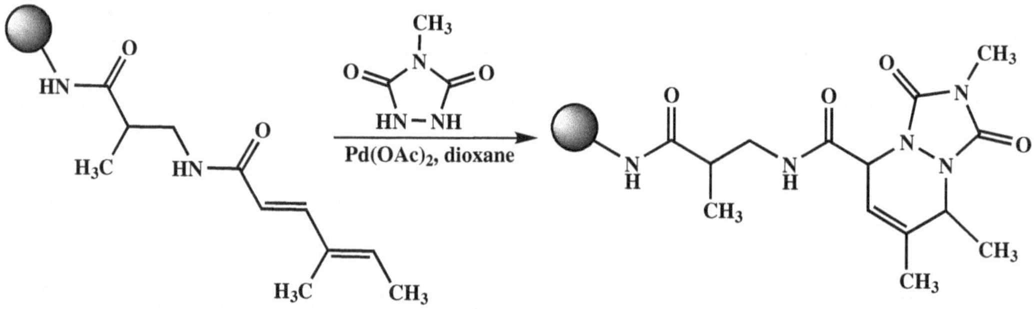

Scheme-49

Melnyk [98-99] explained an intramolecular cyclization of a bromopyridine and an indole in high yield and C-2-selectivity **(Scheme 50)**. The NH-bearing substrate provided a complex mixture of products therefore the protection as tertiary amide was needed to afford good yields. Authors also performed a tandem C-2 cyclization/C-3 Heck reaction during cyclization in the presence of acrylate. Unfortunately, only cyclized product was obtained in low yields when catalytic amounts of Pd were employed. The tandem cyclization/Heck reaction product was formed in modest yields (63%) using stoichiometric amounts of catalyst along with an excess of acrylate (15 eq.).

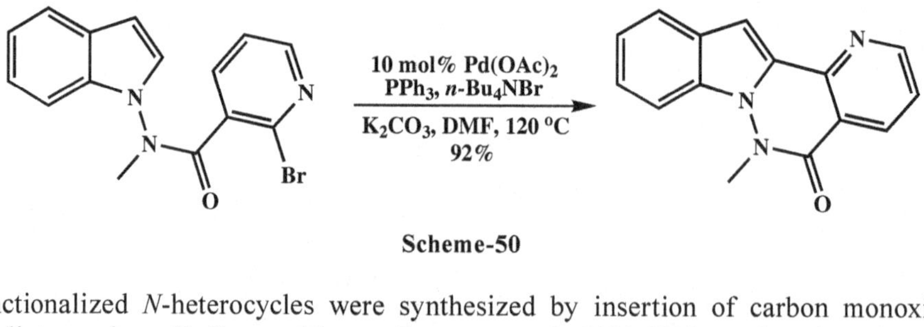

Scheme-50

Functionalized *N*-heterocycles were synthesized by insertion of carbon monoxide into intermediate aminopalladium adducts. Tamaru et al. [100-102] produced pyrimidinones, imidazolidinones, and related *N*-heterocycles under Wacker-type conditions using a number of unsaturated carbamates and ureas as nitrogen nucleophiles **(Scheme 51)**. Both nitrogen atoms acted as nucleophiles when urea derivatives were employed as substrates [50, 103].

The acylation with *o*-nitrobenzoyl chloride synthesized 1,4-benzodiazepinedione derivative, which was reduced to provide high yield of *N*-benzylsclerotigenin **(Scheme 52)** [104].

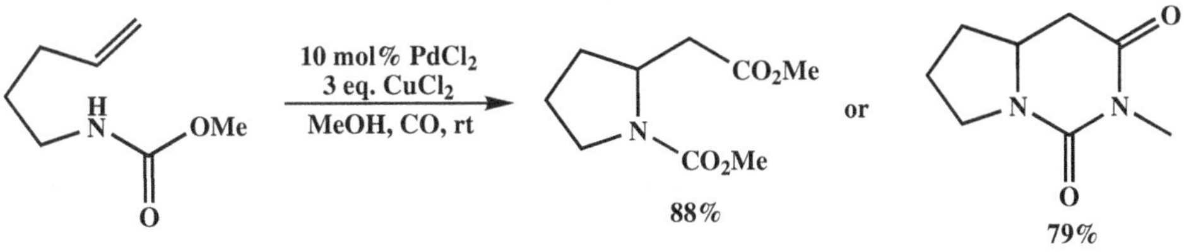

Scheme-51

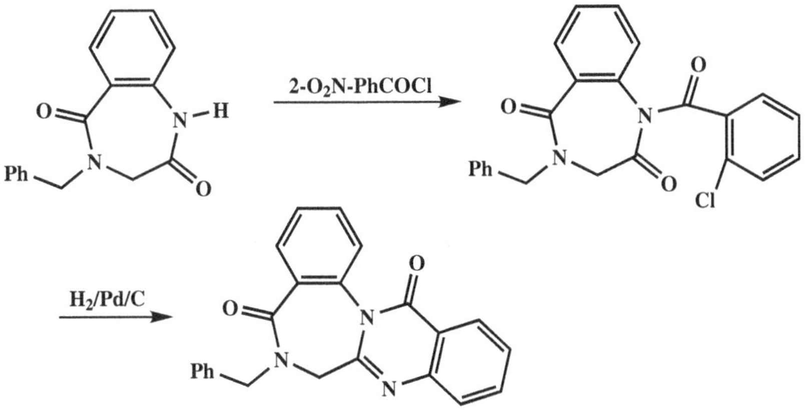

Scheme-52

Through a Suzuki coupling reaction aromatic substituents were introduced at C5. Calderwood and co-workers [105] synthesized a series of pyrrolo[2,3-*d*]pyrimidines bearing N-7 substituents as potent inhibitors of lck, a src family tyrosine kinase expressed primarily in T lymphocytes. The key step was Suzuki coupling of 4-phenoxyphenylboronic acid and iodo derivative for the synthesis of pyrrolo[2,3-*d*]pyrimidines **(Scheme 53)** [106].

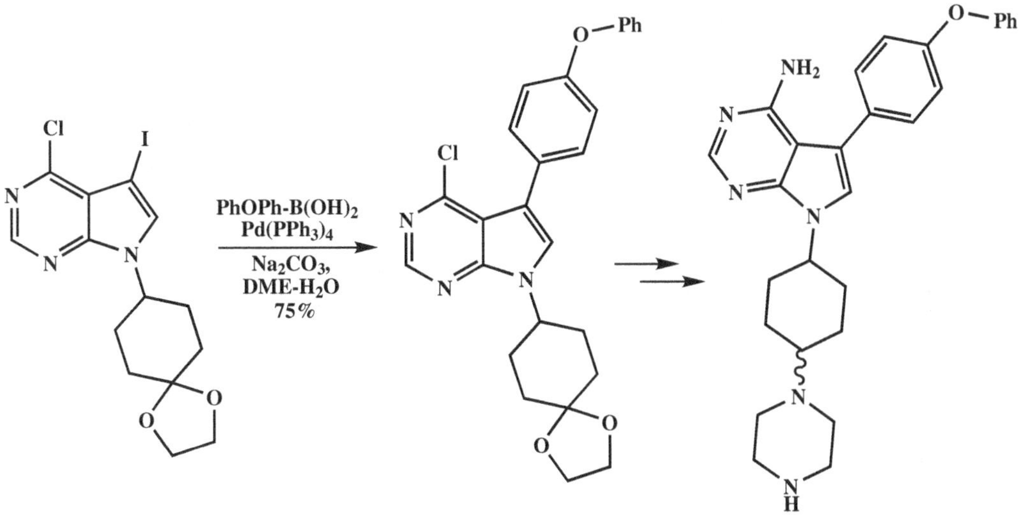

Scheme-53

The initial cycloadducts were prevented from further fragmentation by using a nitroaryl moiety at 3-position of azirine ring **(Scheme 54)**. The cleavage of desired carbon-nitrogen bond was triggered by a subsequent release (by NO$_2$ group reduction and protection) of anilide. Depending on the nature of ester-protecting group these conditions led to both azacepham derivatives [107].

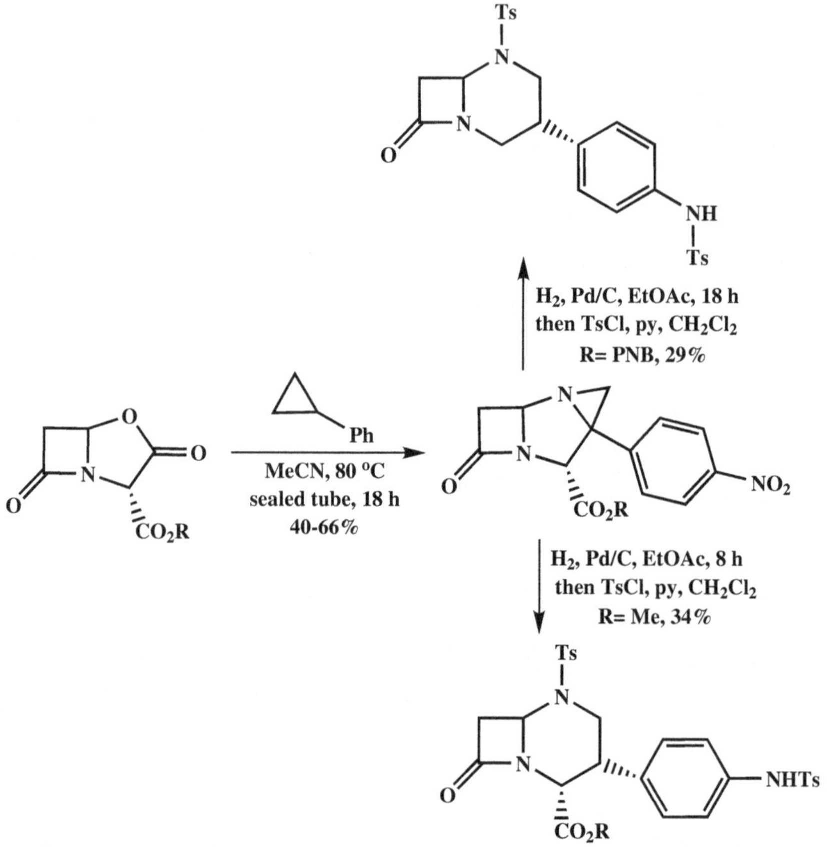

Scheme-54

Furstner and Weintritt [108] described the synthesis of heterobiaryl-pyridoquinazolinone derivative *via* 3-lithio-derivative, which was generated by metal-halogen exchange reaction and subsequent reaction with 3,3′,5,5′-tetramethylbenzidine, followed by appropriate work-up to yield the desired boronic acid. They did not purify this acid and reacted it directly in a Suzuki cross-coupling reaction aimed at the synthesis of a heterobiaryl-pyridoquinazolinone derivative **(Scheme 55)**, which is a potential anti-cancer agent.

The reactions were extended to *o*-dibromovinyl funtionalized isocyanatobenzenes. The reactions occurred efficiently in the presence of *N*-alkyl aromatic amines, to provide masked indoles through cuprous iodide-catalyzed nucleophilic displacement and *N*-vinylation process, and indoles which are very important precursors for one-pot fusion of multicyclic scaffolds *via* a subsequent carbon-hydrogen activation in the presence of palladium catalyst **(Scheme 56)** [109-110].

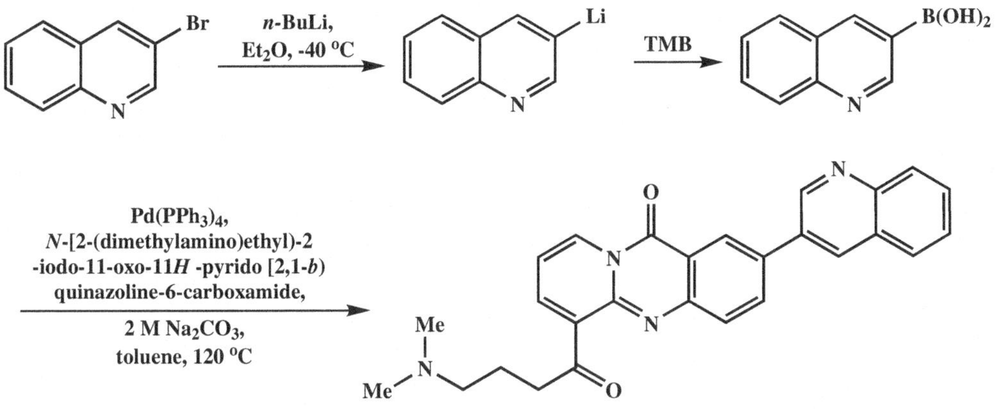

Scheme-55

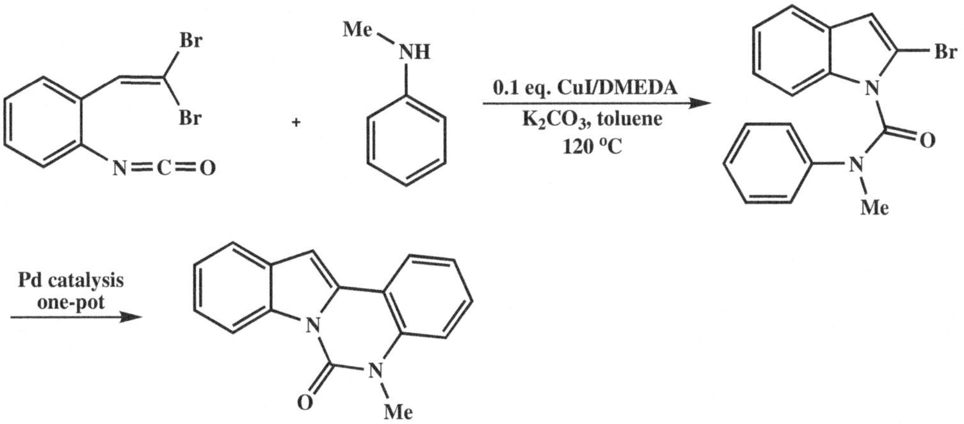

Scheme-56

Zhu [111] explained a domino process involving intramolecular *N*-arylation/direct arylation in the presence of Pd catalyst. The bisaryl diiodide was subjected to 5 mol% of PdCl$_2$-(dppf) and carbon for the preparation of fused macrocyclic dihydroazaphenanthrenes and other medium-ring heterocyclic compounds **(Scheme 57)**.

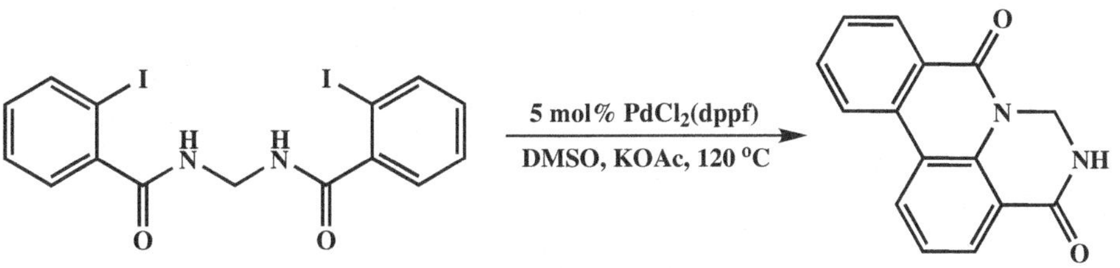

Scheme-57

This protocol afforded a variety of alkaloids, like indoles [112-115], indazoles [116-117], benzimidazoles [118-119], benazepines [120-121], phenazines [122], carbapenems [123], the mitomycin ring system [124], carbolines [125] and polyheterocycles **(Scheme 58)**.

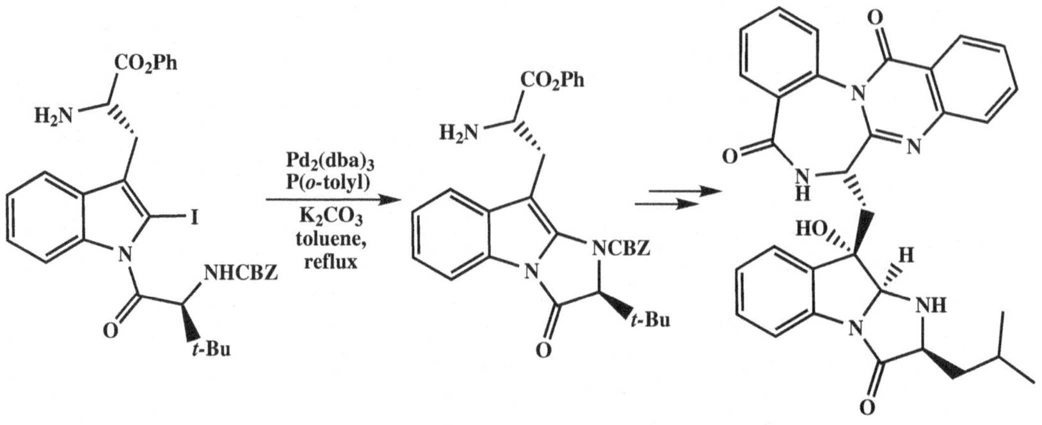

Scheme-58

Arcadi and co-workers [126] synthesized indole[1,2-c]quinazolines in high yields by cyclization of bis(o-trifluoroacetamidophenyl)acetylene with vinyl and aryl halides in the presence of Pd catalyst **(Scheme 59)**. The reaction occurred *via* aminopalladation-reductive elimination. The tetracyclic heterocyclic compound was formed by cyclization of resulting 3-arylinodole derivatives.

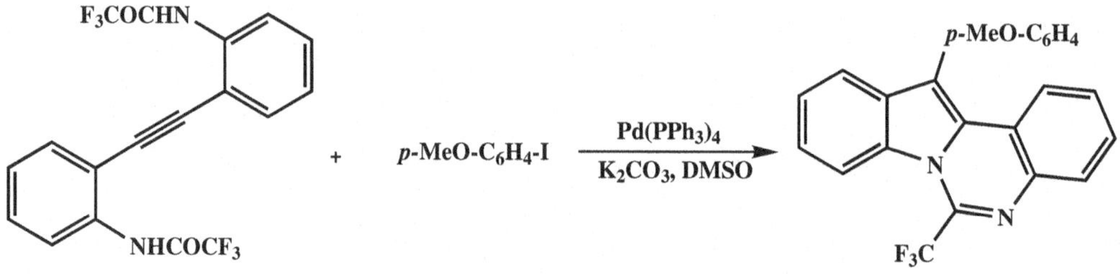

Scheme-59

Arcadi and co-workers [126] synthesized 2,3-substituted indoles when *N*-trifluoromethyl aniline was reacted with alkenyltriflates or aryl halides in the presence of Pd(PPh$_3$)$_4$. The 3-carbomethoxyindole derivative was formed when same reaction was performed in the presence of CO and MeOH [127-128]. Cacchi and co-workers [129-130] carried out Pd-catalyzed cyclocarbonylation of bis(o-trifluoroacetamidophenyl)acetylene with vinyl or aryl halides to form 12-acylindolo[1,2-c]quinazolines **(Scheme 60)** [131].

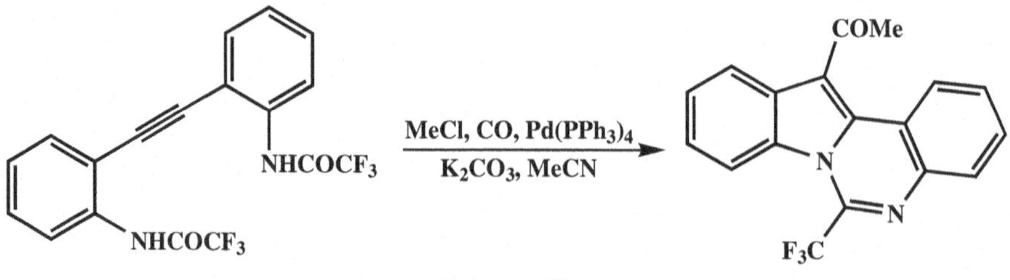

Scheme-60

The 4,6-dichloro-5-nitropyrimidine was displaced with a fluorous aminoester for the formation of *N*-alkylated dihydropteridinones. The formed compounds were then treated with secondary amines. The NO$_2$ group of produced product was reduced by hydrogenation with palladium on charcoal as a catalyst. The cyclization reactions were carried out under MWI. The monobenzylated products *N*-alkylated dihydropteridinones were formed in high selectivity when cyclized products underwent *N*-alkylation reaction with benzyl halides. All the final products and intermediate were purified by crystallization or fluorous solid-phase extraction **(Scheme 61)** [132-133].

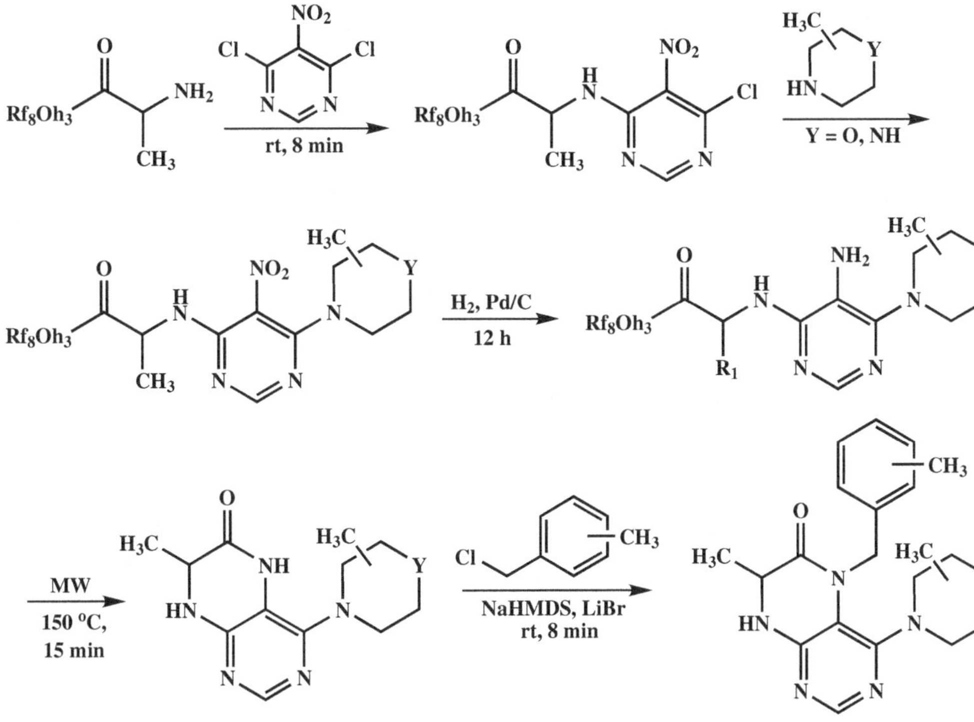

Scheme-61

The complex heterocyclic systems were synthesized by transition metal-catalyzed intra-molecular methods [134-145]. An arylative palladium-catalyzed cyclization of *N*-allyl-pyrrole-2-carboxamides was performed to provide pyrrolo[2,3-*c*]pyridines or pyrrolo[1,2-*a*]pyrazines **(Scheme 62)** [146]. The isomeric pyrrolo[3,2-*c*]pyridines were also produced in this reaction arising from 1,2-migration of amide moiety. Having recently broadened their studies toward Au catalysis, Manzo et al. [147-148] investigated Au-catalyzed intramolecular hydroarylation of alkynyl-tethered pyrrole-2-carboxamides to afford pyrrolo-fused pyridine skeletons in order to have an alternative method. The biological importance of pyrrolo[3,2-*c*]pyridine and pyrrolo[2,3-*c*] pyridine derivatives [149-161] justifies new efforts to synthesize them [162].

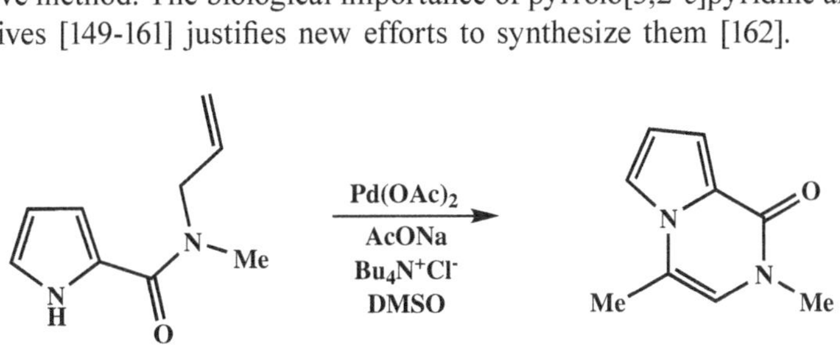

Scheme-62

An intramolecular amidation of 1-allyl-2-indolecarboxamides afforded pyrazino[1,2-*a*] indole derivatives in high yields **(Scheme 63)** [163]. The reaction occurred by cyclization of a Pd-complex intermediate and subsequent double-bond isomerization [50].

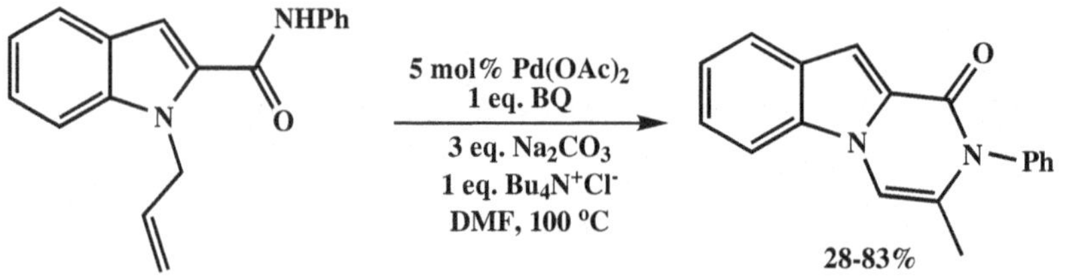

Scheme-63

To reach a better insight about hydroamination process, Meguro [164] found that presence of both palladium catalyst and MWI were necessary for the formation of tarry products. Only a tarry mixture of degradation products was obtained without MW activation. The hydroxy-substituted pyrazino[1,2-*a*]indole was formed in 41% yield in the absence of Pd catalyst **(Scheme 64)** [142].

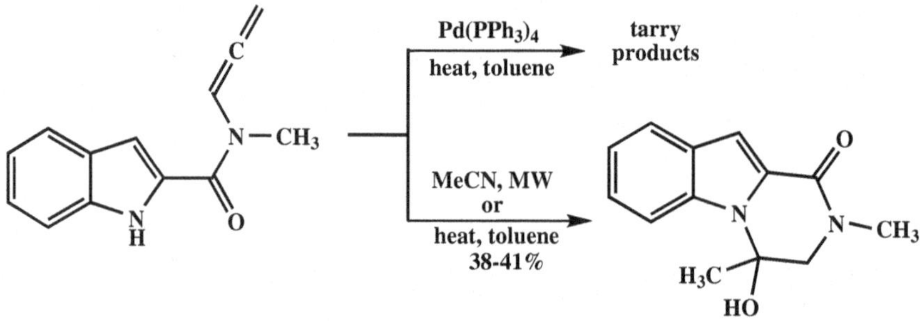

Scheme-64

Palladium-catalyzed asymmetric allylic substitution reactions have also emerged as an efficient method for the construction of carbon-carbon and carbon-heteratom bonds. A wide range of nucleophiles can be employed and a variety of functional groups can be tolerated [165-166]. Trost reported an enantioselective desymmetrization reaction of Boc-activated cyclopenten-1,4-diol for the synthesis of piperazone *via* successive palladium-catalyzed asymmetric amination reactions in one-pot **(Scheme 65)** [167]. Treatment of cyclopenten-1,4-diol and *N*-methoxyamide

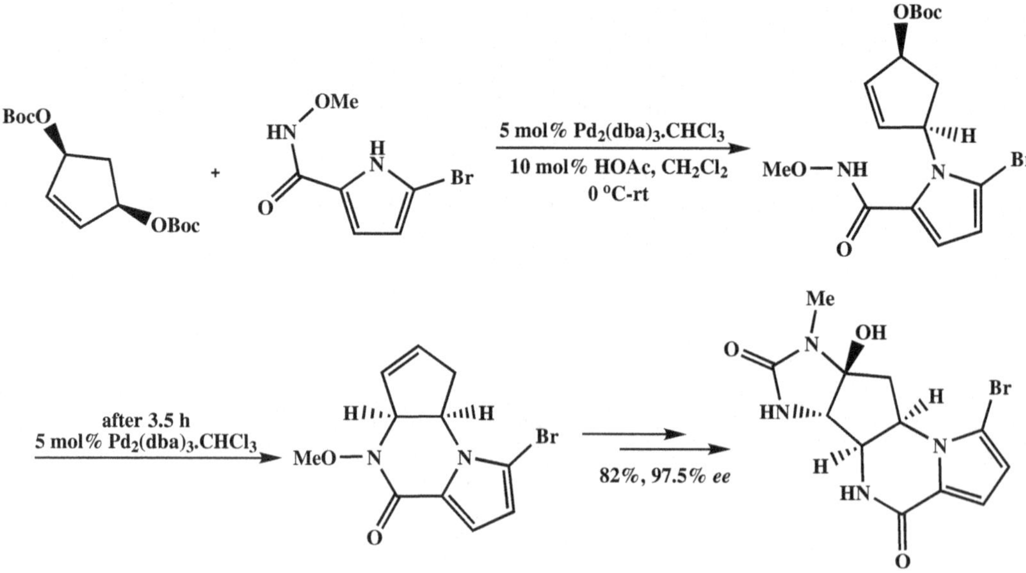

Scheme-65

with catalytic Pd$_2$(dba)$_3$, and acetic acid in dichloromethane facilitated desymmetrization of cyclopenten-1,4-diol to form intermediate. After 3.5 h, another portion of Pd$_2$(dba)$_3$ was added to catalyze a subsequent intramolecular allylic amination reaction. Piperazone was prepared in 82% yield and 97.5% *ee*, and subsequently served as an intermediate in the synthesis of agelastatin A.

REFERENCES

[1]   X. Zhang, H. Wang and Y.L.R. Cao. 2013. Novel substituted heteroaromatic piperazine and piperidine derivatives as inhibitors of human enterovirus 71 and coxsackievirus A16. Molecules 18: 5059-5071.

[2]   (a) N. Kaur. 2015. Microwave-assisted synthesis: fused five-membered *N*-heterocycles. Synth. Commun. 45: 789-823.
      (b) N. Kaur. 2015. Six-membered heterocycles with three and four *N*-heteroatoms: microwave-assisted synthesis. Synth. Commun. 45: 151-172.
      (c) N. Kaur. 2015. Application of microwave-assisted synthesis in the synthesis of fused six-membered heterocycles with *N*-heteroatom. Synth. Commun. 45: 173-201.
      (d) N. Kaur. 2015. Microwave-assisted synthesis of fused polycyclic six-membered *N*-heterocycles. Synth. Commun. 45: 273-299.
      (e) N. Kaur. 2015. Review of microwave-assisted synthesis of benzo fused six-membered *N,N*-heterocycles. Synth. Commun. 45: 300-330.
      (f) N. Kaur and D. Kishore. 2014. Synthetic strategies applicable in the synthesis of privileged scaffold: 1,4-benzodiazepine. Synth. Commun. 44: 1375-1413.

[3]   (a) N.T. Patil and Y. Yamamoto. 2008. Coinage metal-assisted synthesis of heterocycles. Chem. Rev. 108: 3395-3442.
      (b) N. Kaur. 2015. Palladium-catalyzed approach to the synthesis of *S*-heterocycles. Catal. Rev. Sci. Eng. 57: 478-564.

[4]   L. Jimenez-Gonzalez, S. Garcia-Munoz, M. Alvarez-Corral, M. Munoz-Dorado and I. Rodriguez-Garcia. 2006. Silver-catalyzed asymmetric synthesis of 2,3-dihydrobenzofurans: a new chiral synthesis of pterocarpans. Chem. Eur. J. 12: 8762-8779.

[5]   A.R. Dick and M.S. Sanford. 2006. Transition metal catalyzed oxidative functionalization of carbon-hydrogen bonds. Tetrahedron 62: 2439-2463.

[6]   Z. Li and C. He. 2006. Recent advances in silver-catalyzed nitrene, carbene, and silylene-transfer reactions. Eur. J. Org. Chem. 19: 4313-4322.

[7]   H.M.L. Davies and J.R. Manning. 2008. Catalytic C-H functionalization by metal carbenoid and nitrenoid insertion. Nature 451: 417-424.

[8]   M.M. Diaz-Requejo and P.J. Perez. 2008. Coinage metal catalyzed C-H bond functionalization of hydrocarbons. Chem. Rev. 108: 3379-3394.

[9]   P. Muller and C. Fruit. 2003. Enantioselective catalytic aziridinations and asymmetric nitrene insertions into CH bonds. Chem. Rev. 103: 2905-2919.

[10] O.A. Attanasi, G. Favi, P. Filippone, F. Mantellini, G. Moscatelli and F.R. Perrulli. 2010. Copper(II)/copper(I)-catalyzed aza-Michael addition/click reaction of *in situ* generated azidohydrazones: synthesis of novel pyrazolone-triazole framework. Org. Lett. 12: 468-471.

[11] B.C.G. Soderberg. 2000. Synthesis of heterocycles *via* intramolecular annulation of nitrene intermediates. Curr. Org. Chem. 4: 727-764.

[12] S. Fantauzzi, A. Caselli and E. Gallo. 2009. Nitrene transfer reactions mediated by metallo-porphyrin complexes. Dalton Trans. 28: 5434-5443.

[13] S. Cenini, E. Gallo, A. Caselli, F. Ragaini, S. Fantauzzi and C. Piangiolino. 2006. Coordination chemistry of organic azides and amination reactions catalyzed by transition metal complexes. Coord. Chem. Rev. 250: 1234-1253.

[14]   T. Katsuki. 2005. Azide compounds: nitrogen sources for atom-efficient and ecologically benign nitrogen-atom-transfer reactions. Chem. Lett. 34: 1304-1309.

[15]   R. Mishra, K.K. Jha, S. Kumar and I. Tomer. 2011. Synthesis, properties and biological activity of thiophene: a review. Der Pharma Chemica 3: 38-54.

[16]   S.K. Chattopadhyay, S. Karmakar, T. Biswas, K.C. Majumdar, H. Rahaman and B. Roy. 2007. Formation of medium-ring heterocycles by diene and enyne metathesis. Tetrahedron 63: 3919-3952.

[17]   L.F. Tietze, G. Kettschau, J.A. Gewert and A. Schuffenhauer. 1998. Hetero-Diels-Alder reactions of 1-oxa-1,3-butadienes. Curr. Org. Chem. 2: 19-62.

[18]   L.F. Tietze and G. Kettschau. 1997. Hetero-Diels-Alder reactions in organic chemistry. Top. Curr. Chem. 189: 1-120.

[19]   D.A. Evans, J.S. Johnson and E.J. Olhava. 2000. Enantioselective synthesis of dihydropyrans. Catalysis of hetero-Diels-Alder reactions by bis(oxazoline) copper(II) complexes. J. Am. Chem. Soc. 122: 1635-1649.

[20]   R.A. Batey, D.A. Powell, A. Acton and A.J. Lough. 2001. Dysprosium(III) catalyzed formation of hexahydrofuro[3,2-c]quinolines *via* 2:1 coupling of dihydrofuran with substituted anilines. Tetrahedron Lett. 42: 7935-7939.

[21]   W. Zhang and T. Nagashima. 2006. Palladium-catalyzed Buchwald-Hartwig type amination of fluorous arylsulfonates. J. Fluorine Chem. 127: 588-591.

[22]   W. Zhang, T. Nagashima, Y. Lu and C.H.-T. Chen. 2004. A traceless perfluorooctylsulfonyl tag for deoxygenation of phenols under microwave irradiation. Tetrahedron Lett. 45: 4611-4613.

[23]   A.S. Karpov and T.J.J. Muller. 2003. New entry to a three-component pyrimidine synthesis by TMS-ynones *via* Sonogashira coupling. Org. Lett. 5: 3451-3454.

[24]   A.S. Karpov, E. Merkul, F. Rominger and T.J.J. Muller. 2005. Concise syntheses of meridianins *via* carbonylative alkynylation and a novel four-component pyrimidine synthesis. Angew. Chem. Inter. Ed. 44: 6951-6956.

[25]   B. Willy, F. Rominger and T.J.J. Muller. 2008. Novel microwave-assisted one-pot synthesis of isoxazoles by a three-component coupling-cycloaddition sequence. Synthesis 2: 293-303.

[26]   D.M. D'Souza and T.J.J. Muller. 2007. Multi-component syntheses of heterocycles by transition-metal catalysis. Chem. Soc. Rev. 36: 1095-1108.

[27]   V.A. Timoshchuk and R.I. Hogrefe. 2009. The "Corey's reagent," 3,5-di-*tert*-butyl-1,2-benzoquinone, as a modifying agent in the synthesis of fluorescent and double-headed nucleosides. Nucleosides, Nucleotides Nucleic Acids 28: 464-472.

[28]   S. Nag and S. Batra. 2011. Applications of allylamines for the syntheses of aza-heterocycles. Tetrahedron 67: 8959-9061.

[29]   T. Pilarcik, J. Havlicek and J. Hajicek. 2005. Towards schizozygine: synthesis of 15α-hydroxystrempeliopine. Tetrahedron Lett. 46: 7909-7911.

[30]   B. Ferber, G. Prestat, S. Vogel, D. Madec and G. Poli. 2006. Synthesis of 3,5-disubstituted piperazinones *via* palladium(II)-catalyzed amination. Synlett 13: 2133-2135.

[31]   (a) J.S. Nakhla, D.M. Schultz and J.P. Wolfe. 2009. Palladium-catalyzed alkene carboamination reactions for the synthesis of substituted piperazines. Tetrahedron 65: 6549-6570.
        (b) J.S. Nakhla, J.W. Kampf and J.P. Wolfe. 2006. Intramolecular Pd-catalyzed carboetherification and carboamination. Influence of catalyst structure on reaction mechanism and product stereochemistry. J. Am. Chem. Soc. 128: 2893-2901.

[32]   J.S. Nakhla and J.P. Wolfe. 2007. A concise asymmetric synthesis of *cis*-2,6-disubstituted *N*-aryl piperazines *via* Pd-catalyzed carboamination reactions. Org. Lett. 9: 3279-3282.

[33]   B.M. Cochran and F.E. Michael. 2008. Synthesis of 2,6-disubstituted piperazines by a diastereoselective palladium-catalyzed hydroamination reaction. Org. Lett. 10: 329-332.

[34]   G.J. Mercer and M.S. Sigman. 2003. Diastereoselective synthesis of piperazines by manganese-mediated reductive cyclization. Org. Lett. 5: 1591-1594.

[35]   M. Yamashita and J.F. Hartwig. 2004. Synthesis, structure, and reductive elimination chemistry of three-coordinate arylpalladium amido complexes. J. Am. Chem. Soc. 126: 5344-5345.

[36] L.E. Overman. 1976. A general method for the synthesis of amines by the rearrangement of allylic trichloroacetimidates. 1,3 Transposition of alcohol and amine functions. J. Am. Chem. Soc. 98: 2901-2910.

[37] D.A. Cogan, G. Liu and J. Ellman. 1999. Asymmetric synthesis of chiral amines by highly diastereo-selective 1,2-additions of organometallic reagents to *N-tert*-butanesulfinyl imines. Tetrahedron 55: 8883-8904.

[38] J. Pawlas, Y. Nakao, M. Kawatsura and J.F. Hartwig. 2002. A general nickel-catalyzed hydroamination of 1,3-dienes by alkylamines: catalyst selection, scope, and mechanism. J. Am. Chem. Soc. 124: 3669-3679.

[39] A.M. Johns, M. Utsunomiya, C.D. Incarvito and J.F. Hartwig. 2006. A highly active palladium catalyst for intermolecular hydroamination. Factors that control reactivity and additions of functionalized anilines to dienes and vinylarenes. J. Am. Chem. Soc. 128: 1828-1839.

[40] (a) S. Husinec, M. Petkovic, V. Savic and M. Simic. 2012. Synthesis of allyl acetates *via* palladium-catalyzed functionalization of allenes and 1,3-dienes. Synthesis 44: 399-408.
    (b) T. Lu, Z. Lu, Z.-X. Ma, Y. Zhang and R.P. Hsung. 2013. Allenamides: a powerful and versatile building block in organic synthesis. Chem. Rev. 113: 4862-4904.

[41] R. Grigg, V. Sridharan, M. Shah, S. Mutton, C. Kilner, D. MacPherson and P. Milner. 2008. Regioselective synthesis of *N*-aminoisoindolones and mono-*N*- and di-*N,N'*-substituted phthalazones utilizing hydrazine nucleophiles in a palladium-catalyzed three-component cascade process. J. Org. Chem. 73: 8352-8356.

[42] D. Bouyssi, N. Monteiro and G. Balme. 2011. Amines as key building blocks in Pd-assisted multicomponent processes. Beilstein J. Org. Chem. 7: 1387-1406.

[43] R. Grigg, V. Sridharan and L-.H. Xu. 1995. Palladium-catalyzed cyclization-amination of allenes-effect of base on regioselectivity of formation of allylic amines. J. Chem. Soc. Chem. Commun. 18: 1903-1904.

[44] A.E. Kummerle, M.M. Vieira, M. Schmitt, A.L.P. Miranda, C.A.M. Fraga and J.-J. Bourguignon. 2009. Design, synthesis and analgesic properties of novel conformationally-restricted *N*-acylhydrazones (NAH). Eur. J. Med. Chem. 19: 4963-4966.

[45] N.M. Nascimento-Junior, A.E. Kummerle, E.J. Barreiro and C.A.M. Fraga. 2011. MAOS and medicinal chemistry: some important examples from the last years. Molecules 16: 9274-9297.

[46] S. Brase, S. Dahmen and J. Heuts. 1999. Solid-phase synthesis of substituted cinnolines by a Richter type cleavage protocol. Tetrahedron Lett. 40: 6201-6203.

[47] M.R.J. Ife, T.H. Brown, P. Blurton, D.J. Keeling, C.A. Leach, M.L. Meeson, I.E. Parsons and C.J. Theobald. 1995. Reversible inhibitors of the gastric (H^+/K^+)-ATPase. Substituted 2,4-diamino-quinazolines and thienopyrimidines. J. Med. Chem. 38: 2763-2773.

[48] F. Li, Y. Feng, Q. Meng, W. Li, Z. Li, Q. Wang and F. Tao. 2007. An efficient construction of quinazolin-4(3H)-ones under microwave irradiation. ARKIVOC (i): 40-50.

[49] E.M. Beccalli, G. Broggini, G. Paladino, A. Penoni and C. Zoni. 2004. Regioselective formation of six- and seven-membered ring by intramolecular Pd-catalyzed amination of *N*-allyl-anthranilamides. J. Org. Chem. 69: 5627-5630.

[50] E.M. Beccalli, G. Broggini, M. Martinelli and S. Sottocornola. 2007. C-C, C-O, C-N Bond formation on sp^2 carbon by Pd(II)-catalyzed reactions involving oxidant agents. Chem. Rev. 107: 5318-5365.

[51] A.K.A. Persson, E.V. Johnston and J.-E. Bäckvall. 2009. Copper-catalyzed *N*-allenylation of allylic sulfonamides. Org. Lett. 11: 3814-3817.

[52] G. Abbiati, E. Beccalli, G. Broggini, M. Martinelli and G. Palladino. 2006. Pd-catalyzed cyclization of 1-allyl-2-indolecarboxamides by intramolecular amidation of unactivated ethylenic bond. Synlett 1: 73-76.

[53] J. Muzart. 2005. Palladium-catalyzed reactions of alcohols. Formation of C-C and C-N bonds from unsaturated alcohols. Tetrahedron 61: 4179-4212.

[54] S. Bienz, P. Bisegger, A. Guggisberg and M. Hesse. 2005. Polyamine alkaloids. Nat. Prod. Rep. 22: 647-658.

[55] C. Markert, M. Neuburger, K. Kulicke, M. Meuwly and A. Pfaltz. 2007. Palladium-catalyzed allylic substitution: reversible formation of allyl-bridged dinuclear palladium(I) complexes. Angew. Chem. Int. Ed. 46: 5892-5895.

[56] J.E.R. Sadig, R. Foster, F. Wakenhut and M.C. Willis. 2012. Palladium-catalyzed synthesis of benzimidazoles and quinazolinones from common precursors. J. Org. Chem. 77: 9473-9486.

[57] A.C. Tadd, A. Matsuno, M.R. Fielding and M.C. Willis. 2009. Cascade palladium-catalyzed alkenyl aminocarbonylation/intramolecular aryl amidation: an annulative synthesis of 2-quinolones. Org. Lett. 11: 583-586.

[58] C.J. Ball and M.C. Willis. 2013. Cascade palladium- and copper-catalyzed aromatic heterocycle synthesis: the emergence of general precursors. Eur. J. Org. Chem. 3: 425-441.

[59] M.C. Willis, R.H. Snell, A.J. Fletcher and R.L. Woodward. 2006. Tandem palladium-catalyzed urea arylation-intramolecular ester amidation: regioselective synthesis of 3-alkylated 2,4-quinazolinediones. Org. Lett. 8: 5089-5091.

[60] A. Balazs, A. Hetenyi, Z. Szakonyi, R. Sillanpaeae and F. Fueloep. 2009. Solvent-enhanced diastereo- and regioselectivity in the Pd(II)-catalyzed synthesis of six- and eight-membered heterocycles *via cis*-aminopalladation. Chem. Eur. J. 15: 7376-7381.

[61] K. Utimoto. 1983. Palladium catalyzed synthesis of heterocycles. Pure Appl. Chem. 55: 1845-1852.

[62] M. Mori. 2009. Synthesis of nitrogen heterocycles utilizing molecular nitrogen as a nitrogen source and attempt to use air instead of nitrogen gas. Heterocycles 78: 281-318.

[63] T.H. Althuis and J.J. Hess. 1977. Synthesis and identification of the major metabolites of prazosin formed in dog and rat. J. Med. Chem. 20: 146-149.

[64] K. Matsuno, J. Ushiki, T. Seishi, M. Ichimura, N.A. Giese, J.C. Yu, S. Takahashi, S. Oda and Y. Nomoto. 2003. Potent and selective inhibitors of platelet-derived growth factor receptor phosphorylation. Replacement of quinazoline moiety and improvement of metabolic polymorphism of 4-[4-(*N*-substituted (thio)carbamoyl)-1-piperazinyl]-6,7-dimethoxyquinazoline derivatives. J. Med. Chem. 46: 4910-4925.

[65] M.S.R. Murty, B. Jyothirmai, P.R. Krishna and J.S. Yadav. 2003. Zinc mediated alkylation of cyclic secondary amines. Synth. Commun. 33: 2483-2486.

[66] W. Deng, Y. Xu and Q.X. Guo. 2005. Solvent-less Friedel-Crafts acylation under microwave activation. Chin. Chem. Lett. 16: 327-330.

[67] O.O. Ajani, C.A. Obafemi, C.O. Ikpo, K.O. Ajanaku, K.O. Ogunniran and O.O. James. 2009. Comparative study of microwave assisted and conventional synthesis of novel 2-quinoxalinone-3-hydrazone derivatives and its spectroscopic properties. Int. J. Phys. Sci. 2009. 4: 156-164.

[68] A. Bensari and N.T. Zaveri. 2003. Titanium(IV) chloride-mediated *o*-acylation of phenols and naphthols. Synthesis 2: 267-271.

[69] T. Choi and E. Ma. 2007. Simple and regioselective bromination of 5,6-disubstitutedindan-1-ones with Br_2 under acidic and basic conditions. Molecules 12: 74-85.

[70] V.N. Bochatay, P.J. Boissarie, J.A. Murphy, C.J. Suckling and S. Lang. 2013. Mechanistic exploration of the palladium-catalyzed process for the synthesis of benzoxazoles and benzothiazoles. J. Org. Chem. 78: 1471-1477.

[71] G.A. Molander and C.R. Bernardi. 2002. Suzuki-Miyaura cross-coupling reactions of potassium alkenyltrifluoroborates. J. Org. Chem. 67: 8424-8429.

[72] B. Das, K. Venkateswarlu, K. Suneel and A. Majhi. 2007. An efficient and convenient protocol for the synthesis of quinoxalines and dihydropyrazines *via* cyclizationoxidation process using $HClO_4 \cdot SiO_2$ as heterogeneous recyclable catalyst. Tetrahedron Lett. 48: 5371-5374.

[73] T.F. Murray, E.G. Samsel, V. Varma and J.R. Norton. 1981. Palladium-catalyzed cyclocarbonylation of acetylenic alcohols to methylene lactones. Scope and synthesis of appropriate substrates. J. Am. Chem. Soc. 103: 7520-7528.

[74] J. Muzart. 2005. Palladium-catalyzed reactions of alcohols. Formation of ether linkages. Tetrahedron 61: 5955-6008.

[75] B.C. Soderberg, J.M. Wallace and J. Tamariz. 2002. A novel palladium-catalyzed synthesis of 1,2-dihydroquinoxalines and 3,4-dihydroquinoxalinones. Org. Lett. 4: 1339-1342.

[76] T.L. Scott and B.C.G. Soderberg. 2002. Novel palladium-catalyzed synthesis of 1,2-dihydro-4(3*H*)-carbazolones. Tetrahedron Lett. 43: 1621-1624.

[77] L. Zhang, B. Qiu, X. Li, X. Wang, J. Li, Y. Zhang, J. Liu, J. Li and J. Shen. 2006. Preparation of 6-substituted quinoxaline JSP-1 inhibitors by microwave accelerated nucleophilic substitution. Molecules 11: 988-999.

[78] D.E. Kim, C. Choi, I.S. Kim, S. Jeulin, V. Ratovelomanana-Vidal, J.-P. Genet and N. Jeong. 2007. Electronic and steric effects of atropisomeric ligands and BINAPs in Rh(I)-catalyzed asymmetric Pauson-Khand reaction. Adv. Synth. Catal. 349: 1999-2006.

[79] E. Merisor, J. Conrad, I. Klaiber, S. Mika and U. Beifuss. 2007. Triethyl phosphite mediated domino reaction: direct conversion of ω-nitroalkenes into *N*-heterocycles. Angew. Chem. Int. Ed. 46: 3353-3355.

[80] E. Merisor, J. Conrad, S. Mika and U. Beifuss. 2007. Microwave-assisted reductive cyclization of *N*-allyl 2-nitroanilines: a new approach to substituted 1,2,3,4-tetrahydroquinoxalines. Synlett 13: 2033-2036.

[81] I. Kadota, A. Shibuya, L.M. Lutete and Y. Yamamoto. 1999. Palladium/benzoic acid catalyzed hydroamination of alkynes. J. Org. Chem. 64: 4570- 4571.

[82] L.M. Lutete, I. Kadota, A. Shibuya and Y. Yamamoto. 2002. Hydroamination of alkynes catalyzed by palladium/benzoic acid. Heterocycles 58: 347-357.

[83] I. Kadota, L.M. Lutete, A. Shibuya and Y. Yamamoto. 2001. Palladium/benzoic acid-catalyzed hydroalkoxylation of alkynes. Tetrahedron Lett. 42: 6207-6210.

[84] E. Merisor and U. Beifuss. 2007. From the study of naturally occurring *N*-allylated phenazines towards new Pd-mediated transformations. Tetrahedron Lett. 48: 8383-8387.

[85] M. Parisien, D. Valette and K. Fagnou. 2005. Direct arylation reactions catalyzed by Pd(OH)$_2$/C: evidence for a soluble palladium catalyst. J. Org. Chem. 70: 7578-7584.

[86] L.-C. Campeau, M. Parisien, A. Jean and K. Fagnou. 2006. Catalytic direct arylation with aryl chlorides, bromides, and iodides: intramolecular studies leading to new intermolecular reactions. J. Am. Chem. Soc. 128: 581-590.

[87] L.-C. Campeau, P. Thanssandote and K. Fagnou. 2005. High-yielding intramolecular direct arylation reactions with aryl chlorides. Org. Lett. 7: 1857-1860.

[88] W.A. Herrmann. 2002. *N*-Heterocyclic carbenes: a new concept in organometallic catalysis. Angew. Chem. Int. Ed. 41: 1290-1309.

[89] L.-C. Campeau, M. Parisien and K. Fagnou. 2004. Biaryl synthesis *via* direct arylation: establishment of an efficient catalyst for intramolecular processes. J. Am. Chem. Soc. 126: 9186-9187.

[90] A. Sharifi, R. Hosseinzadeh and M. Mirzaei. 2002. Rapid microwave induced palladium catalyzed amination of aryl bromides. Monatsh. Chem. 133: 329-332.

[91] Y. Wan, M. Alterman and A. Hallberg. 2002. Palladium-catalyzed amination of aryl bromides using temperature-controlled microwave heating. Synthesis 11: 1597-1600.

[92] P. Nilsson, K. Olofsson and M. Larhed. 2006. Microwave-assisted and metal-catalyzed coupling reactions. Top. Curr. Chem. 266: 103-144.

[93] A.R. Muci and S.L. Buchwald. 2002. Practical palladium catalysts for C-N and C-O bond formation. Top. Curr. Chem. 219: 131-209.

[94] J.F. Hartwig. 1998. Filtering algorithm for noise reduction in phase-map images with 2π phase jumps. Angew. Chem. Int. Ed. 37: 2046-2050.

[95] M. Tietze, A. Iglesias, E. Merisor, J. Conrad, I. Klaiber and U. Beifuss. 2005. Efficient methods for the synthesis of 2-hydroxyphenazine based on the Pd-catalyzed *N*-arylation of aryl bromides. Org. Lett. 7: 1549-1552.

[96] W.K. Anderson and G. Lai. 1995. Boron trifluoride-diethyl ether complex catalyzed aromatic amino-Claisen rearrangements. Synthesis 10: 1287-1290.

[97] A.M. Boldi, R.C.R. Charles Johnson and H.O. Eissa. 1999. Solid-phase library synthesis of triazolopyridazines *via* [4+2] cycloadditions. Tetrahedron Lett. 40: 619-622.

[98] P. Melnyk, J. Gasche and C. Thai. 1993. Heck reaction to a new heterocyclic system: pyrido[2′,3′-*d*] pyridazino[2,3-*a*]indole. Tetrahedron Lett. 34: 5449-5450.

[99]   P. Melnyk, B. Legrand, J. Gasche, P. Ducrot and C. Thal. 1995. Synthesis of new annelated indole systems: new entry in the E-azaeburnane series. Tetrahedron 51: 1941-1952.

[100] Y. Tamaru, M. Hojo, H. Higashimura and Z.-I. Yoshida. 1988. Urea as the most reactive and versatile nitrogen nucleophile for the palladium(2+)-catalyzed cyclization of unsaturated amines. J. Am. Chem. Soc. 110: 3994-4002.

[101] Y. Tamaru, H. Tanigawa, S. Itoh, M. Kimura, S. Tanaka, K. Fugami, T. Sekiyama and Z. Yoshida. 1992. Palladium(II)-catalyzed oxidative aminocarbonylation of unsaturated carbamates. Tetrahedron Lett. 33: 631-634.

[102] H. Harayama, A. Abe, T. Sakado, M. Kimura, K. Fugami, S. Tanaka and Y. Tamaru. 1997. Palladium(II) -catalyzed intramolecular aminocarbonylation of *endo*-carbamates under Wacker-type conditions. J. Org. Chem. 62: 2113-2122.

[103] T. Tsujihara, T. Shinohara, K. Takenaka, S. Takizawa, K. Onitsuka, M. Hatanaka and H. Sasai. 2009. Enantioselective intramolecular oxidative aminocarbonylation of alkenylureas catalyzed by palladium-spiro bis(isoxazoline) complexes. J. Org. Chem. 74: 9274-9279.

[104] H.A. Naim and N.I. Zakariyya. 2005. Synthesis of *N*-substituted quinazolino[1,4]benzodiazepine: a facial route to *N*-benzylsclerotigenin. Acta Chim. Slov. 52: 328-331.

[105] C.J. Calderwood, D.N. Johnston, R. Munschauer and P. Rafferty. 2002. Pyrrolo[2,3-*d*]pyrimidines containing diverse N-7 substituents as potent inhibitors of Lck. Bioorg. Med. Chem. Lett. 12: 1683-1686.

[106] T.Y.H. Wu, P.G. Schultz and S. Ding. 2003. One-pot two-step microwave-assisted reaction in constructing 4,5-disubstituted pyrazolopyrimidines. Org. Lett. 5: 3587-3590.

[107] D. Brown, G.A. Brown, M. Andrews, J.M. Large, D. Urban, C.P. Butts, N.J. Hales and T. Gallagher. 2002. The azomethine ylide strategy for *β*-lactam synthesis. Azapenams and 1-azacephams. J. Chem. Soc. Perkin Trans. 1 17: 2014-2021.

[108] A. Furstner and H. Weintritt. 1998. Total synthesis of roseophilin. J. Am. Chem. Soc. 120: 2817-2825.

[109] Z.J. Wang, J.G. Yang, F. Yang and W.L. Bao. 2010. One-pot synthesis of pyrimido[1,6-*a*]indol-1(2*H*)-one derivatives by a nucleophilic addition/Cu-catalyzed *N*-arylation/Pd-catalyzed C-H activation sequential process. Org. Lett. 12: 3034-3037.

[110] Y. Liu and J.-P. Wan. 2011. Tandem reactions initiated by copper-catalyzed cross-coupling: a new strategy towards heterocycle synthesis. Org. Biomol. Chem. 9: 6873-6894.

[111] G. Cuny, M. Bois-Choussy and J. Zhu. 2003. One-pot synthesis of polyheterocycles by a palladium-catalyzed intramolecular *N*-arylation/C-H activation/aryl-aryl bond-forming domino process. Angew. Chem. Int. Ed. 42: 4774-4777.

[112] J.A. Brown. 2000. Synthesis of *N*-aryl indole-2-carboxylates *via* an intramolecular palladium-catalyzed annulation of didehydrophenylalanine derivatives. Tetrahedron Lett. 41: 1623-1626.

[113] M. Watanabe, T. Yamamoto and M. Nishiyama. 2000. A new palladium-catalyzed intramolecular cyclization: synthesis of 1-aminoindole derivatives and functionalization of their carbocyclic rings. Angew. Chem. Int. Ed. 39: 2501-2504.

[114] H. Siebeneicher, I. Bytschkov and S. Doye. 2003. A flexible and catalytic one-pot procedure for the synthesis of indoles. Angew. Chem. Int. Ed. 42: 3042-3044.

[115] R. Omar-Amrani, A. Thomas, E. Brenner, R. Schneider and Y. Fort. 2003. Efficient nickel-mediated intramolecular amination of aryl chlorides. Org. Lett. 5: 2311-2314.

[116] J.J. Song and N.K. Yee. 2000. A novel synthesis of 2-aryl-2*H*-indazoles *via* a palladium-catalyzed intramolecular amination reaction. Org. Lett. 2: 519-521.

[117] J.J. Song and N.K. Yee. 2001. Synthesis of 1-aryl-1*H*-indazoles *via* the palladium-catalyzed cyclization of *N*-aryl-*N'*-(*o*-bromobenzyl)hydrazines and [*N*-aryl-*N'*-(*o*-bromobenzyl)-hydrazinato-*N'*] -triphenylphosphonium bromides. Tetrahedron Lett. 42: 2937-2940.

[118] C.T. Brain and S.A. Brunton. 2002. An intramolecular palladium-catalyzed aryl amination reaction to produce benzimidazoles. Tetrahedron Lett. 43: 1893-1895.

[119] C.T. Brain and J.T. Steer. 2003. An improved procedure for the synthesis of benzimidazoles, using palladium-catalyzed aryl-amination chemistry. J. Org. Chem. 68: 6814-6816.

[120] M. Catellani, C. Catucci, G. Celentano and R. Ferraccioli. 2001. Palladium-catalyzed synthesis of enantiopure 1,2,4,5-tetrahydro-1,4-benzodiazepin-3-(3*H*)-one derivatives. Synlett 6: 803-805.

[121] B.J. Margolis, J.J. Swidorski and B.N. Rogers. 2003. An efficient assembly of heterobenzazepine ring systems utilizing an intramolecular palladium-catalyzed cycloamination. J. Org. Chem. 68: 644-647.

[122] T. Emoto, N. Kubosaki, Y. Yamagiwa and T. Kamikawa. 2000. A new route to phenazines. Tetrahedron Lett. 41: 355-358.

[123] Y. Kozawa and M. Mori. 2002. Synthesis of 3-alkoxycarbonyl-1β-methylcarbapenem using palladium-catalyzed amidation of vinyl halide. Tetrahedron Lett. 43: 111-114.

[124] R.S. Colemen and W. Chen. 2001. A convergent approach to the mitomycin ring system. Org. Lett. 3: 1141-1144.

[125] A. Abouabdellah and R.H. Dodd. 1998. A new approach to the synthesis of functionalized pyrido[2,3-*b*]indoles by way of a palladium-catalyzed ring closing reaction between the N-1 and C-9a positions. Tetrahedron Lett. 39: 2119-2122.

[126] A. Arcadi, S. Cacchi, L. Cascia, G. Fabrizi and F. Marinelli. 2001. Preparation of 2,5-disubstituted oxazoles from *N*-propargylamides. Org. Lett. 3: 2501-2504.

[127] C.H. Cho, B. Neuenswander and R.C. Larock. 2010. Diverse methyl sulfone-containing benzo[*b*] thiophene library *via* iodocyclization and palladium-catalyzed coupling. J. Comb. Chem. 12: 278-285.

[128] Y. Kondo, F. Shiga, N. Murata, T. Sakamoto and H. Yamanaka. 1994. Condensed heteroaromatic ring systems. Palladium-catalyzed cyclization of 2-substituted phenylacetylenes in the presence of carbon monoxide. Tetrahedron 50: 11803-11812.

[129] G. Battistuzzi, S. Cacchi, G. Fabrizi, F. Marinelli and L.M. Parisi. 2002. 12-Acylindolo[1,2-*c*] quinazolines by palladium-catalyzed cyclocarbonylation of *o*-alkynyltrifluoroacetanilides. Org. Lett. 4: 1355-1358.

[130] S. Cacchi and G. Fabrizi. 2011. Palladium-catalyzed reactions. Chem. Rev. 111: 215-283.

[131] G. Kirsch, S. Hesse and A. Comel. 2004. Synthesis of five- and six-membered heterocycles through palladium-catalyzed reactions. Curr. Org. Synth. 1: 47-63.

[132] T. Nagashima and W. Zhang. 2004. Solution-phase parallel synthesis of an *N*-alkylated dihydropteridinone library from fluorous amino acids. J. Comb. Chem. 6: 942-949.

[133] F.E. Michael, P.A. Sibbald and B.M. Cochran. 2008. Palladium-catalyzed intramolecular chloroamination of alkenes. Org. Lett. 10: 793-796.

[134] G. Broggini, G. Molteni, A. Terraneo and G. Zecchi. 2003. Transition metal complexation in 1,3-dipolar cycloadditions. Heterocycles 59: 823-858.

[135] E.M. Beccalli, G. Broggini, M. Martinelli, G. Paladino and C. Zoni. 2005. Synthesis of tricyclic quinolones and naphthyridones by intramolecular Heck cyclization of functionalized electron-rich heterocycles. Eur. J. Org. Chem. 10: 2091-2096.

[136] G. Abbiati, E.M. Beccalli, G. Broggini, G. Paladino and E. Rossi. 2005. A valuable synthesis of pyrrolo[1,2-*a*]quinoxalines, indolo[1,2-*a*]quinoxalines and their aza-analogues by palladium-catalyzed intramolecular carbon-nitrogen bond formation. Synthesis 17: 2881-2886.

[137] E.M. Beccalli, G. Broggini, M. Martinelli, N. Masciocchi and S. Sottocornola. 2006. New 4-spiroannulated tetrahydroisoquinolines by a one-pot sequential procedure. Isolation and characterization of σ-alkylpalladium Heck intermediates. Org. Lett. 8: 4521-4524.

[138] E.M. Beccalli, E. Borsini, G. Broggini, M. Rigamonti and S. Sottocornola. 2008. Intramolecular palladium-catalyzed oxidative coupling on thiophene and furan rings: determinant role of the electronic availability of the heterocycle. Synlett 7: 1053-1057.

[139] E.M. Beccalli, G. Broggini, F. Clerici, S. Galli, C. Kammerer, M. Rigamonti and S. Sottocornola. 2009. Palladium-catalyzed domino carbopalladation/5-*exo*-allylic amination of α-amino allenamides: an efficient entry to enantiopure imidazolidinones. Org. Lett. 11: 1563-1566.

[140] L. Basolo, E.M. Beccalli, E. Borsini and G. Broggini. 2009. Efficient palladium-catalyzed direct arylation of azines and diazines using ligand-free conditions. Tetrahedron 65: 3486-3491.

[141] E.M. Beccalli, E. Borsini, S. Brenna, S. Galli, M. Rigamonti and G. Broggini. 2010. σ-Alkylpalladium intermediates in intramolecular Heck reactions: isolation and catalytic activity. Chem. Eur. J. 16: 1670-1678.

[142] E.M. Beccalli, A. Bernasconi, E. Borsini, G. Broggini, M. Rigamonti and G. Zecchi. 2010. Tunable Pd-catalyzed cyclization of indole-2-carboxylic acid allenamides: carboamination vs microwave-assisted hydroamination. J. Org. Chem. 75: 6923-6932.

[143] G. Broggini, E.M. Beccalli, E. Borsini, A. Fasana and G. Zecchi. 2011. Intramolecular oxidative Pd(II)-catalyzed alkoxylation of 3-aza-5-alkenols with O_2 as sole oxidant: mild conditions for the synthesis of 1,4-oxazine derivatives. Synlett 2: 227-230.

[144] E. Borsini, G. Broggini, F. Colombo, M. Khansaa, A. Fasana, S. Galli, D. Passarella, E. Riva and S. Riva. 2011. Enantiopure 2-piperidylacetaldehyde as a useful building block in the diversity-oriented synthesis of polycyclic piperidine derivatives. Tetrahedron: Asymmetry 22: 264-269.

[145] E. Borsini, G. Broggini, A. Fasana, S. Galli, M. Khansaa, U. Piarulli and M. Rigamonti. 2011. Intramolecular palladium-catalyzed aminocarboxylation of olefins as a direct route to bicyclic oxazolidinones. Adv. Synth. Catal. 353: 985-994.

[146] E.M. Beccalli, G. Broggini, M. Martinelli and G. Paladino. 2005. Pd-catalyzed intramolecular cyclization of pyrrolo-2-carboxamides: regiodivergent routes to pyrrolo-pyrazines and pyrrolo-pyridines. Tetrahedron 61: 1077-1082.

[147] A.M. Manzo, A.D. Perboni, G. Broggini and M. Rigamonti. 2009. Gold-catalyzed intramolecular hydroamination of α-amino allenamides as a route to enantiopure 2-vinylimidazolidinones. Tetrahedron Lett. 50: 4696-4699.

[148] A.M. Manzo, A.D. Perboni, G. Broggini and M. Rigamonti. 2011. An alternative synthesis of 2-alkylidene-3,4-dihydro-2H-1,4-benzoxazines by intramolecular gold-catalyzed hydroalkoxylation of 2-(prop-2-yn-1-ylamino)phenols. Synthesis 1: 127-132.

[149] J.-M. Chezal, J. Paeshuyse, V. Gaumet, D. Canitron, A. Maisonial, C. Lartigue, A. Gueiffier, E. Moreau, J.-C. Teulade, O. Chavignon and J. Neyts. 2010. Synthesis and anti-viral activity of an imidazo[1,2-a]pyrrolo[2,3-c]pyridine series against the bovine viral diarrhea virus. Eur. J. Med. Chem. 45: 2044-2047.

[150] G.M.P. Giblin, A. Billinton, M. Briggs, A.J. Brown, I.P. Chessell, N.M. Clayton, A.J. Eatherton, P. Goldsmith, C. Haslam, M.R. Johnson, W.L. Mitchell, A. Naylor, A. Perboni, B.P. Slingsby and A.W. Wilson. 2009. Discovery of 1-[4-(3-chlorophenylamino)-1-methyl-1H-pyrrolo[3,2-c]pyridin-7-yl]-1-morpholin-4-ylmethanone (GSK554418A), a brain penetrant 5-azaindole CB$_2$ agonist for the treatment of chronic pain. J. Med. Chem. 52: 5785-5788.

[151] E. Vanotti, R.R. Amici, A. Bargiotti, J. Berthelsen, R. Bosotti, A. Ciavolella, A. Cirla, C. Cristiani, R. D'Alessio, B. Forte, A. Isacchi, K. Martina, M. Menichincheri, A. Molinari, A. Montagnoli, P. Orsini, A. Pillan, F. Roletto, A. Scolaro, M. Tibolla, B. Valsasina, M. Varasi, D. Volpi and C. Santocanale. 2008. Cdc7 kinase inhibitors: pyrrolopyridinones as potential anti-tumor agents. Synthesis and structure-activity relationships. J. Med. Chem. 51: 487-501.

[152] F. Ni, S. Kota, V. Takahashi, A.D. Strosberg and J.K. Snyder. 2011. Potent inhibitors of hepatitis C core dimerization as new leads for anti-hepatitis C agents. Bioorg. Med. Chem. Lett. 21: 2198-2202.

[153] V.V. Vintonyak, H. Waldmann and D. Rauh. 2011. Using small molecules to target protein phosphatases. Bioorg. Med. Chem. 19: 2145-2155.

[154] G.-B. Li, L.-L. Yang, S. Feng, J.-P. Zhou, Q. Huang, H.-Z. Xie, L.-L. Li and S.-Y. Yang. 2011. Discovery of novel mGluR1 antagonists: a multistep virtual screening approach based on an SVM model and a pharmacophore hypothesis significantly increases the hit rate and enrichment factor. Bioorg. Med. Chem. Lett. 21: 1736-1740.

[155] J. Chen, T. Liu, R. Wu, J. Lou, X. Dong, Q. He, B. Yang and Y. Hu. 2011. Design, synthesis, and biological evaluation of novel γ-carboline ketones as anti-cancer agents. Eur. J. Med. Chem. 46: 1343-1347.

[156] E. Martini, L.C. Mannelli, G. Bartolucci, C. Bertucci, S. Dei, C. Ghelardini, L. Guandalini, D. Manetti, S. Scapecchi, E. Teodori and M.N. Romanelli. 2011. Synthesis and biological evaluation of 3,7-diazabicyclo[4.3.0]nonan-8-ones as potential nootropic and analgesic drugs. J. Med. Chem. 54: 2512-2516.

[157] D. Simard, Y. Leblanc, C. Berthelette, M.H. Zaghdane, C. Molinaro, Z. Wang, M. Gallant, S. Lau, T. Thao, M. Hamel, R. Stocco, N. Sawyer, S. Sillaots, F. Gervais, R. Houle and J.-F. Lévesque. 2011. Azaindoles as potent CRTH2 receptor antagonists. Bioorg. Med. Chem. Lett. 21: 841-845.

[158] T.W. Johnson, S.P. Tanis, S.L. Butler, D. Dalvie, D.M. DeLisle, K.R. Dress, E.J. Flahive, Q. Hu, J.E. Kuehler, A. Kuki, W. Liu, G.A. McClellan, Q. Peng, M.B. Plewe, P.F. Richardson, G.L. Smith, J. Solowiej, K.T. Tran, H. Wang, X. Yu, J. Zhang and H. Zhu. 2011. Design and synthesis of novel *N*-hydroxy-dihydronaphthyridinones as potent and orally bioavailable HIV-1 integrase inhibitors. J. Med. Chem. 54: 3393-3417.

[159] W. Bi, Y. Bi, P. Xue, Y. Zhang, X. Gao, Z. Wang, M. Li, M. Baudy-Floc'h, N. Ngerebara, M.K. Gibson and L. Bi. 2011. A new class of β-carboline alkaloid-peptide conjugates with therapeutic efficacy in acute limb ischemia/reperfusion injury. Eur. J. Med. Chem. 46: 1453-1462.

[160] M.-L. Yang, P.-C. Kuo, T.-L. Hwang, W.-F. Chiou, K. Qian, C.-Y. Lai, K.-H. Lee and T.-S. Wu. 2011. Synthesis, *in vitro* anti-inflammatory and cytotoxic evaluation, and mechanism of action studies of 1-benzoyl-β-carboline and 1-benzoyl-3-carboxy-β-carboline derivatives. Bioorg. Med. Chem. 9: 1674-1682.

[161] J.-X. Duan, X. Cai, F. Meng, J.D. Sun, Q. Liu, D. Jung, H. Jiao, J. Matteucci, B. Jung, D. Bhupathi, D. Ahluwalia, H. Huang, C.P. Hart and M. Matteucci. 2011. 14-Aminocamptothecins: their synthesis, preclinical activity, and potential use for cancer treatment. J. Med. Chem. 54: 1715-1723.

[162] E. Borsini, G. Broggini, A. Fasana, C. Baldassarri, A.M. Manzo and A.D. Perboni. 2011. Access to pyrrolo-pyridines by gold-catalyzed hydroarylation of pyrroles tethered to terminal alkynes. Beilstein J. Org. Chem. 7: 1468-1474.

[163] N. Kaur. 2018. Photochemical mediated reactions in five-membered *O*-heterocycles synthesis. Synth. Commun. 48: 2119-2149.

[164] M. Al-Masum, M. Meguro and Y. Yamamoto. 1997. The two component palladium catalyst system for intermolecular hydroamination of allenes. Tetrahedron Lett. 38: 6071-6074.

[165] Z. Lu and S. Ma. 2008. Metal-catalyzed enantioselective allylation in asymmetric synthesis. Angew. Chem. Int. Ed. 47: 258-297.

[166] C. Schneider. 2006. Synthesis of 1,2-difunctionalized fine chemicals through catalytic, enantioselective ring-opening reactions of epoxides. Synthesis 23: 3919-3944.

[167] B.M. Trost and G. Dong. 2006. New class of nucleophiles for palladium-catalyzed asymmetric allylic alkylation. Total synthesis of agelastatin A. J. Am. Chem. Soc. 128: 6054-6055.

CHAPTER 11

Seven-Membered Heterocycles

11.1 Introduction

Seven-membered heterocyclic compounds are important structural moieties found in a number of medicinal compounds [1-2]. Azepanes have attracted the much attention of chemists and their preparation is subject of intensive study [3]. Because of their importance in pharmaceutical chemistry, seven-membered nitrogen-bearing heterocycles are important molecules. They are inherently non-aromatic and, therefore, represent useful non-flat scaffolds for drug discovery. Some of them, especially benzodiazepines, are known as "privileged scaffolds" [4-8]. However, seven-membered nitrogen-containing heterocyclic compounds, their wide potential structural diversity not withstanding (relative position of two heteroatoms, different unsaturation state, many possibilities of fusion with heterocyclic or benzenoid rings), still seem unexplored in medicinal chemistry, as compared to four-, five-, and six-membered heterocyclic compounds. It has been reported that among all FDA approved drugs only 33 possess 7- or 8-membered *N*-heterocycles. In contrast to this, the number of drugs which contain 5- or 6-membered rings are 250 and 379 respectively [9-14]. A reason for this is the scarcity of general conventional protocols for their preparation in a diversity-oriented manner. Many methods have been developed for the construction of *N*-containing heterocyclic compounds, most of them led to five- and six-membered ring systems, while the synthesis of seven-membered and larger heterocyclic compounds is still quite limited. Most of the existing ring-forming protocols are based on metal-catalyzed reactions [15-18].

11.2 Palladium assisted synthesis of seven-membered heterocycles

11.3 Synthesis of seven-membered heterocycles with one nitrogen heteroatom

Wu and co-workers [19] synthesized seven-membered heterocyclic compounds regioselectively by a Bronsted base-modulated intramolecular oxidative amination in the presence of palladium catalyst **(Scheme 1)**. The activation of sp^2 carbon-hydrogen bonds was less difficult and there have been reported intermolecular and intramolecular aminations as well as intermolecular oxidation [20].

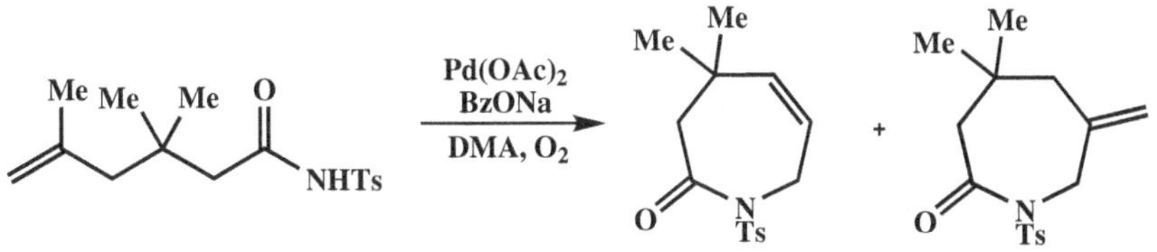

Scheme-1

This protocol was employed for the preparation of drugs to combat schizophrenia, which exerted their anti-pyschotic effects by blocking DOPA receptors **(Scheme 2)** [21].

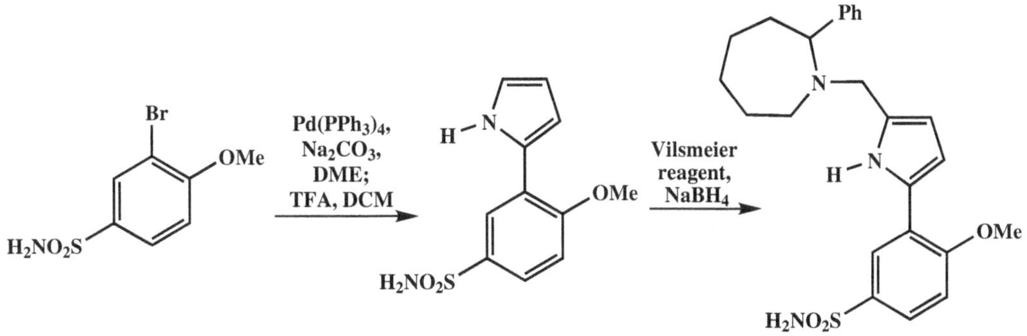

Scheme-2

The product was obtained when nitromethane was added to diester and the formed product underwent reduction of NO_2 group and ester hydrolysis to afford pyrrolidinone **(Scheme 3)** [22]. The pyrrolidinone acid was converted into bicyclo-γ-lactam easily in a few steps. The bicyclo-γ-lactam acts as an inhibitor of penicillin-binding proteins. The optically active pyrrolidinone was produced in both enantiomeric forms upon dissymmetric hydrolysis of racemic pyrrolidinone in the presence of two enantio-complementary enzymes [23-24].

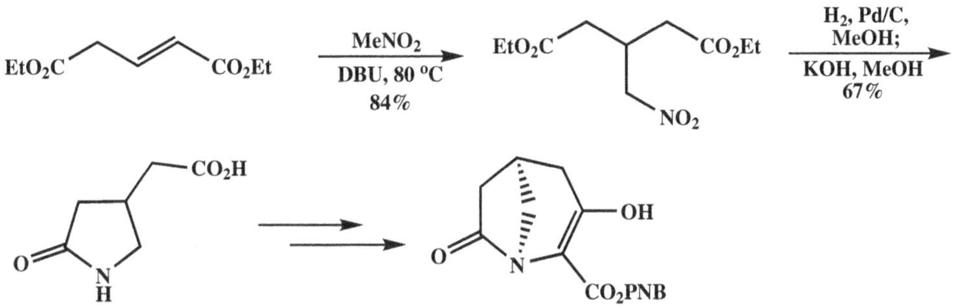

Scheme-3

Habib-Zhamani and co-workers [25] utilized simple cyclic β-ketoamides for the preparation of spiroheterocycles *via* a sequential selective three-component reaction and a carbocyclization in the presence of palladium catalyst **(Scheme 4)** [26].

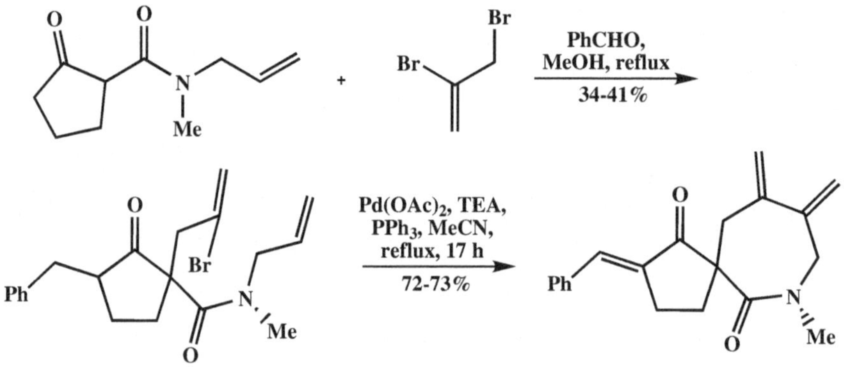

Scheme-4

The azepane derivative was formed in 48% yield by an intramolecular hydroamination of methylenecyclopropane tethered to an amino group with Pd catalyst **(Scheme 5)** [27]. The allylpalladium intermediate was produced by a distal bond cleavage of cyclopropane ring with Pd catalyst. The formed intermediate then produced azepane by reductive elimination of palladium(0) [28].

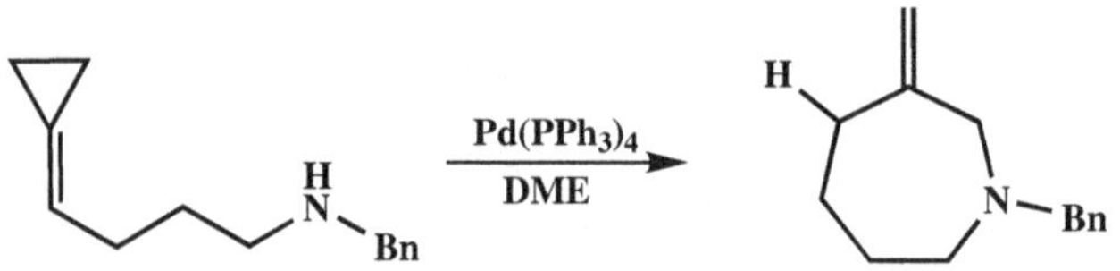

Scheme-5

Buchwald et al. [29] developed a coupling reaction of aryl halides and amines with Pd catalyst, and this reaction was extended to intramolecular version to afford a number of aza-heterocycles **(Scheme 6)**.

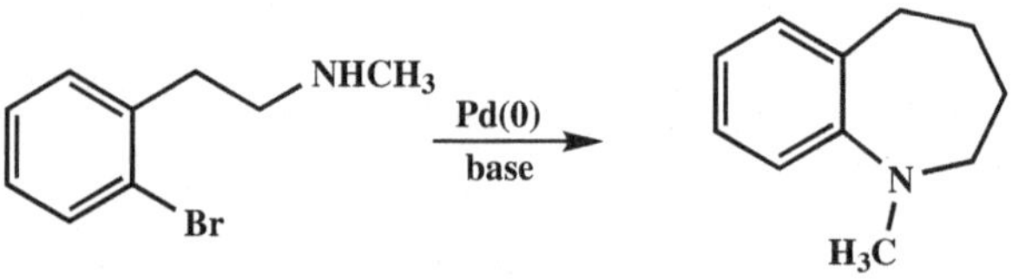

Scheme-6

The *exo*-methylenepyrrolidines were afforded in excellent yields by a palladium-catalyzed [3+2]-cycloaddition of trimethylenemethane to imines. Fused ring azepine was formed from α, β-unsaturated imine in the presence of trimethylenemethane-palladium species in [4+3] manner **(Scheme 7)** [30-32].

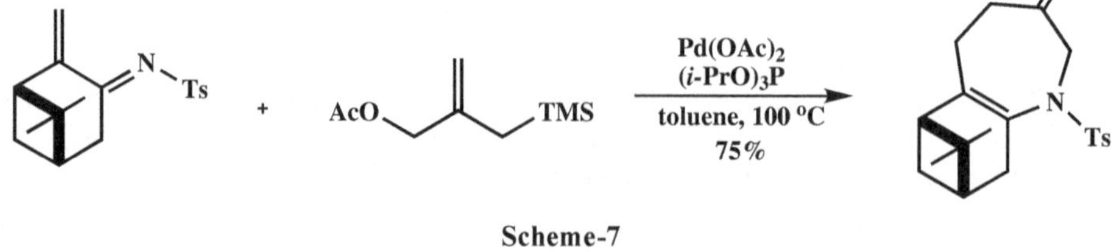

Scheme-7

Stewart and co-workers [33] synthesized seven-membered ring aza-heterocycle, 3-benzazepine with an exocyclic double bond, from allylamine derivative through palladium-catalyzed 8-*endo-trig* cyclizations **(Scheme 8)** [26].

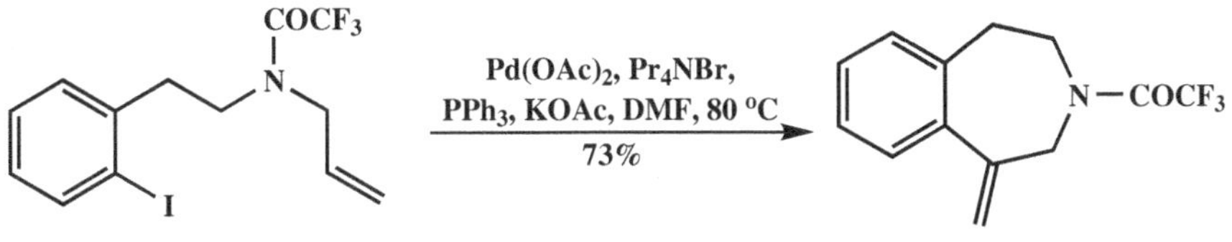

Scheme-8

A further approach to benzoazepine preparation involved the utilization of Friedel-Crafts chemistry. Treatment of *N*-(2-arylethyl)-*N*-(2,2-dimethoxyethyl)amines with TFAA effected amine protection and enabled intramolecular Friedel-Crafts cyclization and MeOH elimination in a single pot to afford dihydrobenzoazepine. Catalytic hydrogenation of dihydrobenzoazepine led to tetrahydrobenzoazepine **(Scheme 9)** [34].

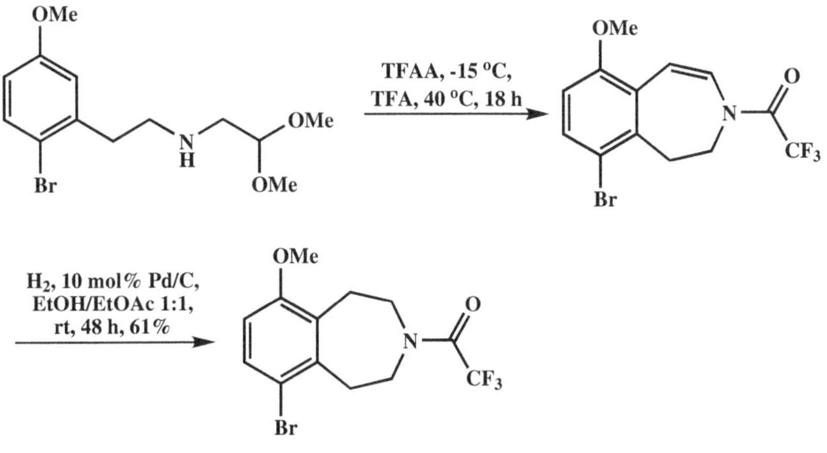

Scheme-9

The 3-benzazepine is present in many natural compounds and pharmaceuticals. The benzazepinones were generated in up to 90% yields *via* an intramolecular Mizoroki-Heck cyclization under MWI [35]. The intramolecular Mizoroki-Heck reaction was performed with palladium acetate, triphenylphosphine, and triethylamine in CH₃CN with 98% yield **(Scheme 10)**. The reaction was carried out on solid-phase (binding the substrate to a resin) and in solution. Both Mizoroki-Heck and Ugi reaction were performed on support [10].

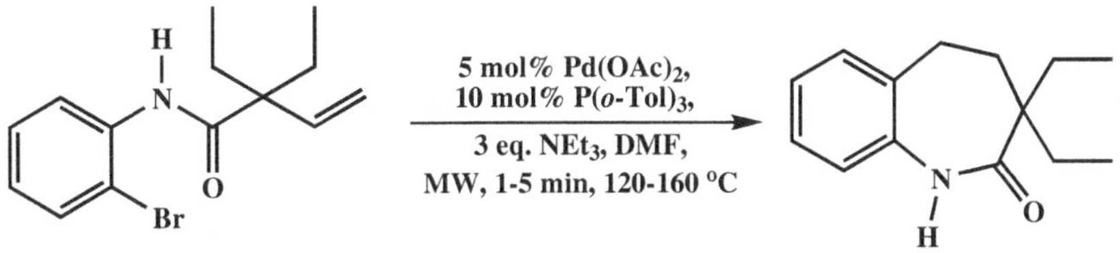

Scheme-10

Recent examples of Pd-catalyzed reactions include an intramolecular Heck reaction, the ring-closing reactions of *o*-(2′-bromophenyl)anilide enolates to afford dibenzoazepinones and intra-molecular reductive arylations of propargylamines to give benzoazepinylidenes **(Scheme 11)** [36].

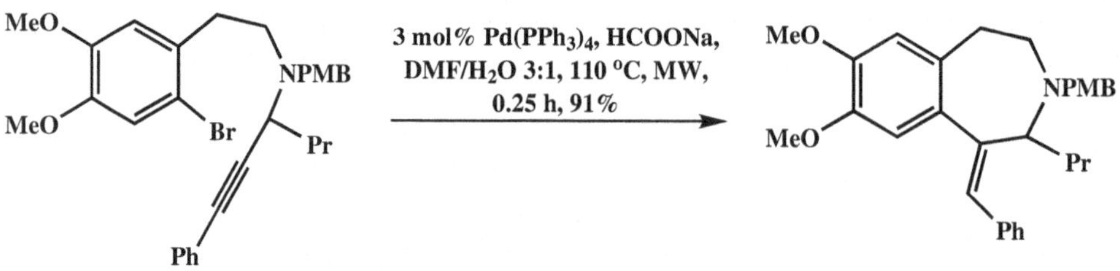

Scheme-11

Bolton and Hodges [37] produced benzazepines through intramolecular Heck cyclization **(Scheme 12)**. The secondary amine was synthesized cleanly following de-protection of immobilized allylglycine ester and reductive amination with benzaldehyde. Bicyclic lactam was produced following acidic cleavage and esterification upon subsequent acylation with 2-iodobenzoyl chloride and Heck cyclization.

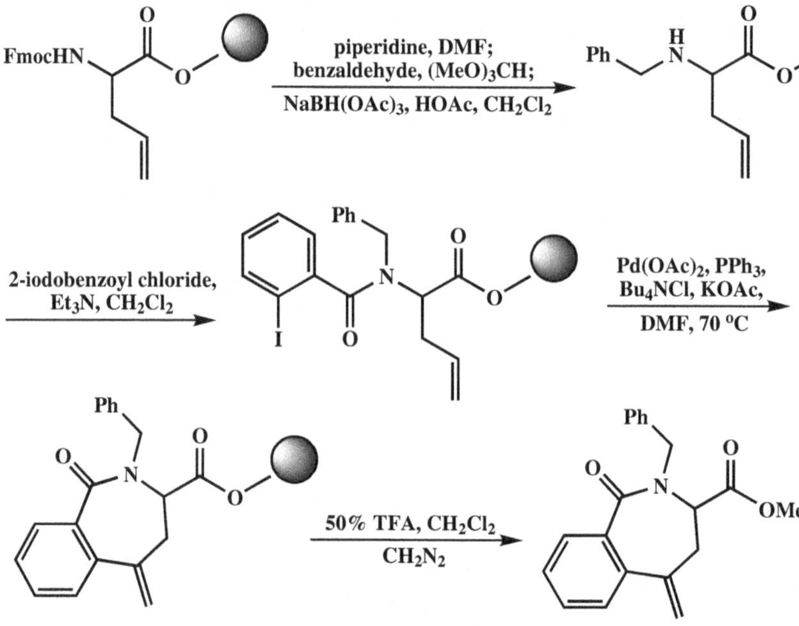

Scheme-12

Gracias and co-workers [38] reported a synthetically useful application of an intramolecular MW-assisted Heck reaction. The initial product of an Ugi four-component reaction underwent an intramolecular Heck cyclization in the presence of 5 mol% palladium acetate/triphenylphosphine catalytic system for the preparation of seven-membered nitrogen heterocycles. The product was afforded in 98% yield under MWI in CH_3CN at 125 °C for 1 h. Many sequential Ugi reaction/ Heck cyclizations were reported with aryl bromides instead of iodides. Addition to powerful MW Heck chemistry was the development of a general procedure for performing oxidative Heck couplings, *i.e.* the C-C coupling of aryl boronic acids with alkenes using palladium(II) catalyst and copper acetate as a re-oxidant (5-30 min, 100-170 °C) **(Scheme 13)** [10, 39-40].

In a paper by Schreiber et al. [41], a B/C/P strategy that relies on an organocatalyzed *syn*-diastereoselective Mannich reaction, as the couple phase, was described. In their work several different skeletons can be achieved in 3-4 steps starting from commercially available reagents **(Scheme 14)**. During the couple phase, commercially available building blocks were coupled *via* a Mannich reaction to form *syn*-diastereomeric aminoaldehyde. Derivatization of aldehyde functionality in *syn*-diastereomeric aminoaldehyde *via* a Wittig reaction afforded *syn* product.

Following alkylation reactions yielded densely functionalized templates poised for subsequent intramolecular functional group pairing reactions.

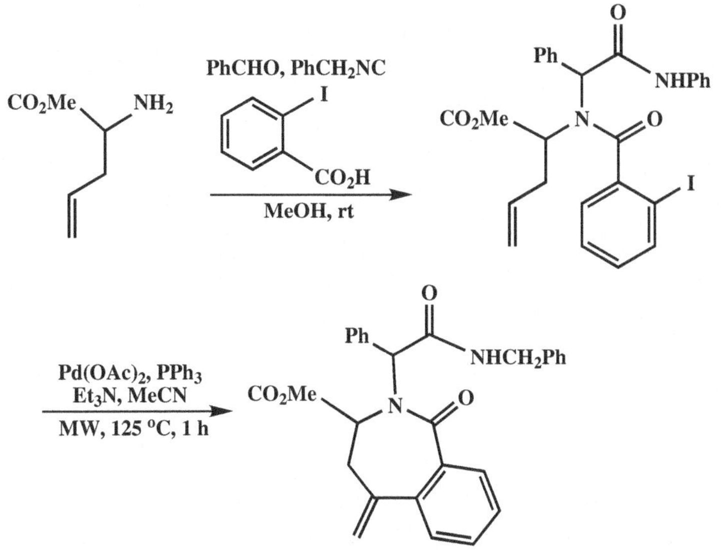

Scheme-13

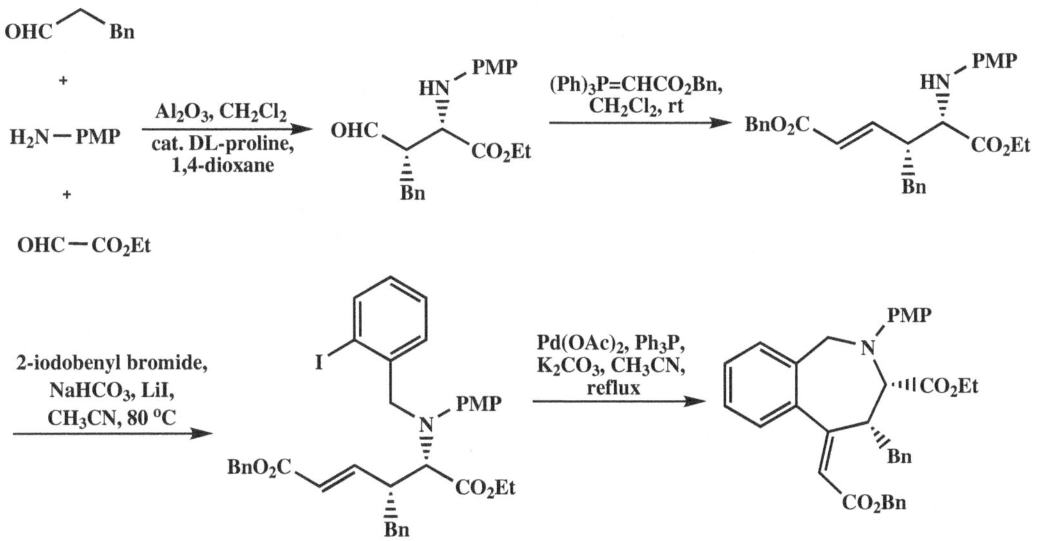

Scheme-14

Akaji and Kiso also carried out a macrocyclization on solid-support using Heck reaction when a cyclic tetrapeptide derivative was produced. Bolton and Hodges **(Scheme 15)** performed an intramolecular Heck cyclization on solid-phase for the preparation of substituted benzazepines [42].

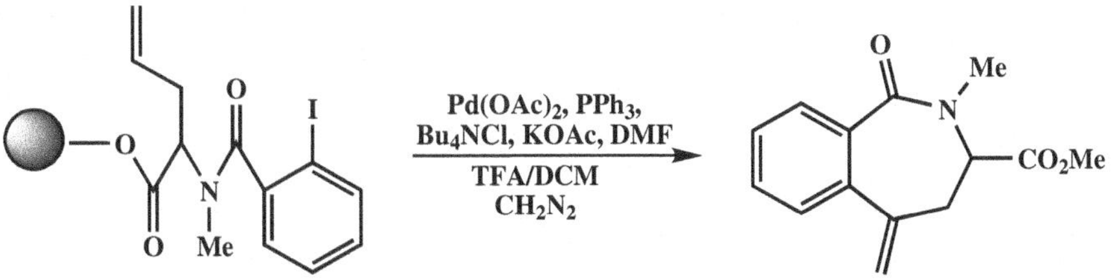

Scheme-15

Alper et al. [43-44] reported many multi-component reactions based on a Pd-catalyzed carbonylation reaction for the preparation of *N*-heterocyclic compounds. The Baylis-Hillman adduct containing an aryl bromide group was reacted with primary amines and CO for the synthesis of unsaturated seven-membered ring lactams. The allylic amines were formed by a selective amination on Baylis-Hillman acetates with primary amines and Pd(0) catalyst. Then there was an oxidative addition of Pd species to aryl bromide, which upon carbon monoxide insertion generated an acylpalladium species, which in turn was intercepted by allylamine to form seven-membered ring lactams (good to excellent yields) after reductive elimination. A variety of amine components were compatible in this one-pot synthetic protocol **(Scheme 16)** [45].

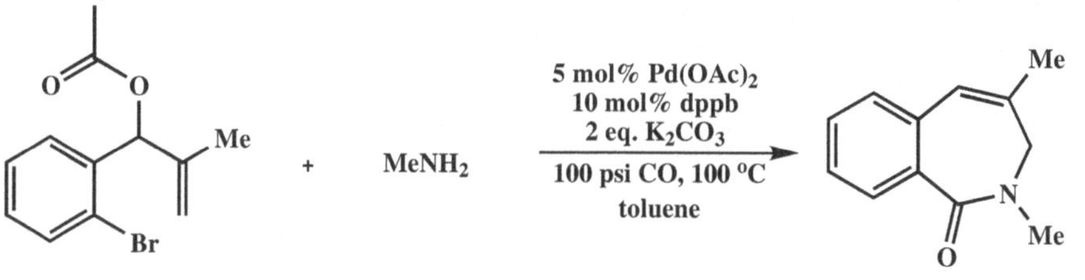

Scheme-16

The 1-substituted 3-benzazepine constitutes the core of several NMDA receptor antagonists. An intramolecular Heck reductive cyclization under MWI synthesized 1-substituted 3-benzazepinones regio- and stereoselectively. The propynoic acid amides were cyclized rapidly into seven-membered 3-benzazepinones with the help of Pd(PPh$_3$)$_4$, sodium formate in dimethylformamide/water in merely 15 min at a ceiling temperature of 110 °C. Same reaction under conventional heating required a longer reaction time (3 h) and proceeded in lower yields **(Scheme 17)** [10, 46].

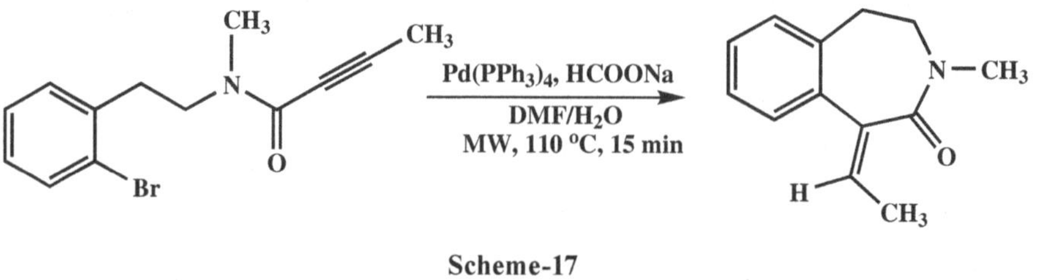

Scheme-17

The poly(ethylene glycols) are non-volatile, highly polar, and non-flammable solvents which are increasingly used in MW-assisted reactions. Lamaty et al. [47] produced benzazepines from 2-(trimethylsilyl)-ethanesulfonyl (SES)-protected β-amino esters through an intramolecular Heck reaction with palladium acetate, potassium carbonate in poly(ethylene glycol) for 30 min at a ceiling temperature of 100 °C **(Scheme 18)**. The same reaction was carried out under thermal conditions and it was found to be low yielding and sluggish [10].

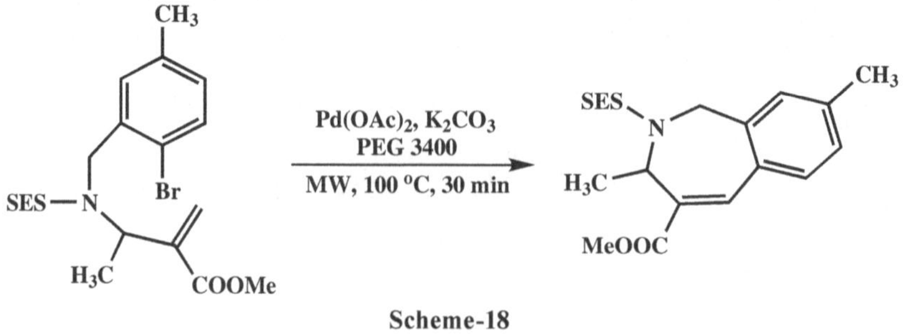

Scheme-18

The 3-benzazepine alkaloid aphanorphine and its analogues were generated by an intramolecular Heck reaction of an acrylamide substrate under MWI in the presence of Pd(dppf) Cl$_2$, TEA in acetonitrile at 110 °C in 15 min. The tricyclic core of aphanorphine was produced from 3-benzazepinone through an intramolecular radical cyclization **(Scheme 19)** [10, 48].

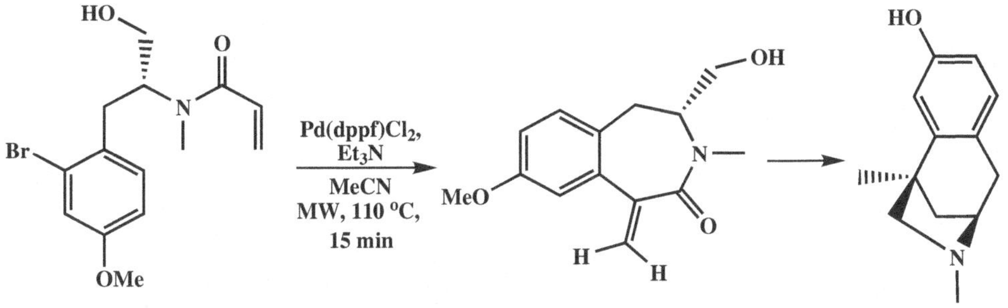

Scheme-19

The tricycle compound was formed by a domino allene amidation/intramolecular Heck-type reaction. The reaction of bromoenyne involved a (*p*-allyl)palladium intermediate. The allenepalladium complex was produced initially and there was a nucleophilic attack by bromide to form a *s*-allylpalladium intermediate, which rapidly equilibrates to (*p*-allyl)palladium intermediate. Then, (*p*-allyl)palladium complex underwent an intramolecular amidation reaction for the formation of bromoenyne intermediate. Heck-type coupling reaction of bromoenyne afforded a tricycle. The alkenylpalladium intermediate was produced from bromoenyne through 7-*exo-dig* cyclization. Subsequently, alkenylpalladium intermediate was trapped by bromide anion to deliver the fused tricycle **(Scheme 20)**. Thus, two different but sequential catalytic cycles were promoted with same catalytic system [49-51].

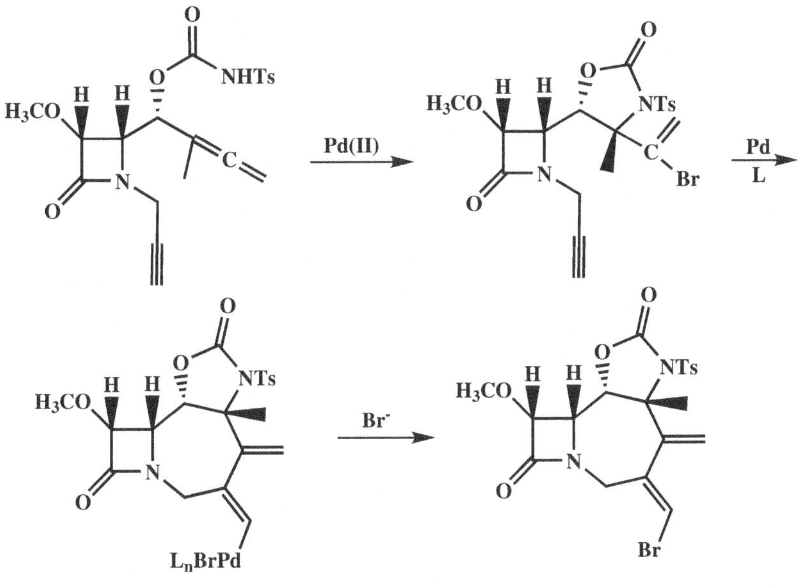

Scheme-20

This method involved a 1,2-functionalization of allene functionality in 2-azetidinone-tethered allenynol derivatives [52]. For Pd(II)-catalyzed reaction, the carbamate worked as starting substrate. The α-allenic alcohol was reacted with tosyl isocyanate to form carbamate. The reaction of carbamate was conducted in CH$_3$CN at rt in the presence of 10 mol% palladium acetate, LiBr (5 eq.), copper acetate (2 eq.) and potassium carbonate (1.2 eq.) under an atmospheric pressure of O_2. The tricycle compound was obtained as only isomer in moderate yield with extremely high regio- and stereoselectivity **(Scheme 21)**.

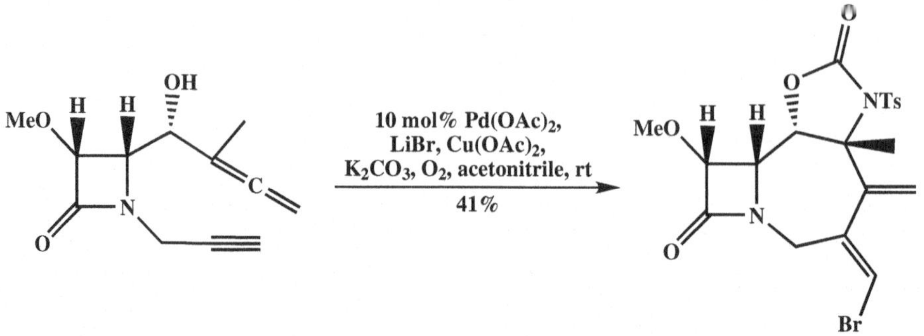

Scheme-21

Under these cascade conditions allenynol moiety was reactive [52]. Interestingly, moderate yields of bridged medium-sized ring tricycles as single isomers were reported when allenynols were reacted under Pd-catalyzed domino reaction conditions **(Scheme 22)** [53a-b]. Thin layer chromatography and 1H NMR analysis of crude reaction mixtures have confirmed the complete transformation but modest yields were obtained due to high polarity of tricycle adducts. These tricycle adducts were remarkable because they contain an unusual pyramidalized bridgehead structure.

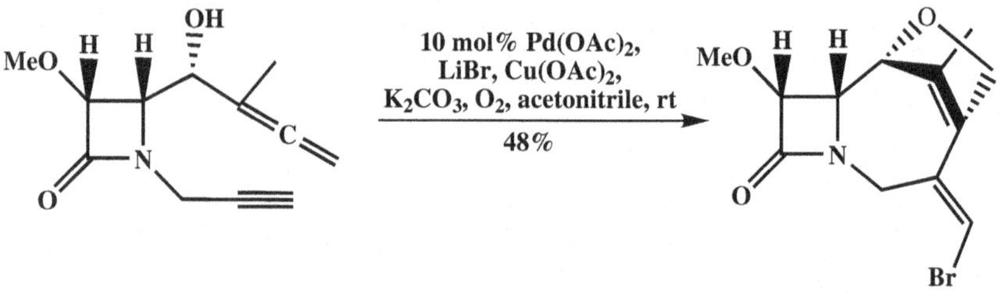

Scheme-22

The Pd-catalyzed cyclization of iodoaryl β-lactams afforded tricyclic β-lactams in the presence of a catalyst system comprising 10 mol% of palladium acetate, 20 mol% of triphenylphosphine, and thallium carbonate [54]. The 7-*endo-trig* cyclization of methallyl β-lactam provided a mixture of double bonds isomers (8:1) **(Scheme 23)** [52].

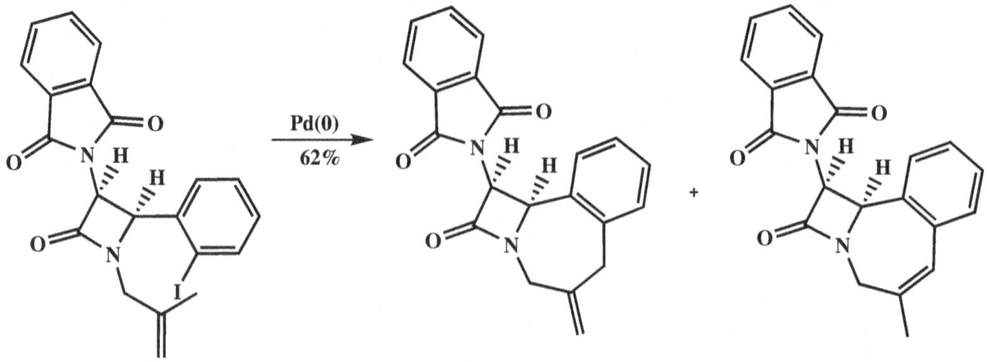

Scheme-23

Similar results were observed in intramolecular arylation of thiophenes and furans. Thiophene and furan underwent direct arylation at most reactive C2 site over C4, even though both were equally kinetically accessible **(Scheme 24-25)** [55]. When C2 was blocked or was the site of intramolecular tether, the arylation was then at C3 over C5, forming a 7-membered ring rather than a disfavored 8-membered ring.

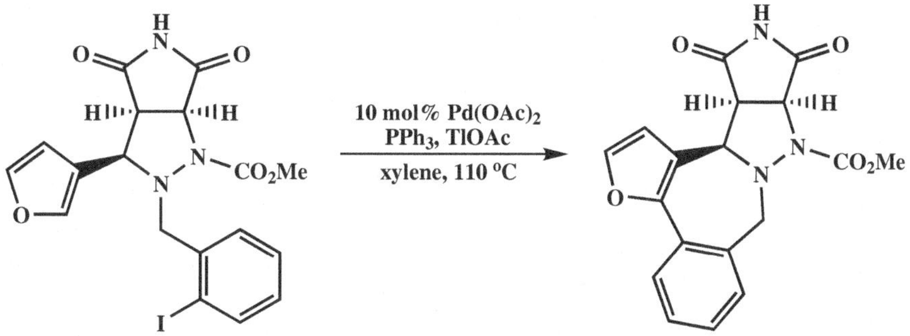

Scheme-24

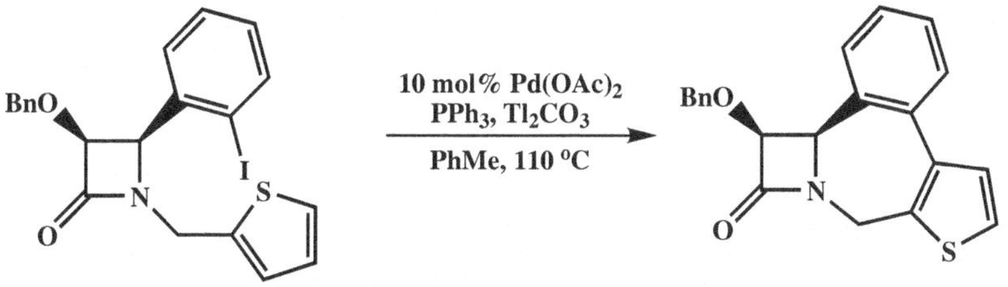

Scheme-25

Six- and seven-membered ring-annulated indoles were synthesized [56-57]. A variety of bromoalkyl indoles with electron-withdrawing or electron-donating substituents were produced. Moderate to good yields of a number of annulated indoles were afforded when substrates were reacted with both electron-poor and electron-rich aryl iodides **(Scheme 26)**. Under these reaction conditions many substituents such as amine, ester, OMe, Me, Cl, and NO_2 were tolerated. The product yields were not much influenced upon changing electronic nature of substituents. However, only 38% yield was observed when *N*-methyl tosyl substituent was present at *meta*-position of PhI due to steric interactions. Lautens [58] reported a highly modular one-pot tandem reaction which involved a direct arylation of indoles. A number of fused tricyclic indole derivatives were synthesized when (bromoalkyl)indoles were reacted with PhI in the presence of a Pd catalyst and norbornene [59-61].

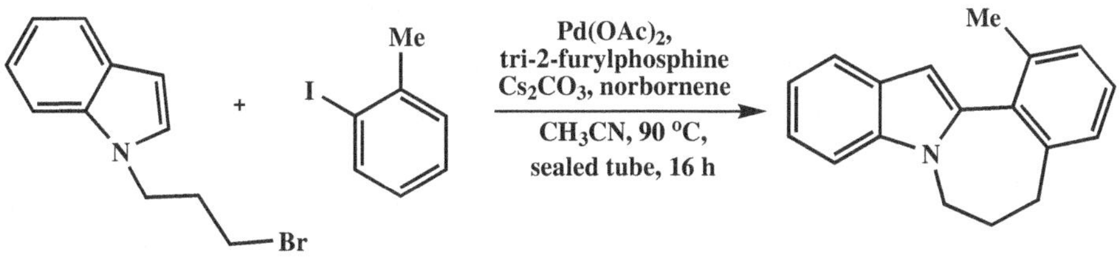

Scheme-26

A number of paullone derivatives were synthesized from many *N*-protected indoles and ArI *via* rapid intramolecular direct arylation reactions [62]. Regardless of position of amide tether the yields of cyclized products were excellent **(Scheme 27-28)**.

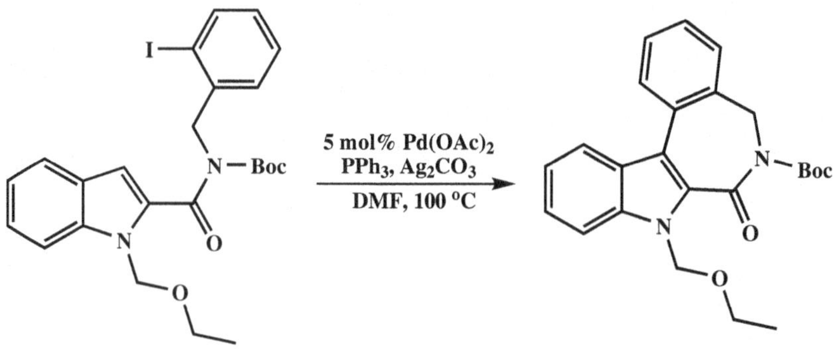

Scheme-27

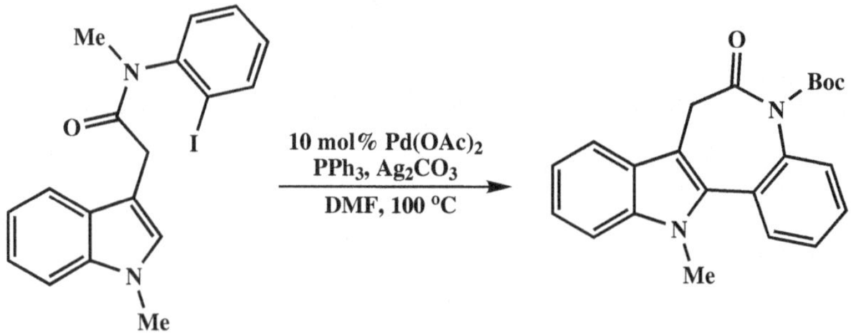

Scheme-28

The core structure of latonduine was synthesized successfully by this protocol **(Scheme 29)**. The intramolecular coupling of ArI onto protected pyrrole occurred in 70% yield [62].

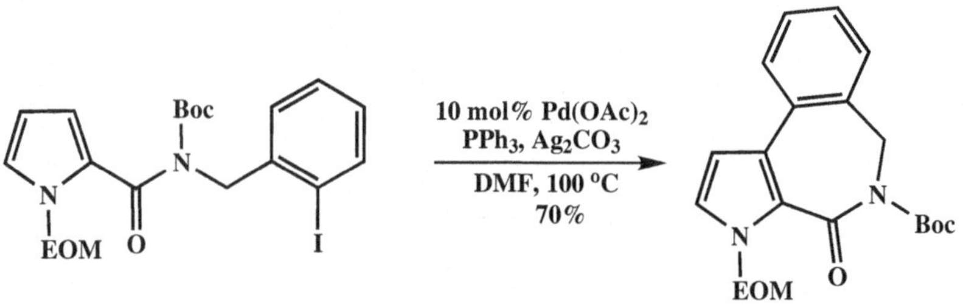

Scheme-29

The seven-membered benzazepinone ring systems were constructed by cyclization onto C-3 position of benzothiophene **(Scheme 30)** [62].

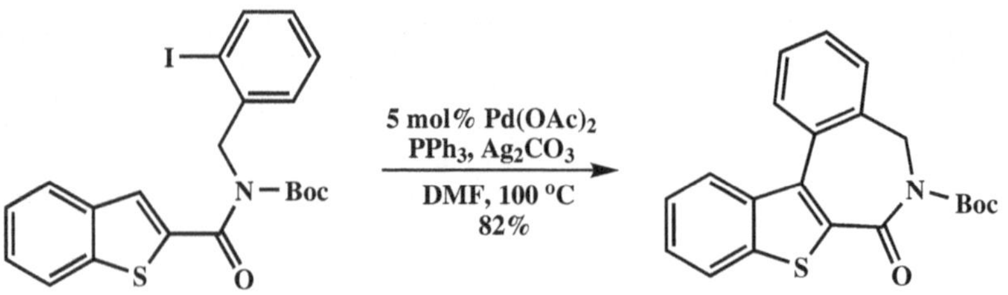

Scheme-30

Beccalli et al. [63] synthesized a family of paullone derivatives under Jeffery's conditions. Modest to excellent yields of seven-, eight-, and nine-membered ring systems were delivered using this highly reactive catalyst system **(Scheme 31)**. To avoid the Pd complexation, *N*-methylation of amide was necessary.

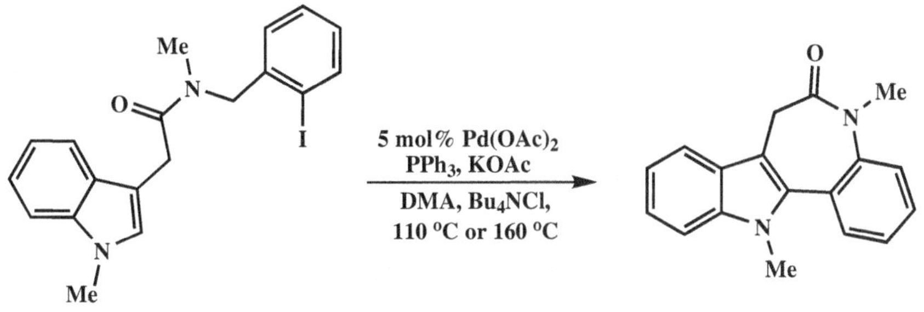

Scheme-31

During the preparation of a maxonine precursor a similar C-7 cyclization of indole and pyridine functionalities was reported as a competing side reaction in a Heck cyclization **(Scheme 32)** [64].

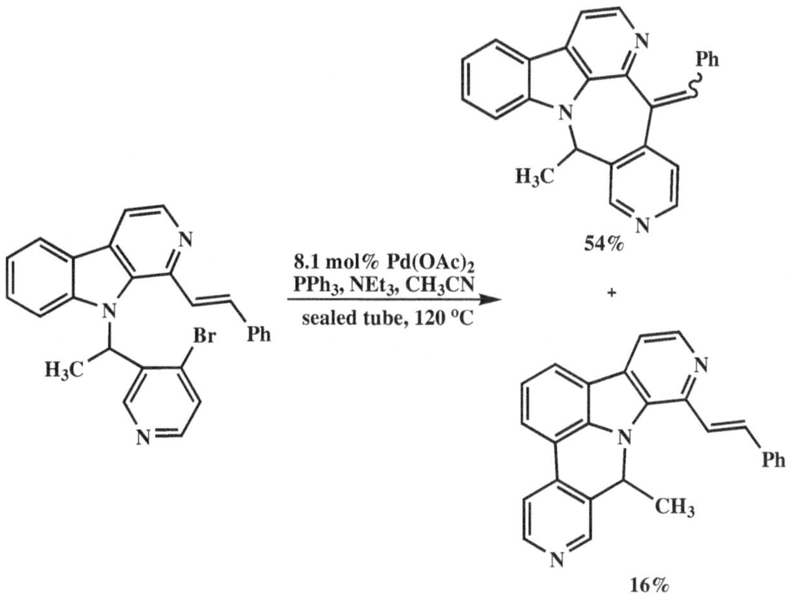

Scheme-32

The Pd-catalyzed Stille coupling of an indole-stannane to afford tryptamines functionalized at indole-2-position was reported in 1993 by Palmisano and Santagostino [65]. Initially, to extend the scope of this reaction, several vinyl-bromides were tethered from *N*10-amine of a tryptamine-tin derivative. Subsequent treatment with Pd(0) facilitated an intramolecular Stille cross-coupling reaction to afford the polycyclic ring systems **(Scheme 33)**.

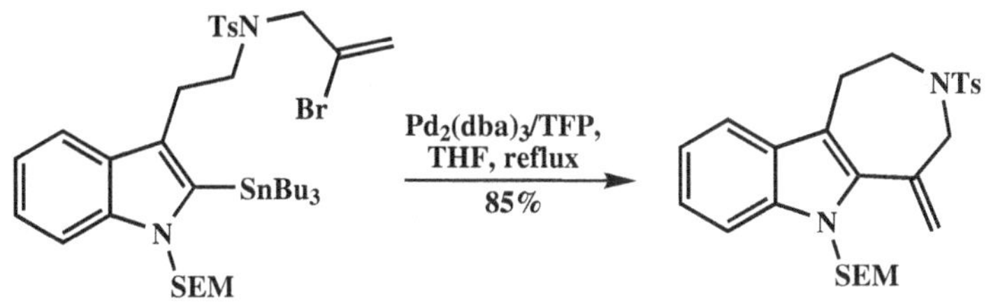

Scheme-33

New methodology for the synthesis of azepinoindoles could be accomplished employing allenes. One reaction sequence would involve a Pd-mediated carbon-carbon cross-coupling reaction at indole-2-position followed by addition of N10-amine, providing access to a series of functionalized azepinoindoles (Scheme 34) [66]. Similarly, by first tethering an allene to N10-amine of tryptamine, followed by Pd-catalyzed cross-coupling at indole-2-position, functionalized 7-membered heterocycles would be produced. A similar strategy, using these allenamide intermediates, was employed in the synthesis of functionalized indoles [67].

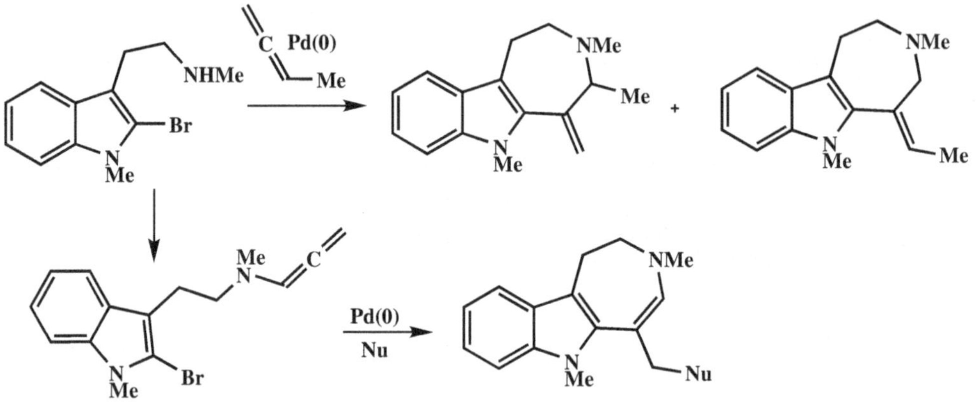

Scheme-34

A stepwise cyclization was reported in case of 2,5-asymmetrically substituted dibromo derivatives. Only benzylic substituent was activated which synthesized 7-membered ring in 62% yield. A second cyclization under forced reaction conditions (24 h, 110 °C) led to pentacyclic compound (61%). The dibromo compounds were utilized for the synthesis of pentaheterocycles in 50-56% yield under same conditions. These condensed heterocycles were not formed easily when cross-coupling protocol was performed under conventional reaction conditions (Scheme 35-36) [68].

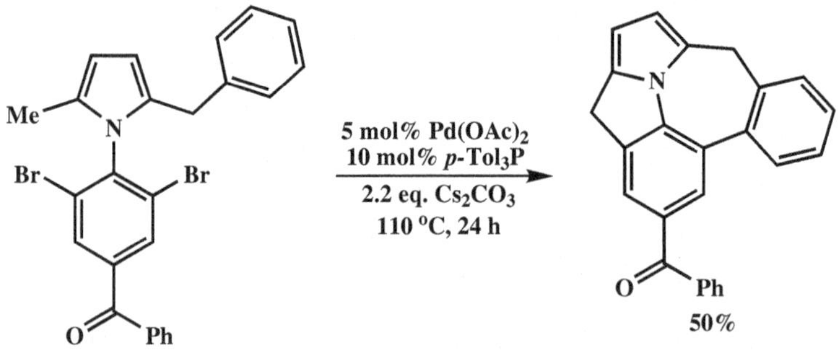

Scheme-35

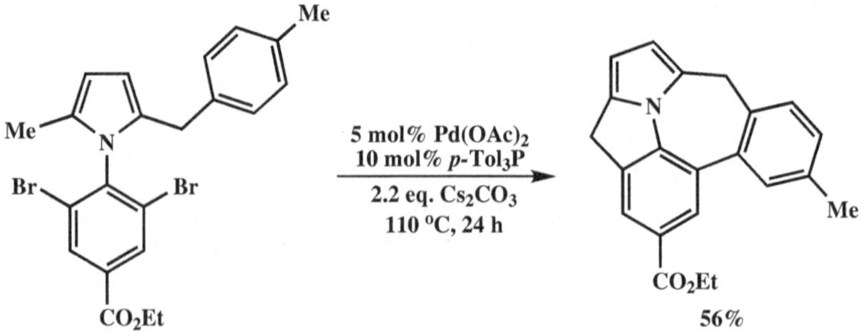

Scheme-36

The propargylamine substrates were prepared by a Cu(I)-catalyzed coupling of an aldehyde, alkyne and amine, otherwise known as A3 coupling [69]. Elsewhere, MW-assisted intramolecular A3 coupling was used as ring-forming step in the preparation of dibenzoazepines. As a further example of Pd catalysis, the syntheses of natural products (-)-aurantioclavine and clavicipitic acid involved one-pot Heck/*N*-alkylation reactions of reactants to form the indoloazepine intermediate [70]. (-)-Aurantioclavine was produced by intramolecular reaction of a sulfinamide with an alkyl tosylate **(Scheme 37)** [71].

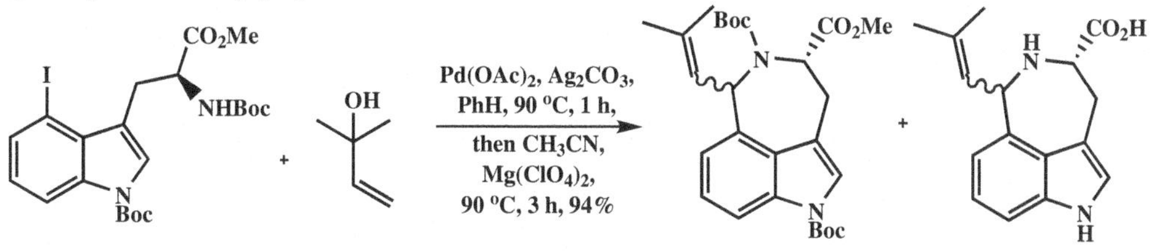

Scheme-37

To date this domino Tsuji-Trost/Heck reaction sequence had only proved successful with unsubstituted allyl bromide. As such, it was envisaged that access to more highly functionalized indole scaffolds could be realized by applying a similar domino process to substituted allyl bromides. The domino precursor for first series of reactions was prepared in accordance to method recently published by Stewart and co-workers [33]. The synthesis of an azepino[4,5-*b*] indole using a Pd-catalyzed single step or domino Tsuji-Trost/Heck reaction was reported by Stewart and co-workers [33] in 2009. The 2-bromoindole domino precursor was then subjected to previously identified domino conditions using crotyl bromide or methyl-4-bromocrotonate. This carefully controlled reaction sequence involved initial functionalization of trifluoroacetate protected *N*10-amine of tryptamine through palladation of allyl bromide, known as Tsuji-Trost reaction. Following the installation of olefin, an additional portion of base was added and temperature was increased to allow intramolecular Heck reaction at indole-2-position, forming new 7-membered *N*-heterocycle in good yield. As the Heck reaction at indole-2-position appeared to occur at a slower rate than that of other aryl halides, the use of Pd catalysis for first reaction in this domino sequence allowed the allylation step to proceed much faster, allowing sufficient time for intramolecular Heck reaction to take place **(Scheme 38)**.

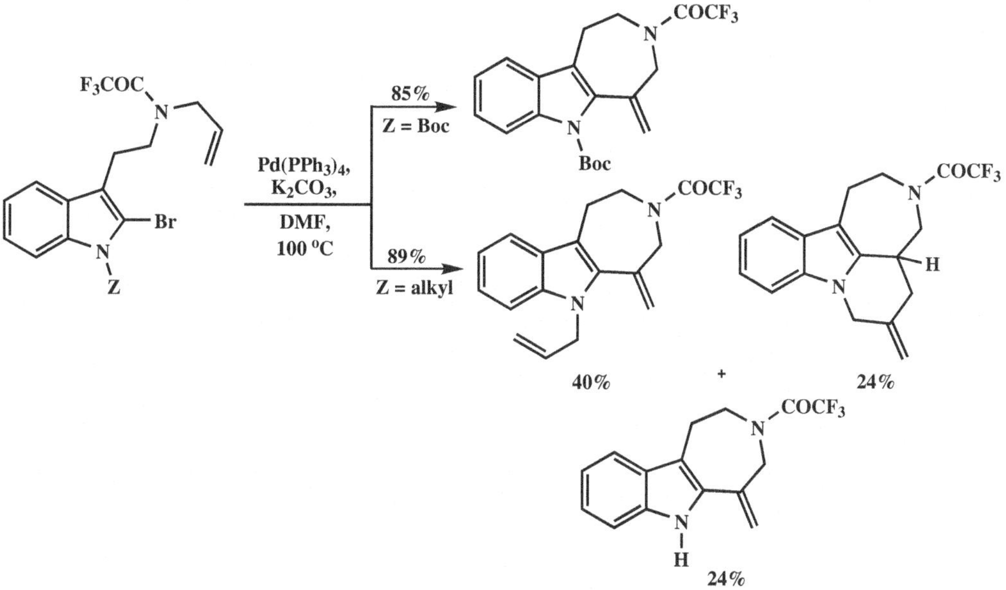

Scheme-38

The benzonaphthazepines were synthesized regioselectively **(Scheme 39-40)** [72-73]. Cyclization occurred selectively at 8-, rather than 2-position with substrates bearing an unsubstituted naphthyl moiety. The reaction involved an oxidative addition of Pd(0) to aryl bromide, followed by amine coordination to Pd(II) and regioselective electrophilic substitution of Pd(II) at 8-position. The product was formed upon subsequent reductive elimination. With the exception of bulky substituents like 7-isopropoxynaphthalene, other substituents on naphthyl rings showed the same regioselectivity. In former case cyclization occurred to provide the 2-cyclized product exclusively.

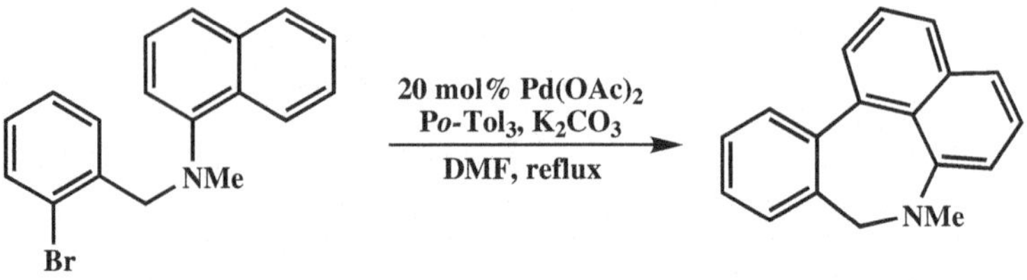

Scheme-39

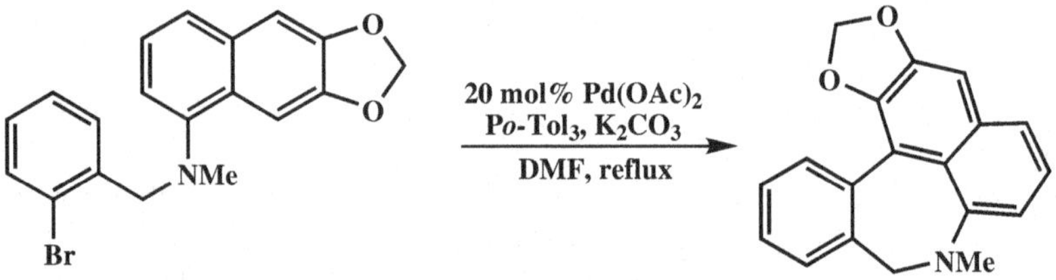

Scheme-40

In contrast, in a number of publications Stahl group [74-76] and Ney and Wolfe [77-78] have presented noteworthy examples demonstrating that aza-Wacker-type oxidative cyclization of alkenes can proceed *via cis-* or *trans*-aminopalladation/β-hydride elimination pathway, *cis* addition being preferred. An early, yet outstanding example was a report by Isomura and co-workers [79] on cyclization of 1-aminohexatrienes with palladium chloride **(Scheme 41)**. It was found that, while the *Z* substrate readily furnished desired benzofuro[2,3-*d*]azepine derivative under stoichiometric palladium catalysis, the *E* substrate provided only palladium-σ-complex, which could be isolated and characterized. Since β-hydride elimination generally proceeded with *cis* stereochemistry, and in case of *E* substrate there was no hydrogen *cis* to Pd, the reaction stopped after addition step. Furthermore, the demonstrated *cis* arrangement of Pd and methyl groups can originate from an initial *cis* addition to *E* double bond.

The pyrido-[2,3-*d*]pyrazino[2,3-*a*]indole derivative and ethyl acrylate were reacted to produce a pentacyclic *E*-azaeburnane [80]. An ergot alkaloid clavicipitic acid was synthesized by coupling reaction of 4-bromoindole and dehydroalanine methyl ester **(Scheme 42)** [81]. The use of Pd avoided the need of chloranil as oxidant. The 2-substituted indoles were easily coupled with electron-poor alkenes to afford 3-alkenyl derivatives in the presence of palladium acetate/silver acetate catalytic system at reflux in acetic acid [82-83].

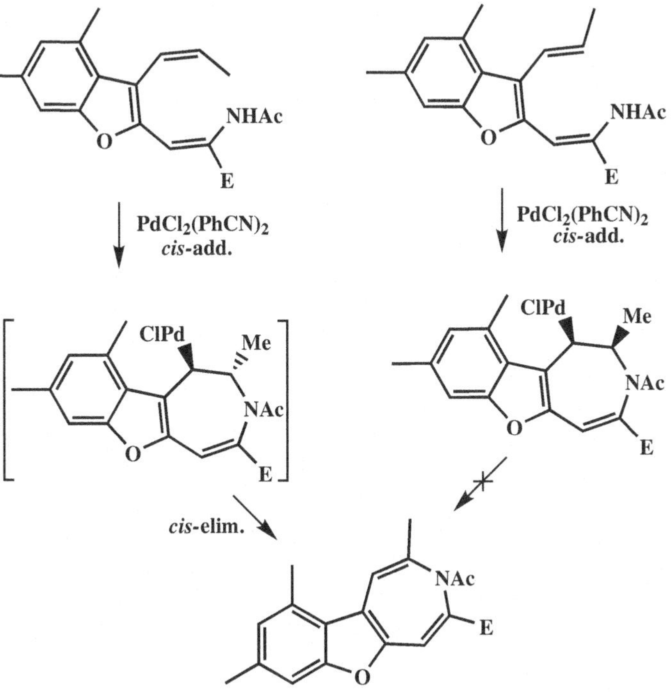

Scheme-41

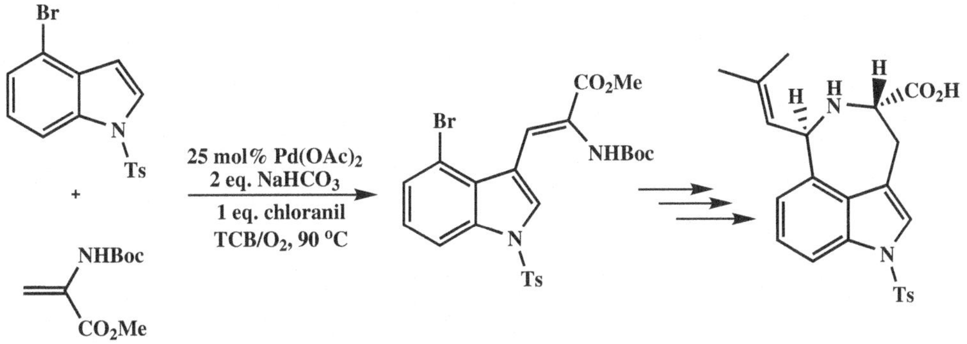

Scheme-42

The reaction of Baylis-Hillman acetate with 2-substituted benzimidazoles in dimethylformamide and potassium carbonate at rt gave benzimidazole-attached Baylis-Hillman adducts in 67-89% yields. The tetracyclic compounds bearing eight-membered ring; benzoazocinobenzimidazole derivatives were formed, in 36-48% yields, from intramolecular Pd-catalyzed cyclization of benzimidazole-attached Baylis-Hillman adducts. Similarly, seven-membered ring compounds were obtained from the reaction of Baylis-Hillman acetate with 2-unsubstituted benzimidazoles in dimethylformamide and potassium carbonate at room temperature to give adducts. Intramolecular palladium-catalyzed cyclization of adducts resulted in the formation of benzo[3,4]azepino[1,2-a]benzimidazole derivatives in reasonable yields. The latter results showed that 2-position of benzimidazole was more reactive than that of 7-position **(Scheme 43)** [84-85].

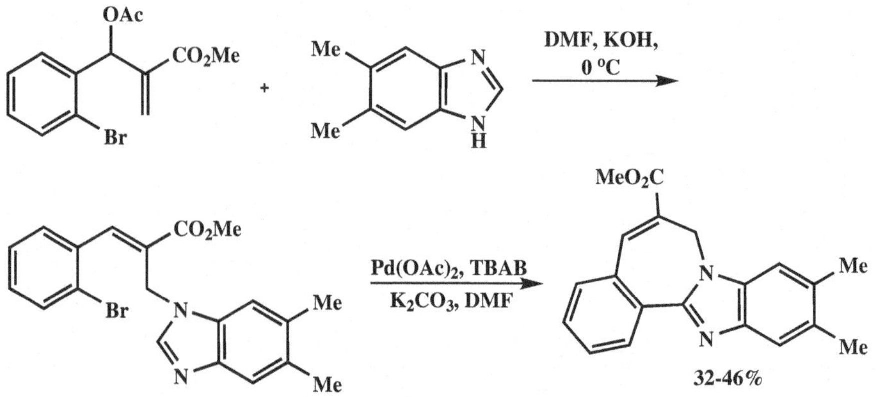

Scheme-43

Several naturally occurring compounds contain a benzazepine moiety. For example, the rare *Cephalotaxus* alkaloids possess a benzazepine scaffold which was fused to a pentacyclic skeleton. The naturally occurring esters of these alkaloids are used for the treatment of acute human leukemia. Riva et al. [86] generated tricyclic compounds resembling *Cephalotaxus* alkaloids in one-pot synthetic protocol. The pyrrolidine intermediates were formed by a method comprised sequential Ugi condensation-S_N2 cyclization. The pyrrolidine intermediates underwent intramolecular Heck reaction under MWI in the presence of Pd(PPh$_3$)$_4$, 1,2-bis(diphenylphosphino) ethane and cesium carbonate in dimethylformamide for 60 min at 120 °C (**Scheme 44**).

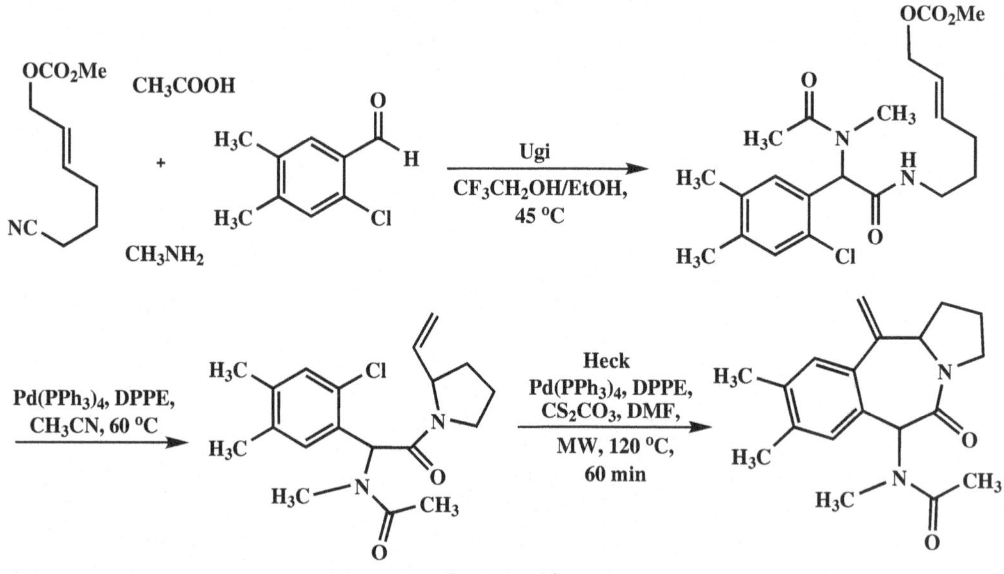

Scheme-44

11.4   Synthesis of seven-membered heterocycles with two nitrogen heteroatoms

Reductive amination of Garner aldehyde with amino ester hydrochlorides followed by divergent functional group manipulation produced azide and alcohol. Intramolecular alkylation reactions of amine derived from azide or alcohol resulted in chiral perhydro-1,4-diazepines or perhydro-1,4-oxazepines, respectively (**Scheme 45**) [87-88].

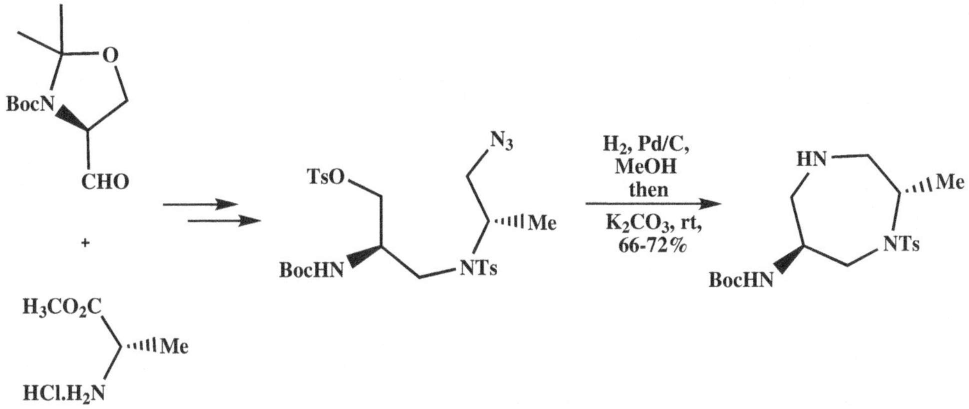

Scheme-45

In this study, seven-membered heterocycles were formed exclusively or in a pronounced excess over five-membered ones. Among chosen substrates, α-amino acid derivatives were also cyclized to corresponding diazepinones in good yields **(Scheme 46)** [89].

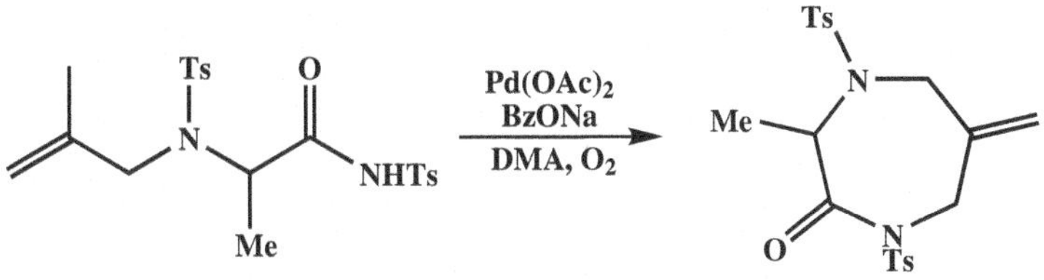

Scheme-46

The results indicated that tosyl group was protecting group of choice to extend the protocol **(Scheme 47)**. Under optimized phosphine-free conditions, the scope of domino sequence was examined with many aryl iodides on a 0.1 mmol scale. The desired benzodiazepinones were afforded in 73%, 63% and 63% yields from electron-rich 2-, 3- and 4-iodoanisoles smoothly, respectively. Reactions of 4-nitro, 4-methoxycarbonyl, and 4-acetyl iodobenzene provided satisfactory yields of 71%, 61%, and 68%. The simple iodobenzene formed benzodiazepinone in 67% yield. Heteroaromatic iodides also gave good yields, as 3-iodopyridine afforded the expected product in 70% yield. The same protocol was also shown to be able to sustain substitutions onto aromatic ring, since the 3-methyl anthranilic allenylamide afforded corresponding benzodiazepinone in good yield (75%) [90-91a, b].

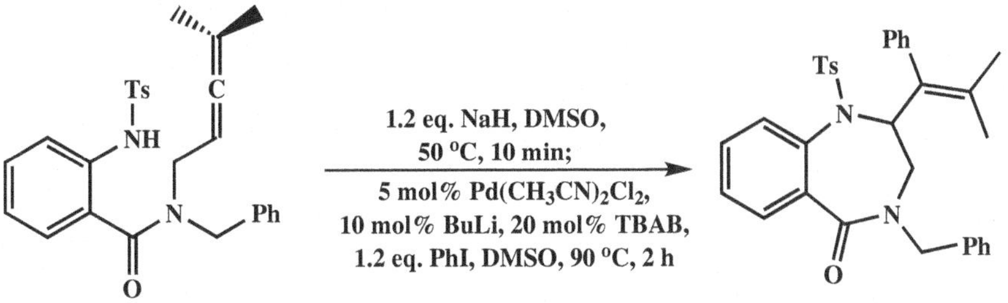

Scheme-47

The 1,4-benzodiazepin-5-ones and 1,4-benzodiazepines were synthesized. Good yield of heterocyclic products was obtained by coupling of *N*-allyl-2-aminobenzylamine derivatives with aryl bromides in the presence of palladium catalyst. Although many attempts were made for the synthesis of unsaturated 1,4-benzodiazepines, fewer protocols were developed for the construction of saturated derivatives [92]. The 1,4-benzodiazepine was provided by a palladium-catalyzed coupling with 4-bromobiphenyl **(Scheme 48)** [93].

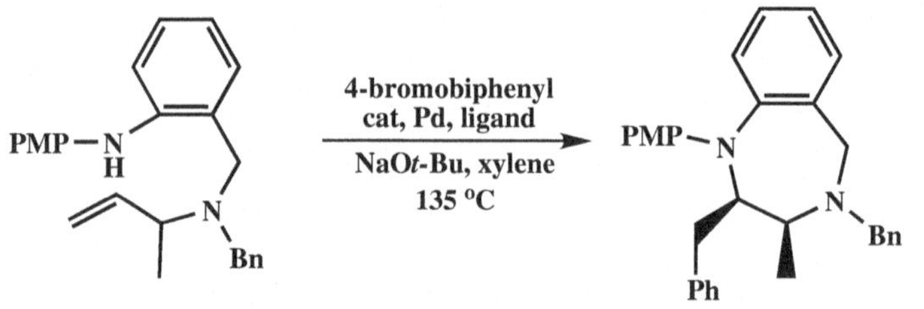

Scheme-48

The [[2-(4-biphenyl)isopropyl]oxy]carbonyl (Boc)-protected (aminoaryl)stannane was produced in solution in four steps, which was subsequently coupled to solid support through HMP linker. Stille coupling was performed with a variety of acid chlorides and $Pd_2(dba)$/ chloroform catalyst **(Scheme 49)** [94].

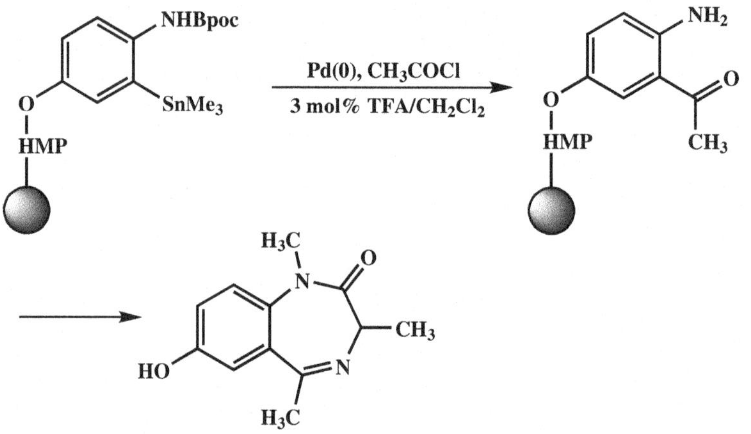

Scheme-49

Plunkett and Ellman [94] synthesized 1,4-benzodiazepine derivatives in an excellent protocol using Stille coupling on solid-support. Structurally diverse derivatives were produced. The authors used Stille coupling for the formation of new traceless linkers to be used in SPS **(Scheme 50)** [95].

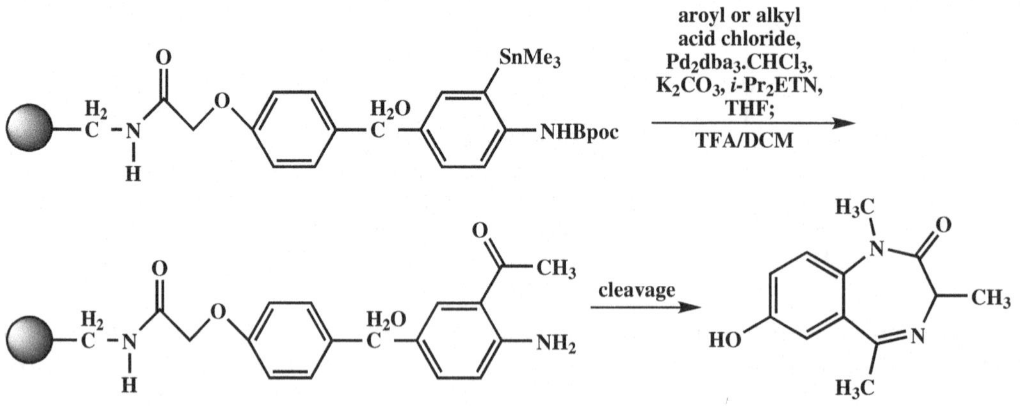

Scheme-50

An anilide derived from Cbz-Val-OH underwent Fries rearrangement. Substrate with benzylic carbamate prevented the photochemical reaction and formed many by-products. Acceptable yields of an intermediate were formed under standard conditions when reaction was performed on anilide derived from *N*-Boc-Ala-OH (R1) Me, (R2) H. This compound was then coupled with Cbz-Gly-OH in DCC (*N,N'*-dicyclohexylcarbodiimide)/4-dimethylaminopyridine. Benzodiazepines were formed in 70% yield after treatment with HCOONH$_4$ in palladium hydroxide/carbon and isopropyl alcohol in a MW monomode cavity **(Scheme 51)** [96].

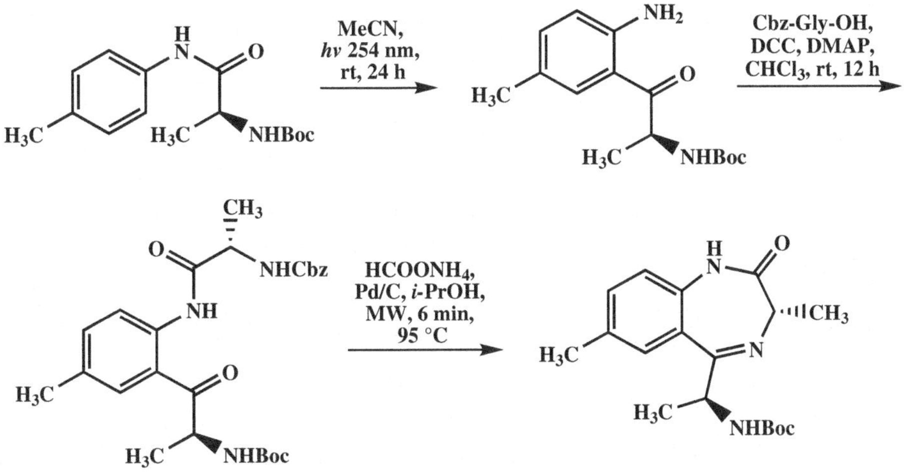

Scheme-51

The ring closure of (*S*)-2-amino-*N*-butyl-*N*-(2-iodobenzyl)propanamide was promoted to synthesize 1,4-benzodiazepine-3-one at 85 °C in PhMe in the presence of 10 mol% Pd$_2$(dba)$_3$/ chloroform, cesium carbonate or potassium *tert*-butoxide, as base, and bidentate phosphine ligand BINAP **(Scheme 52)** [97-98].

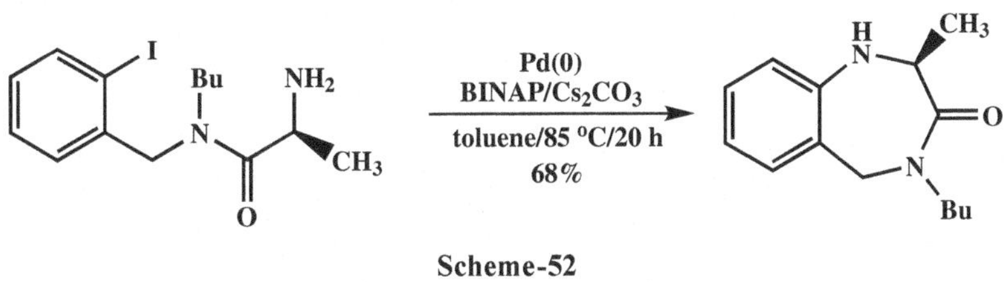

Scheme-52

The carbonylation of *N*1-(2-iodophenyl)-*N*1-methylbenzene-1,2-diamine afforded 5-methyl-5*H*-dibenzo[*b,e*][1,4]diazepin-11(10*H*)-one in the presence of palladium catalyst complexed to a silica-based dendrimer ligand **(Scheme 53)** [99].

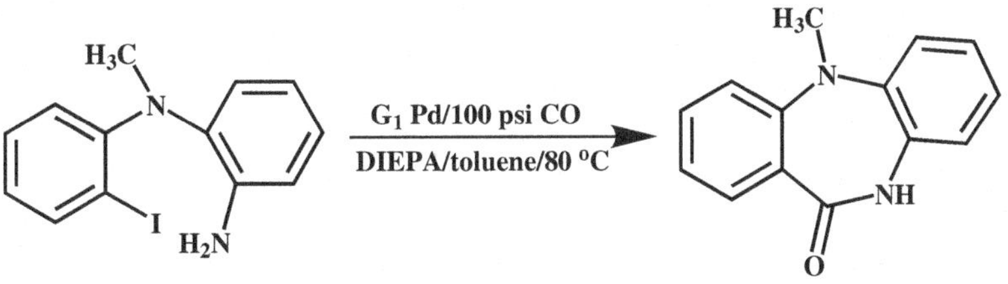

Scheme-53

The peptidic coupling of 2-aminobenzophenone with suitably protected lysine or alanine occurred by *in situ* formed acyl-fluoride compounds with the help of TFFH. Cbz and Boc protecting groups were removed completely by palladium-catalyzed hydrogenolytic cleavage and by treatment with 20% TFA in CH_2Cl_2. The diazepine core was formed by cyclization in the presence of 5 mol% of CH_3COOH in CH_2Cl_2 **(Scheme 54)** [100].

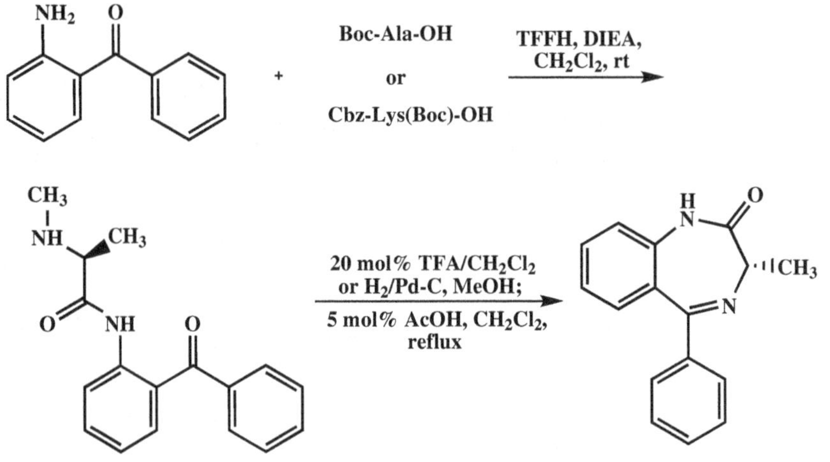

Scheme-54

The *o*-phenylene diamines were reacted with *in situ* formed alkynones to generate seven-membered heterocyclic compounds. The 1,5-benzodiazepines obtained by this coupling addition-cyclocondensation sequence were biologically active **(Scheme 55)** [101-102]. These azepines were essentially nonfluorescent in solution at rt, however, highly fluorescent in solid state. Cryofluorescence was reported upon cooling the solutions due to freezing of ring flip and aggregation. This thermoresponsive behavior of fluorophores as a consequence of restricted conformational changes opens new avenues for the fluorescence labeling of mesoporous materials or surfaces, biomolecules and for the development of tailor-made emitters in thermosensors [103].

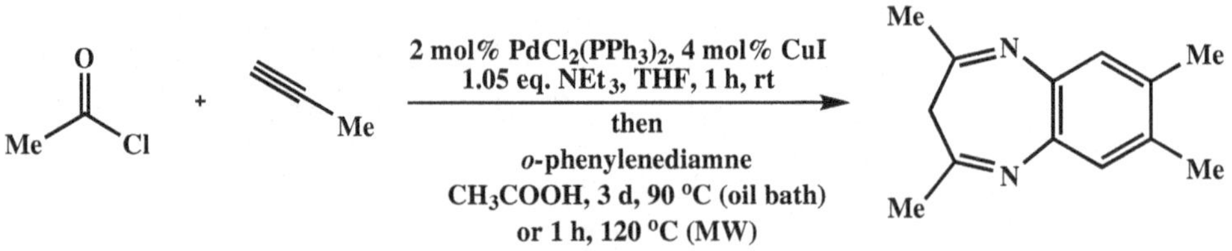

Scheme-55

Neukom and co-workers [104] performed palladium-catalyzed carboamination reactions, using xylene as a solvent and *t*-BuONa as a base at refluxing condition, for the preparation of saturated 1,4-benzodiazepines. For exploring the scope of benzodiazepine-forming reactions, the amides were used as substrates for carboamination reactions. The coupling of amides and 4-bromobiphenyl under optimized conditions transformed the diamine substrates into benzodiazepine in good yields, although regioisomer of benzodiazepine was also obtained in small amounts **(Scheme 56)**. Slightly improved selectivities were obtained using $P(4\text{-}F\text{-}C_6H_4)_3$ as a ligand. These modified conditions were useful for the coupling of amides with a variety of aryl bromides. However, efforts were unsuccessful when an amide substrate containing an allylic methyl group was employed and a complex mixture of regioisomers was observed [93, 105].

The synthetic precursors acylnitroso-derived hetero-Diels-Alder cycloadducts were utilized for the preparation of *N*-4-hydroxy-1,4-benzodiazepines in a single step. The anthranilic acid

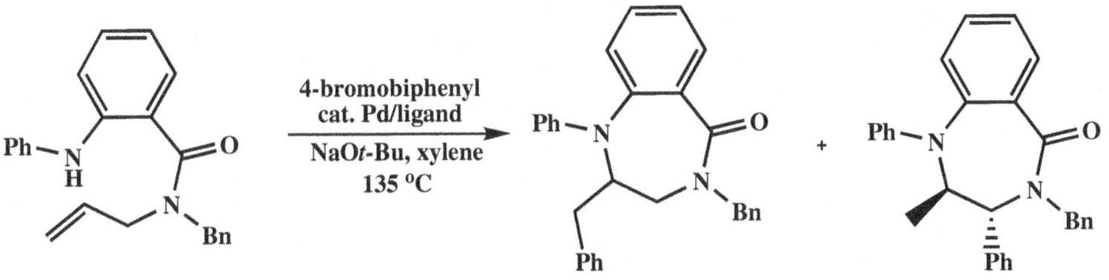

Scheme-56

based cycloadduct was treated with Pd(0) for inducing a cycloadduct ring-opening, subsequently 1,4-benzodiazepine core was constructed by an intramolecular nucleophilic attack on palladium allyl complex. *N*-tosyl cycloadduct was utilized for the synthesis of benzodiazepine. Cycloadduct was produced from anthranilic acid. The *N*-tosyl anthranilic acid was produced by introduction of tosyl group upon reacting with *p*-toluenesulfonyl chloride and Na_2CO_3. The desired *N*-tosyl cycloadduct was afforded by EDC coupling of acid and acylnitroso hetero-Diels-Alder reaction. The targeted benzodiazepine was produced when cycloadduct was treated with Pd(0). The pKa was lowered by introducing a NO_2 group onto sulfonamide to increase the yield of benzodiazepine. The hydroxamic acid was afforded upon coupling of acid with *O*-TBDMS hydroxylamine followed by removal of silyl protecting group. The desired cycloadduct was formed in 81% yield when hydroxamic acid was oxidized with cyclopentadiene. The benzodiazepine was afforded upon treatment of cycloadduct with Pd(0) **(Scheme 57)** [106].

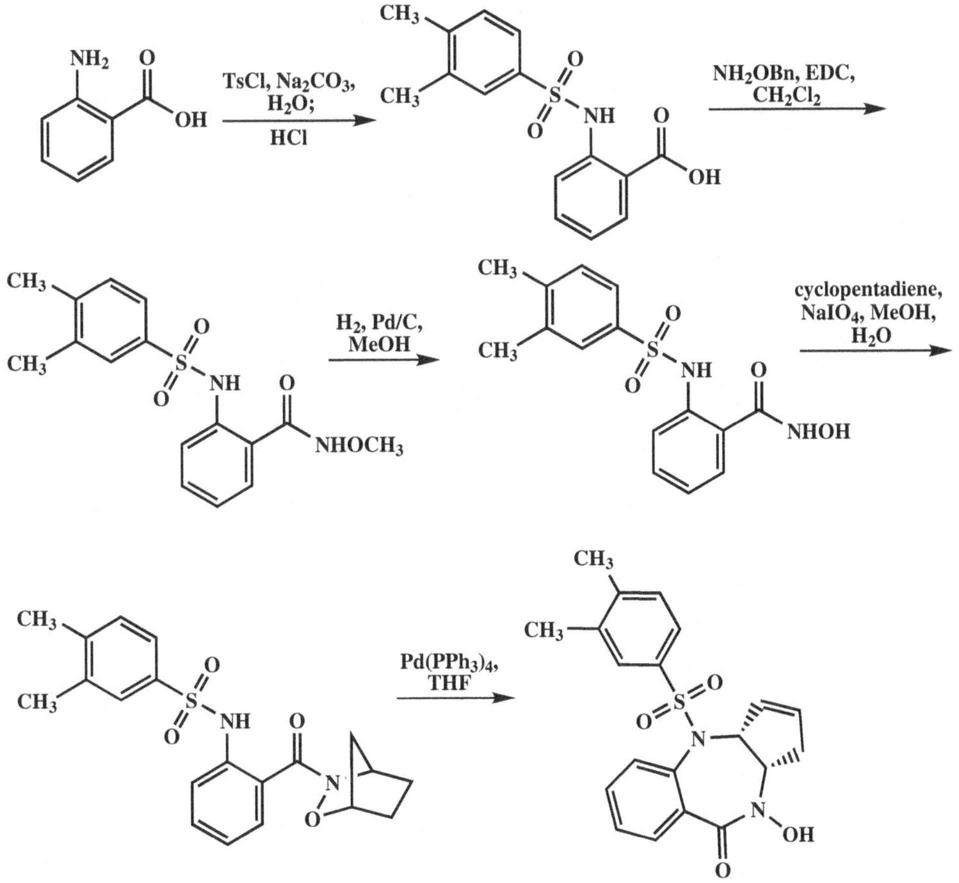

Scheme-57

An acylnitroso-derived cycloadduct underwent an intramolecular palladium(0)-mediated ring-opening to produce hydroxamic acid bearing benzodiazepines. The amide analogues were afforded upon subsequent N-O bond reduction of hydroxamate. Nitrone was generated when cycloadduct was treated with palladium acetate and triphenylphosphine for 10 min at 40 °C. The oxazoline *N*-oxides were important synthons in [3+2]-cycloadditions. The nitrone was re-subjected, after isolation and purification, to palladium acetate and triphenylphosphine in refluxing tetrahydrofuran to afford benzodiazepine. Among many Pd reagents the polymer-bound PPh$_3$-palladium(0) was the most practical reagent because of easy product isolation and increased yield **(Scheme 58)** [107].

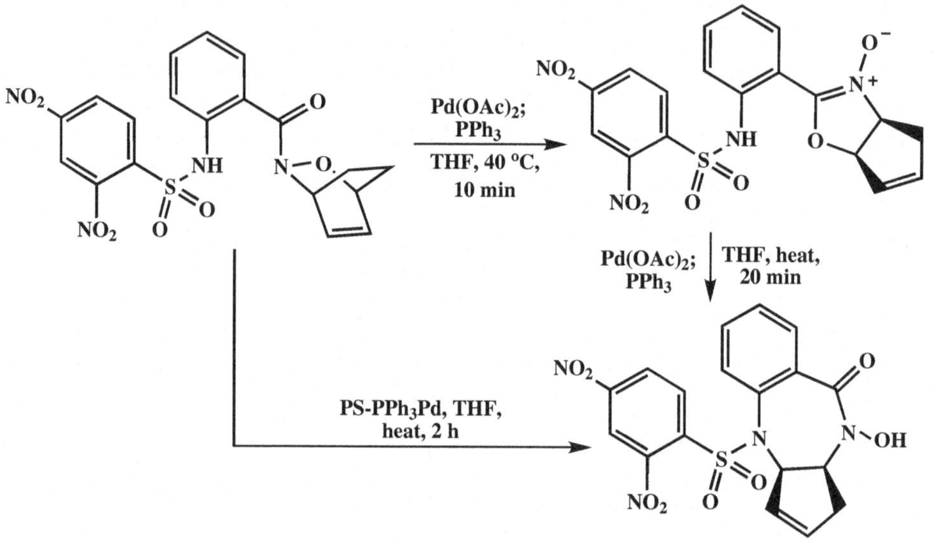

Scheme-58

Some interesting examples of Pd- and Cu-catalyzed *N*-arylation reactions have emerged for diazepine synthesis. Intramolecular Pd-catalyzed amidation of chloroamide afforded pyridopyrrolo-1,4-diazepinone **(Scheme 59)** [108-118].

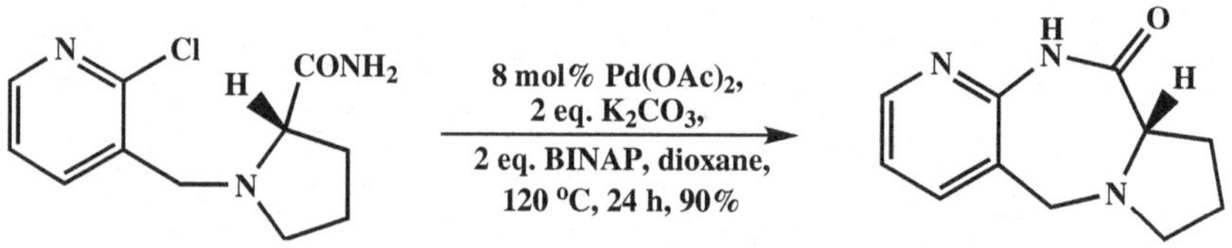

Scheme-59

Acylnitroso-derived hetero-Diels-Alder cycloadducts were valuable synthetic intermediates for the preparation of biologically important molecules, natural products [119-127] and carbocyclic nucleosides [128-129]. An appropriate functionalized cycloadduct was utilized for one-pot synthesis of 1,4-benzodiazepine. An anthranilic acid based cycloadduct was treated with Pd(0) to induce a cycloadduct ring-opening, followed by an intramolecular nucleophilic attack on Pd allyl complex to synthesize 1,4-benzodiazepine core **(Scheme 60)** [106, 130].

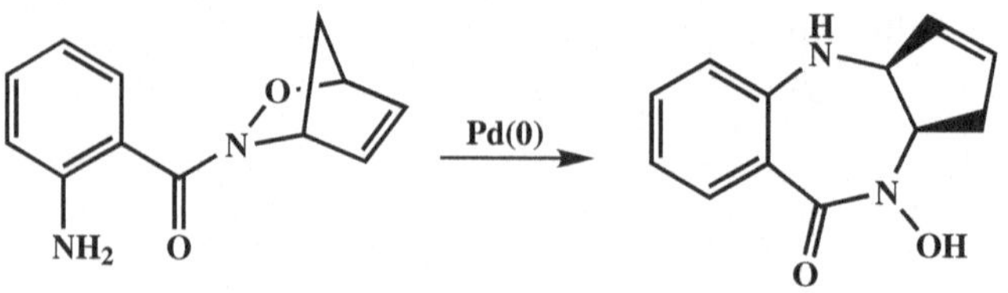

Scheme-60

11.5 Synthesis of seven-membered *O*-heterocycles

The α-ketoesters and unsaturated α-ketoamides underwent a Pd-catalyzed intramolecular oxidative cyclization under aerobic conditions in the presence of Yb(OTf)$_3$ [131-132]. The Yb(OTf)$_3$ acted as a Lewis acid for the enhancement of its nucleophilicity towards palladium(II)-activated olefin and for the promotion of enolization of substrate **(Scheme 61)**. A number of six-, seven-, and eight-membered nitrogen- and oxygen-heterocycles were synthesized regioselectively under very mild conditions in good yields [83].

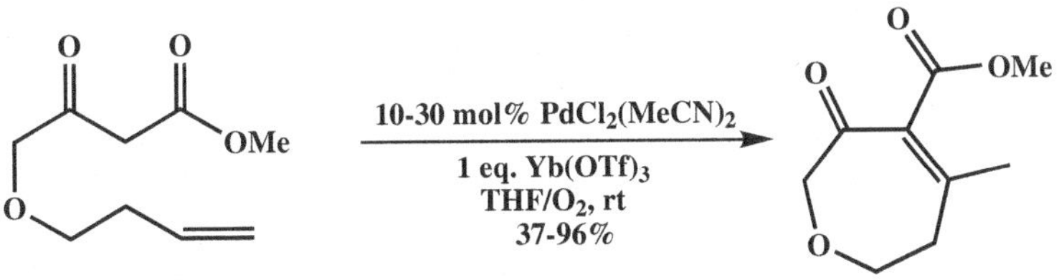

Scheme-61

The palladium(0) catalyst was either produced *in situ* from 5-10 mol% of preformed palladium(0) [Pd[PPh$_3$], Pd$_2$(dba$_3$)$_3$ or triphenylphosphine. Many sources of hydride ion were investigated and formate salts (sodium formate, formic acid) of piperidine were found to be the most effective and suppressed the shunt pathway. The scope of cyclization-anion capture protocol was explored by anion capture agent and ring size **(Scheme 62)** [133].

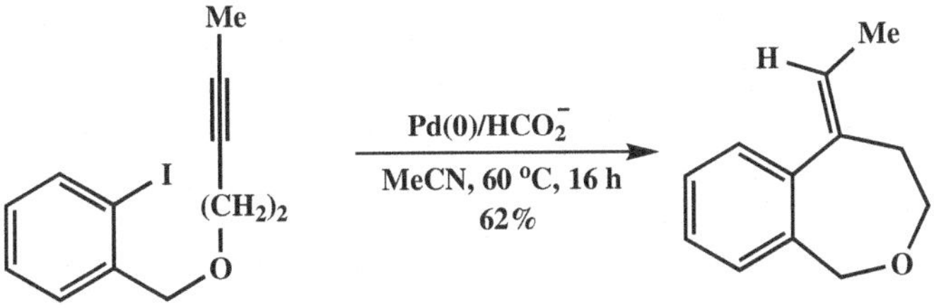

Scheme-62

Lautens et al. [134] utilized aryl bromides containing *O*-containing alkyl side-chains for the preparation of seven-membered heterocyclic benzonitriles under MWI **(Scheme 63)**. This one-pot aryl alkylation-cyanation sequence occurred in the presence of palladium acetate, triphenylphosphine, Zn(CN)$_2$, norbornene, cesium carbonate at 150 °C in dimethoxyethane.

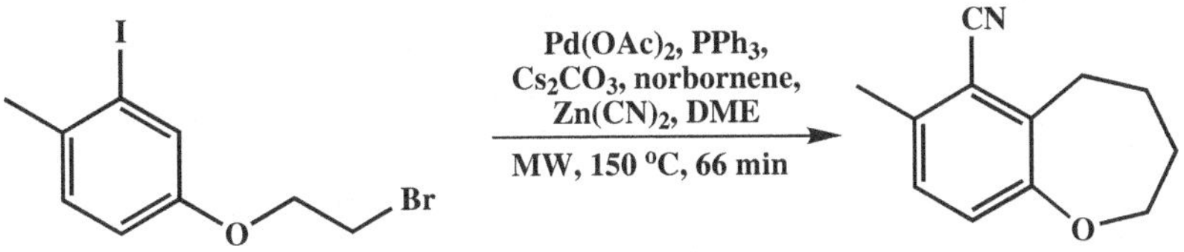

Scheme-63

The valuable heterocyclic or carbocyclic scaffolds were synthesized *via* an intramolecular coupling between allyl and aryl halide moieties in the presence of Pd catalyst. Lautens et al. [135] produced seven-membered *O*-containing heterocyclic compounds when allyl acetates and carbonates underwent an intramolecular coupling with ArI under MWI **(Scheme 64)**. The desired cyclized products were obtained in low yield when allyl carbonates were refluxed in the presence of Pd$_2$(dba)$_3$, *N,N*-dimethylbutylamine, and tri-*o*-tolylphosphine in acetonitrile-water. Under MWI there was an enhancement in yield from 49 to 72%.

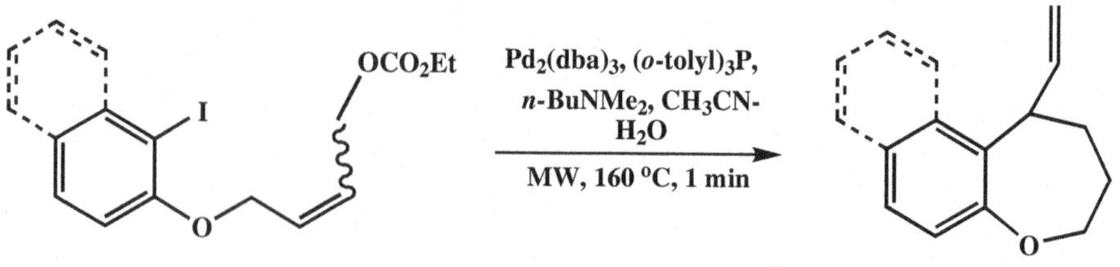

Scheme-64

A number of fused bicyclic β-lactams of non-conventional structure were synthesized by combination of bromoallylation reaction and Heck cyclization [136]. The reaction occurred from acetate substrates using dimethylformamide as solvent, Pd acetate as Pd source, K_2CO_3 as base and PPh_3 (**Scheme 65**).

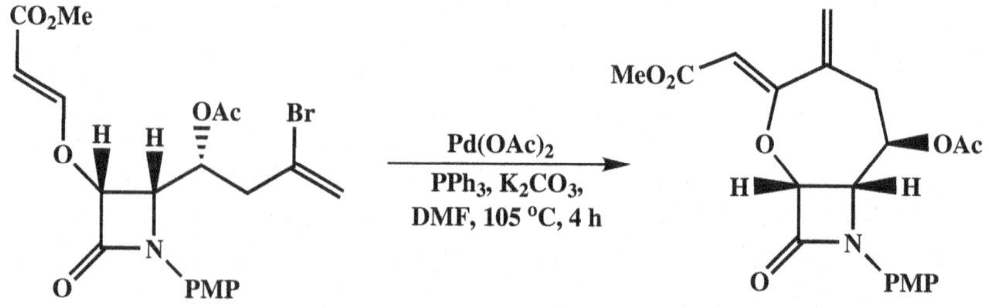

Scheme-65

The desired seven-membered adducts were obtained in impressive yields (up to 94%) as sole products, resulting from a 7-*endo* oxycyclization from cyclizative coupling reaction of allenols with allyl halides in the presence of palladium(II) catalyst (**Scheme 66**) [137]. The ring size (five, six, or seven) of fused oxacycle was modulated with judicious choice of catalyst (lanthanum, Au, or palladium). Having found a solution for 5-*exo* selective hydroalkoxylation, it was next examined that more intricate heterocyclizative problem associated with tuning the regioselectivity of γ-allenols [51, 138].

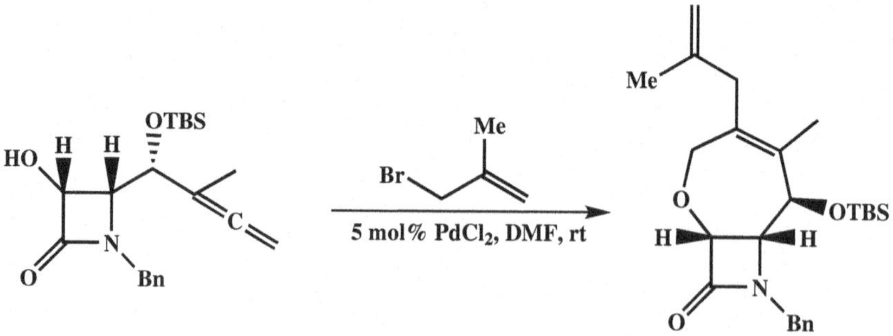

Scheme-66

11.6 Synthesis of seven-membered O,N-heterocycles

The N-arylated five-, six- and seven-membered N-heterocycles were generated by sequential Pd-catalyzed intra- followed by intermolecular aryl amination in the presence of sodium *tert*-butoxide as base and SIPr as a ligand (**Scheme 67**) [139].

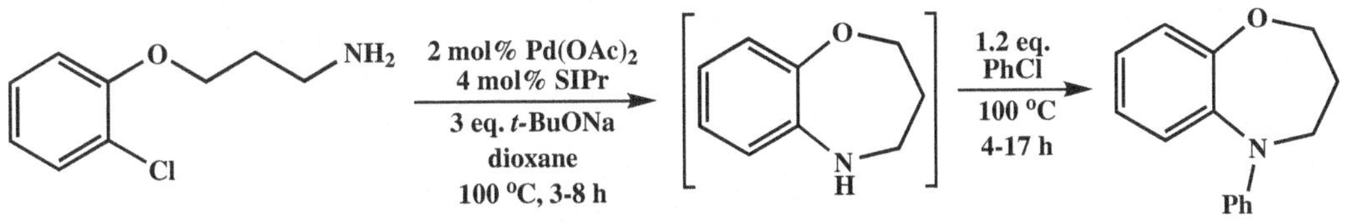

Scheme-67

White and co-workers [140-142] reported allylic amination reactions which use palladium(II) catalysts in dimethylsulphoxide. The homoallyl ether substrate was treated under oxidative cyclization conditions to differentiate between two mechanisms. The major product of reaction was seven-membered ring as expected from aminopalladation. The allylic carbon-hydrogen activation product was detected only in small amount; however, this product was formed probably from aminopalladation (formed *in situ* through isomerization of homoallyl ether substrate). These results suggested that product was synthesized predominantly *via* aminopalladation strategy **(Scheme 68)** [143].

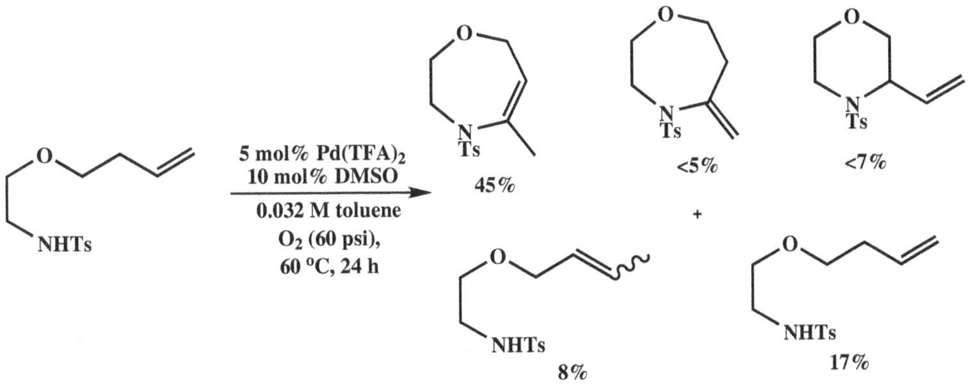

Scheme-68

Nevertheless, two facts have attracted the attention of people after cyclization reaction from epoxide: (a) the presence of two isomers was indicated by 1H NMR spectrum of mixture, as demonstrated by several sets of signals, each one composed of two splitting patterns (b) two compounds were obtained [144]. The minor isomer was identified as 3,4-dihydro-2*H*-3-hydroxymethyl-1,4-benzoxazine and the major one was 2,3,4,5-tetrahydro-1,5-benzoxazepine-3-ol. A mixture of compounds was synthesized in this shorter one-pot synthesis starting from *o*-aminophenol and epichlorohydrin under microwave irradiation conditions (30 min, 160 °C) **(Scheme 69)** [145].

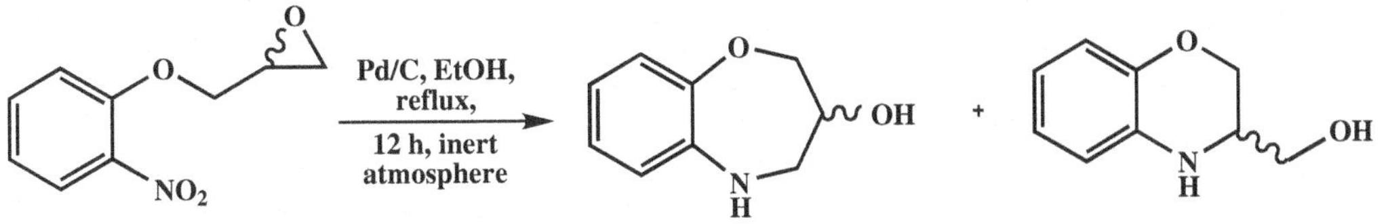

Scheme-69

Hepatitis C is one of the most serious public health problems, among diseases caused by viruses, affecting about 3% of World's population, which represents about 170 million infected people [146]. The hepatitis C virus (HCV) was treated using pegylated interferon-α in combination with ribavirin [147]. However, this therapy is associated with serious side effects and is only effective in about 50% of patients. So, there is a need to search out better tolerated and more efficacious anti-viral lead compounds. Therefore, Zhu et al. [148] constructed novel acyclic 1,2,4-triazole nucleosides with many ethynyl moieties containing triazole nucleobase. The bromotriazole acyclonucleoside synthesized desired molecules efficiently in yields ranging from 75 to 99% in one-pot Sonogashira reaction under MWI in aqueous solution **(Scheme 70)**. Optimized reaction conditions, comprising $Pd(PPh_3)_4$/cuprous iodide and lithium carbonate in water/dioxane (1:3) solvents at 100 °C for 25 min, were developed to avoid the synthesis of intramolecular cyclization by-product under basic conditions. One of the compounds inhibited HCV subgenomic replication with a 50% effective concentration (EC50) and did not inhibit proliferation of host cell [149-150].

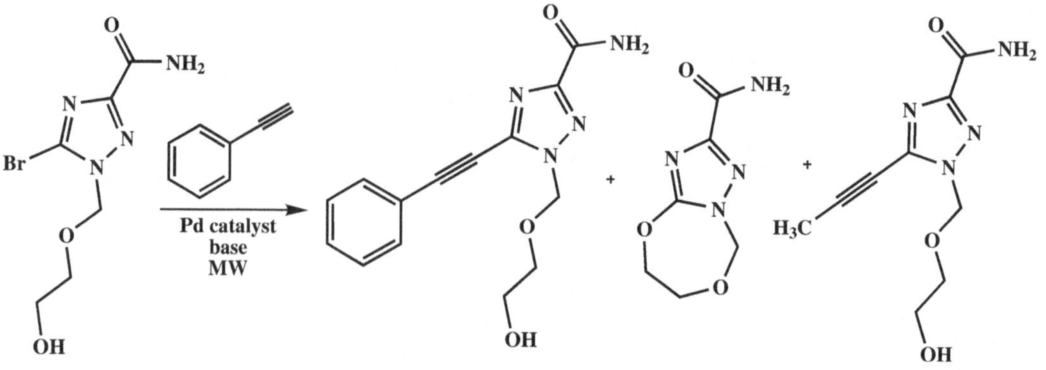

Scheme-70

11.7   Synthesis of seven-membered S-heterocycles

The cyclic sulfamides acts as HIV-1 protease inhibitors. These cyclic inhibitors contain seven-membered rings where sulfonyl oxygen displaced a structural H_2O in enzyme when the inhibitors bind to active site. The seven-membered symmetric ureas showed a symmetric binding while the cyclic sulfamides display an unsymmetric binding to C2-symmetric HIV protease [151]. The design was guided by elegant work of Lam and co-workers [152] for the synthesis of phenyl alanine-derived carbanalogs. For the rationalization of complex structure-activity relationships of this class of compounds a CoMFA (comparative molecular field analysis) model was developed **(Scheme 71)** [153a-b].

Simple and readily accessible *o*-iodothiophenols and *N*-tosyl aziridines were reacted in domino process for the preparation of 1,4-benzothiazepin-5-ones. The aziridine ring was opened with *o*-iodothiophenols, followed by Pd-catalyzed intramolecular carboxamidation. The reaction was performed using many aziridines and *o*-iodothiophenols under optimized reaction conditions to explore the scope and limitation of this conversion. The 1,4-thiazepinone was formed in 93% yield when *N*-tosyl aziridine of cyclohexene was reacted with 2-iodothiophenol, showing that this conversion tolerated both electron-withdrawing (*p*-Cl) and electron-donating (*p*-Me) groups on phenyl group of thiophenol. The yields of desired products decreased slightly (64%-79%), with five- and seven-membered ring-fused aziridines. However, the desired product was not produced, when eight-membered ring-fused aziridine was utilized, only providing the intermediate in 25% yield. The different behavior in comparison to *o*-iodothiophenol was because of lower rate of oxidative addition of Ph-Br moiety to *in situ* formed Pd(0) species. The 1,4-thiazepinone moieties were produced in good yields from same transformations of 2-iodothiophenol with acyclic aziridine and unsaturated ring-fused aziridines **(Scheme 72)** [43, 154].

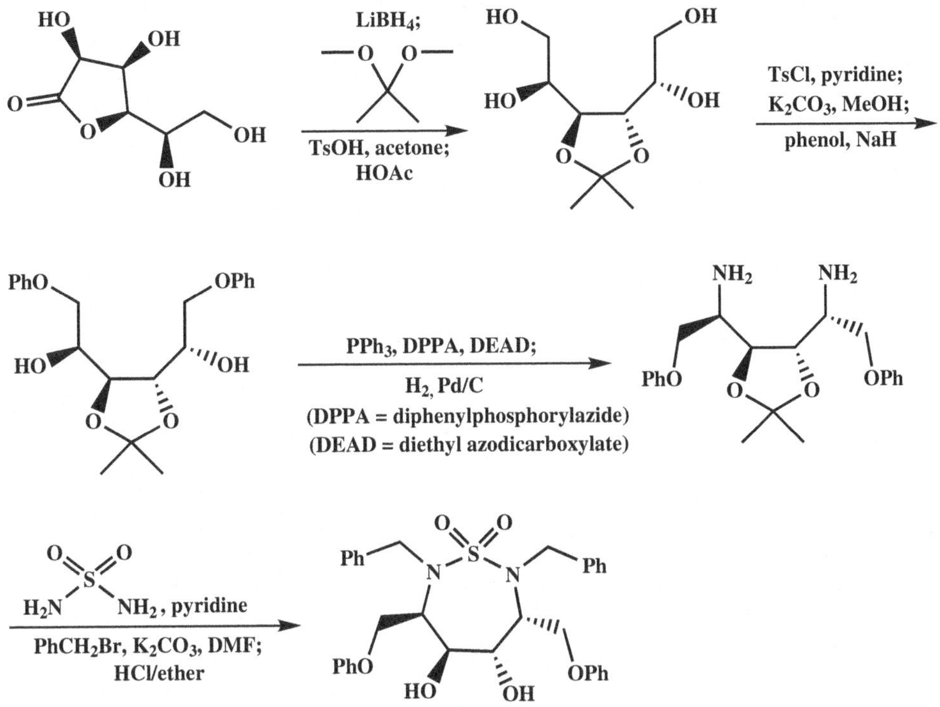

Scheme-71

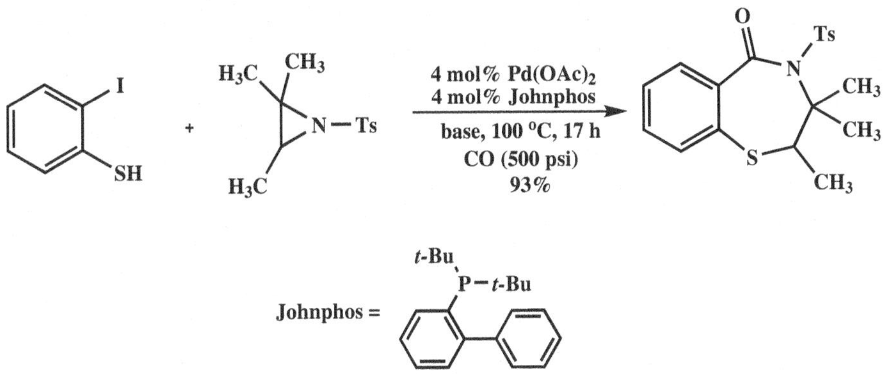

Scheme-72

The indoloazocines were synthesized using this strategy. A similar process for the formation of 7-membered heterocycle was used by Hanson et al. [155] for the synthesis of benzofused sultams **(Scheme 73)**. The σ-alkyl Pd(II) complex was formed at the terminal end of electron rich alkene, eventually resulting in the formation of 8-membered indole-based *N*-heterocyclic ring (the α-substituted product as observed in the synthesis of sultams).

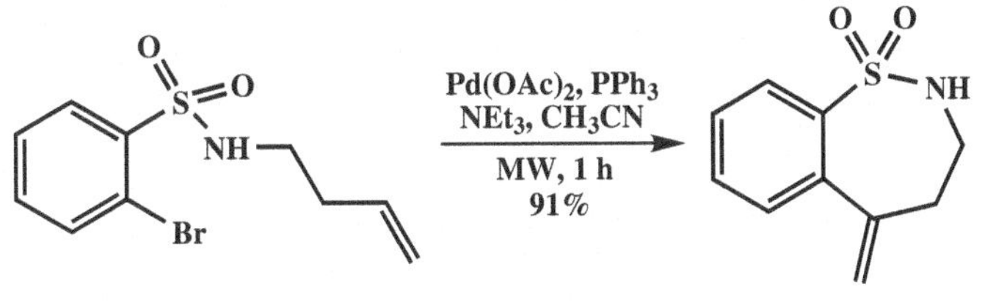

Scheme-73

The desired alkynone was formed when *p*-chlorobenzoyl chloride was reacted with phenyl acetylene under Sonogashira conditions at rt for 1 h. Subsequently, *o*-aminothiophenol and CH_3COOH (upon varying time and reaction temperature under MWI) were added to alkynone for the synthesis of benzothiazepine (**Scheme 74**). Dielectric heating was superior over conductive heating as shown by optimization of hitherto-cyclization. As compared to other multi-component reaction the formation of benzo[*b*][1,5]diazepines was just converse. Although for electronically diverse substitution the Michael addition and cyclo-condensation were completed at 60 °C after 10 min in MW cavity and the optimal condition was chosen to be reaction time of 30 min at 60 °C. Many 2,4-disubstituted benzo[*b*][1,5]thiazepines were synthesized under this optimization from a number of acid chlorides, alkynes, and 2-amino-4-chlorobenzenethiol or *o*-aminothiophenol derivatives *via* coupling-addition/cyclo-condensation sequence (**Scheme 75**) [156a-b].

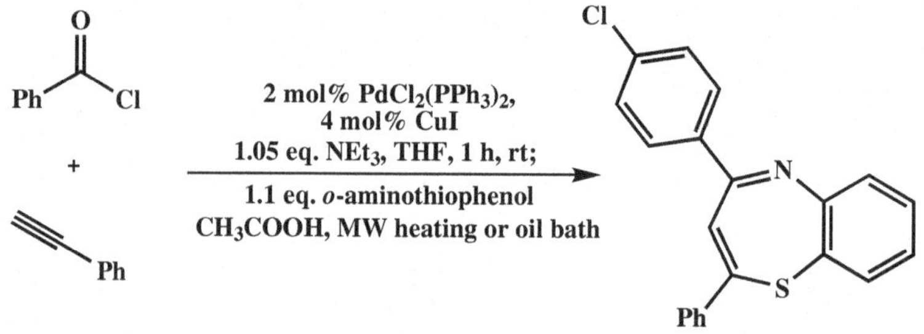

Scheme-74

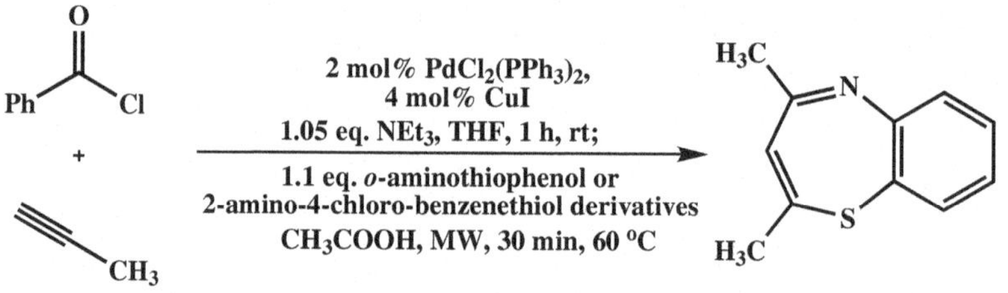

Scheme-75

Vasudevan et al. [157] explained that bromo substituted aza-Baylis-Hillman adducts were useful substrates for the preparation of benzo-fused thiazepine-1,1-dioxides. The aza-Morita-Baylis-Hillman adducts of 2-halosulfonamides were successfully converted into highly constrained bicyclic 6,7-dihydro-5-thia-6-aza-benzocycloheptene 5,5-dioxides through an intramolecular Heck reaction. These adducts underwent an intramolecular Heck cyclization for the synthesis of substituted benzothiazepine-1,1-dioxides in the presence of palladium acetate, P(*o*-tolyl)$_3$ and TEA under MWI in tetrahydrofuran for 60 min at a ceiling temperature of 160 °C (**Scheme 76**) [158a-b].

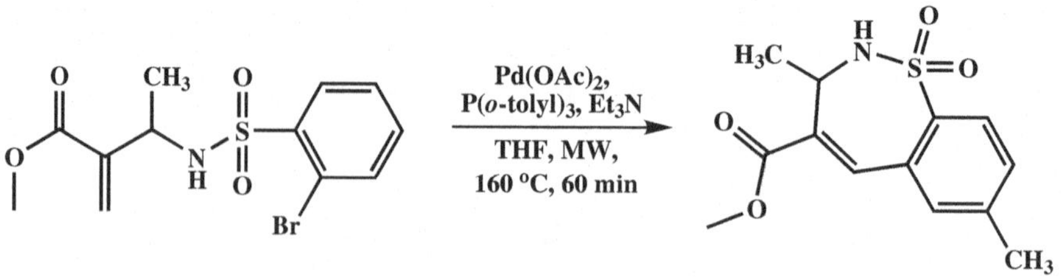

Scheme-76

The *N*-tosylaziridines and *o*-iodothiophenols were reacted through an efficient domino pathway involving one-pot Pd-catalyzed tandem aziridine ring-opening-intramolecular carboxamidation for the construction of 1,4-benzothiazepin-5-ones. In these reactions products were formed in high yields in the presence of (2-biphenyl)di-*t*-butylphosphine (Johnphos) ligand. The *N*-tosylaziridines and halopyridinols or halophenols underwent one-pot sequential phase transfer-catalyzed ring-opening/carboxamidation reactions to synthesize pyrido- or 1,4-benzo-oxazepinones respectively. A series of substituted 1,4-thiazepin-5-ones was synthesized by the reaction of alkylidene monothiosuccinic anhydride with 2-mercaptoethylamine. Interestingly, upon ring-closure of amine onto proximal carbonyl group followed by conjugate addition only 1,4-thiazepin-5-one regioisomer was obtained. The reaction of nitro-enones with *o*-aminobenzenethiol afforded 2-aryl-4-methyl-3-nitro-2,3-dihydro-1,5-benzothiazepines under mild conditions. To investigate the efficiency and feasibility of new domino method the reaction of 2-iodothiophenol with *N*-tosyl aziridine of cyclohexene was selected as a model reaction. Only trace amounts of desired product 1,4-thiazepinone were obtained in the presence of 3.0 eq. of triethylamine, 4 mol% of palladium acetate, and 1,1'-bis(diphenylphosphino)ferrocene, under 500 psi of carbon monoxide for 17 h at 100 °C. The yield of 1,4-thiazepinone was increased to 93% when same reaction was performed using (2-biphenyl)di-*tert*-butylphosphine (Johnphos) as a ligand. The efficiency of reaction was hampered at lower pressure of CO or at lower loading of Pd precursors. Surprisingly, the inorganic base, cesium carbonate, was found to be inferior to other bases, such as potassium carbonate and triethylamine **(Scheme 77)** [43, 159-161].

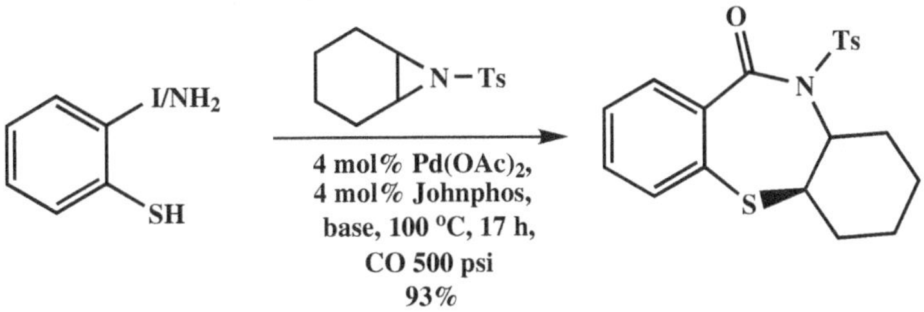

Scheme-77

The use of Bronsted acids as organocatalysts in asymmetric reactions is an expanding area of research. New ligands are often reported for improved catalysis of individual reactions, such as L-proline-substituted binaphthyl sulfonimide for the enantioselective Michael addition of ketones to nitroalkenes. An interesting general approach for the synthesis of optically pure 3,3'-diaryl chiral disulfonimides from racemic BINOL (1,1'-bi-2-naphthol) has been developed that provided an enantiopure 3,3'-dihalide which could serve as common precursor for a range of aryl-substituted chiral disulfonimides **(Scheme 78)** [162-163].

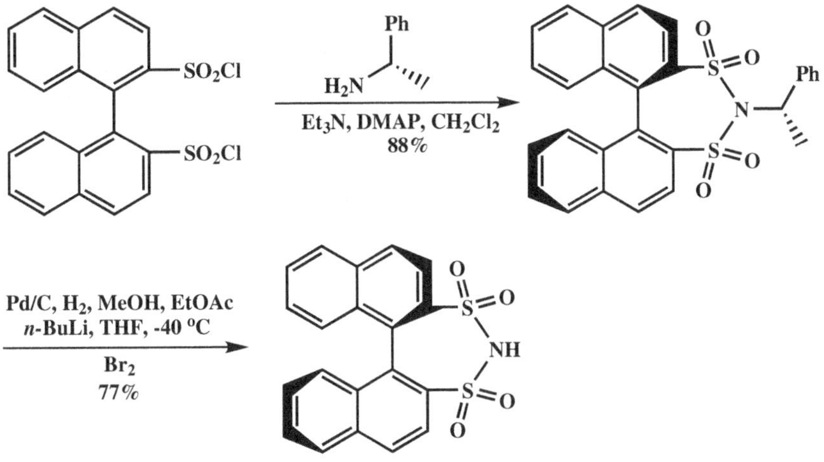

Scheme-78

Appropriate *o*-substitutions of benzyl groups will span the pockets and thereby interacted to two binding sites with one side-chain as suggested by computer modeling and X-Ray structures of enzyme-inhibitor complexes [164]. A new cyclic sulfamide scaffold was synthesized from l-dimethyltartrate in four steps **(Scheme 79)**. The protected aryl bromide was used as a starting substrate in the presence of Pd(0) catalyst under MWI. The type of spacers and length that would allow for optimal interactions of aromatic rings with both sites of enzyme was examined using Heck, Negishi, and Suzuki reactions. Disappointingly, the different linker lengths synthesized compounds that were roughly equipotent and the inhibitors were only moderately active.

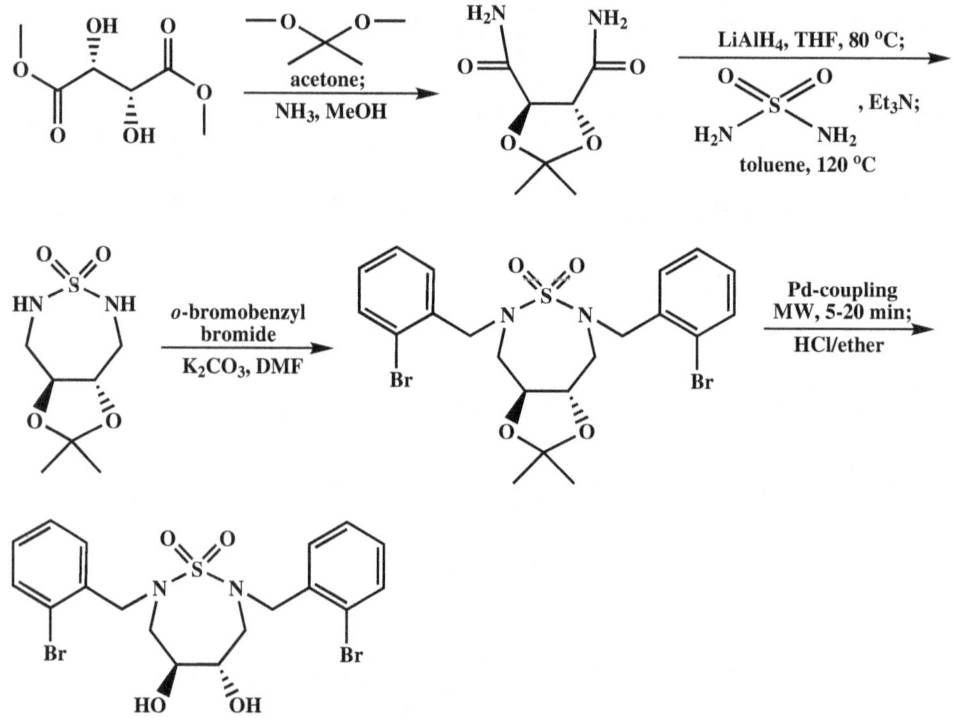

Scheme-79

The 5-aryl-2,4-bis(arylmethylidene)dihydro-3-thiophenones were heated with *o*-amino-thiophenol in a 1:1.5 molar ratio under reflux for 45-60 min in acetic acid for the synthesis of benzothiazepines in 55-91% yields. The benzothiazepines were provided in moderate yields (42-62%) when thiophenone and *o*-aminothiophenol were utilized in the same molar ratio and acetic acid catalyst under MWI at maximum 84 °C for 2-3 min. Therefore, the reaction rates were fast under MWI but yield of desired benzothiazepine products was lower when compared to thermal method **(Scheme 80)** [165].

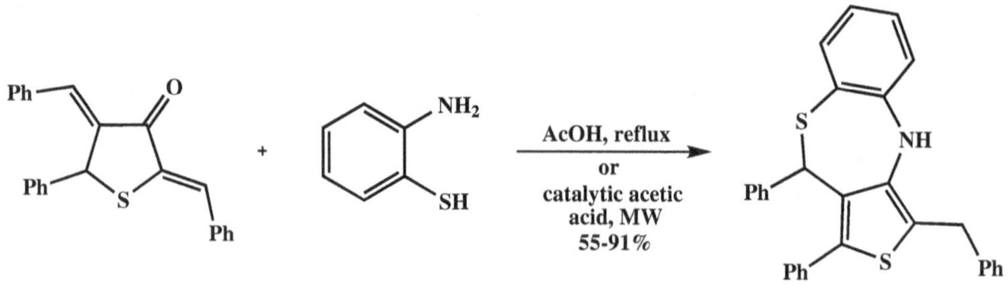

Scheme-80

REFERENCES

[1]   F. Sim, I. Sweetman, S. Kapur and M.X. Patel. 2015. Re-examining the role of benzodiazepines in the treatment of schizophrenia: a systematic review. J. Psychopharmacol. 29: 212-223.

[2]   T.A. Reekie, M.E. Kavanagh, M. Longworth and M. Kassiou. 2013. Synthesis of biologically active seven-membered-ring heterocycles. Synthesis 45: 3211-3227.

[3]   T.A. Katte, T.A. Reekie, W.T. Jorgensen and M. Kassiou. 2016. The formation of seven-membered heterocycles under mild Pictet-Spengler conditions: a route to pyrazolo[3,4]benzodiazepines. J. Org. Chem. 81: 4883-4889.

[4]   B.E. Evans, K.E. Rittle, M.G. Bock, R.M. Dipardo, R.M. Freidinger, W.L. Whitter, G.F. Lundell, D.F. Veber, P.S. Anderson, R.S.L. Chang, V.J. Lotti, D.J. Cerino, T.B. Chen, P.J. Kling, K.A. Kunkel, J.P. Springer and J. Hirshfield. 1988. Methods for drug discovery: development of potent, selective, orally effective cholecystokinin antagonists. J. Med. Chem. 31: 2235-2246.

[5]   D. Saha, G. Jain and A. Sharma. 2015. Benzothiazepines: chemistry of a privileged scaffold. RSC Adv. 5: 70619-70639.

[6]   M.E. Welsch, S.A. Snyder and B.R. Stockwell. 2010. Privileged scaffolds for library design and drug discovery. Curr. Opin. Chem. Biol. 14: 347-361.

[7]   E. Vitaku, D.T. Smith and J.T. Njardarson. 2014. Analysis of the structural diversity, substitution patterns, and frequency of nitrogen heterocycles among U.S. FDA approved pharmaceuticals. J. Med. Chem. 57: 10257-10274.

[8]   L. Banfi, A. Basso, C. Lambruschini, L. Moni and R. Riva. 2017. Synthesis of seven-membered nitrogen heterocycles through the Ugi multicomponent reaction. Chem. Heterocycl. Comp. 53: 382-408.

[9]   G. Mehta and V. Sing. 1999. Progress in the construction of cyclooctanoid systems: new approaches and applications to natural product syntheses. Chem. Rev. 99: 881-930.

[10]   N. Kaur. 2015. Benign approaches for the microwave-assisted synthesis of five-membered 1,2-N,N-heterocycles. J. Heterocycl. Chem. 52: 953-973.

[11]   L. Yet. 2000. Metal-mediated synthesis of medium-sized rings. Chem. Rev. 100: 2963-3008.

[12]   H. Li, Y. Blériot, C. Chantereau, J. Mallet, M. Sollogoub, Y. Zhang, E. Rodríguez-García, P. Vogel, J. Jiménez-Barbero and P. Sinaÿ. 2004. The first synthesis of substituted azepanes mimicking monosaccharides: a new class of potent glycosidase inhibitors. Org. Biomol. Chem. 2: 1492-1499.

[13]   G.I. Georg, X. Guan and J. Kant. 1991. Asymmetric synthesis of α-alkylated α-amino acids: azepane-2-carboxylic acids. Bioorg. Med. Chem. Lett. 1: 125-128.

[14]   P.A. Evans and A.B. Holmes. 1991. Medium ring nitrogen heterocycles. Tetrahedron 47: 9131-9166.

[15]   J.J. Barluenga. 2002. Fischer carbene complexes. A new tool for heterocyclic synthesis. Pure Appl. Chem. 74: 1317-1325.

[16]   S.J. Lee and P. Beak. 2006. Asymmetric synthesis of 4,5,6- and 3,4,5,6-substituted azepanes by a highly diastereoselective and enantioselective lithiation-conjugate addition sequence. J. Am. Chem. Soc. 128: 2178-2179.

[17]   S.A. Reed and M.C. White. 2008. Catalytic intermolecular linear allylic C-H amination *via* heterobimetallic catalysis. J. Am. Chem. Soc. 130: 3316-3318.

[18]   H. Du, W. Yuan, B. Zhao and Y. Shi. 2007. A Pd(0)-catalyzed diamination of terminal olefins at allylic and homoallylic carbons *via* formal C-H activation under solvent-free conditions. J. Am. Chem. Soc. 129: 7496-7497.

[19]   L. Wu, S. Qiu and G. Liu. 2009. Brønsted base-modulated regioselective Pd-catalyzed intramolecular aerobic oxidative amination of alkenes: formation of seven-membered amides and evidence for allylic C-H activation. Org. Lett. 11: 2707-2710.

[20]   C.J. Engelin and P. Fristrup. 2011. Palladium catalyzed allylic C-H alkylation: a mechanistic perspective. Molecules 16: 951-969.

[21]   D. Bolton, I. Boyfield, M.C. Coldwell, M.S. Hadley, A. Johns, C.N. Johnson, R.E. Markwell, D.J. Nash, G.J. Riley, E.E. Scott, S.A. Smith, G. Stemp, H.J. Wadsworth and E.A. Watts. 1997. 2-[(Substituted)phenyl]-[1-(2-phenylazacycloheptyl)methyl]-1H-pyrroles with high affinity and selectivity for the dopamine D3 receptor. Bioorg. Med. Chem. Lett. 7: 485-488.

[22] J. Aszodi, D.A. Rowlands, P. Mauvais, P. Collette, A. Bonnefoy and M. Lampilas. 2004. Design and synthesis of bridged γ-lactams as analogues of β-lactam anti-biotics. Bioorg. Med. Chem. Lett. 14: 2489-2492.

[23] F. Felluga, V. Gombac, G. Pitacco and E. Valentin. 2004. A convenient chemoenzymatic synthesis of (R)-(-) and (S)-(+)-homo-β-proline. Tetrahedron: Asymmetry 15: 3323-3327.

[24] R. Ballini and M. Petrini. 2009. Nitroalkanes as key building blocks for the synthesis of heterocyclic derivatives. ARKIVOC (ix): 195-223.

[25] H. Habib-Zahmani, J. Viala, S. Hacini and J. Rodriguez. 2007. Synthesis of functionalized spiro-heterocycles by sequential multicomponent reaction/metal catalyzed carbocylizations from simple β-ketoesters and amides. Synlett 7: 1037-1042.

[26] S. Nag and S. Batra. 2011. Applications of allylamines for the syntheses of aza-heterocycles. Tetrahedron 67: 8959-9061.

[27] I. Nakamura, H. Itagaki and Y. Yamamoto. 2001. Palladium-catalyzed inter- and intramolecular hydroamination of methylenecyclopropanes with amines. Chem. Heterocycl. Compd. 12: 1684-1692.

[28] I. Nakamura, T. Sato, M. Terada and Y. Yamamoto. 2008. Chirality transfer in gold-catalyzed carbothiolation of o-alkynylphenyl 1-arylethyl sulfides. Org. Lett. 10: 2649-2651.

[29] J.P. Wolfe, R.A. Rennels and S.L. Buchwald. 1996. Intramolecular palladium-catalyzed aryl amination and aryl amidation. Tetrahedron 52: 7525-7546.

[30] B.H. Yang and S.L. Buchwald. 1999. Palladium-catalyzed amination of aryl halides and sulfonates. J. Organomet. Chem. 576: 125-146.

[31] B.M. Trost and C.M. Marrs. 1993. A [3+2] cycloaddition and [4+3] cycloaddition approach to N-heterocycles via palladium-catalyzed TMM reactions with imines. J. Am. Chem. Soc. 115: 6636-6664.

[32] I. Ojima, M. Tzamarioudaki, Z. Li and R.J. Donovan. 1996. Transition metal-catalyzed carbocyclizations in organic synthesis. Chem. Rev. 96: 635-662.

[33] S.G. Stewart, C.H. Heath and E.L. Ghisalberti. 2009. Domino or single-step Tsuji-Trost/Heck reactions and their application in the synthesis of 3-benzazepines and azepino[4,5-b]indole ring systems. Eur. J. Org. Chem. 12: 1934-1943.

[34] J.T. Liang, J. Liu, B.T. Shireman, V.T. Tran, X. Deng and N.S. Mani. 2010. A practical synthesis of regioisomeric 6- and 7-methoxytetrahydro-3-benzazepines. Org. Process Res. Dev. 14: 380-385.

[35] D.M. Garrido, D.F. Corbett, K.A. Dwornik, A.S. Goetz, T.R. Littleton, S.C. McKeown, W.Y. Mills, T.L. Smalley, C.P. Briscoe and A.J. Peat. 2006. Synthesis and activity of small molecule GPR40 agonists. Bioorg. Med. Chem. Lett. 16: 1840-1845.

[36] X. Pan and C. Wilcox. 2010. Synthesis of dibenzazepinones by palladium-catalyzed intramolecular arylation of o-(2′-bromophenyl)anilide enolates. J. Org. Chem. 75: 6445-6451.

[37] G.L. Bolton and J.C. Hodges. 1999. Solid-phase synthesis of substituted benzazepines via intramolecular Heck cyclization. J. Comb. Chem. 1: 130-133.

[38] V. Gracias, J.D. Moore and S.W. Djuric. 2004. Sequential Ugi/Heck cyclization strategies for the facile construction of highly functionalized N-heterocyclic scaffolds. Tetrahedron Lett. 45: 417-420.

[39] L.F. Tietze, J.M. Wiegand and C. Vock. 2003. Synthesis of enantiopure nor-steroids by multiple Pd-catalyzed transformations. J. Organomet. Chem. 687: 346-352.

[40] M.M.S. Andappan, P. Nilsson and M. Larhed. 2003. Arylboronic acids as versatile coupling partners in fast microwave promoted oxidative Heck chemistry Mol. Divers. 7: 97-106.

[41] T. Uchida, M. Rodriquez and S.L. Shreiber. 2009. Skeletally diverse small molecules using a build/couple/pair strategy. Org. Lett. 11: 1559-1562.

[42] J.H. van Maarseveen, H.J.A.J. Den, V. Engelen, E. Finner, G. Visser and C.G. Kruse. 1996. Solid phase ring-closing metathesis: cyclization/cleavage approach towards a seven-membered cycloolefin. Tetrahedron Lett. 37: 8249-8252.

[43] F. Zeng and H. Alper. 2010. One-step synthesis of quinazolino[3,2-a]quinazolinones via palladium-catalyzed domino addition/carboxamidation reactions. Org. Lett. 12: 3642-3644.

[44] H. Cao, T.O. Vieira and H. Alper. 2011. Synthesis of unsaturated seven-membered ring lactams through palladium-catalyzed amination and intramolecular cyclocarbonylation reactions of amines and Baylis-Hillman acetates. Org. Lett. 13: 11-13.

[45] D. Bouyssi, N. Monteiro and G. Balme. 2011. Amines as key building blocks in Pd-assisted multicomponent processes. Beilstein J. Org. Chem. 7: 1387-1406.

[46] P.A. Donets and E.V. Eycken. 2007. Efficient synthesis of the 3-benzazepine framework *via* intramolecular Heck reductive cyclization. Org. Lett. 9: 3017-3020.

[47] V. Declerck, P. Ribiere, Y. Nedellec, H. Allouchi, J. Martinez and F. Lamaty. 2007. A microwave-assisted Heck reaction in poly(ethylene glycol) for the synthesis of benzazepines. Eur. J. Org. Chem. 307: 201-208.

[48] P.A. Donets, J.L. Goeman, J.V. Eycken, K.L. Robeyns, V. Meervelt and E.V. Eycken. 2009. An asymmetric approach towards (-)-aphanorphine and its analogues. Eur. J. Org. Chem. 6: 793-796.

[49] J.S. Prasad and L.S. Liebeskind. 1988. Silver mediated cyclizations of 4-allenyl-and 4-(2-propynyl) azetidinones. A stereoselective synthesis of 3-substituted δ1-carbapenems *via* N-C3 closure. Tetrahedron Lett. 29: 4253-4256.

[50] J.S. Prasad and L.S. Liebeskind. 1988. Palladium mediated formation of δ^{1}- and δ^{2}-carbapenems by cyclofunctionalization of 4-allenylazetidinones and 4-(2-propynyl)azetidinones. Tetrahedron Lett. 29: 4257-4260.

[51] B. Alcaide and P. Almendros. 2011. Allenyl-β-lactams: versatile scaffolds for the synthesis of heterocycles. Chem. Rec. 11: 311-330.

[52] B. Alcaide, P. Almendros and C. Aragoncillo. 2002. Additions of allenyl/propargyl organometallic reagents to 4-oxoazetidine-2-carbaldehydes: novel palladium-catalyzed domino reactions in allenynes. Chem. Eur. J. 8: 1719-1729.

[53] (a) B. Alcaide, P. Almendros and T. Martinez Campo. 2007. Metal-catalyzed regiodivergent cyclization of γ-allenols: tetrahydrofurans versus oxepanes. Angew. Chem. Int. Ed. 46: 6684-6687.
(b) B. Alcaide and P. Almendros. 2002. Recent advances in the stereocontrolled synthesis of bi- and tricyclic-β-lactams with non-classical structure. Curr. Org. Chem. 6: 245-264.

[54] M. Burwood, B. Davies, I. Diaz, R. Grigg, P. Molina, V. Sridharan and M. Hughes. 1995. Sequential and cascade [2+2]-cycloaddition-palladium catalyzed cyclization: bicyclic β-lactams. Tetrahedron Lett. 36: 9053-9056.

[55] C.W.G. Fishwick, R. Grigg, V. Sridharan and J. Virica. 2003. Sequential azomethine imine cycloaddition-palladium catalyzed cyclization processes. Tetrahedron 59: 4451-4468.

[56] G.R. Humphrey and J.T. Kuethe. 2006. Practical methodologies for the synthesis of indoles. Chem. Rev. 106: 2875-2911.

[57] S. Cacchi and G. Fabrizi. 2005. Synthesis and functionalization of indoles through palladium-catalyzed reactions. Chem. Rev. 105: 2873-2920.

[58] C. Bressy, D. Alberico and M. Lautens. 2005. A route to annulated indoles *via* a palladium-catalyzed tandem alkylation/direct arylation reaction. J. Am. Chem. Soc. 127: 13148-13149.

[59] G. Dyker. 1993. Pd-catalyzed C-H activation of methoxy groups by aryl-tomethoxy 1,4-migration. J. Org. Chem. 58: 6426-6428.

[60] G. Dyker. 1992. Transition-metal-catalyzed annulation reactions. Palladium-catalyzed activation of the carbon-hydrogen bond of methoxy groups: simple synthesis of substituted 6*H*-dibenzo[*b,d*] pyrans. Angew. Chem. Int. Ed. Engl. 31: 1023-1025.

[61] C. Blaszykowski, E. Aktoudianakis, D. Alberico, C. Bressy, D.G. Hulcoop, F. Jafarpour, A. Joushaghani, B. Laleu and M. Lautens. 2008. A palladium-catalyzed alkylation/direct arylation synthesis of nitrogen-containing heterocycles. J. Org. Chem. 73: 1888-1897.

[62] L. Joucla, A. Putey and B. Joseph. 2005. Synthesis of fused heterocycles with a benzazepinone moiety *via* intramolecular Heck coupling. Tetrahedron Lett. 46: 8177-8179.

[63] E.M. Beccalli, G. Broggini, M. Martinelli, G. Paladino and E. Rossi. 2006. Practical and efficient palladium-promoted synthesis of indole systems containing medium- and large-ring-fused heterocycles. Synthesis 14: 2404-2412.

[64] T.R. Kelly, W. Xu and J. Sundaresan. 1993. Maxonine: structure correction and synthesis. Tetrahedron Lett. 34: 6173-6176.

[65] G. Palmisano and M. Santagostino. 1993. Modified tryptamines by Sn-Pd transmetalation-coupling process. Synlett 10: 771-773.

[66] R.C. Larock, N.G. Berriospena and C.A. Fried. 1991. Regioselective, palladium-catalyzed hetero-annulation and carboannulation of 1,2-dienes using functionally substituted aryl halides. J. Org. Chem. 56: 2615-2617.

[67] H. Fuwa and M. Sasaki. 2007. A strategy for the synthesis of 2,3-disubstituted indoles starting from N-(o-halophenyl)allenamides. Org. Biomol. Chem. 5: 2214-2218.

[68] M. Toyata, A. Ilangovan, R. Okamoto, T. Masaki, M. Arakawa and M. Ihara. 2002. Simple construction of bicyclo[4.3.0]nonane, bicyclo[3.3.0]octane, and related benzo derivatives by palladium-catalyzed cycloalkenylation. Org. Lett. 4: 4293-4296.

[69] V.A. Peschkov, O.P. Pereshivko, P.A. Donets, V.P. Mehta and E.V. van der Eycken. 2010. Diversity-oriented microwave-assisted synthesis of the 3-benzazepine framework. Eur. J. Org. Chem. 25: 4861-4867.

[70] Z. Xu, W. Hu, Q. Liu, L. Zhange and Y. Jia. 2010. Total synthesis of clavicipitic acid and aurantioclavine: stereochemistry of clavicipitic acid revisited. J. Org. Chem. 75: 7626-7635.

[71] K. Brak and J.A. Ellman. 2010. Total synthesis of (-)-aurantioclavine. Org. Lett. 12: 2004-2007.

[72] T. Harayama, T. Sato, A. Hori, H. Abe and Y. Takeuchi. 2003. Novel synthesis of naphthobenzazepines from N-bromobenzylnaphthylamines by regioselective C-H activation utilizing the intramolecular coordination of an amine to Pd. Synlett 8: 1141-1144.

[73] T. Harayama, T. Sato, A. Hori, H. Abe and Y. Takeuchi. 2004. Novel synthesis of a new skeletal compound benzonaphthazepine by regioselective C-H activation utilizing the intramolecular coordination of an amine to Pd. Synthesis 9: 1446-1456.

[74] G. Liu and S.S. Stahl. 2007. Two-faced reactivity of alkenes: *cis-* versus *trans*-aminopalladation in aerobic Pd-catalyzed intramolecular aza-Wacker reactions. J. Am. Chem. Soc. 129: 6328-6335.

[75] M.M. Rogers, V. Kotov, J. Chatwichien and S.S. Stahl. 2007. Palladium-catalyzed oxidative amination of alkenes: improved catalyst reoxidation enables the use of alkene as the limiting reagent. Org. Lett. 9: 4331-4334.

[76] V. Kotov, C.C. Scarborough and S.S. Stahl. 2007. Palladium-catalyzed aerobic oxidative amination of alkenes: development of intra- and intermolecular aza-Wacker reactions. Inorg. Chem. 46: 1910-1923.

[77] J.E. Ney and J.P. Wolfe. 2004. Palladium-catalyzed synthesis of N-aryl pyrrolidines from γ-(N-arylamino) alkenes: evidence for chemoselective alkene insertion into Pd-N bonds. Angew. Chem. Int. Ed. 43: 3605-3608.

[78] J.E. Ney and J.P. Wolfe. 2005. Selective synthesis of 5- or 6-aryl octahydrocyclopenta[b]pyrroles from a common precursor through control of competing pathways in a Pd-catalyzed reaction. J. Am. Chem. Soc. 127: 8644-8651.

[79] K. Isomura, N. Okada, M. Saruwatari, H. Yamasaki and H. Taniguchi. 1985. Firm evidnce for *cis*-aminopalladation in the reaction of 1-aminohexatrienes with palladium dichloride. Chem. Lett. 14: 385-388.

[80] P. Melnyk, B. Legrand, J. Gasche, P. Ducrot and C. Thal. 1995. Synthesis of new annelated indole systems: new entry in the E-azaeburnane series. Tetrahedron 51: 1941-1952.

[81] Y. Yokoyama, T. Matsumoto and Y. Murakami. 1995. Optically active total synthesis of clavicipitic acid. J. Org. Chem. 60: 1486-1487.

[82] U. Pindur and A. Reinhard. 1990. Thermal 1,6-electrocyclization reactions of acceptor-substituted 2,3-divinyl-1H-indoles yielding functionalized carbazoles. Helv. Chim. Acta 73: 827-838.

[83] E.M. Beccalli, G. Broggini, M. Martinelli and S. Sottocornola. 2007. C-C, C-O, C-N Bond formation on sp^2 carbon by Pd(II)-catalyzed reactions involving oxidant agents. Chem. Rev. 107: 5318-5365.

[84] H.S. Lee, S.H. Kim, S. Gowrisankar and J.N. Kim. 2008. Palladium-mediated synthesis of poly-fused heterocycles from Baylis-Hillman adducts. Tetrahedron 64: 7183-7190.

[85] K.M. Dawood and B.F. Abdel-Wahab. 2010. Synthetic routes to benzimidazole-based fused polyheterocycles. ARKIVOC (i): 333-389.

[86] R. Riva, L. Banfi, A. Basso, G. Cerulli, G. Guanti and M. Pani. 2010. A highly convergent synthesis of tricyclic N-heterocycles coupling an Ugi reaction with a tandem S(N)2′-Heck double cyclization. J. Org. Chem. 75: 5134-5143.

[87] S.K. Das, A.K. Srivastava and G. Panda. 2010. A new route to 1,4-oxazepanes and 1,4-diazepanes from Garner aldehyde. Tetrahedron Lett. 51: 1483-1485.

[88] Z. Qian, I.R. Baxendale and S.V. Ley. 2010. A flow process using microreactors for the preparation of a quinolone derivative as a potent 5HT1B antagonist preparation of a potent $5HT_{1B}$. Synlett 4: 505-508.

[89] J.L. Brice, J.E. Harang, V.I. Timokhin, N.A. Anastasi and S.S. Stahl. 2005. Aerobic oxidative amination of unactivated alkenes catalyzed by palladium. J. Am. Chem. Soc. 127: 2868-2869.

[90] E. Negishi, T. Takahashi and K. Akiyoshi. 1986. 'Bis(triphenylphosphine)palladium:' its generation, characterization, and reactions. J. Chem. Soc. Chem. Commun. 17: 1338-1339.

[91] (a) M. Bottex, M. Cavicchioli, B. Hartmann, N. Monteiro and G. Balme. 2001. A versatile palladium-mediated three-component reaction for the one-pot synthesis of stereodefined 3-arylidene-(or 3-alkenylidene-)tetrahydrofurans. J. Org. Chem. 66: 175-179.
   (b) C. Kammerer, G. Prestat, D. Madec and G. Poli. 2009. Phosphine-free palladium-catalyzed allene carbopalladation/allylic alkylation. Domino sequence: a new route to 4-(α-styryl) γ-lactams. Chem. Eur. J. 15: 4224-4227.

[92] J.S. Nakhla, D.M. Schultz and J.P. Wolfe. 2009. Palladium-catalyzed alkene carboamination reactions for the synthesis of substituted piperazines. Tetrahedron 65: 6549-6570.

[93] N. Kaur. 2018. Photochemical reactions for the synthesis of six-membered *O*-heterocycles. Curr. Org. Synth. 15: 298-320.

[94] M.J. Plunkett and J.A. Ellman. 1995. Stille coupling in the solid-phase synthesis of structurally diverse 1,4-benzodiazepine derivatives. J. Am. Chem. Soc. 117: 3306-3307.

[95] R. Franzen. 2000. The Suzuki, Heck, and Still reactions: three versatile methods for the introduction of C-C bonds on solid support. Can. J. Chem. 78: 957-962.

[96] S. Ferrini, F. Ponticelli and M. Taddei. 2006. Rapid approach to 3,5-disubstituted 1,4-benzodiazepines *via* the photo-Fries rearrangement of anilides. J. Org. Chem. 71: 9217-9220.

[97] M. Catellani, C. Catucci, G. Celentano and R. Ferraccioli. 2001. Palladium-catalyzed synthesis of enantiopure 1,2,4,5-tetrahydro-1,4-benzodiazepin-3-(3*H*)-one derivatives. Synlett 6: 803-805.

[98] E.M. Beccalli, G. Broggini, G. Paladino, A. Penoni and C. Zoni. 2004. Regioselective formation of six- and seven-membered ring by intramolecular Pd-catalyzed amination of *N*-allyl-anthranilamides. J. Org. Chem. 69: 5627-5630.

[99] S.M. Lu and H. Alper. 2005. Intramolecular carbonylation reactions with recyclable palladium-complexed dendrimers on silica: synthesis of oxygen, nitrogen, or sulfur-containing medium ring fused heterocycles. J. Am. Chem. Soc. 127: 14776-14784.

[100] D. Jennifer, L. Wang-Qing, G. Nohad and G. Christiane. 2007. Novel 1,4-benzodiazepine derivatives with anti-proliferative properties on tumor cell lines. Bioorg. Med. Chem. Lett. 17: 2527-2530.

[101] B. Willy, T. Dallos, F. Rominger, J. Schönhaber and T.J.J. Müller. 2008. Three-component synthesis of cryo-fluorescent 2,4-disubstituted 3*H*-benzo[*b*][1,4]diazepines-conformational control of emission properties. Eur. J. Org. Chem. 28: 4796-4805.

[102] S.S. Palimkar, R.J. Lahoti and K.V. Srinivasan. 2007. A novel one-pot three-component synthesis of 2,4-disubstituted-3*H*-benzo[*b*][1,4]diazepines in water. Green Chem. 9: 146-152.

[103] B. Willy and T.J.J. Muller. 2008. Consecutive multi-component syntheses of heterocycles *via* palladium-copper catalyzed generation of alkynones. ARKIVOC (i): 195-208.

[104] J.D. Neukom, A.S. Aquino and J.P. Wolfe. 2011. Synthesis of saturated 1,4-benzodiazepines *via* Pd-catalyzed carboamination reactions. Org. Lett. 13: 2196-2199.

[105] A. Correa, I. Tellitu, E. Dominguez and R. SanMartin. 2006. An advantageous synthesis of new indazolone and pyrazolone derivatives. Tetrahedron 62: 11100-11105.

[106] M.D. Surman, M.J. Mulvihill and M.J. Miller. 2002. Novel 1,4-benzodiazepines from acylnitroso-derived hetero-Diels-Alder cycloadducts. Org. Lett. 4: 139-141.

[107] L.P. Tardibono and M.J. Miller. 2009. Synthesis and anti-cancer activity of new hydroxamic acid containing 1,4-benzodiazepines. Org Lett. 11: 1575-1578.

[108] L. Legeren and D. Dominguez. 2010. Intramolecular *N*-arylation in heterocyclization: synthesis of new pyrido-fused pyrrolo [1,2-*a*][1,4] diazepinones. Tetrahedron Lett. 51: 4053-4057.

[109]   G. Cuny, M. Bois-Choussy and J. Zhu. 2004. Palladium- and copper-catalyzed synthesis of medium-
        and large-sized ring-fused dihydroazaphenanthrenes and 1,4-benzodiazepine-2,5-diones. Control of
        reaction pathway by metal-switching. J. Am. Chem. Soc. 126: 14475-14484.

[110]   J.A. Brown. 2000. Synthesis of N-aryl indole-2-carboxylates via an intramolecular palladium-
        catalyzed annulation of didehydrophenylalanine derivatives. Tetrahedron Lett. 41: 1623-1626.

[111]   M. Watanabe, T. Yamamoto and M. Nishiyama. 2000. A new palladium-catalyzed intramolecular
        cyclization: synthesis of 1-aminoindole derivatives and functionalization of their carbocylic rings.
        Angew. Chem. Int. Ed. 39: 2501-2504.

[112]   H. Siebeneicher, I. Bytschkov and S. Doye. 2003. A flexible and catalytic one-pot procedure for
        the synthesis of indoles. Angew. Chem. Int. Ed. 42: 3042-3044.

[113]   R. Omar-Amrani, A. Thomas, E. Brenner, R. Schneider and Y. Fort. 2003. Efficient nickel-mediated
        intramolecular amination of aryl chlorides. Org. Lett. 5: 2311-2314.

[114]   J.J. Song and N.K. Yee. 2000. A novel synthesis of 2-aryl-2*H*-indazoles *via* a palladium-catalyzed
        intramolecular amination reaction. Org. Lett. 2: 519-521.

[115]   J.J. Song and N.K. Yee. 2001. Synthesis of 1-aryl-1*H*-indazoles *via* the palladium-catalyzed cyclization
        of *N*-aryl-*N'*-(*o*-bromobenzyl)hydrazines and [*N*-aryl-*N'*-(*o*-bromobenzyl)-hydrazinato-*N'*]-
        triphenylphosphonium bromides. Tetrahedron Lett. 42: 2937-2940.

[116]   C.T. Brain and S.A. Brunton. 2002. An intramolecular palladium-catalyzed aryl amination reaction
        to produce benzimidazoles. Tetrahedron Lett. 43: 1893-1895.

[117]   C.T. Brain and J.T. Steer. 2003. An improved procedure for the synthesis of benzimidazoles, using
        palladium-catalyzed aryl-amination chemistry. J. Org. Chem. 68: 6814-6816.

[118]   B.J. Margolis, J.J. Swidorski and B.N. Rogers. 2003. An efficient assembly of heterobenzazepine ring
        systems utilizing an intramolecular palladium-catalyzed cycloamination. J. Org. Chem. 68: 644-647.

[119]   T. Emoto, N. Kubosaki, Y. Yamagiwa and T. Kamikawa. 2000. A new route to phenazines.
        Tetrahedron Lett. 41: 355-358.

[120]   Y. Kozawa and M. Mori. 2002. Synthesis of 3-alkoxycarbonyl-1β-methylcarbapenem using palladium
        -catalyzed amidation of vinyl halide. Tetrahedron Lett. 43: 111-114.

[121]   R.S. Colemen and W. Chen. 2001. A convergent approach to the mitomycin ring system. Org. Lett.
        3: 1141-1144.

[122]   A. Abouabdellah and R.H. Dodd. 1998. A new approach to the synthesis of functionalized
        pyrido[2,3-*b*]indoles by way of a palladium-catalyzed ring closing reaction between the N-1 and
        C-9a positions. Tetrahedron Lett. 39: 2119-2122.

[123]   G. Cuny, M. Bois-Choussy and J. Zhu. 2003. One-pot synthesis of polyheterocycles by a palladium-
        catalyzed intramolecular *N*-arylation/C-H activation/aryl-aryl bond-forming domino process. Angew.
        Chem. Int. Ed. 42: 4774-4777.

[124]   F. He, B.M. Foxman and B.B. Snider. 1998. Total syntheses of (-)-asperlicin and (-)-asperlicin C.
        J. Am. Chem. Soc. 120: 6417-6418.

[125]   B.M. Trost and D.L. van Vranken. 1993. A general synthetic strategy toward aminocyclopentitol
        glycosidase inhibitors. Application of palladium catalysis to the synthesis of allosamizoline and
        mannostatin A. J. Am. Chem. Soc. 115: 444-458.

[126]   S.B. King and B. Ganem. 1991. Enantioselective synthesis of mannostatin A: a new glycoprotein
        processing inhibitor. J. Am. Chem. Soc. 113: 5089-5090.

[127]   B.E. Ledford and E.M. Carreira. 1995. Total synthesis of (+)-trehazolin: optically active spirocy-
        cloheptadienes as useful precursors for the synthesis of amino cyclopentitols. J. Am. Chem. Soc.
        117: 11811-11812.

[128]   A.R. Ritter and M.J. Miller. 1994. Amino acid-derived chiral acyl nitroso compounds: diastereo-
        selectivity in intermolecular hetero-Diels-Alder reactions. J. Org. Chem. 59: 4602-4611.

[129]   D. Zhang and M.J. Miller. 1998. Total synthesis of (±) carbocyclic polyoxin C and its α-epimer.
        J. Org. Chem. 63: 755-759.

[130]   L.M. Pardo, I. Tellitu and E. Dominguez. 2010. A versatile PIFA-mediated approach to structurally
        diverse pyrrolo (benzo) diazepines from linear alkynylamides. Tetrahedron 66: 5811-5818.

[131] D. Yang, J.-H. Li, Q. Gao and Y.-L. Yan. 2003. Lanthanide triflate-promoted palladium-catalyzed cyclization of alkenyl β-keto esters and amides. Org. Lett. 5: 2869-2871.

[132] K.-T. Yip, J.-H. Li, O.-Y. Lee and D. Yang. 2005. Aerobic oxidative cyclization under Pd(II) catalysis: a regioselective approach to heterocycles. Org. Lett. 7: 5717-5719.

[133] R. Grigg and V. Sridharan. 1998. Heterocycles *via* Pd catalyzed molecular queuing processes. Relay switches and the maximization of molecular complexity. Pure Appl. Chem. 70: 1047-1057.

[134] B. Mariampillai, D. Alberico, V. Bidau and M. Lautens. 2006. Synthesis of polycyclic benzonitriles *via* a one-pot aryl alkylation/cyanation reaction. J. Am. Chem. Soc. 128: 14436-14437.

[135] M. Lautens, E. Tayama and C. Herse. 2005. Palladium-catalyzed intramolecular coupling between aryl iodides and allyl moieties *via* thermal and microwave-assisted conditions. J. Am. Chem. Soc. 127: 72-73.

[136] B. Alcaide, P. Almendros and R. Rodriguez-Acebes. 2005. Novel carbonyl bromoallylation/Heck reaction sequence. Stereocontrolled access to bicyclic β-lactams. J. Org. Chem. 70: 2713-2719.

[137] B. Alcaide, P. Almendros, T. Martinezdel Campo, E. Soriano and J.L. Marco-Contelles. 2009. Regioselectivity control in the metal-catalyzed O-C functionalization of γ-allenols: experimental study. Chem. Eur. J. 15: 1901-1908.

[138] S. Ma and W. Gao. 2002. Efficient synthesis of 4-(2′-alkenyl)-2,5-dihydrofurans and 5,6-dihydro-2*H*-pyrans *via* the Pd-catalyzed cyclizative coupling reaction of 2,3- or 3,4-allenols with allylic halides. J. Org. Chem. 67: 6104-6112.

[139] R. Omar-Amrani, R. Schneider and Y. Fort. 2004. Novel synthetic strategy of *N*-arylated heterocycles *via* sequential palladium-catalyzed intra- and inter-arylamination reactions. Synthesis 15: 2527-2534.

[140] M.S. Chen and M.C. White. 2004. A sulfoxide-promoted, catalytic method for the regioselective synthesis of allylic acetates from monosubstituted olefins *via* C-H oxidation. J. Am. Chem. Soc. 126: 1346-1347.

[141] M.S. Chen, N. Prabagaran, N.A. Labenz and M.C. White. 2005. Serial ligand catalysis: a highly selective allylic C-H oxidation. J. Am. Chem. Soc. 127: 6970-6971.

[142] K.J. Fraunhoffer and M.C. White. 2007. *syn*-1,2-Amino alcohols *via* diastereoselective allylic C-H amination. J. Am. Chem. Soc. 129: 7274-7276.

[143] Z. Lu and S.S. Stahl. 2012. Intramolecular Pd(II)-catalyzed aerobic oxidative amination of alkenes: synthesis of six-membered *N*-heterocycles. Org. Lett. 14: 1234-1237.

[144] P.-F. Jiao, B.-X. Zhao, W.-W. Wang, Q.-X. He, M. Wan, D.-S. Shin and J.-Y. Miao. 2006. Design, synthesis, and preliminary biological evaluation of 2,3-dihydro-3-hydroxymethyl-1,4-benzoxazine derivatives. Bioorg. Med. Chem. Lett. 16: 2862-2867.

[145] E. Garca-Rubino, M.C. Nunez, M.A. Gallo and J.M. Campos. 2012. Synthesis, unambiguous chemical characterization, and reactivity of 2,3,4,5-tetrahydro-1,5-benzoxazepines-3-ol. RSC Adv. 2: 12631-12635.

[146] U. Weiss. 2005. Hepatitis C. Nature 436: 929-929.

[147] J.J. Feld and J.H. Hoofnagle. 2005. Mechanism of action of interferon and ribavirin in treatment of hepatitis C. Nature 436: 967-972.

[148] R. Zhu, M. Wang, Y. Xia, F. Qu, J. Neyts and L. Peng. 2008. Arylethynyltriazole acyclonucleosides inhibit hepatitis C virus replication. Bioorg. Med. Chem. Lett. 18: 3321-3327.

[149] R. Zhu, F. Qu, G. Quelever and L. Peng. 2007. Direct synthesis of 5-aryltriazole acyclonucleosides *via* Suzuki coupling in aqueous solution. Tetrahedron Lett. 48: 2389-2393.

[150] N.M. Nascimento-Junior, A.E. Kummerle, E.J. Barreiro and C.A.M. Fraga. 2011. MAOS and medicinal chemistry: some important examples from the last years. Molecules 16: 9274-9297.

[151] K. Backbro, S. Lowgren, K. Osterlund, J. Atepo, T. Unge, J. Hulten, N.M. Bonham, W. Schaal, A. Karlen and A. Hallberg. 1997. Unexpected binding mode of a cyclic sulfamide HIV-1 protease inhibitor. J. Med. Chem. 40: 898-902.

[152] P.Y.S. Lam, P.K. Jadhav, C.J. Eyermann, C.N. Hodge, Y. Ru, L.T. Bacheler, O.M.J. Meek and M.M. Rayner. 1994. Rational design of potent, bioavailable, nonpeptide cyclic ureas as HIV protease inhibitors. Science 263: 380-384.

[153] (a) R.D. Cramer, D.E. Patterson and J.D. Bunce. 1988. Comparative molecular field analysis (CoMFA). Effect of shape on binding of steroids to carrier proteins. J. Am. Chem. Soc. 110: 5959-5967.

(b) J. Wannberg, K. Ersmark and M. Larhed. 2006. Microwave-accelerated synthesis of protease inhibitors. Top. Curr. Chem. 266: 167-198.

[154] F. Zeng and H. Alper. 2010. Palladium-catalyzed domino ring-opening/carboxamidation reactions of N-tosyl aziridines and 2-iodothiophenols: a facile and efficient approach to 1,4-benzothiazepin-5-ones. Org. Lett. 12: 5567-5569.

[155] D.K. Rayabarapu, A. Zhou, K.O. Jeon, T. Samarakoon, A. Rolfe, H. Siddiqui and P.R. Hanson 2009. α-Haloarylsulfonamides: multiple cyclization pathways to skeletally diverse benzofused sultams. Tetrahedron 65: 3180-3188.

[156] (a) B. Willy and T.J.J. Muller. 2010. Three-component synthesis of benzo[1,5]thiazepines *via* coupling-addition-cyclocondensation sequence. Mol. Divers. 14: 443-453.

(b) K.A.M. El-Bayouki. 2013. Benzo[1,5]thiazepine: synthesis, reactions, spectroscopy, and applications. Org. Chem. Int. 2013: 1-71.

[157] A. Vasudevan, P.S. Tseng and S.W. Djuric. 2006. A post aza Baylis-Hillman/Heck coupling approach towards the synthesis of constrained scaffolds. Tetrahedron Lett. 47: 8591-8593.

[158] (a) A. Sharma, P. Appukkuttana and E.V. Eycken. 2012. Microwave-assisted synthesis of medium-sized heterocycles. Chem. Commun. 48: 1623-1637.

(b) V. Singh and S. Batra. 2008. Advances in the Baylis-Hillman reaction-assisted synthesis of cyclic frameworks. Tetrahedron 64: 4511-4574.

[159] G. Chouhan and H. Alper. 2010. Domino ring-opening/carboxamidation reactions of N-tosyl aziridines and 2-halophenols/pyridinol: efficient synthesis of 1,4-benzo- and pyrido-oxazepinones. Org. Lett. 12: 192-195.

[160] D. Crich and M.Y. Rahaman. 2010. Dihydro-3-(triphenylphosphoranylidene)-2,5-thiophendione: a convenient synthon for the preparation of substituted 1,4-thiazepin-5-ones and piperidinones *via* the intermediacy of thioacids. Tetrahedron 66: 6383-6390.

[161] R.I. Baichurin, N.I. Aboskalova and V.M. Berestovitskaya. 2010. One-pot synthesis of 2-aryl-4-methyl-3-nitro-2,3-dihydro-1,5-benzothiazepines. Russ. J. Org. Chem. 46: 1590-1591.

[162] S. Ban, D.M. Du, H. Liu and W. Yang. 2010. Synthesis of binaphthyl sulfonimides and their application in the enantioselective Michael addition of ketones to nitroalkenes. Eur. J. Org. Chem. 27: 5160-5164.

[163] H. He, L.Y. Chen, W.Y. Wong, W.H. Chan and A.W.M. Lee. 2010. Practical synthetic approach to chiral sulfonimides (CSIs)- chiral Brønsted acids for organocatalysis. Eur. J. Org. Chem. 22: 4181-4184.

[164] A. Ax, W. Schaal, L. Vrang, B. Samuelsson, A. Hallberg and A. Karlen. 2005. Cyclic sulfamide HIV-1 protease inhibitors, with sidechains spanning from P2/P2′ to P1/P1′. Bioorg. Med. Chem. 13: 755-764.

[165] S.V. Karthikeyan and S. Perumal. 2007. A facile tandem protocol for the regioselective synthesis of novel thienobenzothiazepines. Tetrahedron Lett. 48: 2261-2265.

Index

Biography

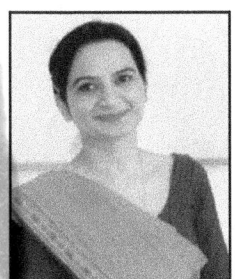

Dr. Navjeet Kaur received her B.Sc. degree from Punjab University Chandigarh, Punjab, India (2008). She did her M.Sc. in chemistry from Banasthali University (2010). She was awarded PhD in 2014 by the same university under the supervision of **Prof. D. Kishore**. Presently, she has been working as an assistant professor in the Department of Chemistry, Banasthali University. She entered into a specialized research career focused on the synthesis of 1,4-benzodiazepine based heterocyclic compounds (Organic Synthetic and Medicinal Chemistry). With 8 years of teaching experience, she has published 120 scientific research papers, review articles, book chapters and monographs in the field of organic synthesis in national and international reputed journals. She obtained Prof. G. L. Telesara Award 2011 by Indian Council of Chemists, Agra, UP, at Osmania University, Hyderabad and Best Paper Presentation Award in National Conference on "Emerging Trends in Chemical and Pharmaceutical Sciences" Banasthali University, Rajasthan. She has attended around 40 conferences/workshops/seminars. She is working as NSS Program Officer since 2016 and delivered many radio talks.

Dr. Navjeet finds interests in Sikh literature. She has completed two year Sikh Missionary course from Sikh Missionary College, Ludhiana, Punjab.